Clinical pharmacology
in dental practice

Clinical pharmacology in dental practice

Edited by

SAM V. HOLROYD

**B.S., D.D.S., M.S.(Pharmacology),
M.S.(Periodontics), F.A.C.D.**

Captain, Dental Corps, United States Navy;
Head, Department of Educational Program Development,
Naval Health Sciences Education and Training Command,
National Naval Medical Center, Bethesda, Maryland;
Consultant in Pharmacology and Consultant in Periodontics,
National Naval Dental Center,
Bethesda, Maryland

SECOND EDITION

Illustrated

THE C. V. MOSBY COMPANY

Saint Louis   1978

SECOND EDITION

Copyright © 1978 by The C. V. Mosby Company

All rights reserved. No part of this book may be reproduced in any manner without written permission of the publisher.

Previous edition copyrighted 1974

Printed in the United States of America

Distributed in Great Britain by Henry Kimpton, London

The C. V. Mosby Company
11830 Westline Industrial Drive, St. Louis, Missouri 63141

Library of Congress Cataloging in Publication Data

Holroyd, Samuel V   1931-
    Clinical pharmacology in dental practice.

    Bibliography: p.
    Includes index.
    1. Dental pharmacology.   I. Title. [DNLM:
1. Dentistry. 2. Pharmacology.   QV50 C641]
RK701.H64   1978   615'.1'0246176   77-22265
ISBN 0-8016-2241-7

GW/CB/CB   9 8 7 6 5 4 3 2 1

Contributors

RONALD D. BAKER, D.D.S., M.A.(Ed.), F.A.C.D.

Professor, Department of Oral Surgery, University of North Carolina School of Dentistry, Chapel Hill, North Carolina; Consultant in Oral Surgery to the National Naval Dental Center, Bethesda, Maryland; Dorothea Dix State Psychiatric Hospital, Raleigh, North Carolina; Veterans Administration Hospital, Fayetteville, North Carolina

K. W. BESLEY, D.D.S.

Captain, Dental Corps, United States Navy; Chief of the Dental Service, Naval Hospital, Key West, Florida

WILLIAM K. BOTTOMLEY, B.S., M.S.(Chemistry), D.D.S., M.S.(Oral Diagnosis), F.A.C.D.

Chairman, Department of Oral Diagnosis, Georgetown University School of Dentistry, Washington, D.C.

SEBASTIAN G. CIANCIO, D.D.S.

Professor and Chairman, Department of Periodontics-Endodontics; Clinical Professor of Pharmacology, State University of New York at Buffalo Schools of Dentistry and Medicine, Buffalo, New York

TOMMY W. GAGE, B.S., D.D.S., Ph.D.

Professor and Chairman, Department of Pharmacology, Baylor College of Dentistry, Dallas, Texas

J. MAX GOODSON, D.D.S., Ph.D.

Head, Department of Pharmacology, Forsyth Dental Center, Boston, Massachusetts

SAM V. HOLROYD, B.S., D.D.S., M.S.(Pharmacology), M.S.(Periodontics), F.A.C.D.

Captain, Dental Corps, United States Navy; Head, Department of Educational Program Development, Naval Health Sciences Education and Training Command, National Naval Medical Center, Bethesda, Maryland; Consultant in Pharmacology and Consultant in Periodontics, National Naval Dental Center, Bethesda, Maryland

GEORGE B. PELLEU, Jr., A.A., B.S., M.S., Ph.D.

Chairman, Research Department, Naval Graduate Dental School, National Naval Medical Center, Bethesda, Maryland

BARBARA REQUA-GEORGE, Pharm.D.

Associate Professor of Dentistry (Pharmacology), School of Dentistry, University of Missouri–Kansas City, Kansas City, Missouri

BARBARA F. ROTH-SCHECHTER, B.S., Ph.D.

Maitre de Conference Associé, Centre de Neurochimie, Centre National de la Recherche Scientifique, Strasbourg, France

R. C. TERHUNE, B.S., M.S., D.M.D.

Captain, Dental Corps, United States Navy; Fleet Liaison Officer and Preventive Dentistry Officer, Navy Regional Dental Center, San Diego, California

RICHARD L. WYNN, B.S., M.S., Ph.D.

Associate Professor and Chairman, Department of Oral Biology, University of Kentucky School of Dentistry, Lexington, Kentucky

I was once asked why most authors and editors
dedicate their books to their wives and children.
I answered that I guessed that most people dedicate what they do
to those they love. Although this is surely true,
I now know another reason. The legion of pressures inherent
in producing a book are conducive to the development of a
demeanor not unlike that of a wounded rhinoceros.

And so, I dedicate this book to my wife
Davene
and to our children
Eveann, Melissa, and Samuel
for their patience and understanding
during their residence with a wounded
but recovering rhinoceros

Preface

I have often wondered why anyone writes a preface. They are frequently meaningless, usually dull, and generally ignored. The degree to which they are ignored is probably proportional to their length. Consequently, I will be as brief as possible in making a comment or so about the second edition.

The basic approach and objectives of this revision are the same as those for the first edition. Since the ultimate objective of studying pharmacology is to relate the acquired knowledge to the treatment of patients, the fundamental objective in the preparation of this book has been to apply the science of pharmacology to the art of clinical practice. With the dental student in mind, a special effort has been made to relate pharmacology to clinical dentistry. With the busy practitioner in mind, the effort has been to provide a condensed and practical source for facile review and rapid reference.

I do not intend that this book be used as a substitute for a complete reference source. A number of excellent encyclopedic pharmacology texts are available for that purpose. The intention is that this book serve as a dentally oriented supplement to the more voluminous reference texts. We have avoided nonclinical details and in-depth pharmacology in order to be more concise in emphasizing material of *practical* importance in dental practice. I hope that the superficiality in some areas will thus be an advantage rather than a disadvantage to the dental student and clinician.

Although all major drug groups are covered, the points of emphasis differ to some extent. In chapters concerning drugs that the dentist actively prescribes or employs, the emphasis has been placed on information that will allow the dentist to make the *safest* and *most effective* use of these agents. In discussing drugs that the dentist normally does not prescribe, the principal effort has been to present information relative to how these drugs modify a patient's function and how these modifications are reflected in the proper handling of patients in a dental practice. I am emphasizing at this point that dental pharmacology cannot be limited to the drugs a dentist prescribes. A large percentage of our patients are taking medically prescribed agents. No patient should be treated unless the dental practitioner is fully aware of the effect these drugs are having on his patient. Additionally, in consultation with our medical colleagues it is essential that we have at least conversant knowledge of the drugs that *they* may be prescribing for *our* patients. The dentist who believes he can limit his knowledge of pharmacology to only those drugs he prescribes or uses not only deprives his patients of the safest and most effective pharmacologic management but also compromises the status of his profession.

In this edition a continuing effort has been made to strike a proper balance between basic pharmacology and information with a more direct clinical application. The fundamentals, on which all "practical" knowledge is based and which allow clinical decisions based on understanding rather than on a mechanical response, must lead into and blend with knowledge that permits the safest and most effective efforts in patient management. In this revision we have continued in our efforts to bring these areas together in a condensed and readable manner. One specific effort in this area has been to have chapters written by clinicians in the first edition carefully reviewed or coauthored by basic pharmacologists for the second edition and to have chapters written by basic pharmacologists in the first edition carefully reviewed or coauthored by clinicians for the second edition.

Important chapters on antineoplastic drugs, vitamins, and pharmacology of intravenous sedation have been added. Chapters appearing in the first edition have been updated by either revision or total rewriting. Our efforts have been not only to make the revision current but also to increase the readability and clarity and, above all, to make this book *useful* to both student and practitioner.

Although the coverage of basic pharmacology has been increased, we have continued to avoid nonclinical details in order to be more concise in emphasizing material of practical importance in dental practice. As Andres Goth said in *Medical Pharmacology*, "Omission of unimportant details should be interpreted as kindness to the reader rather than a tendency to be superficial."

I would like to acknowledge again the United States Navy Dental Corps for providing me with the educational and inspirational opportunities that have made my academic efforts possible. I would also like to express my most sincere gratitude to Dr. Daniel T. Watts, who led me into the world of pharmacology, to Dr. George D. Selfridge, for his leadership, guidance, and support, and to Mrs. Elizabeth Graeff, for helping me see writing and editing as a cooperative art. More specifically, relative to this book, I thank the collaborative authors for their interest and cooperation in applying their considerable talents to *Clinical Pharmacology in Dental Practice*. Only through their dedicated efforts has this book been possible.

Sam V. Holroyd

Contents

Appendices

Board review questions, 356

PART ONE
General pharmacology

1

Introduction

SAM V. HOLROYD
BARBARA REQUA-GEORGE

DEFINITIONS

Pharmacology (Gr. *pharmakon*, "drug"; L. *-logia*, "study of," from Gr. *logos*, "discourse") is the study of drugs. The extensive scope of this discipline is obvious when one considers that a drug may be broadly defined as any chemical substance that affects biologic systems. For convenience of reference, pharmacology may be divided into pharmacodynamics and pharmacotherapeutics. *Pharmacodynamics* is a basic medical science that deals with the effect, mechanism of action, and metabolism of drugs. *Pharmacotherapeutics* (Gr. *pharmakon*, "drug"; *therapeia*, "treatment") is applied or clinical pharmacology that is concerned with the use of drugs in the treatment and prevention of disease. Other related disciplines include the following:

Pharmacy deals with the procurement, preparation, and dispensing of drugs.

Pharmacognosy (Gr. *pharmakon*, "drug"; *gnōsis*, "knowledge") is concerned with the identification of crude or naturally occurring drugs. When most drugs were of natural origin, the subject of pharmacognosy was usually termed *materia medica*.

Posology (Gr. *posos*, "how much"; L. *-logia*, "study of") is the study of dosage.

Toxicology is the study of poisons.

HISTORY

Pharmacologic thought had its beginning when early man began to wonder why the chewing of certain plant roots or leaves altered his awareness and/or functions. As experience in root and leaf chewing progressed into therapeutic berry picking and smoke smelling, the experiences were shared and

☐ The opinions or assertions contained herein are the private ones of the writers and are not to be construed as official or as reflecting the views of the Navy Department or the naval service at large.

spread. As time went on, some individuals naturally became more astute in observing and more absorptive in remembering that certain plant products affected his fellowman in a rather predictable manner. Thus the first pharmacologist was born. He probably began the practice of medicine, extracted an occasional tooth, and had one of the finest trees in the forest. This clearly humble beginning has evolved through the years into a huge industrial and academic community that is concerned with the study and development of drugs. Drugs that are evolved are then prescribed and dispensed through the practice of medicine, dentistry, and pharmacy.

The progress of pharmacology is marked by the accomplishments of many scientists. Specific historic milestones are discussed in the appropriate chapters that follow. One may refer to Krantz and Carr[2] for condensed and interesting historic detail concerning various drugs and to Cutting[6] for a similar presentation in outline form.

PHARMACOLOGY IN DENTAL PRACTICE

The dentist must be concerned with two areas of drug use. *First*, he should be able to obtain the maximum advantage from available drugs while inducing minimal disadvantages. This requires a knowledge of what drugs can do therapeutically and a knowledge of what adverse potentialities exist. *Second*, an essential aspect of drug information in dental practice concerns medically prescribed or self-prescribed (over-the counter, OTC) drugs. An ever-increasing number of dental patients are taking drugs. It behooves the dentist to know how these drugs have modified the physiology of the patient he is treating. This modification may be insignificant, but, on the other hand, it may contraindicate certain dental procedures, change intended therapy, or alter one's approach to treatment.

The dentist should never use a drug with which he is not thoroughly familiar. He should never begin treatment of a patient who is taking a drug the nature of which is unknown to him. This requires more than a basic knowledge of pharmacology. No one can remember everything that should be known about all drugs. New drugs are developed so frequently that what is competent knowledge one year is not the next. Consequently, the practitioner must be able to expand his understanding of pharmacology by ready referral to reference material. Knowing where to look for quick answers is very important, and a knowledge of certain publications in pharmacology is essential.

PUBLICATIONS IN PHARMACOLOGY

The periodic literature provides the clinician with reports of recent pharmacologic developments. This information, when sufficiently documented, becomes incorporated into textbooks, pharmacopeias, and clinical references. An up-to-date textbook of general pharmacology is a fundamental reference and should be a part of every clinician's library. Several helpful pharmacology texts are listed in the references.[1-8]

The United States Pharmacopeia (USP) is issued every 5 years by the US Pharmacopeial Convention, Inc., which is composed of representatives from schools of medicine and pharmacy, the American Medical Association, state medical societies, the American Pharmaceutical Association, the American Chemical Society, and other scientific organizations and federal agencies. A Dental Advisory Committee to the USP was established in 1972. This compendium lists single-entity drugs* of established merit. It sets official chemical and physical standards that relate essentially to strength and purity.

The National Formulary (NF) is issued every 5 years and published by the USP convention. Like the USP it is also recognized by federal law and further establishes official standards for drugs not described in the USP. The inclusion of a drug in the *National For-*

mulary is based on extent of use and therapeutic value.

Beginning with the 1980 USP (USPXX), expert medical opinion will determine the basis for inclusion in the compendium. The new edition will include all drugs from USP-XIX and NF 14 as well as new drugs discovered before 1980. Standards set by the USP are enforced under federal law, notably the Federal Food, Drug, and Cosmetic Act. The importance of the USP and the NF in dental practice is indirect in that they are not so much clinical references but rather set manufacturing standards for drugs of known value.

The British Pharmacopoeia (BP) is the English equivalent of the *United States Pharmacopeia* and is official in Great Britain and Canada. An international pharmacopeia, *Pharmacopoeia Internationalis* (PhI) is issued by the World Health Organization.

AMA Drug Evaluations (AMA-DE), formerly *New and Non-Official Remedies* (NNR) and *New Drugs* (ND), is prepared by the Department of Drugs of the American Medical Association. The first edition became available in 1971. This publication provides authoritative, unbiased information on all single-entity drugs introduced during the preceding 10 years and all single-entity drugs or mixtures commonly prescribed in the United States. Other drugs of unusual toxicity or special importance are evaluated, and pharmacologic action, uses, and adverse reaction are discussed. The principal importance of this publication in dentistry is that it will provide authoritative and unbiased information on all drugs of current medical use.

Accepted Dental Therapeutics (ADT), formerly *Accepted Dental Remedies* (ADR), is a biennial publication of the Council on Dental Therapeutics (CDT) of the American Dental Association. Drugs of recognized value in dentistry that are labeled and advertised in accordance with the CDT are included. ADT is primarily a handbook of dental pharmacotherapeutics and is intended to assist the dental practitioner in selecting the appropriate drugs for the treatment of oral diseases. The "status" of drugs, as determined by the CDT, is presented. All dentists should have immediate access to this publication.

Physician's Desk Reference (PDR) is published annually by some 200 manufacturers whose products are listed. Product descrip-

---

*Single-entity drugs are those containing only one active ingredient, whereas multiple-entity drugs are those containing more than one active ingredient.

tions that cover clinically related pharmacology in some detail are prepared by the manufacturer. Almost all currently available single- or multiple-entity preparations are included. The special value of the PDR is twofold: (1) it is published annually and thereby includes relatively up-to-date information, and (2) it is cross-indexed to include the use of proprietary names. The latter facilitates reference when only the proprietary name of a drug is known. It is important at this point that consideration be given to the various names that are applied to drugs.

DRUG NOMENCLATURE[9-12]

Unfortunately, all drugs have more than one name. This fact perplexes the teacher, confuses the clinician, and irritates the student.

During the time that a compound is being investigated for possible clinical use, it is identified by a *chemical name* that conveys the chemical structure of the compound. For convenience, or if the structure is not yet known, a code number may be assigned to the compound by the investigating company or activity. If the chemical is determined to be therapeutically useful and is to be marketed commercially, the company gives the drug their *trade name (proprietary name)*. This trade name is registered as a trademark under Federal Trade-Mark Law and becomes the property of the registering company. The trade name is generally short and amenable to commercial promotion. *Brand name* has been used to mean trade or proprietary name; however, it technically is the name of the company marketing the product. At this point the product is usually patented under Federal Patent Law, which gives the company exclusive right to manufacture the drug for 17 years.

Before any drug can be marketed, it must be given a generic name (nonproprietary name). This becomes the "official" name of the drug and is the one used in the USP or NF. Although additional trade names may come, go, and accumulate, there is only one generic name and it seldom changes.

Generic names are selected by the USAN (US Adopted Name) Council. This council is sponsored by the American Medical Association, the American Pharmaceutical Association, and the US Pharmacopeial Convention,

Inc. The council is made up of one member from the AMA one from the APA, one from the USP Convention, one from the FDA, and one at-large member selected by the sponsors. The manufacturer of a new drug usually submits a proposal for a generic name to the council. The council considers recommendations by respective pharmaceutical manufacturers, the FDA, and other foreign and international agencies in selecting a generic name that will be simple and meaningful and will not conflict with other drug names. Once the generic name is selected, it is published by the AMA Department of Drugs in the *Journal of the American Medical Association.*

Examples of names for two products are as follows:

CHEMICAL NAME: 2-diethylamino-2,6-acetoxylidide
GENERIC NAME: lidocaine
TRADE NAMES: Xylocaine
Lidocaton
Doricaine
ProLido
Octocaine

CHEMICAL NAME: N-acetyl-p-aminophenol
GENERIC NAME: acetaminophen
TRADE NAMES: Tylenol
Tempra
Nebs
Tenlap
Temlo
Datril
Phenaphen
Valadol
Tapar

This problem in drug nomenclature really begins when the original manufacturer's exclusive rights to market a product expire. Other companies may now put their brands on the market under different trade names. Thus it becomes more difficult to determine the nature of a drug a patient is taking or to which he has had an adverse reaction.

For 17 years there was only one lidocaine; this was Xylocaine. Now there are Lidocaton, Doricaine, and Octocaine. If a patient told his dentist that he was allergic to Octocaine, there is a strong probability that the dentist would not know that Octocaine was lidocaine. The problem with medically prescribed drugs is particularly acute because of the large number of drugs being used and the fact that most are marketed under two or more trade names. Unfortunately, when a patient tells his dentist that he is taking a drug prescribed by his physician, he will usually identify it by its trade name. As in the case of lidocaine, if the patient told you he was taking chloramphenicol, this would mean much more to you than if he said he was taking Amphicol or Mychel, which are trade names for chloramphenicol.

More confusion is thrown into drug nomenclature when multiple-entity drugs are considered. Many new names are added when new trade names are created for combination products. For example, the 1976 edition of the *Physician's Desk Reference* lists over 80 names for preparations containing chlorpheniramine maleate, over 60 names for preparations containing phenylephrine, and over 90 names for preparations containing iron.

There are two important disadvantages of trade names: (1) they make the problem of drug identification complex, and (2) if a practitioner writes a prescription using a trade name, in many states the pharmacist must dispense that particular product despite the fact that less expensive generic preparations may be available. Some state laws allow substitution of a generic equivalent unless the prescriber specifically forbids it. There may be an advantage to prescribing a specific proprietary brand, and this will be discussed later, but the disadvantage of the cost differential should be known by the practitioner.

There are some advantages to using trade names: (1) they are convenient and save time when writing prescriptions for multiple-entity drugs; for instance, if a preparation contains more than one ingredient, the use of the product's *trade name* will avoid the necessity of listing each ingredient and its amount separately in a prescription; (2) trade names are usually shorter and easier to remember than are generic names; and (3) the use of a trade name demands the product of a specific manufacturer in whose products the practitioner may have special confidence.

This raises an important question: Does "generic equivalence," as now determined, accurately indicate "therapeutic equivalence"? As previously noted, after a drug company's exclusive right to manufacture a product expires, other companies frequently produce and market it. The latter companies may add their trade names to the product or simply market the drug under its generic name. In either case they usually sell the drug at less than the original producer's prices. In recent years foreign products under generic names have been imported into the United States at relatively low prices. It has been contended that the basis of determining *generic equivalence* (chemical and physical standards as required by the USP) does not necessarily establish therapeutic equivalence.[13]

In considering the question of prescribing by generic or trade name, we may conclude the following:

1. Most generic preparations are significantly less expensive than trade preparations.
2. Infrequently, some generic products may be more expensive than some trade products.
3. Although generic preparations are generally accepted to be as therapeutically effective as trade name preparations, there are apparently some instances where this is not true.[13,14]

Although these conclusions may be enlightening, they unfortunately do not provide a complete basis for determining the merit of using generic names instead of trade names when writing prescriptions.

Although the advantages and disadvantages of using generic names in prescription writing may be argued, *there is no question that both student and practitioner must relate drug information to generic names, not trade names.* The Kefauver-Harris amendments (1962) to the Food, Drug, and Cosmetic Act require that all drug labels list the generic names and quantities of all ingredients. The generic name must also appear in all advertising and labeling wherever the trade name appears. Consequently, if what one knows about a drug is associated with its generic name, it is unnecessary to learn a large number of trade names.

FEDERAL REGULATORY AGENCIES

The production, marketing, advertising, labeling, and prescribing of drugs are under certain controls imposed and enforced by the federal government. Following are the principal agencies involved.

The Food and Drug Administration (FDA)

The Food and Drug Administration of the Department of Health, Education, and Welfare determines what drugs can be marketed in the United States. It considers data relative to safety and effectiveness for drug entities, and physical and chemical standards for specific products. It requires quality control in United States manufacturing plants, determines what drugs must be sold by prescription only, and controls the labeling and advertising of prescription drugs. The legal authority of the FDA in these matters is the Food, Drug and Cosmetic Act of 1938 and its amendments, which include the Durham-Humphrey Law of 1952 and the Kefauver-Harris Bill of 1962.

The Federal Trade Commission (FTC)

The Federal Trade Commission is not a part of the Department of Health, Education, and Welfare. This independent commission has the responsibility to regulate trade practices and prohibit false advertising of foods, nonprescription drugs, and cosmetics. Its authority is granted by the Federal Trade Commission Act.

Drug Enforcement Administration (DEA)

The Drug Enforcement Administration (DEA) of the Department of Justice administers the Controlled Substance Act of 1970, which replaced the Harrison Narcotic Act. It enforces the federal control of narcotics and other drugs considered to have a potential for abuse.

REFERENCES

1. Goodman, L. S., and Gilman, A.: The pharmacological basis of therapeutics, ed. 5, New York, 1975, The Macmillan Co.
2. Krantz, J. C., Jr., and Carr, C. J.: The pharmacologic principles of medical practice, ed. 7, Baltimore, 1969, The Williams & Wilkins Co.
3. Goth, A.: Medical pharmacology, ed. 8, St. Louis, 1976, The C. V. Mosby Co.
4. DiPalma, J. R., editor: Basic pharmacology in medicine, New York, 1976, McGraw-Hill Book Co.
5. Sutherland, V. C.: A synopsis of pharmacology, ed. 2, Philadelphia, 1970, W. B. Saunders Co.
6. Cutting, W. C.: Handbook of pharmacology, ed. 5, New York, 1972, Appleton-Century-Crofts.
7. Meyers, F. H., Jawetz, E., and Goldfien, A.: Review of medical pharmacology, ed. 5, Los Altos, Calif., 1976, Lange Medical Publications.
8. American Medical Association Department of Drugs: AMA drug evaluations, ed. 3, Acton, Mass., 1977, Publishing Sciences Groups, Inc.
9. Holroyd, S. V.: Pharmacotherapeutics in dental practice (NAVPERS 10486), Washington, D.C., 1969, Bureau of Naval Personnel.
10. Pettit, W.: Manual of pharmaceutical law, New York, 1957, The Macmillan Co.
11. Martin, E. W., editor: Remington's pharmaceutical sciences, ed. 13, Easton, Pa., 1965, Mack Publishing Co.
12. American Medical Association Council on Drugs: New names, J.A.M.A. 206:118-119, 1968.
13. Varley, A. B.: The generic inequivalence of drugs, J.A.M.A. 206:1745-1748, 1968.
14. Mindel, J. S.: Bioavailability and generic prescribing, Surv. Ophthal. 21:262-275, 1976.

2

General principles of drug action

RICHARD L. WYNN

Drugs are chemical substances that are used for the diagnosis, prevention, or treatment of disease and the prevention of pregnancy. Most drugs are differentiated from inert chemicals and chemicals necessary for the maintenance of life processes by their ability to act *selectively* in biologic systems to accomplish a desired effect. This selective action of drugs with regard to their use in diagnosing, preventing, and treating disease is the basis of *pharmacotherapeutics*.

Historically, drugs were found by random searching for active components among plants, animals, minerals, and the soil. Today the search for new drugs involves a different approach. Systematic screening techniques are utilized to discover therapeutic agents from natural sources. Also, the rise of organic synthetic chemistry in this century has witnessed the development of thousands of new synthetic drugs. *Screening tests* are necessary to determine if natural and synthetic compounds elicit biologic activity. Once activity is established for a compound, more exacting quantitative evaluations are performed in studies known as *biologic assays*. This type of assay compares the activity of a drug with that of a preparation eliciting similar activity at a known strength—commonly referred to as a *reference standard*. If the drug eventually becomes available in a pure form, it is also standardized by *chemical assay*.

Chemical modifications of the structure of parent compounds exhibiting known pharmacologic activity have resulted in the production of congeners, or analogs—many of which have become useful members of a variety of drug classes. Local anesthetics, antihistamines, cholinergic agents, and the phenothiazine type of tranquilizers are some examples of these classes. The technique of modifying a chemical molecule for the purposes of producing more useful therapeutic agents evolved from studies of the relationship between chemical structure and biologic activity (*structure activity relationships*). For example, the naturally occurring cholinergic agent acetylcholine is not a useful drug, since it is rapidly hydrolyzed by plasma enzymes. On the addition of a methyl group to the beta carbon atom to form acetyl-β-methylcholine (methacholine), the acetylcholine is transformed into a cholinergic compound resistant to plasma hydrolytic enzymes, as follows:

$$CH_3-\overset{\overset{\displaystyle CH_3}{|}}{\underset{\underset{\displaystyle CH_3}{|}}{N^+}}-\underset{\alpha}{CH_2}-\underset{\beta}{CH_2}-O-\overset{\overset{\displaystyle O}{\|}}{C}-CH_3$$

Acetylcholine

$$CH_3-\overset{\overset{\displaystyle CH_3}{|}}{\underset{\underset{\displaystyle CH_3}{|}}{N^+}}-\underset{\alpha}{CH_2}-\underset{\beta}{\overset{\overset{\displaystyle CH_3}{|}}{CH}}-O-\overset{\overset{\displaystyle O}{\|}}{C}-CH_3$$

Methacholine

CHARACTERIZATION OF DRUG ACTION

Drugs are classified according to their biochemical actions, their physiologic effects, or the organ system on which they exert their therapeutic action. For example, drugs are described as hypoglycemic agents, antihypertensive agents, central nervous system stimulants, and so on.

All drugs exert some effect on biologic systems, and in most instances a given effect can be related to drug dosage in a quantitative fashion. If the dose of a drug is plotted on a logarithmic scale against intensity of effect, a sigmoid log dose–effect curve is obtained (Fig. 1). From this curve two important expressions of drug action can be dem-

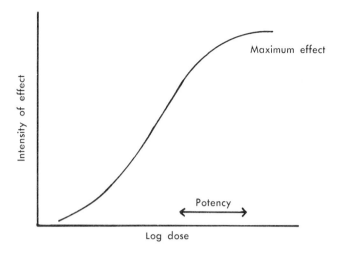

Fig. 1. Log dose-effect curve. A representative dose-effect curve indicating potency and efficacy.

onstrated—*potency* and maximum effect, or *efficacy*.

Potency is indicated by the location of the curve along the log dose axis. For example, the curve, if shifted to the right, would indicate that higher doses of a drug are necessary to attain similar intensities of effect. A shift to the left would indicate that lower doses of a drug are needed to attain the same intensities of effect. Different drugs eliciting similar effects can be compared in potency by comparing the dose that gives 50% of the total or maximum effect. The maximum effect would be the effect attained at a certain dose of a drug that cannot be further increased with higher doses of the drug. A drug requiring less of a dose to elicit a 50% maximum effect of a drug requiring a greater dose would be the more potent of the two.

Potency is a relative term when the action of two similar drugs is compared, and it merely indicates that the less potent drug must be administered in higher doses to attain the desired effect. The absolute potency of any drug matters little as long as its appropriate dose is utilized. A clinical example may be cited to describe potency. Both meperidine HCl and morphine HCl elicit similar effects therapeutically in that they induce analgesia in even the most severe types of pain. A dose of 80 to 100 mg meperidine HCl parenterally, however, is required to elicit the equivalent analgesic response attained by 10 mg morphine HCl.

The log dose–effect curve in Fig. 1 also indicates a maximum intensity of effect, or efficacy, as shown by the plateau of the curve. The efficacy of any drug is a major descriptive characteristic indicating some degree of its action. For example, the efficacy of meperidine HCl and morphine HCl is about the same, since both drugs relieve severe pain. Other analgesics, however, such as propoxyphene HCl and salicylates, are less efficacious in that they relieve only mild to moderate pain. The dose of a drug required to produce a specific intensity of effect in an individual is regarded as the effective dose for that individual. If the percentage of individuals who exhibit an effect is plotted as a function of logarithm dose, a dose-percent curve is obtained. The dose-percent curve is not a dose-effect curve but is a means to express individual variability for a single effect. The dose of a drug required to produce a specified intensity of effect in 50% of individuals is known as the median effective dose, or ED50.

If a given dose of drug is administered to many individuals, variations in response and effect will occur among those individuals. These variations are due to individual variations to the general factors that characterize the actions of all drugs and that determine the effective level of any therapeutic agent at its site of action. These factors are (1) the route by which a drug may be administered, (2) passage across body membranes, (3) absorption, (4) transport and distribution, (5) molecular mechanisms of action and the termination of activity through, (6) metabolism, and (7) elimination. Most of this chapter includes a discussion of these processes in relation to variations in individual drug response and the time course of drug action.

ROUTES OF DRUG ADMINISTRATION

The route by which a drug is administered will affect the time required for the drug to enter the bloodstream. Since most drugs must be distributed throughout the body in the water phase of blood plasma before a response is elicited, the route of administration will affect the time of onset of drug action and to a lesser extent its duration of action. The routes of drug entry into a patient can be conveniently classified as *enteral* and *parenteral*. Enteral routes are those by which a drug is placed directly into the gastrointestinal tract from where absorption occurs across the enteric membranes, and this method includes oral and rectal administration. Parenteral administration bypasses the gastrointestinal tract and includes injections, inhalation, and topical routes.

Oral route

The simplest way to introduce a drug into the body is by the oral route, which allows the use of many different dose forms to attain desired results. Tablets, capsules, liquids, and preparations eliciting prolonged action are all conveniently given orally.[1,2] It is the most frequently used route and is convenient for self-administration. The large absorbing area that the intestine presents is considered an advantage to this route. Oral administration is associated with a longer onset time of drug action compared with many parenteral routes, since absorption takes place relatively slowly. Many agents can cause stomach and intestinal irritation that results in nausea and vomiting. Other drugs such as certain penicillins and protein preparations (for example, insulin) are inactivated by gastrointestinal tract acidity or enzymes. One must remember that most drugs given orally are initially perfused into the hepatic portal circulation—a process that will rapidly deactivate some drugs in the liver such as testosterone propionate.

The presence of food in the stomach slows drug absorption. Variability in the presence and absence of food, various pathologic conditions of the gastrointestinal tract, and the effect of gastric acidity and hepatic portal circulation make blood levels obtained after oral administration less predictable than levels obtained parenterally.

Rectal route

Drugs may be given rectally by way of suppositories or creams. Agents that cause irritation when given orally may be well tolerated in the anal canal. Nausea and unconsciousness in the patient will not prevent the rectal administration of a drug. Both local effects and systemic absorption are obtained by this route. Most drugs, however, are not as well absorbed rectally as from the upper intestine, and absorption of many drugs is often irregular and incomplete.

Intravenous route

The most rapid method of eliciting a drug response in a patient is by the intravenous (IV) route, since the onset of drug action is immediate after intravenous injection. Of the several injectable routes available, this route can accommodate the largest volume of drug solution. Also, when compared with the oral route, a more predictable drug response can be obtained, since many of the factors affecting absorption have been eliminated. This is the route of choice for emergency administration of agents during crisis situations, for example, the injection of diazepam to counteract convulsions resulting from systemic toxicity of local anesthetics.[3] Constant plasma levels of drugs may be maintained by intravenous infusion.

Disadvantages of this route include the occurrence of hazardous reactions because of high local concentrations of drugs that can result on injection. Also, drugs cannot be recalled once injected, whereas a stomach pump or emetic can be utilized to recall drugs after oral administration. Too rapid an injection rate may cause untoward effects on the circulation and respiration.

Intramuscular route

Rapid absorption of drugs occurs after intramuscular (IM) injection, since blood flow through skeletal muscle even while an individual is at rest is very high (0.02 to 0.07 ml/min/per gram tissue).[4] Large amounts of solution may be given by this route, and many irritating drugs are well tolerated, since less pain is associated with this route compared with subcutaneous injection. Intramuscular injection is an inconvenient method for repetitive drug administration. Injections are usually made in the deltoid region or gluteal mass underlying the upper outer quadrant of each buttock.

Subcutaneous route

Although blood flow is poorer and absorption rates are said to be slower, it has been shown that the rate of subcutaneous absorption of certain drugs is as rapid as intramuscular absorption.[4] Solutions or suspensions of drugs are injected into subcutaneous areolar tissue to gain access to the systemic circulation. However, irritating solutions are painful when injected subcutaneously, and sterile abscesses may develop as a result of irritation. Rates of drug absorption may be modified in subcutaneous regions by inducing peripheral vasoconstriction on cooling of the area or with the local application of epinephrine.

Intradermal route

Drugs such as local anesthetics can be injected in small amounts into the epidermis of the skin. This technique provides an insensitive area through which longer needles can be passed without pain for much deeper injections.

Intrathecal

Spinal anesthesia is accomplished by injecting local anesthetic solutions into the spinal subarachnoid space. Some anti-infective drugs are also injected by this route to treat infections of the meninges.

Intraperitoneal route

Injections may be made into the peritoneal cavity, where absorption of the drug occurs by way of the mesenteric veins. Because of dangers of infection and adhesions, however, this route is seldom employed clinically.

Inhalation

Gaseous, microcrystalline, and volatile drugs may be inhaled. They are then absorbed through the pulmonary endothelium at the alveoli to gain rapid access to the general circulation. Absorption can also take place through the mucous membranes of the respiratory tract. Drugs in solution may be atomized in an aerosol preparation and the fine droplets in the air inhaled.

Topical route

The topical route of drug administration includes application to oral mucous membranes, the skin, and other epithelial surfaces. Topical application may be instituted to obtain local drug effects, such as the use of a topical local anesthetic prior to incision and drainage, or may be used as a route to obtain a systemic blood level. The mucous membranes of the oral cavity provide a convenient absorbing surface for the systemic administrations of drugs, which can be placed under the tongue (sublingual) or on other areas of the oral mucosa. Absorption of many drugs rapidly occurs into the systemic circulation, as exemplified by the fast onset of action of nitroglycerin sublingual tablets to treat anginal pain. Drugs that are susceptible to degradation by the gastrointestinal tract and even the liver, such as testosterone, are safely administered as sublingual tablets. The oral cavity provides an attractive route of topical drug administration that has never been fully taken advantage of.

Most drugs do not penetrate the intact skin, and this route is generally utilized for local drug effects. Systemic toxicities have occurred because of the absorption of highly lipid soluble agents such as organophosphate insecticides. Since absorption through the skin is proportional to the lipid solubility of a drug, lipid insoluble agents and ions penetrate very slowly. Many potentially toxic drugs may be applied topically to the skin without worry of systemic side effects. For example, potent synthetic corticosteroids will relieve various localized skin disorders. Although some of the steroid drug may be absorbed systemically, plasma levels are insufficient to produce systemic effects. Drugs known to induce frequent allergic reactions such as penicillins should not be used topically, since sensitization may occur.

Drugs are applied to the vagina and urethra for their local action. Certain drugs may reach the circulation through the mucous membranes at these sites. However, these routes are not utilized for this purpose. Drugs are applied intravaginally in the form of suppositories or creams and intraurethrally as suppositories or urethral inserts. Drugs applied into the ear and eye as solutions or suspensions are seldom absorbed systemically to any significant extent. In fact, some drugs that are extremely toxic systemically such as the organophosphate derivative echo-thiophate iodide may be safely administered in most patients as a local application to the eye.

Although drugs are applied nasally in the form of solutions or sprays, on occasion it is the systemic effect that results. In fact, certain local anesthetics such as tetracaine achieve similar systemic blood levels after absorption through the pharyngeal mucous membranes as they do after intravenous injection.[5]

PASSAGE OF DRUGS ACROSS BODY MEMBRANES

The amounts of drug moving across body membranes and the rates with which a drug moves have important implications in the time course of action and the variation in individual response. For a drug to be absorbed, transported and distributed to body tissues, metabolized, and subsequently eliminated from the body, it must traverse various membranes such as those of the blood capillaries, cellular membranes, and intracellular membranes. Although these membranes vary considerably in function, they share certain physicochemical characteristics that influence the passage of drugs and other chemical substances. Membranes are composed of lipids, proteins, and carbohydrates. Lipids comprise approximately 40% of the content, proteins 50% to 60%, and carbohydrates the remainder. The membrane lipids are a class of compounds called phospholipids, the presence of which makes the membrane relatively impermeable to ions and polar molecules. Membrane proteins act in a functional capacity as enzymes in transport processes and also make up the structural components of the membrane. Membrane carbohydrates consist of oligosaccharides, which are linked covalently to proteins to form complexes called glycoproteins or to lipids to form glycolipids. In the past it was held that the chemical components of membranes were arranged into a bimolecular lipid sheet bordered on both sides by a monolayer of protein.[6] More recently, Singer and Nicholson[7] have proposed a fluid mosaic model of membrane structure. The phospholipid molecules orient themselves so that they form a fluid bimolecular leaflet structure with the hydrophobic ends of the molecule shielded from the surrounding aqueous environment and the hydrophilic ends in contact with water. The various protein, glycoprotein, and glycolipid molecules are embedded in and layered onto this fluid lipid bilayer, thus forming a mosaic (Fig. 2). Studies on the membrane penetration of substances of varying molecular weights and sizes have also indicated the presence of a system of pores, although this remains to be confirmed by electron microscopy.[8,9]

The physicochemical properties of drugs that influence their passage across biologic membranes are *lipid solubility, degree of ionization,* and *molecular size and shape.* The mechanism of drug transfer across biologic

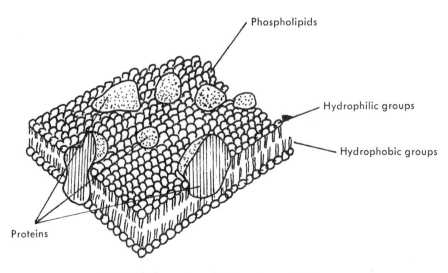

Phospholipids

Hydrophilic groups

Hydrophobic groups

Proteins

Fig. 2. Fluid mosaic model of membrane structure.

membranes is by passive transfer and specialized transport.

Passive transfer

Lipid-soluble substances move across the lipoprotein membrane by a passive transfer process of *simple diffusion.*[10] This type of transfer is directly proportional to the concentration gradient of the drug across the membrane and its degree of lipid solubility. For example, a highly lipid-soluble compound, such as an organic solvent, will attain a high concentration at the membrane site and will diffuse readily across the membrane into an area of lower concentration. Most drugs are partially ionized at physiologic pH, and the degree of lipid solubility of both the ionized and nonionized species determines the degree of passive transfer (although the ionized species is usually poorly lipid soluble).

Water-soluble molecules small enough to pass through the membrane pores (molecular radius of 30 Å for capillary membranes and 4 Å for other cell membranes) may be carried through the pores by the bulk flow of water.[11,12] This process of *filtration* through single cell membranes may occur with drugs of molecular weights of 200 or less. Drugs up to molecular weights of 60,000, however, can "filter" through capillary membranes.

Specialized transport

Certain substances, including small molecular weight ionized drug molecules, are transported across cell membranes by pro-cesses more complex than simple diffusion or filtration. *Active transport* is a process by which a substance is transported against a concentration gradient or electrochemical gradient and which is blocked by metabolic inhibitors. This action is believed to be mediated by transport "carriers" that furnish energy for transportation of the drug to regions of higher concentration.[13]

The transport of some substances such as glucose into cells is also blocked by metabolic inhibitors. This type of transport, however, does not move against a concentration gradient. This phenomenon has been termed *facilitated diffusion.*[14] The process of pinocytosis (the ability of cells to engulf fluids) has been suggested to explain the passage of macromolecular substances into cells.

Those factors remaining to be discussed that cause variations in individual drug response and influence the time course of drug action in the body are depicted schematically in Fig. 3. It should be noted that each of these processes involves the passage of drugs across body membranes. The ultimate goal in drug administration is to achieve adequate concentrations of a drug at its specific sites of action in target tissues. The factors to be discussed (Fig. 3) that influence the time course of drug action will also influence the amount of drug reaching target tissue sites.

ABSORPTION

Absorption is the process by which drug molecules are transferred from the site of

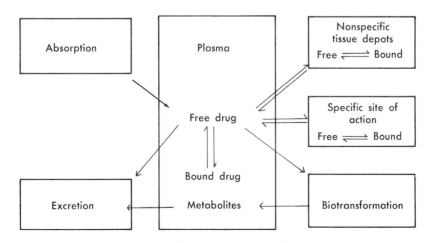

Fig. 3. Absorption and fate of a drug.

administration in the body to the circulating fluids. Since this process requires the drug to pass through biologic membranes, the *physicochemical factors* discussed earlier will influence the absorption rates of drugs. The *site of absorption* will also greatly affect the absorption rate. For example, one of the advantages of oral administration is attributable to the large absorbing area presented by the gastrointestinal mucosa. The route by which a drug is administered determines its site of absorption. *Drug solubility* is another important factor affecting absorption. Drugs in solution are more rapidly absorbed than are insoluble drugs.

Drug absorption with regard to their nature as weak electrolytes

Drugs that are weak electrolytes dissociate in solution as both a nonionized and an ionized form. The nonionized portion behaves as a nonpolar lipid-soluble compound, which readily traverses body membranes. The ionized portion, being less lipid soluble, will traverse these membranes with greater difficulty. The more the compound is ionized at membrane sites the less the amount of absorption will occur and vice versa.

The amount of ionization that any weak electrolyte will undergo depends on the pH at the drug site in the tissues and its dissociation characteristics. The relationship to pH is as follows: For weak acids, the higher the pH, the greater degree of ionization. For weak bases, the lower the pH, the greater the ionization. The dissociation characteristics of a weak electrolyte are given by a dissociation constant (pKa), which is an indication of its tendency to ionize. The pKa of a compound is the same as the pH at which it will be half undissociated and half ionized. Aspirin has a pKa of 3.5. This means that at pH 3.5, aspirin will be 50% ionized. Since aspirin is a weak acid, decreasing the pH below 3.5 as would occur in the stomach would decrease ionization less than 50%, and an increase in the amount of nonionized aspirin absorbed would occur. Conversely, increasing the pH above 3.5 as would occur in the intestine or if the gastric contents were alkalinized would increase the ionization of aspirin above 50% and subsequently decrease the amount absorbed.

Knowing the pKa of a drug, the clinician can calculate the extent to which it will ionize

at any pH. For example, consider the ionization of weakly basic local anesthetics in the plasma. Assuming that the pKa of a typical local anesthetic is 8.4, at plasma pH 7.4:

$$pH = pKa + \log \frac{\text{(nonionized drug)}}{\text{(ionized drug)}}$$

$$7.4 = 8.4 + \log \frac{\text{(nonionized drug)}}{\text{(ionized drug)}}$$

$$\text{Antilog } (7.4 - 8.4) = \frac{\text{(nonionized drug)}}{\text{(ionized drug)}}$$

$$0.1 \text{ or } \frac{1}{10} = \frac{\text{(nonionized drug)}}{\text{(ionized drug)}}$$

Therefore at plasma pH the ratio of nonionized to ionized drug is 1:10, which means that 10% of the drug (nonionized) is available for passage through membranes from the plasma.

Although the calculations of the actual percentage of ionization at a known pH are of greater academic and research importance than of clinical significance, its theoretic basis has important implications in the rational utilization of drugs.

Oral absorption

Aside from those general factors previously mentioned that affect drug absorption, an important factor influencing absorption in the gastrointestinal tract is the dosage form of a drug. Unless administered as a solution, the absorption of a drug in the gastrointestinal tract involves its release from a dose form such as a tablet, capsule, or suspension. This release may involve the initial disruption of a tablet coating or capsule shell, the disintegration of the tablet or capsule contents, the dispersion of the concentrated drug particles, and the dissolution of the drug in gastrointestinal fluids. The process of drug absorption from a particular dose form is referred to as the *bioavailability* of the drug.

Dissolution rate is proportional to the surface area of the dissolving solid, and drugs such as griseofulvin (an antifungal) and spironolactone (a diuretic) are better absorbed in a microcrystalline state. The shape and crystal form of the drug particles also influence dissolution. Drugs such as steroids, barbiturates, and sulfonamides exist as several kinds of molecular arrangements within a crystal—a phenomenon known as polymorphism. These polymorphic forms of the drug differ in their rates of dissolution and subsequent absorption. The incorporation of water into drug crystals (hydrates) induces dissolution rates that differ from those of the original drug crystal. Hydrates are common forms of penicillin preparations. Pronounced differences in dissolution rates may also occur with salts and esters of original drug crystals. Different esters of erythromycin impart varying dissolution rates compared with the base compound, and the absorption rate is affected accordingly.

Absorption at injection sites

Absorption at various sites of injection depends on the solubility of the drug and the blood flow at the site. For example, drugs of low aqueous solubility such as the depot type of penicillins (procaine penicillin G suspension and benzathine penicillin G) are absorbed very slowly after intramuscular injection. Absorption at injection sites is also affected by the dose form. For example, drugs in suspension are absorbed much more slowly than those in solution. This fact is utilized to decrease the absorption rate of certain insulin preparations by formulating them into suspensions.

TRANSPORT AND DISTRIBUTION

For a drug to exert activity, it must be made available to its locus of action in the body, and distribution is the mechanism by which this is accomplished. Distribution is regarded as the passage of drugs into various body fluid compartments such as plasma, interstitial fluids, and intracellular fluids. The patterns of distribution in the body determine how rapidly a drug will elicit a desired response, the duration of the response, and in some cases whether a response will be elicited at all.

The primary purpose of drug distribution is to allow a drug to reach its site of action at specific tissue sites. Many drugs, however, are distributed to nonspecific tissues, which serve as storage depots (Fig. 3). Other drugs cannot be distributed in certain regions of the body. Still other drugs are redistributed from one tissue accumulation site to another.

Transport in plasma

After a drug is absorbed from its site of administration, it is transported to its site of action by the blood plasma. Therefore the biologic activity of a drug is usually related to its concentration in plasma. More specifically, drug activity is related to its concentration in *plasma water*, since a drug exists in this phase only in the free or *unbound state*, that is, not bound to plasma protein. This is the biologically active form of a drug.

The reversible binding of drugs to plasma proteins such as albumin and globulins is a well-known phenomenon that causes an unequal distribution of drugs in the body.[15,16] Since only the unbound species is the biologically active form of a drug, that proportion of drug bound in the plasma does not contribute to intensity of drug action. In fact, the binding process is considered to be a site of drug loss or storage. This binding is reversible, and as unbound drug disappears from plasma water to be distributed to tissue sites, a dynamic equilibrium results in a dissociation of bound to unbound drug—a process that results in an increased supply of unbound drug. In this way the plasma binding process prolongs drug activity. Without such a process most drugs would have to be administered at very frequent intervals to be effective therapeutically.

The biologic half-life ($t_{\frac{1}{2}}$) of a drug is the time necessary for the body to eliminate half the peak quantity of drug present in the circulation. This is greatly affected by the extent of plasma protein binding. Suramin, an agent used to protect against sleeping sickness, has a great affinity for plasma proteins. In fact, a single dose will exert its effect for up to 3 months because plasma protein binding prohibits it from being eliminated from the body. Drugs vary as to the extent of binding in the plasma, and most drugs used in medicine and dentistry do bind to some extent. Phenylbutazone, a nonsteroidal anti-inflammatory agent, is bound to the extent of 98% of its therapeutic dose, whereas pentobarbital, a barbiturate hypnotic, is bound approximately 55%.

Plasma protein binding is characterized by the existence of a limited number of binding sites on albumin—the major plasma protein involved in drug binding. Two drugs having affinity for the same binding sites will compete with one another for binding. If a drug is highly bound, the usual therapeutic dose may become toxic when followed by the administration of a drug that displaces it from its plasma protein storage sites.[16]

Tissue distribution

Along with plasma transport, drugs are simultaneously distributed to organ tissue sites. These sites are conveniently classified as *specific* or *nonspecific*, depending on whether the drug elicits therapeutic activity at the site in question. Tissue distribution from the plasma involves the passage of drugs across cell membranes—a process involving those factors discussed earlier for membranes in general. Tissue distribution of drugs also involves binding to intracellular components such as mucopolysaccharides, nucleoprotein, and phospholipids. Like plasma protein binding, binding to intracellular tissue components affects the half-life of a drug. Without these tissue storage sites many drugs would be rapidly metabolized and eliminated from the body, having little time to exert any effect. Some drugs show a greater affinity for tissue components than for plasma proteins, whereas other drugs prefer localization in one type of tissue rather than in another. Tetracyclines have an unusual affinity for bone and enamel tissue. The antimalarial quinacrine binds selectively to nuclear material in liver and skeletal muscle cells.[17] Guanethidine, a drug useful in treating hypertension, selectively binds to heart and skeletal muscle tissues.[18] Thiopental, a barbiturate hypnotic, has a predisposition for adipose tissue.[19] These "affinity tissues" may be sites of action or areas for transient storage.

Certain tissue sites of the body deserve special consideration in drug distribution. Passage of drugs into and out of the central nervous system involves transfer across the blood-brain barrier. This specialized limiting barrier consists of membranes of the capillary walls and surrounding glial cells. The passage of a drug through this barrier into the cerebrospinal fluid is related to its degree of lipid solubility and ionization. Thiopental, a highly lipid-soluble, nonionized drug, readily penetrates into the cerebrospinal fluid to induce sleep within seconds after intravenous injection. On the other hand, the less lipid-soluble barbiturate phenobarbital takes much longer to induce the same degree of narcosis. Lipid-insoluble drugs such as quaternary ammonium compounds pass a thousand times less rapidly into the cerebrospinal fluid than does thiopental.[20]

Knowledge concerning the passage of chemical substances through the placenta is at present fragmentary. With respect to drug transfer, the placenta is considered to resemble the blood-brain barrier, and the majority of drugs are believed to cross by a process of simple diffusion in accordance with their degree of lipid solubility.[21,22] Thus nonionized drugs of high fat solubility such as anesthetics and barbiturate hypnotics cross the placenta readily and rapidly.

There are indications that the placenta may act as a selective barrier toward certain drugs passing into and out of fetal tissues. After intravenous injection of lidocaine, a large gradient existed between maternal and fetal blood levels, with higher levels of drug existing in fetal tissues for up to 40 minutes.[23] This gradient could not be explained by increased binding to fetal serum protein or transformation in the fetus to a more polar compound, which would prevent its passage out of the fetal tissues. Molecular drug characteristics other than lipid solubility may also influence transplacental transfer. Procaine has been shown to cross the placenta without difficulty but is detected in fetal venous blood only after the maternal injection of 4 mg/kg, whereas mepivacaine, another local anesthetic, can be detected in fetal blood after the injection of a much smaller dose. This phenomenon is explained by the fact that mepivacaine is resistant to enzyme attack in maternal blood, whereas procaine is readily hydrolyzed in maternal blood and is therefore less stable biologically.[24]

Redistribution

Redistribution of a drug from one organ tissue to another can greatly affect its duration of action. For example, if redistribution occurs between tissues at the site of action and nonspecific tissues, termination of drug effect can result. The clinical example of thiopental may be cited. After a single intravenous dose of this hypnotic, plasma levels fall abruptly and subjects awake within 10 minutes. Subsequently, plasma levels decline very slowly, and most of the drug localizes first in muscle, then in fat depots of the body. The rapid termination of the hypnotic action of this agent results from redistribution from the brain and other tissues to adipose tissue.[19] Although a drug may be redistributed to other tissues after an action occurs, its eventual elimination from the body is dependent on biotransformation and excretion mechanisms.

MOLECULAR MECHANISMS OF DRUG ACTION

The three mechanisms by which drugs act to elicit a pharmacologic effect are drug-receptor interactions, physicochemical actions, and enzyme modifications.

Drug receptors

Authorities have postulated for many years that drug actions result from the attachment to specific chemically defined portions of the tissues or cells on which they act. Such a specific cellular component is called a receptor substance, or *drug receptor*. As long ago as 1878, receptor substances were postulated that were capable of forming complexes with substances having proper chemical affinity.[25] Although receptor substances have yet to be isolated from tissues, it has become possible to hope that drug-receptor interactions may be visualized as the interaction of three dimensionally defined chemical entities.[26]

Drugs which have a chemical affinity for a receptor substance so that combination with the receptor produces a functional change in the surrounding tissue cells are called *agonists*. Theories concerning the response of receptor substances to agonists include certain basic assumptions. First, the intensity of agonist effect is not necessarily proportional to the number of receptors occupied in any given tissue. For many years the viewpoint was held that the intensity of response was directly related to the number of receptors occupied by an agonist.[27] However, observations show that a maximum drug effect could be induced with certain drugs when only 1% of the available receptors were occupied.[28] Second, a maximum effect can be produced by an agonist when only a small proportion of the receptors is occupied, and the response is not linearly proportional to the number of receptors occupied.[29] Third, different agonists may have different capacities to induce a response and consequently occupy different proportions of the receptors when producing equal responses.[29] This assumption takes into consideration the *affinity* and *efficacy* of drug action. Affinity is the ability of an agonist to combine with its receptor. Efficacy, as explained previously, is

a descriptive characteristic of drug action and may be thought of as the ability to induce a response subsequent to receptor occupation. Any agonist will exhibit both good affinity and high efficacy at a given receptor. Certain drugs act as weak agonists at certain receptor sites in that they exhibit low efficacy and have the ability to antagonize agonists of greater efficacy. Such drugs are regarded as *partial agonists*. Drugs exhibiting zero efficacy at a given receptor are considered to be *antagonists*.

Drug-receptor interactions may be described as the setting off of a chain of biochemical reactions resulting in increased cellular activity. For example, acetylcholine combines with receptor substances at the membranes of skeletal muscles and nerve cells. The drug-receptor interaction sets off biochemical changes that result in the contraction of muscle cells and impulse propagation in nerve cells. A drug such as atropine is capable of combining with the acetylcholine-receptor substance to form a complex that prevents the access of acetylcholine to the same receptors. The antagonist (atropine) thus competes for the acetylcholine receptor substance—a process known as *competitive antagonism*.

Paton[30] has explained drug-receptor interactions in terms of a rate theory. This hypothesis states that drug effects are not related to the proportion of receptors occupied but are proportional to the rate of drug-receptor combination where each drug-receptor association provides one "quantum" of excitation. Although this theory has been criticized, it still remains popular.

Physicochemical actions and enzyme modifications

Some drugs may affect the structure of essential macromolecules such as membrane components, receptor proteins, or nucleic acids through modifications of the solvent structure surrounding the macromolecule. This action is descriptive of agents such as general anesthetics and hypnotics that induce actions at the cellular level through physicochemical rather than pure chemical means. For example, one mechanism proposed for general anesthetics involves a physical combination with water molecules to form hydrate microcrystals called clathrates,[31] the presence of which may alter the properties of nerve cell membranes to depress nerve cell function.

Some drugs act by affecting the function of cellular enzyme systems. This action is based on the fact that the molecular configuration of the drug so resembles that of the enzyme substrate that an enzyme-drug interaction occurs which modifies or inhibits the normal function of the enzyme. Anticholinesterase drugs such as neostigmine and edrophonium exert pharmacologic effects as a consequence of inhibition of the cholinesterase enzyme. Monoamine oxidase inhibitors such as iproniazid are used therapeutically because of their enzyme-inhibitory properties.

In summary, drugs may act by way of drug-receptor interactions, physicochemical actions, or enzyme modifications. All of these mechanisms result from a drug's ability to seek out cellular tissue components for which it has specific affinity. To be useful for altering cellular functions, this selective action of a drug on cellular components must be reversible.

Mechanisms must exist in the body for the termination of drug action, since most drugs act for only a short period of time after the administration of a single dose. This process occurs by way of (1) biotransformation and (2) elimination of unchanged drug or its metabolites. Knowledge concerning these processes is essential for the intelligent use of drugs. A third mechanism not involving drug elimination has previously been considered and entails the redistribution of drug from active sites to storage sites in the tissues.

DRUG METABOLISM (BIOTRANSFORMATION)

Most drugs undergo metabolic transformation in the body. Metabolism or biotransformation is one of the factors that determine plasma and tissue levels of an active drug. A metabolic product is usually more polar and less lipid soluble than its parent compound. As a result, renal tubular reabsorption of the metabolite will be reduced, since this process favors lipid-soluble compounds. Also, specific secretory mechanisms in proximal renal tubules and parenchymal liver cells operate on highly polar compounds. Therefore kidney and biliary secretion of these polar compounds will be favored. Compared with their parent compounds, metabolites are less likely to bind to plasma or tissue macromolecules and to be stored in fat tissue.

Drug metabolism is an enzyme-dependent process that developed as an adaptation to terrestrial life. Unlike fish, terrestrial vertebrates are unable to excrete lipid-soluble compounds because renal tubular reabsorption favors their retention. Excretion of these substances is accomplished easily across gill membranes of fish into the surrounding water.[32] Although drug metabolism results in the formation of compounds of a more polar nature, it does not always result in the initial production of biologically inactive compounds. Enzymatic modification of a parent drug can be distinguished by three different patterns. First, an inactive parent drug may be transformed to an active compound, for example:

6-Mercaptopurine → 6-Mercaptopurine ribonucle-
(inactive)   (active)   otide

6-Mercaptopurine is useful as an antineoplastic agent but is inactive until converted to the corresponding ribonucleotide through conjugation in body tissues.[33] Also, parathion, a cholinesterase inhibitor, is inactive until converted to paraoxon by oxidative desulfuration in mammalian liver.[34]

Second, an active parent drug may be converted to a second active compound, which is subsequently converted to an inactive product, for example:

Phenacetin
(active)

Acetaminophen
(active)

Acetaminophen
glucuronide
(inactive)

Phenacetin, a mild analgesic-antipyretic, is initially converted to acetaminophen, another analgesic-antipyretic, through an oxidative mechanism. Acetaminophen is then inactivated through the formation of a second metabolite.[35]

Third, an inactive compound may be formed from an active parent drug, for example:

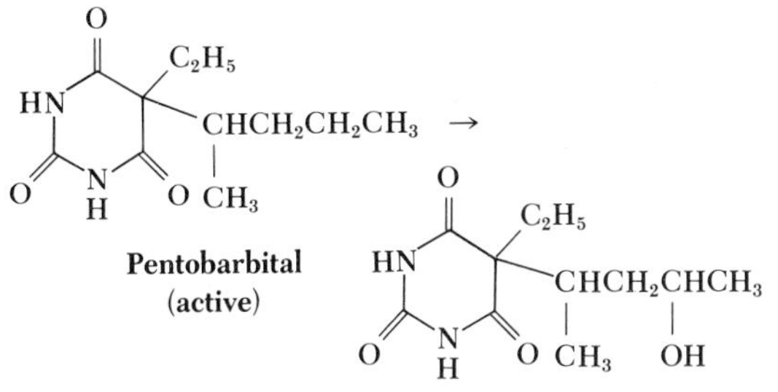

Pentobarbital
(active)

Pentobarbital alcohol
(inactive)

Pentobarbital, a barbiturate hypnotic, is converted to its inactive alcoholic derivative, which will be subsequently transformed into other inactive products. Reactions of this third general type are the most common in drug biotransformation. Drug metabolism rates and pathways may vary, depending on the species. Most studies indicate, however, that drug biotransformation in laboratory animals (the most studied population) is similar to that in humans.

Conjugations

One way the body converts lipid-soluble drugs to more polar compounds is through the synthesis of a conjugated compound. This is achieved by the attachment of a molecule of an acid normally present in the body to the drug in question. Both the parent compound and those metabolites formed by other reactions can be conjugated—a process mediated by enzymes called *transferases.*

Glucuronic acid, a normally occurring substance in the body, may be transferred to any drug molecule possessing an appropriate functional group to accept it, for example:

Uridine diphosphoglucuronic acid (UDPGA) serves as a donor of glucuronic acid to the phenolhydroxyl group of acetaminophen to form an ether glucuronide. Some other acceptor substances with which glucuronic acid will combine to form a conjugate include alcohols, aromatic amines, and carboxylic acids.

Other synthetic mechanisms of drug metabolism include the acetylation of aromatic amines, the synthesis of mercapturic acids and of sulfuric acid esters, glutamine conjugation, and methylation. Table 2-1 summarizes these synthetic mechanisms and indicates the type of compound that is detoxified by each mechanism and the activated compound responsible for the donation of the molecule with which a particular compound conjugates.

Liver microsomal drug-metabolizing system

The body is faced with a more difficult problem if a drug molecule lacks appropriate functional groups suitable for conjugation. An enzyme system located in the hepatic endoplasmic reticulum is responsible for the oxidative metabolism of many drugs. These enzymes are known as *microsomal enzymes,* since they are located in the microsomal fraction as prepared from liver homogenates. A variety of oxidative reactions occur in the hepatic microsomes. A common occurrence, however, is that most of the oxidations consist of the hydroxylation of substrate or the direct incorporation of oxygen into the substrate molecule.[36] The specific metabolic reactions include the following:

Aromatic ring and side-chain hydroxylation
N- and O-dealkylation
Sulfoxide formation
N-oxidation and N-hydroxylation
Deamination of primary and secondary amines

The hepatic microsomal oxidative enzyme system is characterized by a requirement for reduced nicotine adenine diphosphate (NADPH) and molecular oxygen. The oxida-

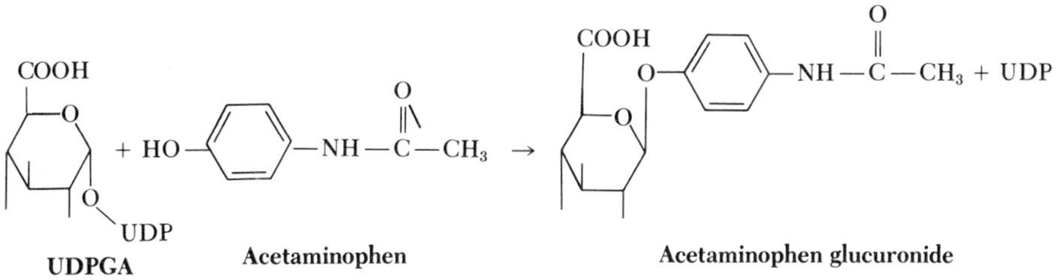

UDPGA　　　**Acetaminophen**　　　**Acetaminophen glucuronide**

Table 2-1. Synthetic mechanisms of drug metabolism

Mechanism	Compounds detoxicated	Active donor compound
Glucuronic acid conjugation	Compounds having: Phenolic OH Alcoholic OH COOH Aromatic amines	Glucuronic acid as uridine diphosphoglucuronic acid (UDPGA)
Acetylation	Aromatic amines	Acetyl CoA
Mercapturic acid formation	Aromatic hydrocarbons Halogenated aromatic hydrocarbons Halogenated nitrobenzenes	Activated glutathione
Sulfuric acid ester formation	Aromatic OH Aliphatic OH	3'-phosphoadenosine-5'-phosphosulfate (PAPS)
Glutamine conjugation	Aromatic acids	CoA derivative of the acid to be conjugated
Methylation	Compounds having: Two phenolic OH >NH —NH$_2$	S-adenosylmethionine

tive processes of drug metabolism also involve an electron transport chain. The oxidative mechanisms may be summarized. A drug substrate binds with oxidized cytochrome P-450 (so called because it absorbs light at 450 mm when exposed to carbon monoxide).[38] The resulting drug-cytochrome P-450 complex is reduced by the flavoprotein NADPH–cytochrome C reductase, and the reduced complex then combines with molecular oxygen. A second electron and two hydrogen ions are acquired from a flavoprotein donor system, and the resulting products are oxidized drug and water. Oxidized cytochrome P-450 is subsequently regenerated (Fig. 4).

The rate of drug biotransformation appears to be related to the amounts of cytochrome P-450 present in the microsomes. In fact, there is a direct correlation between the stimulation of drug oxidation by various substances and an increase in the amounts of cytochrome P-450.[37]

Other oxidations

Enzymes other than those of the hepatic microsomal system can mediate oxidative reactions of selected pharmacologic compounds. Alcohol is dehydrogenated by alcohol dehydrogenase to the corresponding aldehyde. Naturally occurring amines and a few drugs are oxidatively deaminated by monoamine and diamine oxidases located in mitochondria of liver, kidney, and nervous tissue. Halogenated compounds (such as insecticides and industrial solvents) are dehalogenated by specific oxidative enzymes.

Hydrolysis

The hydrolysis of the local anesthetic procaine (an ester type of compound) by plasma cholinesterase is illustrative of this type of drug transformation:

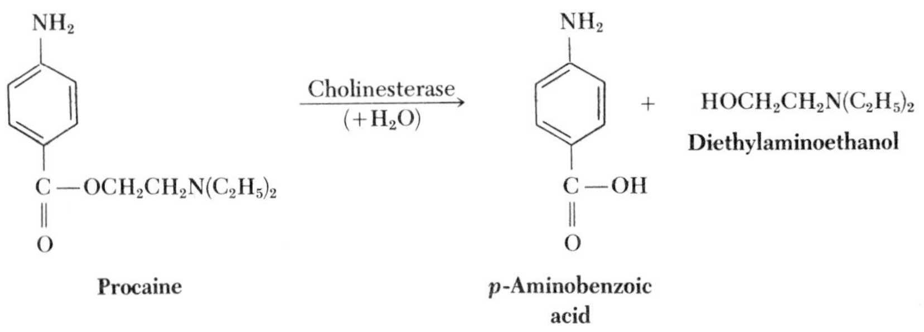

NH$_2$ (benzene ring) C—OCH$_2$CH$_2$N(C$_2$H$_5$)$_2$ ‖ O **Procaine**

$$\xrightarrow[\text{(+H}_2\text{O)}]{\text{Cholinesterase}}$$

NH$_2$ (benzene ring) C—OH ‖ O **p-Aminobenzoic acid**

+ HOCH$_2$CH$_2$N(C$_2$H$_5$)$_2$ **Diethylaminoethanol**

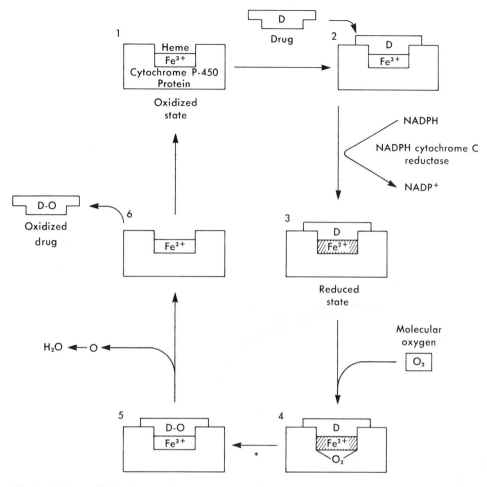

Fig. 4. Oxidation of a drug by cytochrome P-450. Cytochrome P-450 is a complex of protein and heme that contains an atom of iron initially in the ferric (Fe^{3+}) or oxidized state (*1*). The cytochrome complex binds the drug (*2*). The enzyme NADPH cytochrome C reductase, utilizing NADH, reduces the heme iron to the ferrous form (Fe^{2+}) (*3*), the form which then binds molecular oxygen (*4*). One atom of the molecular oxygen then oxidizes the drug (D-O) and one forms water, with the cytochrome P-450 reverting to its oxidized form (*5*). Oxidized drug is released (*6*), and cytochrome P-450 is regenerated. The asterisk denotes the contribution of a second electron and two hydrogen ions from a flavoprotein donor system.

Drug metabolism by mechanisms of hydrolysis is limited to ester compounds. Hydrolytic enzymes such as cholinesterases are found in plasma and a variety of tissues.

Reduction

An example of this type of metabolic transformation is the reduction of chloral hydrate, a hypnotic agent, to trichloroethanol.

$$
\underset{\substack{|\\ OH}}{\overset{\substack{H\\|}}{Cl_3C - C - OH}} \quad \rightarrow \quad \underset{\substack{|\\ H}}{\overset{\substack{H\\|}}{Cl_3C - C - OH}}
$$

Alcohol dehydrogenase, found in the nonmicrosomal portion of hepatic cells, catalyzes this reduction of chloral hydrate. Another common reduction reaction is the nitro reduction of the antibiotic chloramphenicol. This reductive reaction is mediated by enzymes found in hepatic microsomes.

Clinical aspects of hepatic microsomal enzyme drug metabolism

Microsomal enzyme activity is influenced by the administration of various drugs. The experimental drug SKF525-A (β-diethylaminoethyl-2,2-diphenylpentanoate) is a well-known inhibitor of microsomal enzymes in animals. Clinically, coumarin anticoagulants inhibit the metabolic inactivation of tolbutamide and phenytoin through an effect on microsomal enzymes. The simultaneous administration of the anticoagulant with the former drug resulted in a hypoglycemic crisis, whereas administration with the latter drug resulted in toxic manifestations.[39,40]

It is a well-known fact that the activities of hepatic microsomal oxidative enzymes are decidedly increased when animals are treated with various drugs. The increased enzymatic activity is caused by an increase in the concentration of enzyme protein—a phenomenon referred to as *enzyme induction*.[37] These stimulatory effects of drugs on microsomal enzymes also have been found to occur in humans. The administration of 30 mg phenobarbital three times every 24 hours decreased the anticoagulant response to bishydroxycoumarin in hospitalized patients.[41] This effect was attributable to the stimulatory effects of phenobarbital on the hepatic microsomal enzymatic metabolism of the anticoagulant.[42]

Griseofulvin (an antifungal agent) was observed to stimulate the hepatic microsomal metabolism of the anticoagulant warfarin, and simultaneous therapy with the two drugs resulted in a decreased anticoagulant response.[43] Phenobarbital stimulates the metabolism of phenytoin and griseofulvin, an action that resulted in decreased plasma levels of the two drugs.[42,44] Also, phenylbutazone has been observed to cause an increase in the metabolic deactivation of the analgesic aminopyrine through a similar mechanism.[45] Certain drugs can stimulate their own metabolism when administered over a long period of time to humans. Patients who become tolerant to the hypnotic effects of glutethimide were found to have an increased capacity to metabolize the drug.[37]

EXCRETION

Drugs may be excreted by any route in the body that has direct access to the environment. Renal excretion is the most important route. Extrarenal routes include the lungs, bile and gastrointestinal tract, sweat, saliva, and milk. Drugs may be excreted unchanged or as a more polar, less lipid-soluble metabolite. Body excretion mechanisms favor the elimination of the latter compounds.

Renal route

Elimination of substances in the kidney is dependent on glomerular filtration, active tubular secretion, and passive tubular diffusion. Molecules of unchanged drug or its metabolites are first filtered through the glomeruli and are concentrated in the renal tubular fluid. Many drugs are added to the amount in the glomerular filtrate by active secretion that transports the drug from the blood across renal tubular epithelial cells into renal tubular fluid. Penicillin, an organic acid, is excreted rapidly by glomerular filtration and tubular secretion.

With most drugs, passive tubular diffusion plays a part in regulating the amount of drug in the tubular fluid. This is a reabsorption process that favors nonionized lipid-soluble compounds. On filtration of these compounds through the glomerulus into the tubular fluid, passive diffusion of the substance will occur into the plasma through the epithelial cell membranes that line the tubules. More ionized, less lipid-soluble metabolites are less able to penetrate these cell membranes by passive diffusion and are more likely to be retained in the tubular fluid to be eventually eliminated in the urine.

Most drugs are weakly ionized acids or bases, and urinary pH has an influence on the renal excretion rates of these compounds. When tubular urinary pH is more alkaline than plasma, weak acids are excreted more rapidly. When tubular urine is more acid, weak acids are excreted more slowly. With weak bases, the effects of urinary pH are the opposite. Thus, in aspirin or barbiturate poisoning greater quantities of these weakly acidic drugs can be eliminated by simply making the tubular urine more alkaline than plasma. This is often accomplished by injecting sodium bicarbonate intravenously.

Extrarenal routes

Gaseous and volatile liquids such as those used in general anesthesia are absorbed and excreted across pulmonary alveolar membranes by the process of simple diffusion. Some drugs taken orally such as paraldehyde may also be partially eliminated by way of the lungs.

Biliary excretion is the major route by which systemically absorbed drugs enter the gastrointestinal tract where elimination in the feces occurs, unless the drug is reabsorbed through the enteric membranes of the intestine. Many organic acids, which exist in an ionized state at physiologic pH, and also charged quaternary ammonium compounds can be recovered in the bile. This is believed to occur through specific carrier-mediated transport mechanisms. On the other hand, substances such as insulin and sucrose passively diffuse into the bile. Drugs such as erythromycin, estradiol, and testosterone have been shown to be excreted in bile in amounts greater than 10% of an administered dose in humans.[46]

Excretion of drugs in milk and sweat are considered minor routes of elimination. Drugs excreted in milk may be potential sources of undesired effects to the nursing infant. Drugs such as nicotinamide, quinine, and sulfanilamide have been recovered from human sweat after oral administration.[47-49]

Salivary drug excretion is of interest to dentistry and has been adequately reviewed by Afonsky.[50] Most of the information concerning salivary drug excretion has been obtained in animal studies. High concentrations of phenytoin, an anticonvulsant agent, have been found in the rat salivary gland and cat saliva in the form of the unmetabolized drug.[51] It is interesting to speculate on a possible relationship between salivary secretion of the drug and the development of gingival hyperplasia. Sulfonamides and barbiturates have been recovered in human saliva but in levels well below their unbound levels in plasma.[52] Penicillins, dihydrostreptomycin, and tetracyclines have also been recovered from saliva.[53] With penicillin G there is evidence for an active secretory mechanism similar to its active secretion in renal tubular cells.

CONSIDERATIONS IN DRUG ADMINISTRATION

Most of this chapter has been concerned with those factors which affect the availability of a drug to its site of action in the body and their relation to the time course of drug action and variation in individual drug response. The remaining discussion involves some factors that have considerations in drug administration.

Tolerance

Drug tolerance is defined as the need for increasingly larger doses of drug to obtain the effects observed with the original dose or,

conversely, when, after repeated administration, a given dose of drug produces a decreasing effect. Tolerance is commonly acquired with narcotic analgesics, sedatives and hypnotics, and nitrate coronary vasodilators. When a patient becomes tolerant to one drug, a cross tolerance may develop to the actions of pharmacologically related drugs. Increasing the drug dosage is one method utilized to overcome this condition. If tolerance to a drug exists, normal sensitivity to the drug effect can usually be reestablished by suspending the administration of the drug.

Pathologic state

The pathologic condition of a patient may influence his response to medication. The hyperthyroid patient is extremely sensitive to the therapeutic and toxic effects of epinephrine. Patients with intracranial pressure are unusually sensitive to the actions of morphine. Hepatic and renal disease will have much influence on the hepatic metabolism and renal excretion of drugs.

Age and weight

Age is only rarely considered in determining drug dosage for adults. Weight, however, is the usual basis for determining drug dosage, and optimum therapeutic doses are generally identified in terms of amount of drug per kilogram of body weight of the patient.

Children's dosage presents a special problem in therapeutics. Traditionally, a child's dose has been adjusted in accordance with formulas based on body weight or age. With many drugs, however, the manufacturer issues suggested pediatric dose schedules usually in terms of amount of drug per pound of body weight per 24 hours. This is particularly common with antibiotic agents. The following formulas have been suggested for dose calculation in infants and preschool children:

CLARK'S RULE
$$\frac{\text{Weight (lb)} \times \text{Adult dose}}{150} = \text{Infant dose}$$

FRIED'S RULE
$$\frac{\text{Age (mo)} \times \text{Adult dose}}{150} = \text{Infant dose}$$

Clark's rule is based on the child's weight; Fried's rule is based on the child's age. The former rule assumes that an average adult weight is 150 pounds, and the latter rule assumes that by the 150th month, a child has reached a time in age when an adult dose can be tolerated. Two other formulas have been suggested to be used for children ranging from preschool to adolescent years.

YOUNG'S RULE

$$\frac{\text{Age (yr)} \times \text{Adult dose}}{\text{Age (yr)} + 12} = \text{Child dose}$$

COWLING'S RULE

$$\frac{\text{Age (at next birthday)} \times \text{Adult dose}}{24} = \text{Child dose}$$

Both of these formulas are based on the age of the child, and Young's rule seems to be the more popular of the two. Since weight may vary according to different children and infants of the same age, and in many cases the dose based on age is underestimated, a better method for the estimation of a child or infant's dose is based on body surface area.

$$\frac{\text{Surface area} \times \text{Adult dose}}{2.00} = \text{Child dose}$$

This formula assumes that the body surface area of a 6-foot, 175-pound adult is 200 square meters. Tables are available indicating the body surface area of a child in square meters given his height and weight. At present it is believed that the pediatric doses based on the manufacturer's or prescriber's experience are much better than those calculated from any of the above rules.

REFERENCES

1. Campbell, J. A., and Morrison, A. B.: Oral prolonged-action medication, J.A.M.A. 181:102-105, 1962.
2. Nelson, E.: Pharmaceuticals for prolonged action, Clin. Pharmacol. Ther. 4:283-292, 1963.
3. Feinstein, M. B., Lenard, W., and Mathias, J.: The antagonism of local anesthetic induced convulsions by the benzodiazepine derivative diazepam, Arch. Int. Pharmacodyn. Ther. 187:144-154, 1970.
4. Goldstein, A., Aronow, L., and Kalman, S. M.: Principles of drug action: the basis of pharmacology, New York, 1968, Harper & Row, Publishers, p. 111.
5. Adriani, J., and Campbell, B.: Fatalities following topical application of local anesthetics to mucous membranes, J.A.M.A. 162:1527-1530, 1956.
6. Robertson, J. D.: The ultrastructure of cell membranes and their derivatives, Biochem. Soc. Symp. 16:3-43, 1959.
7. Singer, S. J., and Nicolson, G. L.: A fluid mosaic model of cell membranes, Science 175:720-731, 1972.
8. Goldstein, A., Aronow, L., and Kalman, S. M.: Principles of drug action: the basis of pharmacology, New York, 1968, Harper & Row, Publishers, pp. 149-150.
9. Pappenheimer, J. R., Renkin, E. M., and Borrero, L. M.: Filtration, diffusion and molecular sieving through peripheral capillary membranes: a contribution to the pore theory of capillary permeability, Am. J. Physiol. 167:13-46, 1951.
10. Schanker, L. S.: Passage of drugs across body membranes, Pharmacol. Rev. 14:501-550, 1962.
11. Pappenheimer, J. R.: Passage of molecules through capillary walls, Physiol. Rev. 33:387-423, 1953.
12. Solomon, A. K.: The permeability of red cells to water and ions, Ann. N.Y. Acad. Sci. 75:175-181, 1958.
13. Wilbrandt, W., and Rosenberg, T.: The concept of carrier transport and its corollaries in pharmacology, Pharmacol. Rev. 13:109-183, 1961.
14. Danielli, J. F.: Morphological and molecular aspects of active transport, Symp. Soc. Exp. Biol. 8:502-516, 1954.
15. Goldstein, A.: The interaction of drugs and plasma proteins, Pharmacol. Rev. 1:102-165, 1949.
16. Meyer, M. S., and Guttman, D. E.: The binding of drugs by plasma proteins, J. Pharm. Sci. 57:895-918, 1968.
17. Shannon, J. A., Earle, D. P., Jr., Brodie, B. B., Taggart, J. V., and Berliner, R. W.: The pharmacological basis for the rational use of atabrine in the treatment of malaria, J. Pharmacol. Exp. Ther. 81:307-330, 1944.
18. Schanker, L. S., and Morrison, A. S.: Physiological disposition of guanethidine in the rat and its uptake by heart slices, Int. J. Neuropharmacol. 4:27-39, 1965.
19. Brodie, B. B.: Physicochemical and biochemical aspects of pharmacology, J.A.M.A. 202:600-609, 1967.
20. Mayer, S., Maickel, R. P., and Brodie, B. B.: Kinetics of penetration of drugs and other foreign compounds in cerebrospinal fluid and brain, J. Pharmacol. Exp. Ther. 127:205-211, 1959.
21. Ginsburg, J.: Placental drug transfer, Ann. Rev. Pharmacol. 11:387-408, 1971.
22. Moya, F., and Thorndike, V.: Passage of drugs across the placenta, Am. J. Obstet. Gynecol. 84:1778-1798, 1962.
23. Shnider, S. M., and Way, E. L.: The kinetics of transfer of lidocaine (Xylocaine^R) across the human placenta, Anesthesiology 29:944-950, 1968.
24. Usubiaga, J. E., Iuppa, M. L., Moya, F., Wikinski, J. A., and Velazco, R.: Passage of procaine hydrochloride and para-aminobenzoic acid across the human placenta, Am. J. Obstet. Gynecol. 100:918-923, 1968.
25. Langley, J. N.: On the mutual antagonism of atropine and pilocarpine, having special reference to their relations in the sub-maxillary gland of the cat, J. Physiol. 1:339-369, 1878.
26. Mautner, H. G.: The molecular basis of drug action, Pharmacol. Rev. 19:107-144, 1967.
27. Clark, A. J.: General pharmacology. In Heffter, A., editor: Handbuch der experimentellen Pharmakologie, Berlin, 1937, Julius Springer-Verlag, Vol. 4, p. 63.
28. Nickerson, M.: Receptor occupancy and tissue response, Nature (Lond.) 178:697-698, 1956.
29. Stephenson, R. P.: A modification of receptor theory, Br. J. Pharmacol. Chemother. 11:379-393, 1956.
30. Paton, W. D. M.: A theory of drug action based on

the rate of drug-receptor combination, Proc. R. Soc., Ser. B. **154:**21-69, 1961.

31. Pauling, L.: A molecular theory of general anesthesia, Science **134:**15-21. 1961.
32. Brodie, B. B., and Maickel, R. P.: Comparative biochemistry of drug metabolism. In Brodie, B. B., and Erdös, E. G., editors: Metabolic factors controlling duration of drug action, Proceedings of First International Pharmacological Meeting, New York, 1962, The Macmillan Co., Vol. 6, p. 299.
33. Allan, P. W., Schnebli, H. P., and Bennett, L. L., Jr.: Conversion of 6-mercaptopurine and 6-mercaptopurine ribonucleotide to 6-methylmercaptopurine ribonucleotide in human epidermoid carcinoma cells in culture, Biochim. Biophys. Acta **114:**647-650, 1966.
34. Davison, A. N.: The conversion of Schradan (OMPA) and Parathion into inhibitors of cholinesterase by mammalian liver, Biochem. J. **61:**203-209, 1955.
35. Brodie, B. B., and Axelrod, J.: The fate of acetophenetidin (phenacetin) in man and methods for the estimation of acetophenetidin and its metabolites in biological material, J. Pharmacol. Exp. Ther. **97:**58-67, 1949.
36. Gillette, J. R.: Biochemistry of drug oxidation and reduction by enzymes in hepatic endoplasmic reticulum. In Garattini, S., and Shore, P. A., editors: Advances in pharmacology, New York, 1966, Academic Press Inc., Vol. 4.
37. Conney, A. H.: Pharmacological implications of microsomal enzyme induction, Pharmacol. Rev. **19:**317-366, 1967.
38. Omura, J., Sato, R., Cooper, D. Y., Rosenthal, O., and Estabrook, R. W.: Function of cytochrome P-450 of microsomes, Fed. Proc. **24:**1181-1189, 1965.
39. Hansen, J. M., Kristensen, M., Skovsted, L., and Christensen, L. K.: Dicumarol induced diphenylhydantoin intoxication, Lancet **2:**265-266, 1966.
40. Kristensen, M., and Hansen, J. M.: Potentiation of the tolbutamide effect of dicumarol, Diabetes **16:**211-214, 1967.
41. Corn, M., and Rockett, J. F.: Inhibition of bishydroxycoumarin activity by phenobarbital, Med. Ann. D.C. **34:**578-579, 1965.
42. Cucinell, S. A., Conney, A. H., Sansur, M., and Burns, J. J.: Drug interactions in man: 1. Lowering effect of phenobarbital on plasma levels of bishydroxycoumarin (dicumarol) and diphenylhydantoin (Dilantin), Clin. Pharmacol. Ther. **6:**420-429, 1965.
43. Catalano, P. M., and Cullen, S. I.: Warfarin antagonism by griseofulvin, Clin. Res. **14:**266, 1966.
44. Busfield, D., Child, K. J., Atkinson, R. M., and Tomich, E. G.: An effect of phenobarbitone on blood-levels of griseofulvin in man, Lancet **2:**1042-1043, 1963.
45. Chen, W., Vrindten, P. A., Dayton, P. G., and Burns, J. J.: Accelerated aminopyrine metabolism in human subjects pretreated with phenylbutazone, Life Sci. **1:**35-42, 1962.
46. Stowe, C. M., and Plaa, G. L.: Extrarenal excretion of drugs and chemicals, Ann. Rev. Pharmacol. **8:**337-356, 1968.
47. Comaish, J. S., and Shelley, W. B.: Fluorometric determination of quinine and fluorescein excretion in human sweat, J. Invest. Dermatol. **44:**279-281, 1965.
48. Sargent, F., Robinson, P., and Johnson, R. E.: Water soluble vitamins in sweat, J. Biol. Chem. **153:**285-294, 1944.
49. Thaysen, J. H., and Schwartz, I. L.: The permeability of human sweat glands to a series of sulfonamide compounds, J. Exp. Med. **98:**261-268, 1953.
50. Alfonsky, D.: Saliva and its relation to oral health, University, Ala., 1961, University of Alabama Press.
51. Noach, E. L., Woodbury, D. M., and Goodman, L. S.: Studies on the absorption, distribution, fate and excretion of 4C^{14}-labeled diphenylhydantoin, J. Pharmacol. Exp. Ther. **122:**301-314, 1958.
52. Killmann, S. A., and Thaysen, J. H.: Permeability of human parotid gland to series of sulfonamide compounds, paraaminohippurate and inulin, Scand. J. Clin. Lab. Invest. **7:**86-91, 1955.
53. Borzelleca, J. F., and Cherrick, H. M.: The excretion of drugs in saliva. Antibiotics, J. Oral Ther. Pharmacol. **2:**180-187, 1965.

3

Adverse drug reactions

RICHARD L. WYNN

Although drugs act selectively in biologic systems to accomplish a desired effect, they lack absolute specificity in that they may act on many different organs or tissues. This lack of absolute specificity is the reason for undesirable or adverse drug reactions. No drug is free of producing some sort of adverse effect in a certain number of patients. This is a problem of importance that one must consider to practice dental therapeutics intelligently. It has been estimated that about 5% of the patients hospitalized annually in the United States are admitted because of adverse reactions to drugs,[1] with some hospitals reporting incidences as high as 20%.[2] Also, a minimum of 15% of hospitalized patients experience at least one adverse drug reaction.[3]

This chapter will summarize those principles of adverse drug effects that are fundamental to rational drug therapy. Definitions and classifications of adverse drug reactions are discussed and descriptions of selected clinical manifestations of those reactions are given. Also, fundamental principles of the toxicologic evaluation of drugs in lower animals and human beings are briefly discussed with regard to the evaluation of drug safety.

DEFINITIONS AND CLASSIFICATION OF ADVERSE DRUG REACTIONS

Unfortunately, all drugs have more than one action. The actions that are clinically desirable are termed *therapeutic effects*, and the undesirable actions are termed *adverse effects*. The fundamental objective in pharmacotherapeutics is to select the drug and dosage that will give maximal therapeutic effects and minimal adverse effects.

The literature does not reflect consistency in definitions related to adverse drug effects. Toxicology has been broadly defined as the study of the adverse effects of chemicals on biologic systems. Under this definition a "toxic effect" would be *any* adverse effect. I believe that some distinction should be made between toxic effects and certain other adverse reactions. In this text, toxic effects are defined as adverse effects that result from the direct action of drugs on the tissues or organ systems or both. Thus allergy, which results from antigen-antibody reactions, and some other undesirable effects will be categorized separately from toxicity. The importance of certain of these semantic distinctions is that a drug such as penicillin G has practically no effect on the tissues or organ systems and consequently should be considered to have a very low toxicity. However, the incidence of adverse reactions to penicillin is high in the form of allergic reactions. As is discussed in the chapters on specific drug groups, the direct toxic effect of drugs on certain tissues or organs represents therapeutic considerations that are different from considerations relative to allergic and certain other adverse potentialities.

"Side effects" are sometimes considered to be any undesirable effect. This is not a useful definition. In this text side effects are considered to be expected actions that occur in addition to the therapeutic effect. These are relatively predictable, generally mild reactions that the practitioner must accept as being rather consistently present when a certain drug is used. For instance, dryness of the mouth after the use of atropine in gastrointestinal tract ulcer therapy may be considered a side effect of the drug. At certain doses, however, atropine will cause a transient glaucoma-like condition in some patients because of its anticholinergic action on the eye. The severity of this effect leads to its categorization as a toxic effect. Obviously the dividing line between a severe side effect and a mild toxic effect is not distinct.

The following classification shows the important types of adverse drug reactions.

1. Toxic reactions
   a. Exaggerated effects on target organs or tissues
   b. Action on nontarget organ or tissues
   c. Effects on fetal development (teratogenic effects)
   d. Local reactions
   e. Drug interactions
2. Sensitization and allergic reactions
   a. Anaphylaxis
   b. Serum sickness
   c. Drug fever
   d. Cytotoxic reaction
   e. Skin reactions
3. Idiosyncrasy
4. Interference with natural defense mechanisms

Included are various toxic reactions, allergic reactions, idiosyncrasies, and interference with natural defense mechanisms. The following discussion will define these adverse effects by describing the clinical manifestations of each. Side effects of individual drugs will not be discussed here and are covered in the chapters devoted to specific drugs.

CLINICAL MANIFESTATIONS OF ADVERSE DRUG REACTIONS
Exaggerated effects on target organs or tissues

Adverse drug reactions may be caused by an exaggerated effect of a drug on its target organ or tissues. These reactions are considered to be an extension of the therapeutic effect caused by overreactions of the patient to the drug or by a drug overdose. For example, patients have experienced an exaggerated hypoglycemia when exposed to therapeutic doses of an oral hypoglycemic agent.[4] Occasionally, this type of drug reaction may result from the presence of an acquired disease condition by the patient. The presence of liver and kidney disorders may inhibit the termination of drug activity, since the mechanisms responsible for drug metabolism or excretion are inhibited. This effect will prolong the action of a drug, which could result in exaggerated responses or drug overdoses.

Effects on nontarget organs or tissues

Effects on nontarget organs or tissues are caused by nontherapeutic actions of a drug that usually appear at high doses or prolonged administration and that can generally be terminated by a reduction in dose. Thus salicylism results from repeated administration of large doses of salicylates and is manifested as headache, dizziness, ringing in the ears, mental confusion, alterations in acid-base balance, hyperventilation, drowsiness, nausea, and vomiting. The damaging effects of chloramphenicol on hematologic tissues, tetracyclines on hepatic tissues, and sulfonamides on renal tissues are other examples.

A preexisting disease condition may intensify this type of adverse drug effect. For example, peptic ulcers of the stomach and duodenum cause enhancement of the ulcerogenic effect of many drugs—an effect that can lead to gastric bleeding and ulcer perforation. Also, congenital anomalies of body metabolism may alter a patient's reaction to many drugs—an area of study known as *pharmacogenetics*. For example, some drugs are capable of inducing hemolysis to red blood cells in subjects who have inadequate levels of reduced glutathione caused by a genetically inherited deficiency of glucose-6-phosphate dehydrogenase—the enzyme responsible for maintaining reduced glutathione levels in red blood cells. Hemolysis occurs because of the inadequate amounts of glutathione present to protect against oxidative destruction of cell constituents. Sulfonamides and the antimalarial primaquine are some of the drugs implicated in this effect.

Effects on fetal development (teratogenic effects)

Karnofsky has stated that "any drug administered at the proper dosage, and at the proper stage of development to embryos of the proper species . . . will be effective in causing disturbances in embryonic development."[5] The human teratogenic effects associated with maternal rubella infection and progestational hormones have been known for some time, but concern over the potential teratogenic effects of other drugs was not evident until the thalidomide disaster of 1962. This seemingly innocuous sedative was shown to be responsible for an incidence of around 20% of abnormal offspring from patients exposed to the drug during critical periods of gestation. Fetal anomalies attributed to thalidomide included, among others, malformed or absent limbs and digits, soft tissue defects, cleft palate, malformed ears, failure of closure of the spinal cord, and skull defects. A limited number of other drugs have now been shown to be teratogenic to the human fetus and include growth-inhibiting anticancer agents and a few steroid hormones. Drugs used in dentistry such as penicillins, salicylates, sulfonamides, and vitamins have been shown to be teratogenic in a variety of animal species. Recently, the minor tranquilizer diazepam has been shown to be teratogenic in mice.[6] An association between ingestion of minor tranquilizers during pregnancy and increased risk of congenital anomalies has been suggested by three recent studies.[7-9] One study showed that the rate of anomalies when meprobamate was prescribed during the first 6 weeks of pregnancy was higher than when no drug was given.[7] For chlordiazepoxide the rate following exposure during the same period was also greater than the rates for other drugs. A second study reported an association of oral clefts with meprobamate and diazepam usage during pregnancy.[8] A third study showed that selected birth defects including cleft lip were associated with the use of diazepam by women during pregnancy.[9] The incorporation of tetracyclines into human fetal ossifying tissues results in irreversible staining of enamel, an action that can be considered teratogenic. The practical implications of the thalidomide tragedy have served as an impetus to reduce the use of drugs during pregnancy and to monitor potential teratogenic agents by way of preclinical testing in animals.

Local reactions

Local reactions are characterized by local tissue irritation and tissue deposition of drug crystals. Injectable drugs on occasion produce irritation, pain, and tissue necrosis in the skin and skeletal muscle. Aspirin readily causes irritation to the gastric mucosa because of its acidic properties. Upper gastrointestinal tract symptoms of many drugs taken orally include nausea, vomiting, dyspepsia, and heartburn. Many of the original sulfonamides caused renal damage attributable to the urinary concentration of these agents and to their properties of urine insolubility at physiologic pH. The synthesis of more soluble derivatives, however, has decreased the incidence of this toxic manifestation.

Drug interactions

The actions of an administered drug on the effectiveness of a second drug administered earlier, simultaneously, or later may result in undesired drug effects and, in many cases, toxicologic manifestations. The implications of drug interactions in dentistry are discussed in another chapter.

Sensitization and allergic reactions

Allergic reactions are considered to be the largest group of drug-induced adverse effects.[10] Drugs produce allergic reactions by acting as an antigen and reacting with antibody in a previously sensitized individual. Drugs can act as an antigen only after combining with large molecular weight compounds present in the body such as proteins.[11] The combination of a reactive drug with protein to form antigen occurs only after metabolic degradation of the drug so that a chemically reactive metabolite is formed. The reactive drug metabolite is referred to as the hapten.

When the antigen combines with antibody to form an antigen-antibody complex, a series of biochemical and physiologic events are triggered that can be extremely damaging. These events occur because of the release of mediators that provide the allergic symptoms. These mediators are present in the body in inactive form and become active when liberated. They include histamine, serotonin, and bradykinin. Antibodies to the drug antigen are formed during the sensitizing portion of the immune mechanism when the individual comes into initial contact with the antigen. The reaction part is seen when the sensitized individual is reexposed to the antigen.

Anaphylaxis

Anaphylaxis is an acute, life-threatening allergic reaction characterized by hypotension, bronchospasm, laryngeal edema, cardiac arrhythmias, and hyperperistalsis occurring in combination or as isolated manifestations. Symptoms most frequently appear after intravenous or intramuscular drug administration, although fatal anaphylaxis has sometimes occurred after a single oral dose of penicillin in highly sensitive individuals.[12,13]

Anaphylaxis occurs within 5 to 30 minutes, with early symptoms including nausea, vomiting, and dyspnea. The reaction usually occurs during the institution of a new course of treatment with a drug to which there has been previous exposure. There may or may not have been allergic symptoms during earlier exposure to the drug. Drugs used in dentistry that have produced fatal anaphylaxis include penicillins, local anesthetics, aspirin, vitamin B_{12}, tetracyclines, and cephalosporins.[14] The occurrence of 1 to 10 deaths per 10 million injections of penicillin attributable to anaphylaxis have been cited.[15] Unexpected anaphylaxis may occur during simple therapeutic procedures. For example, benzocaine has induced respiratory distress leading to the death of a patient who was medicated with a throat lozenge containing the drug.[16]

Serum sickness

Serum sickness is an allergic reaction produced by circulating antigen-antibody complexes characterized by fever, rash, lymphadenopathy, arthritis, edema, and neuritis. Drugs that produce serum sickness include penicillins, sulfonamides, phenytoin, and streptomycin. In the initial exposure to a drug, symptoms of serum sickness develop after 6 days or more with the allergic symptoms lasting for a few days to a week.

Drug fever

Drug allergy may be manifested as fever, particularly in association with treatment using penicillins, anticonvulsants, sulfonamides, and streptomycin. A severe and sustained fever usually occurs, which is associated with small-vessel inflammation. Withdrawal of the drug will cause the fever to subside.

Cytotoxic reactions

Allergic reactions to drugs may result in cellular damage because of a chemical reaction of the drug with the cell, making it susceptible to antibody-mediated cytotoxicity. An example of this type of allergy is penicillin-induced hemolytic anemia. At high penicillin blood levels, red blood cells become altered by penicillin haptens and combine with complementary antibody. As a result, accelerated phagocytosis and lysis of the cells occur, causing an increased red blood cell destruction and anemia. Cephalosporins and phenacetin also have caused immune hemolytic anemia.[17]

Skin reactions

Drug allergy is also manifested as skin reactions, and drugs have produced almost every known cutaneous reaction. These include petechial, maculopapular, bullous, nodular, eczematous, urticarial, erythematous, or photosensitive eruptions. The occurrence of dermatitis in a patient receiving a pharmacologic agent should always raise the possibility of the presence of a drug allergy.

Idiosyncrasy

Idiosyncratic reactions are those which cannot be explained by any known pharmacologic or biochemical mechanisms. For example, barbiturates have caused excitement in some geriatric patients. Obstructive jaundice induced by phenothiazines is also considered to be an idiosyncrasy. Idiosyncratic reactions may involve allergic mechanisms, since the obstructive jaundice condition is believed to result from hepatic sensitization.

Interference with natural defense mechanisms

Drug effects on nonspecific defense mechanisms can result in adverse reactions. Antibiotics have been shown to cause an overgrowth of the intestinal flora with nonphysiologic bacteria and fungi. Also, the long-term systemic administration of corticosteroids results, among other effects, in a depression in the resistance to infection.

TOXICOLOGIC EVALUATION OF DRUGS IN LOWER ANIMALS AND HUMAN BEINGS

Evaluation of the toxic effects of drugs must be based on experiments with lower animals and clinical trials in human beings. The optimum situation is the ability to predict adverse drug reactions in humans from data acquired in animals. Unfortunately, many drug reactions occurring in humans are not manifested in animals or are difficult to observe. Species differences in the physiologic handling of the drug undoubtedly con-

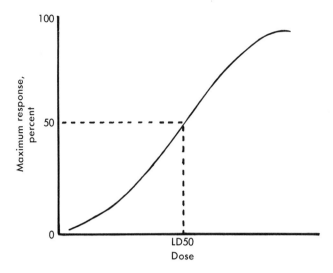

Fig. 5. Asymmetrical dose-response curve. Response is equivalent to death.

tribute to this problem. Also, many effects do not occur with enough frequency to be observed in the limited numbers of animals that are used for testing. The current animal tests utilized, however, are adequate in providing some fundamental information concerning the eventual safety of a drug in humans.

One of the first tests in evaluating the toxicity of any drug is to measure its acute lethality. A variety of approaches may be used to measure this, but the LD50 is by far the most popular. The term *LD50* is that dose of a drug (usually expressed as milligrams per kilogram) which kills 50% of the treated animals. This is determined in a fashion similar to that for the ED50 (Chapter 2). If increasing doses of a drug are administered to groups of animals, the mortality of the groups will be a direct function of the dose administered, and a certain dose of the drug will be lethal to 50% of the animals. For example, Fig. 5 indicates the dose of a drug plotted against the percent maximum response of animals responding (response equivalent to death). An asymmetrical curve known as a *dose-response curve* is then obtained. The dose on the dose axis that corresponds to the 50% response level on the response axis can then be read directly from the curve. This figure is the LD50.

Since all drugs are toxic at some dose, the LD50 is meaningless unless the ED50 is also known. For example, a drug having a lower ED50 (for example, 100 times less)

than its congener may at first appear to be more useful, since it is the more potent of the two. However, if the LD50 of the drug is only twice its ED50 and the LD50 of its congener is ten times its respective ED50, the congener would be the more useful of the two. The original drug, even though more potent than its congener, is much more toxic. The ratio LD50:ED50 is known as the therapeutic index of a drug.

$$\text{Therapeutic index} = \frac{\text{LD50}}{\text{ED50}}$$

This is a useful figure that gives some measure as to how far a therapeutic dose may be exceeded before eliciting toxic effects. For the clinical situation a better measure would be "adverse-effect dose 50/ED50," where a specific adverse effect is considered rather than the median lethal dose. It is difficult, however, to determine what the adverse ED50 is in each case. Theoretically, it would equal the dose of a drug that causes a specific adverse effect in 50% of the treated patients.

The LD50 and the therapeutic index as derived from animal studies are merely two measurements of many that are obtained for the safety evaluation of any drug. The following outline summarizes the various preclinical and clinical tests utilized to evaluate the safety of drugs:

1. Acute toxicity tests
2. Subacute (prolonged) toxicity tests
3. Chronic toxicity tests

4. Special studies
   a. Carcinogenicity
   b. Teratogenicity
   c. Mutagenicity
   d. Potentiation with other drugs
   e. Irritation
   f. Biotransformation
5. Clinical evaluation
   Phase I. Clinical pharmacology
   Phase II. Controlled evaluation phase
   Phase III. Broad trial phase

The preclinical tests are divided into three major phases—acute, subacute or prolonged, and chronic. It is during the acute phase that the LD50 is determined. For this phase single doses of the drug are administered usually on one occasion to two species, one of which is a rodent. Two routes of administration are used, with one being the intended clinical route.

The subacute phase generally consists of a duration of 2 to 13 weeks. The major purpose of this phase of testing is to determine in broad terms the dosages at which physiologic and specific toxicologic effects appear. Administration of the drug is generally by the intended clinical route, with rats and dogs being the usual species of choice. The doses given are based on the LD50 determined during the acute testing and usually consist of three levels. Evaluations are made of the state of health of the animals during the testing, and complete autopsies are performed.

Chronic tests are, of necessity, long in duration (90 days to 2 years). However, the methods are similar to the subacute testing, except that the testing may be carried through several generations of animals. The chronic tests sometimes reveal the need for specific tests requiring special procedures. Included are tests for carcinogenicity, teratogenicity, mutagenicity, drug potentiation, dermal irritation, and biotransformation characteristics of the compound.

Clinical trials performed for drug safety evaluation may also be divided into three phases. Phase I is a pilot study that uses small numbers of human volunteers. Initially, low doses of the drug that are gradually increased are used, and the toxic or exaggerated effects are monitored. Effects looked for are (1) those related to the desired pharmacologic effects but are exaggerated at the recommended dose, (2) those result-ing from actions on wrong target tissues, and (3) those unrelated to desired pharmacologic effects. Phase II is a controlled evaluation study that is required to confirm the data obtained in Phase I. It is during this phase that data concerning biotransformation and mechanisms of action of the drug are usually obtained. During the broad trial phase (Phase III), large-scale testing is performed to confirm data obtained in the first two phases. If the three studies demonstrate effectiveness and safety of the drug to the satisfaction of the Food and Drug Administration, the drug may be approved for distribution and eventual use by drug prescribers.

SUMMARY

One should note that drugs approved for therapeutic use are not necessarily free of adverse effects to the patient, since as previously mentioned, all drugs elicit some undesired effects in a certain percentage of patients. With regard to those reactions that can be predicted from information obtained during safety evaluation studies in animals and humans, however, certain questions can be answered. For example, do the beneficial effects outweigh the adverse effects of the drug to the patient? If not, is the need for the drug in a particular clinical situation great enough to justify subsequent adverse effects to the patient? With regard to unpredictable drug effects, the competency of the clinician to recognize and to treat specific adverse drug reactions is an important factor that will help limit this problem. Finally, by being fully cognizant of the pharmacologic actions, therapeutic use, and adverse effects of each drug, dental and medical practitioners can begin to successfully control those consequences of drug therapy that result from both predictable and unpredictable adverse drug reactions.

REFERENCES

1. Azarnoff, D. L.: Application of metabolic data to to the evaluation of drugs, J.A.M.A. 211:1691, 1970.
2. Miller, L. C.: How good are our drugs? Am. J. Hosp. Pharm. 27:367-374, 1970.
3. Report of the International Conference on Adverse Reactions Reporting Systems, Washington, D.C., 1971, National Academy of Sciences.
4. Sackner, M. A., and Balian, L. J.: Severe hypoglycemia after the ingestion of a sulfonylurea compound, Am. J. Med. 28:135-142, 1960.
5. Karnofsky, D. A.: Drugs as teratogens in animals and man, Ann. Rev. Pharmacol. 5:447-472, 1965.

6. Miller, R. P., and Becker, B. A.: Teratogenicity of oral diazepam and diphenylhydantoin in mice, Toxicol. Appl. Pharmacol. **32:**53-61, 1975.

7. Milkovich, L., and van den Berg, B. J.: Effects of prenatal meprobamate and chlordiazepoxide hydrochloride on human embryonic and fetal development, N. Engl. J. Med. **291:**1268-1271, 1974.

8. Saxen, I.: Associations between oral clefts and drugs taken during pregnancy, Int. J. Epidemiol. **4:**37-44, March, 1975.

9. Safra, M. J., and Oakley, G. P.: Association between cleft lip with or without cleft palate and prenatal exposure to diazepam, Lancet **2:**478-540, 1975.

10. Zbinden, G.: Experimental and clinical aspects of drug toxicity. In Garattini, S., and Shore, P. A., editors: Advances in pharmacology, New York, 1963, Academic Press Inc., vol. 2.

11. Landsteiner, K.: The specificity of serological reactions, Cambridge, Mass., 1945, Harvard University Press.

12. Maganzini, H. C.: Anaphylactoid reaction to penicillins V and G administered orally: report of two cases and brief review of the subject, N. Engl. J. Med. **256:**52-56, 1957.

13. Spark, R. P.: Fatal anaphylaxis due to oral penicillin, Am. J. Clin. Pathol. **56:**407-411, 1970.

14. Parker, C. W.: Drug allergy, N. Engl. J. Med. **292:**511-514, 1975.

15. Carr, E. A., Jr., and Aste, G. A.: Recent laboratory studies and clinical observations on hypersensitivity to drugs and use of drugs in allergy, Ann. Rev. Pharmacol. **1:**105-124, 1961.

16. Hesch, D. J.: Anaphylactic death from the use of a throat lozenge, J.A.M.A. **172:**12-15, 1960.

17. Parker, C. W.: Drug reactions. In Samter, M., and Alexander, H. L., editors: Boston, 1965, Little, Brown & Co., Inc.

4

Prescription writing

SAM V. HOLROYD

BARBARA REQUA-GEORGE

Some years ago, prescription writing was a rather complex and pretentious art. Written in Latin and embellished by the hieroglyphics of the apothecaries' system of weights and measures, the prescription represented clinical virtuosity at its best. Early prescriptions described the compounding of a preparation from various and frequently numerous constituents. In more recent years, four changes have greatly simplified prescription writing:

1. The pharmaceutical industry currently provides drugs in the proper forms and dosages to fill most pharmacotherapeutic needs. Consequently, it is now seldom necessary to detail the compounding of a drug on a prescription form. It is only necessary to indicate the particular liquid, tablet, or capsule one wishes to prescribe, and the drug is dispensed by the pharmacist without the necessity of his mixing the various active and passive ingredients of the preparation.
2. Prescriptions are no longer written in Latin (although currently used abbreviations are generally derived from the Latin).
3. The metric system of weights and measures has to to a great extent replaced the more confusing apothecaries' system in prescription writing.
4. It is no longer considered unsophisticated to limit or eliminate the use of abbreviations in prescription writing.[1]

METRIC SYSTEM

Scientific calculations employ a base of 10. Consequently, the metric system, which is based on 10, is the language of scientific measurement. Metric units are employed in the USP and should always be used in prescription writing.

□ The opinions or assertions contained herein are the private ones of the writers and are not to be construed as official or as reflecting the views of the Navy Department or the naval service at large.

The basic metric unit for the measurement of weight is the kilogram (kg). This unit is standardized as the mass of a metal cylinder kept at the International Bureau of Weights and Measures. The basic metric unit for volume is the liter (L), which was originally standardized as the volume of 1 kilogram of water at 4° C. In 1964[2] the liter was restandardized as 1 cubic decimeter, or 1000 cubic centimeters (cc). Consequently, 1 milliliter (ml) is exactly equivalent to 1 cc. Since the various units of the metric system are based on multiples of 10, several prefixes that apply to units of both weight and volume can be used. (See Table 4-1.)

Solid drugs are dispensed by weight (mg) and liquid drugs by volume (ml). It is rarely necessary to use units other than the milligram or the milliliter in prescription writing. Some practitioners learned and continue to use the apothecaries' system of weights and measures. Although this cumbersome system will in time be completely replaced by the metric system, one should be aware of its units. Table 4-2 shows the approximate equivalents of the metric and apothecaries' systems.

In summary, modern prescription writing is a simple procedure, usually requiring either one of two units of metric measurement, the milligram (mg) or the milliliter (ml). In a few rare cases requiring the microgram (μg, mcg), it is best to spell this out rather than risk any confusion on account of abbreviation.

ABBREVIATIONS

Abbreviations are used in prescription writing to save time. They also make alteration of a prescription by the patient more difficult. In some cases they are necessary to get

Table 4-1. Metric weight and volume

Weight	Volume
*kilo*gram (kg) = 1,000 grams (Gm)	liter (L) = 10 *deci*liters (dl)
	100 *centi*liters (cl)
	1,000 *milli*liters (ml)
	1,000,000 *micro*liters (μl)
1 gram (Gm) = 10 *deci*grams (dg)	
100 *centi*grams (cg)	
1,000 *milli*grams (mg)	
1,000,000 *micro*grams (μg, mcg)	

Table 4-2. Approximate equivalents of metric and apothecaries' systems

Metric	Apothecary
Weight	
0.1 milligram (mg)	1/600 grain (gr)
0.5 mg	1/120 gr
1 mg	**1/60 gr**
30 mg	1/2 gr
60 mg	**1 gr**
100 mg	1 1/2 gr
120 mg	2 gr
1 gram (Gm)	**15 gr**
4 Gm	1 dram (dr, ℨ)
30 Gm	1 ounce (oz, ℥)
1 kilogram (kg)	2.2 pounds (lb)
Volume	
0.06 ml (cc)	1 minim (min, ♏)
1 ml	15 minims (min, ♏)
4 ml	1 fluidram (fl dr, fl ℨ)
15 ml	1/2 fluidounce (fl oz, fl ℥)
30 ml	1 fluidounce (fl oz, fl ℥)
500 ml	1 pint (pt)
1000 ml	1 quart (qt)

all the required information into the space on the prescription form. Historically, abbreviations are of Latin and Greek terminology. Some that may be useful are shown in Table 4-3.

Unless a practitioner writes a large number of prescriptions daily, he saves little time using abbreviations. Since abbreviations are more likely to be misinterpreted by the pharmacist than are terms written in full, the practitioner who uses them should ensure that they are clear. This is of particular importance to the practitioner who does not write prescriptions with great frequency and may not be completely familiar with the use of abbreviations.

HOUSEHOLD MEASURES

Although the clinician will direct the pharmacist to dispense a liquid preparation in milliliters, it is generally necessary to convert this to a convenient household measurement in directions to the patient. For most drugs dispensed in dental practice, the teaspoon or tablespoon is sufficiently accurate (Table 4-4). *The teaspoon holds about 5 ml and the tablespoon about 15 ml.* When greater accuracy is required, the patient may need to use a graduated cylinder or medicine glass. A calibrated dropper is issued with most liquid preparations that require relatively exact measurements. One should be cautioned that the use of a dropper is not particularly accurate if it is *not* calibrated. The size of a drop may vary considerably and depends on the specific gravity, temperature, and viscosity of the drug and on the diameter of the dropper's orifice.

PARTS OF THE PRESCRIPTION

The parts of the prescription have been named and defined classically as follows:

SUPERSCRIPTION: Patient's name, address, and age; date; and the symbol ℞ (L. *recipe*, "[you] take" or "take thou of").

INSCRIPTION: Name of drug, dose form, and amount.

SUBSCRIPTION: Directions to the pharmacist.

TRANSCRIPTION (OR SIGNATURE): Directions to the patient.

The classic categorization serves no particularly useful purpose and is presented here only for reference. It is a more practical approach to consider the parts of a prescrip-

Table 4-3. Common abbreviations

Abbreviation	Latin or Greek	English
a. or $\bar{a}$	ante	before
aa or $\overline{aa}$	ana	of each
a.c.	ante cibum	before food (meals)
ad lib.	ad libitum	as desired, as much as wanted
b.i.d.	bis in die	twice a day
c.	cibus	meal
$\bar{c}$	cum	with
cap.	capsula	capsule
d.	dies	day
disp.	dispensa	dispense
Gm		gram
gr		grain
gtt.	gutta	drop
h.	hora	hour
h.s.	hora somni	at bedtime ("hour of sleep")
no.	numero	number
non rep.	non repetatur	no refill, do not repeat
$\bar{p}$	post	after
p.c.	post cibum	after food
p.o.	per os	by mouth
p.r.n.	pro re nata	as required, if needed
q.d.	quaque die	every day
q.h.	quaque hora	every hour
q.i.d.	quater in die	4 times a day
q.4h.	quaque quarta hora	every 4 hours
repet.	repetatur	to be repeated
$\bar{s}$	sine	without
ss or $\overline{ss}$	semis	one-half
sig.	signa	write (label)
stat.	statim	immediately (now)
tab.	tabella	tablet
t.i.d.	ter in die	3 times a day

tion to consist of the following information, which is shown in Fig. 6.

Heading
Name, address, and phone number of the prescriber. Name, address, age, and phone number of the patient. Date.

Body
The symbol "℞."
Name and dosage unit* or concentration (liquids) of the drug.
Amount to be dispensed.
Directions to the patient.

Closing
Prescriber's signature.
Space for DEA number.
Refill instructions.
"Please place name of drug on label."

---

*"Dosage unit" refers to the size (mg) of the tablet or capsule.

Table 4-4. Common household equivalents

Household measure	Apothecary (approximate)	Metric
1 drop (gtt)	1 minim (min,♏)	0.05 ml
1 teaspoonful (tsp)	1 fluidram (fl dr, fl ℨ)	5 ml
1 tablespoonful (tbsp)	½ fluidounce (fl oz, fl ℥)	15 ml

MECHANICS OF PRESCRIPTION WRITING

The prescription must serve two functions. First, it must tell the pharmacist the specific drug, dosage unit or concentration, and amount to be issued. Second, its directions to the patient, which will be transcribed to the packaged drug, must state precisely how the patient is to take the drug. Thus the essence of prescription writing is that the pharmacist knows exactly which preparation

John J. Doe, D.D.S.
111 State Street
Bethesda, Maryland 20050
Phone: 497-6211

Date _____

Name: _____   Age: _____

Address: _____   Phone: _____

Rx

Please place name of drug on label.

May be refilled _____ time(s)

_____ D.D.S.

DEA Number --

Fig. 6. Typical prescription blank.

to dispense and the patient has explicit written instructions for self-administration.

Heading

Printed on the top of the prescription form is the name, address, and phone number of the prescriber. Spaces for the date and the patient's name, address, age, and phone number are included. Identification of the prescriber is important in cases where the pharmacist must contact the prescribing clinician. The date is particularly important in that it allows the pharmacist to intercept prescriptions that may not have been filled at the time of writing. A patient may withhold filling a prescription until his problem intensifies, at which time a different pharmacotherapeutic regimen may be necessary. Under these conditions most pharmacists will refer the patient to or contact the prescribing clinician. The age of the patient enables the pharmacist to double-check the dose.

Body

The first entry after the Rx symbol must be the name of the drug being prescribed. This is followed by the size (mg) of the tablet or capsule desired. In the case of liquids the name of the drug is followed by its concentration (mg/ml). The second entry is the quantity to be dispensed, that is, the number of capsules or tablets or milliliters of liquid. This should be preceded by "Dispense:" or "Disp:"

> Rx
> Codeine phosphate tablets, 32 mg
> Dispense: 8 (eight) tablets

or

> Rx
> Phenoxymethyl penicillin liquid, 125 mg/5 ml
> Dispense: 120 ml

In the case of tablets and capsules the word "dispense" is frequently replaced with the symbol for a number, "#." When writing prescriptions for narcotics or other drugs that may require special control, it is wise to write out the number of tablets or capsules or put the number in Roman numerals in parentheses after the written number. This avoids the possibility of an intended 8 becoming 18 or 80 at the discretion of an enterprising patient. Directions to the patient now follow and are preceded by the abbreviation "Sig:" (L. *signa*, "write"). The directions to the patient must be completely clear and explicit, and should include the route, amount of medication, time, and frequency of administration. The statement "Use as directed" should not be used because the patient may not understand the clinician's oral directions or may forget the directions after leaving the office. Latin abbreviations that are used in writing the directions will be transcribed on the packaged drug in full and in English by the pharmacist. The completed body of the prescription then becomes the following:

R̸

Codeine phosphate tablets, 32 mg
Dispense: 8 (eight) tablets or 8 (VIII) tablets
Sig: Take 2 tablets every 4 hours for pain

or, if abbreviations are used,

R̸

Codeine phosphate tabs., 32 mg
Disp: 8 (eight) tabs., or # 8 (eight) tabs.
Sig: 2 tabs. q.4h. for pain

Closing

After the body of the prescription is space for the prescriber's signature. In this general area there should also be space for his DEA number and refill instructions as illustrated in Fig. 6. It is good practice to place the name of the drug and the dosage unit on the packaged drug. Some states have laws that require pharmacies to label all medications routinely, but in any state a pharmacist is required to do so by having the statements, "Please place name of drug on label" or "Label" printed on the prescription form. Placing the name of the drug on the package label is important for the following three reasons:

1. In case of overdose or adverse reactions, the drug's identity can be quickly obtained.
2. Other practitioners can identify drugs the patient is taking.
3. In most cases the patient has a right to know what drug he or she is taking.

It is good practice to write out the number of refills, since Arabic numbers can easily be changed and a blank space can be filled in with any number. If no refill is desired, "No" should be written in the refill space to prevent forgery.

Since the practice of printing the DEA number on the prescription blank increases the chances of stolen prescriptions being used, the DEA number should be written in for controlled substances (Schedules II through V).

HINTS FOR PRESCRIPTION WRITING

Although these hints for prescription writing may seem self-evident, many prescribers fail to follow them, and errors may result.

1. Write legibly in ink.
2. Use the metric system.
3. Avoid abbreviations.
4. Keep a copy of each prescription or transcribe the information to the patient's record.
5. Include complete information for the patient.
   a. Never use "Take as directed" unless a written instruction sheet is provided.
   b. Include the intended purpose, for example, "For relief of pain."
   c. Use precautions to remind a patient of a drug's side effects, for example, "Caution: Sedation" or "Caution: May cause drowsiness."
   d. Add reminder phrases to increase the patient's compliance. Studies[3] have shown that over one half of patients fail to take medication properly. One example is to include, "Take until all are gone."

EXAMPLES OF PRESCRIPTIONS

The following are examples of the bodies of prescriptions that are frequently employed in dental practice.[1]

EXAMPLE 1: Prescription for potassium penicillin G tablets as might be used in infections where the oral route was acceptable

R̸

K penicillin G tablets, 250 mg
Disp: 25
Sig: Take 1 tablet at bedtime and 1 hour before meals.

EXAMPLE 2: Example 1 using abbreviations
R̸

K penicillin G tabs., 250 mg
Disp: 25
Sig: 1 tab. h.s. and 1 h.a.c

EXAMPLE 3: Prescription for a liquid preparation of potassium phenoxymethyl penicillin (penicillin V) as might be used for young children who are unable to swallow tablets

R̸

K penicillin V liquid, 125 mg/5 ml
Disp: 150 ml
Sig: 1 teaspoonful 1 h.a.c. and h.s.

EXAMPLE 4: Prescription for penicillin V tablets as might be used in patients with rheumatic heart disease who are appointed for procedures that would be expected to precipitate a bacteremia

℞
Penicillin V tablets, 250 mg
Disp: 24
Sig: Take 8 tablets 30 to 60 minutes before appointment, and 2 tablets every 6 hours thereafter.

EXAMPLE 5: Prescription for a low adult dose of nystatin that might be employed in treating oral moniliasis (thrush)

℞
Nystatin liquid, 100,000 U/ml
Disp: 180 ml
Sig: Swish 4 ml* in mouth for 2 minutes and then swallow q.6h.

EXAMPLE 6: Prescription for tetracycline hydrochloride capsules

℞
Tetracycline HCl capsules, 250 mg
Disp: 25
Sig: Take 1 capsule every 6 hours.

EXAMPLE 7: Example 6 using abbreviations

℞
Tetracycline HCl caps., 250 mg
Disp: 25
Sig: 1 cap. q.6h.

EXAMPLE 8: Prescription for secobarbital sodium that might be used in an adult for preoperative sedation

℞
Secobarbital Na capsules, 100 mg
Disp: 1 (one)
Sig: Take 1 capsule 1 hour before dental appointment. (Caution: Sedation)

EXAMPLE 9: Example 8 using abbreviations

℞
Secobarbital Na caps., 100 mg
Disp: 1 (one)
Sig: 1 cap. 1 h.a. dental appointment. (Caution: Sedation)

EXAMPLE 10: Prescription for pentobarbital in liquid form (elixir), as might be used for the preoperative sedation of a 60-pound child (1 mg/lb to a maximum of 100 mg)

℞
Pentobarbital elixir, 20 mg/5 ml
Disp: 20 ml
Sig: 1 tablespoonful 1 hour before dental appointment (Caution: Sedation)

EXAMPLE 11: Prescription for maximal adult dose of codeine sulfate

℞
Codeine sulfate tabs., 60 mg
Disp: 6 (six)
Sig: 1 tab. q.4h. p.r.n. pain (Caution: Sedation)

EXAMPLE 12: Prescription for low adult dose of codeine sulfate to be taken with aspirin to add analgesic and antipyretic effects

℞
Codeine sulfate tabs., 30 mg
Disp: 6 (six)
Sig: 1 tab. with 2 aspirin tabs. q.4h. p.r.n. pain (Caution: Sedation)

EXAMPLE 13: Prescription for adult dose of meperidine HCl

℞
Meperidine HCl tabs., 100 mg
Disp: 6 (six)
Sig: 1 tab. q.4h. p.r.n. pain (Caution: Sedation)

DRUG LEGISLATION

The *Food and Drugs Act of 1906* was the first federal law to regulate interstate commerce in drugs. It was rewritten and reenacted to become the *Food, Drug and Cosmetic Act of 1938*. This law and its subsequent amendments prohibit interstate commerce in drugs that have not been shown to be safe and effective. They further regulate labeling and packaging and establish standards of strength and purity. The enforcement of the Food, Drug and Cosmetic Act is the responsibility of the Food and Drug Administration of the Department of Health, Education, and Welfare.

The *Durham-Humphrey Law of 1952* is a particularly important amendment to the Food, Drug and Cosmetic Act because it requires that certain types of drugs be sold by prescription only. These preparations include certain habit-forming and addicting drugs and any other agents considered unsafe for lay use. The Durham-Humphrey Law requires that these drugs be labeled as follows: "Caution: Federal law prohibits dispensing without prescription." This law also prohibits the refilling of a prescription unless directions to the contrary are indicated on the prescription. This amendment allows the filling of prescriptions called in by telephone if the pharmacist promptly files a written record of the prescription.

The *Drug Amendments of 1962 (Kefauver-Harris Bill)* made some major changes in the Food, Drug and Cosmetic Law.

---

*The milliliter can be used in the directions here because the drug is dispensed with a dropper calibrated at 1 milliliter.

These amendments require the manufacturer to demonstrate the drug's effectiveness as well as its safety before the drug can receive Food and Drug Administration approval for marketing, to follow stringent rules in preliminary testing, and to submit to FDA any reports of adverse effects and other relevant data on drugs already on the market. The 1962 amendments require that all drug labels list the generic name and quantity of all active ingredients. The generic name must also appear in labeling wherever the proprietary name appears. Advertising for prescription drugs must also list all ingredients by generic name and briefly state the adverse effects, contraindications for use, and efficacy of a drug.[1]

The *Drug Abuse Control Amendments of 1965* required accounting for drugs with a potential for abuse: barbiturates, amphetamines, and any other depressants or stimulants that the U.S. Attorney General designates as having a potential for abuse. These amendments prohibited the refilling of a prescription for these drugs more than five times in 6 months after the date of the prescription.

The *Harrison Narcotic Act of 1914* and its amendments provided federal control over the importation, manufacture, production, compounding, selling, and dispensing of narcotic drugs. It required that all practitioners prescribing narcotics register with the Internal Revenue Service and receive a registration number. This law was administered by the Bureau of Narcotics of U.S. Treasury Department.

The *Controlled Substance Act of 1970* replaced the Harrison Narcotic Act and the Drug Abuse Control Amendments to the federal Food, Drug and Cosmetic Act. This new act is an extremely important one to the clinician. It sets current requirements for writing prescriptions for drugs frequently prescribed in dental practice. The federal law divides the controlled substances into five schedules according to abuse potential. Individual states or local governments may legislate additional requirements concerning controlled substances whenever state and federal laws differ. The most stringent law must be followed. Drugs controlled by the federal law are divided into five schedules as follows.

Schedule I substances. This schedule includes drugs with a high potential for abuse for which there is no accepted medical use in the United States. Examples include heroin,

LSD, marihuana, peyote, mescaline, psilocybin, tetrahydrocannabinols (THC), and other hallucinogens. These substances are not for prescription use but can be obtained for research purposes.

Schedule II substances: This schedule includes drugs with a high potential for abuse (potential for severe psychic or physical dependence) for which there is a currently accepted medical use in the United States. Most of the narcotic drugs in this schedule had been categorized in the past as "Class A narcotic drugs." Examples include narcotics such as opium, morphine, codeine alone, hydromorphone (Dilaudid), meperidine (Demerol), oxycodone (ingredient in Percodan), anileridine (Leritine), oxymorphone (Numorphan), alphaprodine (Nisentil), levorphanol (Levo-Dromoran), and methadone (Dolophine); stimulants such as cocaine, most amphetamines including amphetamine (Benzedrine) and dextroamphetamine (Dexedrine), methylphenidate (Ritalin), and phenmetrazine (Preludin); and sedative-hypnotics such as amobarbital (Amytal), methaqualone (Quaalude, Parest, Sopor), pentobarbital (Nembutal), and secobarbital (Seconal).

Schedule III substances. This schedule includes drugs with a lower potential for abuse than those in Schedules I and II for which there is a currently accepted medical use in the United States. These drugs may lead to moderate or low physical dependence or high psychological dependence. They include those drugs formerly known as "Class B narcotic drugs" plus a number of nonnarcotic agents. Examples include narcotics such as codeine mixtures like Empirin compound with codeine, aspirin with codeine (ASA with codeine, Ascodeen #3*), acetaminophen with codeine (Phenaphen #3,* Tylenol #3*), Fiorinol #3,* and other narcotic mixtures including paregoric; stimulants such as benzphetamine (Didrex), chlorphentermine (Pre-Sate), clortermine (Voranil), mazindol (Sanorex), and phendimetrazine (Plegine); and sedative-hypnotics such as butabarbital (Butisol), butalbital (ingredient in Fiorinal), glutethimide (Doriden), methyprylon (Noludar), and thiopental (Pentothal).

Schedule IV substances. This schedule in-

---

*The #3 is used as an example and designates the presence of 30 mg codeine. These products are also available in other strengths.

cludes drugs with a lower potential for abuse than those in Schedule III for which there is a currently accepted medical use in the United States. Examples include sedative-hypnotic drugs such as chloral hydrate, chlordiazepoxide (Librium), clorazepate (Tranxene), diazepam (Valium), ethchlorvynol (Placidyl), ethinamate (Valmid), flurazepam (Dalmane), meprobamate (Equanil, Miltown), methohexital (Brevital), oxazepam (Serax), paraldehyde, and phenobarbital; and stimulants such as diethylpropion (Tepanil, Tenuate), fenfluramine (Pondimin), pemoline (Cylert), and phentermine (Ionamin).

Schedule V substances. This schedule includes drugs with a lower potential for abuse than those in Schedule IV for which there is a currently accepted medical use in the United States. Drugs in this category were previously known as "exempt narcotics."

It must be remembered that drug entities are continuously being evaluated and moved from schedule to schedule and from being unscheduled to being scheduled. One such drug, dextropropoxyphene (Darvon), has recently been added to Schedule IV.

The *current requirements for prescribing controlled drugs* as promulgated by the Controlled Substance Act of 1970 are as follows:

1. Any prescription for a controlled substance requires a DEA number (Schedules II through V).
2. Schedule I drugs may not be prescribed because they have no medical use.
3. All Schedule II through IV drugs and most schedule V drugs are *prescription drugs.*
4. Schedule II drugs must be written in the prescriber's handwriting, in ink, and cannot be refilled.
5. Schedule III and IV drugs may be telephoned to the pharmacist and may be refilled no more than five times in 6 months if so noted on the prescription.

An application for registration and assignment of a DEA number can be obtained by writing to the U.S. Department of Justice, Drug Enforcement Administration, P.O. Box 28083, Central Station, Washington, D.C. 20005. The prescriber should simultaneously apply to the state to obtain a Controlled Substances number.

REFERENCES

1. Holroyd, S. V.: Pharmacotherapeutics in dental practice (NAVPERS 10486), Washington, D.C., 1969, Bureau of Naval Personnel.
2. Conférence Générale des Poids et Mesures: Comptes rendus des séances de la 12ᵉ Conférence Générale des Poids et Mesures, Paris, 1964, Gauthier-Villars.
3. Stewart, R. B., and Cluff, L. E.: A review of medication errors and compliance in ambulant patients, Clin. Pharmacol. Ther. **13**:463-468, 1972.

PART TWO
Specific drug groups

5

General anesthetics

TOMMY W. GAGE

General anesthetics are a class of drugs that are potent central nervous system depressants. They produce a reversible loss of consciousness and insensibility to painful stimuli. The cortex is the first central nervous system structure to be depressed, followed in order by the brain stem, spinal cord, and medulla. Protective reflexes are abolished by most of these agents, and with increasing doses depression of respiration and many vital organ systems also occurs. For these reasons the constant job of the anesthesiologist throughout the anesthetic period is that of patient evaluation and monitoring of vital signs. General anesthesia is the result of the early efforts of general dentists who were seeking a suitable means of pain control for their patients. Since that time, general anesthesia has become a highly scientific and structured specialty.

A large number of general anesthetic agents have become available for use. Contemporary general anesthetic techniques employ a balanced combination of drugs for the total management of the patient, taking into account the patient's physical status as well as the preanesthetic and postanesthetic needs. Because of the variety of anesthetic agents and techniques employed, special training and complete knowledge of the pharmacology of each anesthetic is essential. The environment of the hospital operating room provides the optimal setting for general anesthesia, since the proper monitors for vital signs, resuscitative equipment and trained anesthesia personnel, are readily available. However, it should be noted that oral surgeons have used general anesthetics in their offices for many years with an excellent safety record. Indeed, dentists should have knowledge of general anesthesia because it is an indispensable tool for the total dental needs of special patients as well as for more extensive oral and maxillofacial surgery.[1]

HISTORY

Dentists have played a significant role in the recognition and use of drugs that could provide relief from pain. Although many drugs such as morphine and alcohol have been used to make surgery more comfortable, and Joseph Priestly is aptly given the credit for describing nitrous oxide, it took the concern of a dentist for his patient to bring the pain-relieving benefits of general anesthesia to the public eye. In December, 1844, Horace Wells, a dentist, observed a demonstration of the effects of nitrous oxide while attending a lecture. During the course of the program, Wells noted that one of the participants inhaling the gas had injured a leg without being aware of the associated pain. Wells was impressed with this observation and asked his associate John Riggs to remove one of his own teeth while he was under the effects of nitrous oxide. The extraction was completed without pain.

Wells persuaded a former dental partner and now Harvard University medical student, William T. G. Morton, to arrange for a demonstration of the use of nitrous oxide. Wells obtained the necessary permission to demonstrate the gaseous agent before the Harvard University medical faculty. Unfortunately, the low potency of nitrous oxide was not known, and the anesthetic attempt failed.

In the months that followed, Morton with the aid of C. T. Jackson demonstrated the use of ether as an effective general anesthetic before the same Harvard University group. Later, Howard W. Long, a Georgia physician, reported his earlier use of ether as an anesthetic for surgical procedures. A tragic conflict developed among these different in-

43

dividuals as each sought recognition for the introduction of general anesthesia. Wells committed suicide, but as years passed, both the dental and medical professions have recognized his contribution.

It should also be pointed out that during this same time period, a noted Scottish surgeon, James Y. Simpson introduced the use of the volatile liquid chloroform for obstetric anesthesia in 1847.[2]

METHODS FOR ADMINISTERING ANESTHETIC AGENTS

The method employed for administering a general anesthetic agent is dictated by the choice of anesthetic agent. Ether and chloroform are volatile liquids at room temperature and were simply dropped onto a gauze-covered wire mask placed over the patient's face. As the liquid volatilized, its vapors mixed with the inspired air. This was a rather slow process and uncomfortable for the patient. Additionally, expiration of carbon dioxide and inspiration of adequate oxygen were uncontrollable. Towels were often draped around the open mask to increase the concentration of anesthetic vapors inhaled. Gas anesthetics are administered from storage cylinders through hoses, metered flow valves, and a face mask.

The demand for patient safety, explosion-free operating rooms, and a more suitable means of volume flow of gases to the patient resulted in the development of sophisticated anesthetic machines. These units are usually self-contained packages consisting of metered flow valves, calibrated vaporizers for volatile anesthetic liquids, gas storage cylinders, a carbon dioxide absorber, and a breathing bag. These units are constructed in a variety of ways with the essential features including an adequate oxygen source that can be mixed with the anesthetic gas. This mixture can then flow through the vaporizer that is adding the volatilized liquid anesthetic. The total anesthetic mixture is then delivered to the patient through a face mask. The system can be designed with a series of valves to allow rebreathing or non-rebreathing of gases. Excess carbon dioxide is removed by the absorber system. Some gases are explosive, requiring a closed-type system. The breathing bag serves as a reservoir for the anesthetic gas mixture, but more importantly, it provides a means for the arti-ficial assistance of the patient's respiration. Most machines are equipped with an oxygen flush valve that allows for the rapid removal of anesthetic gases from the system while providing emergency oxygen to the patient.[3]

The intravenous route is commonly employed in dental offices and for the rapid induction of unconsciousness by the ultrashort-acting barbiturates. Also, muscle relaxants and other support-type drugs are given by this route during anesthesia. Whatever means is chosen, the more important factors to keep in mind would include the patient's comfort and safety and a patent airway. The competent use of anesthetic machines implies a knowledge of the equipment as well as specialized training.

THEORIES ON THE MECHANISM OF ACTION

Many theories have been proposed in an effort to explain the mechanism of action of the various general anesthetic agents, but unfortunately, none of them does so completely. It may seem relatively simple to say that these drugs are central nervous system depressants, but just how they depress the normal neuronal function is a matter complicated by lack of knowledge of the physiologic and biochemical events of arousal and unconsciousness.[4] Some of the more widely discussed theories of mechanism of action follow:

1. *Lipid or Meyer-Overton theory.* This theory resulted from the combined efforts of Meyer[5] and Overton,[6] and basically it relates the potency of anesthetic agents to their lipid solubility. Whereas certain effects of the anesthetics on the lipid neuronal tissues are related to their oil–water partition coefficient, this theory cannot explain the action of many other anesthetic agents.

2. *Inhibition of biochemical actions.* Numerous theories have been described relating the effects of anesthetic agents to the utilization of oxygen by the cell. Early workers suggested that anesthetics produced asphyxiation or antagonized the action of oxygen at the cell level. Quastel[7] sought to explain the role of barbiturate anesthetics by a decreased oxygen uptake. Greig[8] reported that chloroform inhibited respiration in the brain homogenates.

3. *Molecular theories.* At least two investigators, Miller and Pauling, have pro-

posed mechanisms related to the effects anesthetics could have on water. Miller[8a] suggested that the anesthetics cause the formation of "icebergs" around nerves that interferred with their function. Pauling[9] contends that certain inert anesthetic gases (xenon) produce minute crystals or "clathrates," which trap certain electrically charged groups of neuronal protein thus impeding neural transmission.

No attempt has been made to include every theory about how general anesthetics may act at the cellular level. No doubt this area of research will continue to provide provocative and interesting evidence for not only the action of drugs but also new information about arousal and unconsciousness. For the interested reader a review reference is included.[10]

STAGES AND PLANES OF ANESTHESIA

In a relatively short time after the introduction of general anesthesia, anesthesiologists began to describe and identify the various levels of anesthetic depression. John Snow is credited with this early description, which was later amplified by Guedel[11] in 1920. Guedel's classification has become the standard for describing the various stages and planes of central nervous system depression. It is important to note that Guedel's system applied to the administration of ether by the open drop method in a nonpremedicated patient. Modern anesthetic techniques are such that many of these classic signs are not actually observed. It seems important to describe briefly the four stages, since reference to depth of anesthesia is still related to Guedel's system.

State I—Analgesia. This stage is characterized by the development of analgesia. The patient can still respond to command, and reflexes are present. This initial stage will terminate with the loss of consciousness. Some amnesia may also be evident.

State II—Delirium. This stage of anesthesia begins with unconsciousness and is associated with increased muscle tone. The patient moves and shows excitement. As the depth of anesthesia increases, the patient begins to relax and progresses to the next stage. This can be an uncomfortable time for the patient because vomiting and incontinence can occur. The ultrashort-acting barbiturates provide the modern anesthesiologist with a rapid means of inducing unconsciousness, thereby avoiding this stage.

Stage III—Surgical anesthesia. This is the stage associated with the majority of surgical procedures. Its onset is typically characterized by regular respiratory movements, muscular relaxation, and normal heart and pulse rates. Conjunctival and eyelid reflexes are absent. This stage is further divided into four planes that are differentiated on the basis of eye movements, depth of respiration, and muscular relaxation. Plane 3 is associated with decreased skeletal muscle tone and dilated pupils. The progression to plane 4 is characterized by intercostal paralysis, absences of all reflexes, and extreme muscle flaccidity. If the depth of anesthesia is allowed to increase, the patient will rapidly progress to the last stage.

Stage IV—Respiratory paralysis. This stage is characterized by complete cessation of respiration. If it is not reversed immediately, death of the patient will occur.

Modern anesthetic techniques now employ more rapidly acting agents than those associated with the signs of Guedel. Some of the signs associated with the early stages of anesthesia are less obvious, and the anesthesiologist must give undivided attention to the constant evaluation of anesthetic depth as measured by changes in the patient's reflexes, respiration, circulation, and muscular tone. The best depth of anesthesia is that which will include consideration for the patient's well-being in addition to the surgeon's requirements.

A more recent approach to measuring the stages of anesthesia is to consider phases as suggested by Flagg.[12]

Induction. This phase encompasses all the preparation and medication necessary for a patient up to the time the surgeon is ready to begin. Medication for preoperative sedation, adjunctive drugs to anesthesia, as well as those anesthetics required for induction of unconsciousness are included in this phase.

Maintenance phase. This phase begins with the patient at a depth of anesthesia sufficient to allow surgical manipulation and continues until completion of the procedure.

Recovery phase. This phase begins with the termination of the surgical procedure and continues through the postoperative period until the patient is fully responsive to the environment.

These phases are more fully discussed by Bennett.[13] They are important to list because they demonstrate that modern general anesthesia is the result of a balanced combination of drugs and skill, all designed to provide the best care for the patient.

ANESTHETIC AGENTS

The general anesthetic agents are usually categorized according to their route of administration. The two principal classes are the inhalation agents and the intravenous agents. The inhalation type of general anesthetics may be divided into gases and volatile liquids. The volatile liquids are vaporized at or near room temperature and carried in gas form to the patient, usually in combination with other anesthetic gases and oxygen. At least one drug, ketamine, can produce anesthesia when given intramuscularly. Table 5-1 lists the common general anesthetic agents.

Inhalation anesthetics
Physical factors controlling inhalation anesthetics

A number of physical factors influence the ultimate anesthetic concentration in the brain. These factors include the partial pressure of the anesthetic(s) in the inspired gas, the concentration of anesthetic in the lungs at induction, the rate of uptake of anesthetic by the blood (blood/gas solubility), and the rate of uptake of anesthetic by the tissues (tissue/blood solubility). At the time of induction of anesthesia, the percentage of anesthetic gas in the lungs is nil and the anesthetic is taken up rapidly as determined by rapid movement of the anesthetic from a high concentration (inspired air) to a low concentration (lung). The anesthetic is then carried to the blood and tissue by diffusion, moving from higher to lower concentrations.

If the anesthetic agent is poorly soluble in the blood, it will be transported rapidly to the tissues, hence a rapid induction. Conversely, if the anesthetic agent is highly soluble in blood, more of it will have to be dissolved in the blood before the concentration in the tissues can reach a desired level, hence a slow induction. Since the rate of uptake is initially very fast, an adequate volume flow and concentration of anesthetic is required at induction. Induction can be speeded by hyperventilation of the patient, thus increasing the rate at which the gases enter the lung. As the desired level of anesthesia is reached, the rate of exchange of anesthetic gases slows and the concentration of the anesthetic in the inspired gas mixture can be reduced to maintain the desired level.

Recovery from inhalation anesthesia is just the reverse. The anesthetic concentration of the inspired gas is reduced, and the gases diffuse from the tissues to the blood to the alveoli along the concentration gradient. If the anesthetic is highly soluble in body tissues, recovery will be slow. The fact that ether is highly soluble in blood whereas nitrous oxide is not correlates well with their onset and duration of action.

Minimum alveolar concentration

The specific dose of a general anesthetic is not given in a manner similar to that for other drugs. Instead, the term *minimum alveolar concentration* (MAC) has been used to

Table 5-1. Classification of general anesthetics by route of administration

Inhalation anesthetics		Intravenous anesthetics
Gases	Volatile liquids	
Cyclopropane	Chloroform	Fentanyl with droperidol (neurolept) (Innovar)
Ethylene	Diethyl ether (ether)	Ketamine (dissociative) (Ketalar, Ketaject)
Nitrous oxide	Enflurane (Ethrane)	Methohexital sodium (Brevital)
	Ethyl chloride	Thiamylal sodium (Surital)
	Halothane (Fluothane)	Thiopental sodium (Pentothal)
	Methoxyflurane (Penthrane)	
	Trichloroethylene (Trilene, Trimar)	
	Vinyl ether (Vinethene)	

compare the potency of the various general anesthetics. The value is determined by measuring the minimum alveolar concentration of the anesthetic in the dog lung required to prevent a painful response. Potency is given as the reciprocal of the minimum alveolar concentration.

It should be remembered that potency does not necessarily relate to the efficacy of a drug to produce a desired anesthetic response. The MAC of nitrous oxide has been given the value of 100. Halothane has an MAC of 0.77 and methoxyflurane 0.16, whereas ether is 1.92. The lower MAC value indicates a more potent anesthetic effect.[14]

Pharmacologic effects

The general anesthetics are all depressants of the central nervous system. The development of analgesia, reduction in reflex actions, and skeletal muscle relaxation is related to the degree of central nervous system depression. It is fortunate that the medulla is the least susceptible to depression, since all the anesthetic agents are respiratory depressants. Nitrous oxide is unique in that it is not referred to as a respiratory depressant anesthetic except in hypoxic concentrations. The intravenous barbiturates are potent depressants of respiration, and dosage adjustment is more critical with these drugs.

Other body systems such as the cardiovascular system are also depressed by the general anesthetics. A number of general anesthetics also produce liver damage, limiting their usefulness. Included in this group are chloroform and the halogenated volatile anesthetics. Urine output is usually reduced, especially with procedures of long duration. The stress of general anesthesia can be accompanied by release of adrenocorticotrophic hormone (ACTH), antidiuretic hormone, and sympathetic neurotransmitters.

Gas anesthetics

Nitrous oxide. Nitrous oxide (N_2O) was first described by Joseph Priestly in 1771; its historic significance is well documented.[15] It is a colorless gas with little or no odor and is stored in blue cylinders at 750 psi.

As mentioned earlier, nitrous oxide is a low potency general anesthetic agent, and when used alone, it is unsatisfactory as a complete anesthetic. For induction of anesthesia a ratio of 85:15 nitrous oxide to oxygen

is required. The concentration is sustained only briefly, and the depth of anesthesia attained at a more desirable 65:35 ratio is insufficient for most surgery. However, if anesthesia is first induced with a rapidly acting barbiturate and then nitrous oxide–oxygen administered with a low concentration of halothane, a good quality of balanced anesthesia results.

Nitrous oxide is poorly soluble in blood and has a rapid onset of action as a result. Excretion of nitrous oxide is also rapid, and little if any metabolism occurs. During recovery 100% oxygen is administered to prevent diffusion hypoxia. At the usual anesthetic concentrations the respiratory center response to carbon dioxide is not depressed. There is little change in the cardiovascular system during nitrous oxide anesthesia.

The adverse effects associated with the use of nitrous oxide are few and related to its poor quality as an anesthetic. Vomiting may occur in some patients, and there is no muscle relaxation. Toxicity is minimal as long as exposure is not prolonged. Nitrous oxide is more soluble than nitrogen in body tissues and will replace it in body cavities where nitrogen has accumulated.

The use of nitrous oxide for sedation and analgesia in the dental office is discussed in Chapter 26.

Cyclopropane. Cyclopropane was introduced during the 1930s and is the most potent of the gas anesthetics. It is a gas at room temperature and is stored in gas cylinders. However, it is highly explosive and must be administered in a closed anesthetic system. Its chemical structure is as follows:

$$H_2C$$
$$\diagup\diagdown$$
$$H_2C-CH_2$$

Cyclopropane

Induction with cyclopropane occurs rapidly, in 2 or 3 minutes, resulting in complete surgical anesthesia and muscle relaxation without additional muscle relaxant medication. Excessive secretions can be controlled with an anticholinergic drug. A 1% to 3% concentration produces light analgesia, and anesthesia will begin with a 10% concentration. Cyclopropane is rapidly absorbed and excreted through the lungs with very little metabolism.

The adverse effects associated with the use

of cyclopropane include cardiac arrhythmias. Sympathetic nerve activity is increased, and the administration of exogenous catecholamines such as epinephrine or norepinephrine can induce serious cardiac arrhythmias. Because of increased bronchial constriction, patients with asthma are at risk with cyclopropane anesthesia. Other adverse effects include headache with nausea and vomiting during recovery. Although cyclopropane is a very useful anesthetic, its use in dentistry is limited because of the explosive hazard.

Ethylene. Ethylene ($CH_2=CH_2$) is an unsaturated hydrocarbon that was first used for surgical anesthesia in 1923. Its popularity has declined over the years, and it has largely disappeared from use. It is a gas with a disagreeable odor and taste. Concentrations of 25% to 35% produced good analgesia, but higher concentrations, up to 85%, are required for light anesthesia. Its explosiveness, lack of patient acceptability, and low potency have limited its usefulness.

Volatile anesthetics

The volatile general anesthetics are low boiling point liquids that volatilize easily at room temperature. Most of these agents are highly potent anesthetics and are relatively soluble in blood and fat. Vaporization is accomplished by special vaporizers attached to the anesthetic apparatus. There are two general classes of these agents: the ethers and the halogenated hydrocarbons.

Ethers

Diethyl ether. Ether ($CH_3CH_2-O-CH_2CH_3$) has been the most popular volatile liquid anesthetic used since its discovery in the 1840s. Like most of the older liquid agents, its use has diminished and been replaced by the newer type of liquid anesthetics. Nevertheless, ether remains an effective and useful anesthetic agent.

Induction with ether is usually slow and uncomfortable for the patient. Its odor is objectionable, and irritation of mucous membranes produces secretions that have to be controlled with anticholinergic premedication. Ether is a complete anesthetic, providing good analgesia and muscular relaxation for abdominal surgery. The cardiovascular system is depressed but is compensated by release of endogenous catecholamines from the adrenal medulla. As long as anesthetic concentrations are maintained, respiration is not depressed.

The principal disadvantages of ether include slow induction with a following slow recovery, objectionable odor, explosive hazard, and nausea and vomiting on recovery.

Ether is marketed in small copper-lined cans containing a 3% ethyl alcohol additive. The reason for this type of package is to minimize the formation of peroxides that are potentially explosive.

Vinyl ether (Vinethene). Vinyl ether ($CH_2=CH-O-CH=CH_2$) is a potent anesthetic agent introduced in the 1930s. Induction with 2% to 4% vinyl ether is rapid, and surgical anesthesia can be continued with approximately a 4% concentration. Because vinyl ether is more potent, it is easier to produce respiratory depression than with ether. Vinyl ether provides good anesthesia for short procedures of 20 minutes or less, but its use is limited because of resulting liver toxicity.

Halogenated hydrocarbons

Halothane (Fluothane). Halothane was introduced as a general anesthetic in the late 1950s and has become widely used and accepted as a reliable anesthetic agent. Its chemical formula is $CF_3-BrCF-OCH_3$; it has a fruity pleasant odor and is nonflammable and nonexplosive.

Induction is rapid at a 3% concentration, and patients are maintained with a concentration of 0.5% to 1.5% as needed. Recovery is also relatively rapid. Halothane is nonirritating to mucous membranes so that there is little increase in salivary or bronchial secretions, and it is considered a good agent to use for asthmatic patients. However, it is a progressive respiratory depressant, reducing both tidal volume and alveolar ventilation. Therefore the depth of anesthesia must be carefully regulated. Pharyngeal and laryngeal reflexes are rapidly obtunded and bronchodilation occurs.

The effects on the cardiovascular system are manifested in increased vagal activity, with cardiac slowing and peripheral vasodilation lowering the blood pressure. Halothane, unlike ether, does not cause the release of stored catecholamines. It will sensitize the myocardium to the cardiac stimulatory effects of injected epinephrine and norepinephrine, leading to serious cardiac arrhythmias such as ventricular fibrillation.

Halothane provides only moderate muscle relaxation, and muscle relaxants are required during surgery. Because the quality of pain relief is poor during recovery, supplemental analgesics are required. Kidney function is depressed, and uterine relaxation occurs.

The most serious disadvantage to the use of halothane is depression of liver function and resultant necrosis, leading to death in certain individuals. The exact cause is unknown, but since halothane is metabolized to a significant extent, some of the metabolites have been implicated as a possible causative factor. A nationwide survey of deaths associated with halothane anesthesia showed that these cases of liver necrosis occurred at about the expected rate for patients undergoing surgery. Some believe this reaction to be a hypersensitivity to the drug. For these reasons halothane is contraindicated in patients when previous exposure to this agent or other halogenated anesthetics has been followed by evidence of liver disease or damage.[16]

In summary, halothane has proved to be an effective and reliable general anesthetic. It can be used in almost every situation with the exception of obstetric anesthesia, where uterine relaxation is a problem. Its adverse effects include cardiac arrhythmias when exogenous catecholamines are given, postoperative hepatic necrosis especially with multiple exposures, respiratory depression, and nausea and vomiting on recovery. It should be given in combination with oxygen or mixed with oxygen and nitrous oxide.

Methoxyflurane (Penthrane). Methoxyflurane is a volatile nonflammable liquid anesthetic with the chemical formula $Cl_2CH—CF_2—OCH_3$. Concentrations of 1% to 3% produce general anesthesia with good postoperative analgesia that frequently lasts until after the patient has regained consciousness, thereby reducing the need for supplemental analgesia. Muscle relaxation is perhaps better than with halothane, but succinylcholine or *d*-tubocurarine is necessary for good muscle relaxation.

As is the case with halothane, methoxyflurane sensitizes the myocardium to the stimulant effects of injected catecholamines. Bradycardia and a decrease in blood pressure occur with anesthetic doses.

Methoxyflurane is metabolized in the liver, and certain of the metabolic products are believed to be associated with the neuropathy that sometimes occurs during methoxyflurane anesthesia. The effect appears to be dose related. For this reason a caution appears in the product information stating that methoxyflurane should not be administered to patients who have received the drug in the previous month. Additionally, its use should be avoided in patients with a previous history of jaundice occurring with other halogenated hydrocarbons.

Drug interactions appear to be prominent with methoxyflurane. The concurrent intravenous use of tetracycline with methoxyflurane has been implicated in renal toxicity. Other antibiotics may also be suspect, including gentamycin, kanamycin, the polymyxins, and amphotericin B. Enzyme-inducing drugs such as the barbiturates could increase the rate of metabolism, leading to an increase in the amount of toxic metabolites.[17]

As is the case with halothane, methoxyflurane is administered in combination with oxygen and nitrous oxide.

Chloroform. Chloroform ($CHCl_3$) was introduced as a general anesthetic in 1847 in Great Britain, where its use was popular for a number of years. Induction with chloroform is rapid, and anesthesia is maintained by a 1% chloroform concentration. It is a more potent respiratory depressant than ether, and it is likely to produce hypotension during deep anesthesia. The known hepatotoxicity of this agent, the difficulty in regulation of anesthetic depth, plus the development of newer and safer anesthetics have diminished the use of chloroform. Currently, it is of more historic than practical interest.

Ethyl chloride. Ethyl chloride (CH_3CH_2-Cl) has been used as a general anesthetic agent but is no longer employed in this manner because of the occurrence of cardiac arrhythmias and liver toxicity. Its current usefulness is limited to that of a "spray-on" type of local anesthetic. Ethyl chloride is packaged in a small cylinder under pressure, and when released, it produces a form of cryoanesthesia of the skin by rapid evaporation and cooling. The depth of tissue anesthesia is small, and the duration is short. The principal adverse effects of this use include delayed healing and possible tissue slough if administered incorrectly.

Trichloroethylene (Trilene, Trimar). Trichloroethylene ($ClCH=CCl_2$) is a volatile, nonflammable liquid with many properties similar to those of chloroform. Its dangers when used as a general anesthetic include cardiac arrhythmias and tachypnea. Currently, it is used as an inhalation analgesic to control certain pain episodes such as tic douloureux. It is packaged in inhalers for professional or self-administration use. Its self-administration use carries with it the potential for drug abuse. Trichloroethylene has been used to supplement nitrous oxide anesthesia and provide pain relief during labor and childbirth.

Miscellaneous group

A number of halogenated hydrocarbons have been introduced, tried, and subsequently abandoned as general anesthetics. Although these agents are not as important as the others previously mentioned, they will be briefly listed for completeness. Both enflurane (Ethrane) and fluroxene (Fluoromar) are similar to halothane in effect. The explosiveness of fluroxene severely limits its use, and halothane has proved to be superior to enflurane even though greater muscle relaxation is claimed as an advantage. Isoflurane (Forane) is available for research only, whereas the use of tribromoethanol (Avertin) has largely been discontinued as a rectally administered anesthetic.[18]

Intravenous anesthetics

The intravenous general anesthetics include the ultrashort-acting barbiturates and a nonbarbiturate dissociative anesthetic ketamine. The so-called neuroleptanalgesic combination of fentanyl and droperidol will also be included, although the exact position of this combination is hard to fix. The intravenous agents find their greatest usefulness in the rapid induction of unconsciousness so that delirium may be avoided.

Ultrashort-acting barbiturates

The ultrashort-acting barbiturates that are of current interest include methohexital sodium (Brevital) and thiopental sodium (Pentothal). Others such as thiamylal sodium (Surital) and hexobarbital sodium have been used but less frequently in dental anesthesia. Although the basic pharmacology of the barbiturates is discussed in Chapter 6, there are certain pertinent facts about these drugs that need emphasis.

These drugs are ultrashort acting in that intravenous doses have a rapid onset of about 30 to 40 seconds. If repeated doses are given, as is often the case during anesthesia, the drug accumulates in body tissues, resulting in a prolonged recovery. This effect results from a redistribution of the drug from neural tissues to fat depots and muscle so that absolute recovery may take considerable time.

These drugs are sometimes employed as the sole anesthetic for short procedures, and if the degree of central nervous system depression is kept at or near anesthetic levels, the patient will respond to painful stimuli. No analgesia is observed. Doses necessary to reduce the pain stimulus response are very near apneic doses. For this reason the intravenous barbiturates function more effectively in smaller doses when used as part of a balanced anesthetic technique with local anesthesia.

A serious complication in the use of the intravenous barbiturates occurs when the injected solution is accidentally given extravascularly or into an artery. If extravascular infiltration occurs, symptoms ranging from tissue tenderness to necrosis and sloughing can occur. Intra-arterial injection is an extremely dangerous situation. Arteriospasm associated with ischemia of the arm and fingers and severe pain may be observed. The injection should be stopped immediately. An injection of 1% procaine is used to relieve the pain and spasm. If the reaction progresses, it may be necessary in some cases to block the sympathetic response in the brachial plexus. In some cases heparin is given to prevent local thrombus formation, and an alpha-adrenergic blocking agent such as phentolamine should be considered.[19]

Other complications with the ultrashort-acting barbiturates include laryngospasm and bronchospasm. In some patients hiccoughs, increased muscle activity, and delirium occur on recovery. Premedication with atropine has proved reasonably effective in reducing some of these recovery problems. Scopolamine and the opiates are also effective premedicants.[20]

The absolute contraindications to the use of these agents include an absence of suitable veins for administration, status asthmaticus, porphyria, and a known hypersensitivity. Adjustment of dosage and caution should be taken in patients with hepatic, renal, and cardiovascular impairment. Because these drugs are potent anesthetics, they should be administered by qualified individuals only, and resuscitative equipment should be readily available.[21]

Dissociative anesthesia

Ketamine (Ketalar, Ketaject). Ketamine is a newer type of anesthetic agent. It is not related chemically to the barbiturates or the narcotics. The anesthetic state it produces has been given the name dissociative anesthesia. Ketamine appears to disrupt association pathways in the brain and to depress both the reticular activating system and the limbic system. The mechanism of action remains to be described.

Ketamine hydrochloride

Ketamine may be given intravenously or intramuscularly with a rapid onset of action occurring by either route. Even intramuscular doses can produce unconsciousness within 1 or 2 minutes. After administration there is a transient stimulation of both blood pressure and pulse rate that rapidly disappears. Pharyngeal and laryngeal reflexes remain unaffected with little respiratory change. Because excessive salivation is a common finding with ketamine, atropine is a necessary premedication. Muscle tone may increase during its use.

The principal drawback to the use of ketamine is the occurrence of delirium and hallucinations during recovery, most often in adults, older age children, and drug abusers. Emergence reactions of this type may be minimized if visual and auditory stimuli are reduced during recovery. Small doses of the intravenous barbiturates and diazepam have been employed to control the recovery problems, but the success is variable.

Ketamine should be used by those experienced in anesthetic procedures. Specific contraindications include a history of cerebrovascular disease, hypertension, and hypersensitivity to the drug. Since protective reflexes are not obtunded, care should be taken not to stimulate the pharynx.[22]

Neurolept analgesia

The term *neurolept analgesia* was coined by de Castro in 1958 to describe a so-called "wakeful anesthetic state." It is induced by the administration of a combination of a neuroleptic drug and a narcotic type of analgesic. For all practical purposes the patient appears to be awake but is tranquil, catatonic, and free of pain. The proper placement of this type of pain and apprehension control is a puzzle, but reason should dictate their discussion with anesthetic agents.

A neuroleptic drug is one that is a major tranquilizer capable of inducing a catatonic state. It produces a placid and calm patient but has no analgesic effect. This drug also decreases the sensitivity of the patient to epinephrine and norepinephrine, inhibits learned behavioral activity, and is antiemetic. The particular neuroleptic drug used in this technique is the butyrophenone derivative droperidol (Inapsine). It is similar in many respects to the phenothiazine tranquilizers.

The narcotic agent employed in this type of anesthesia is known as fentanyl (Sublimaze). It is a potent central nervous system depressant and a derivative of meperidine. Fentanyl has all the properties of a narcotic, including analgesia and respiratory depression. It is a short-acting narcotic and will cause an increase in muscle tone.

The combination of fentanyl and droperidol is known as Innovar. This combination is usually given intravenously with a rapid onset of action. Although return to consciousness appears to be rapid, the effects of droperidol are long lasting, and complete recovery is slower. The adverse effects can be quite serious and are those which would normally be associated with the narcotics and major tranquilizers. Respiratory depression and CNS damage manifesting as extrapyramidal tremors have occurred. This combination of drugs should be used with great care, especially in patients with pulmonary insufficiency and parkinsonism. A "boardlike" chest reaction, associated with intercostal muscle paralysis and requiring ventilatory support, occurs in some patients. Fentanyl is sometimes employed as a sole agent for sedation.[23]

ANESTHETIC HAZARDS

Surgical anesthesia administered with the goals of good patient control, adequate muscular relaxation, and pain relief has become a safe procedure. However, it should be remembered that to produce anesthesia, potent central nervous system depressants are given in relatively high doses, and many combinations of drugs are employed in balanced anesthesia. Some of the possible interactions encountered are as follows:

1. Adrenergic blocking agents may mask the reflex stimulation of the adrenal medullary release of sympathetic neurotransmitters leading to hypotension.

2. Narcotics used in premedication reduce the amount of anesthetic required but could potentiate respiratory depression.

3. Anticholinergics, such as atropine, reduce the secretions associated with irritating anesthetics as well as block vagal slowing of the heart.

4. Cyclopropane, halothane, ethyl chloride, methoxyflurane, trichloroethylene, and chloroform sensitize the myocardium to the effects of epinephrine, norepinephrine, and isoproterenol. Serious cardiac arrhythmias may result.

5. Ether, cyclopropane, halothane, and methoxyflurane augment the neuromuscular blocking effects of tubocurarine, pancuronium, and gallamine, requiring a dose reduction.

6. The aminoglycoside antibiotics will potentiate the effects of the neuromuscular blocking agents.[24]

A more recent concern regarding anesthetic hazards relates to the attending personnel rather than the patient. Current data seem to support the fact that waste anesthetic gases found to contaminate surgical suites are a potential health hazard. In a survey of operating room personnel, including dentists, an increase of spontaneous abortions in the spouse of the exposed dentist was noted. There was also a significant increase in liver disease in the exposed dentists. Other complaints included headache, fatigue, and irritability. In response to this survey and noting an increase in the use of inhalation agents in the dental office, the American Dental Association has appointed a special committee to study the potential hazard of trace anesthetic gases in the dental office. Until this committee reports, adequate ventilation of the dental operatory and use of good technique and equipment seem prudent.[25]

REFERENCES

1. Driscoll, E. J.: ASOS anesthesia morbidity and mortality survey, ASOS Committee on Anesthesia, J. Oral Surg. **32:**733-738, 1975.
2. Schmiesa, A. A.: The birth of anesthesia, TIC, pp. 10-13, Aug., 1975.
3. Adriani, J.: The pharmacology of anesthetic drugs, ed. 5, Springfield, Ill., 1970, Charles C Thomas, Publisher.
4. Fink, R. B., editor: Molecular mechanisms of anesthesia, New York, 1975, Raven Press, Vol. 1.
5. Meyer, H. H.: Zur Theorie der Alkoholnarkose. I. Welche Eigenschaft der Anästhetika bedingt ihre narkotische Wirkung? Arch. Exp. Path. Pharmak. **42:**109, 1899.
6. Overton, E.: Studien über die Narkose zugleich ein Beitrag zur allgemeinen Pharmakologie, Jena, 1901, G. Fischer.
7. Quastel, J. H.: Biochemical aspects of narcosis, Curr. Res. Anesth. Analg. **31:**151, 1952.
8. Greig, M. E.: The site of action of narcotics on brain metabolism, J. Pharmacol. Exp. Ther. **87:**185, 1946.
8a. Miller, S. L.: Effects of anesthetics on water structure, Fed. Proc. **27:**879, 1968.
9. Pauling, L.: A molecular theory of general anesthesia, Science **134:**15, 1961.
10. Wallace, W. D.: Effects of drugs on the electrical activity of the brain: anesthetics, Annu. Rev. Pharmacol. Toxicol. **16:**413-426, 1976.
11. Guedel, A. E.: Inhalational anesthesia: a fundamental guide, ed. 2, New York, 1951, The Macmillan Co.
12. Flagg, P. J.: The art of anesthesia, ed. 7, Philadelphia, 1944, J. B. Lippincott Co.
13. Bennett, C. R.: Monheim's general anesthesia in dental practice, ed. 4, St. Louis, 1974, The C. V. Mosby Co.
14. Wollman, H., and Smith, T. C.: Uptake, distribution, elimination and administration of inhalation anesthetics. In Goodman, L. S., and Gilman, A., editors: The pharmacological basis of therapeutics, ed. 5, New York, 1975, The Macmillan Co.
15. Schofield, R. E.: A scientific autobiography of Joseph Priestley (1733-1804), Cambridge, Mass., 1966, The Massachusetts Institute of Technology Press, pp. 138-197.
16. Subcommittee on the National Halothane Study of the Committee on Anesthesia, National Academy of Sciences–National Research Council: Summary of national halothane study, J.A.M.A. **197:**775, 1966.
17. American Medical Association Council on Drugs: AMA drug evaluations—1973, Chicago, 1973, American Medical Association.
18. Miller, J. D., and Katz, R. L.: Anesthetic agents. In Bevan, J. A., editor: Essentials of pharmacology, ed. 2, New York, 1976, Harper & Row, Publishers, chap. 27.
19. Physician's Desk Reference, ed. 30, Oradell, N.J., 1976, Medical Economics, Inc.

20. Dundee, J. W.: The influence of preanesthetic medication on thiopental and methohexital anesthesia, J. Oral Ther. **2:**388-389, 1966.

21. Dundee, J. W.: Clinical studies of induction agents. VII. A comparison of eight intravenous anesthetics as main agents for a standard operation, Br. J. Anaesth. **35:**784, 1963.

22. Hellinger, M. J.: Ketamine hydrochloride, a general anesthetic in oral surgery, J.A.D.A. **83:**349-351, 1971.

23. Greenfield, W.: Neuroleptanalgesia and dissociative drugs, Dent. Clin. North Am. **17:**263-274, April, 1973.

24. Evaluations of drug interactions, ed. 2, Washington, D.C., 1976, American Pharmaceutical Association.

25. Cohen, E. N., Brown, B. W., Jr., Bruce, D. L., et al.: A survey of anesthetic health hazards among dentists, J.A.D.A. **90:**1291-1296, 1975.

6

Sedative-hypnotic drugs

SAM V. HOLROYD
TOMMY W. GAGE

The sedative-hypnotic drugs can produce varying degrees of central nervous system (CNS) depression as a function of the dose administered. A small dose will produce a mild degree of CNS depression described as sedation (reduction of activity and simple anxiety). A somewhat larger dose of the same drug will produce a greater CNS depression, resulting in hypnosis (sleep). Thus the same drug may be either a sedative or hypnotic, depending on the dose administered.

Anyone who has practiced dentistry recognizes the value of having a relaxed patient. More often than not patient anxiety is eliminated or sufficiently reduced by a calm, confident, and understanding attitude on the part of the dentist and assisting personnel. Patients approach dentistry with varying degrees of anxiety, ranging from complete calmness when anticipating extensive procedures to severe apprehension about the simplest of procedures. Although most patients lie somewhere between these extremes, dentists should provide their patients with the most pleasant experience possible within the limits of safety. Inducing relaxation in a patient allows the accomplishment of more productive appointments with less nervous strain to both patient and dentist. For this reason and because orally administered sedative-hypnotic drugs are relatively safe, their use may be beneficial in reducing patient anxiety in many cases.

Working with a relaxed patient is not only a matter of pleasantness and convenience but with some patients it may be a matter of life and death. McCarthy[1] has pointed out

□ The opinions of assertions contained herein are the private ones of the writers and are not to be construed as official or as reflecting the views of the Navy Department or the naval service at large.

that sudden unexpected death is not uncommon, even occurs in people who appear to be in good health, and can be brought on by emotional stress. He states that this is strong justification for adequate pain-anxiety control for dental patients.

Prior to a consideration of the sedative-hypnotic drugs, certain generalizations should be made. Although any precise degree of sedation can be obtained by intravenous titration, and inhalation sedation, both require special training and experience on the part of the practitioner. Therefore, for many dentists, oral sedation is the principal method of reducing anxiety in dental patients. This presents a most fundamental problem: Sedation by orally administered drugs will not provide consistent or highly predictable results. As noted in Chapter 2, many factors influence the blood level obtained from orally administered drugs. Additionally, variations are seen in patient responses to similar blood levels. Because of the variations and lack of predictability from oral sedation, many practitioners continually switch from drug to drug, hoping to find the ultimate agent or dose that will provide ideal sedation. Neither the ultimate drug nor dosage is there so that such searching usually is fruitless. The greatest consistency will be found in staying with one or two drugs, knowing these well, and knowing how they affect different types of patients. In the long run this will yield greater benefit than "jumping" from drug to drug.[2]

An important point should be made regarding the extent of patient sedation desired in comparison with the dose employed. Whereas the stated sedative dose of any one sedative-hypnotic drug may be expected to produce a calmness, it may not be a sufficient dose to produce the desired degree of "sedation" in the dental patient. The meaning of a sedative dose for a sedative effect has to be related to the original use of these drugs in medicine. This class of drugs, especially the barbiturates, was used for many years to calm mildly anxious patients, much like the so-called tranquilizers are used today. A sedative dose allowed the patient to function as usual on a day-to-day basis but with less anxiety. A hypnotic dose was designed to provide sufficient amount of drug to allow the patient to drift into sleep. Therefore a patient with apprehension about dentistry may require more than the usual "sedative" dose of the drug. Sedation of dental patients so that they are calm and cooperative about the dental procedure cannot necessarily be equated with the sedative dose of one of these drugs. Indeed, the hypnotic dose may be required more often than not to obtain the degree of patient sedation desired.

Sedative-hypnotic drugs can be categorized as barbiturates or nonbarbiturates and will be discussed on that basis.

BARBITURATES

The barbiturates are effective, safe, and convenient to administer and can provide either short or prolonged durations of action. They have been used in great quantities over many years; consequently, problems associated with their use are well known. Their principal adverse potentialities as sedatives are that they induce both psychic and physical dependence, are a likely source of use in suicides and acute overdosage, and are involved in many drug interactions. In recent years the tranquilizers have largely replaced barbiturates in clinical practice.

Chemistry

Barbituric acid (malonylurea) was formed by the condensation of urea and malonic acid by von Baeyer in 1864. It does not have sedative properties.

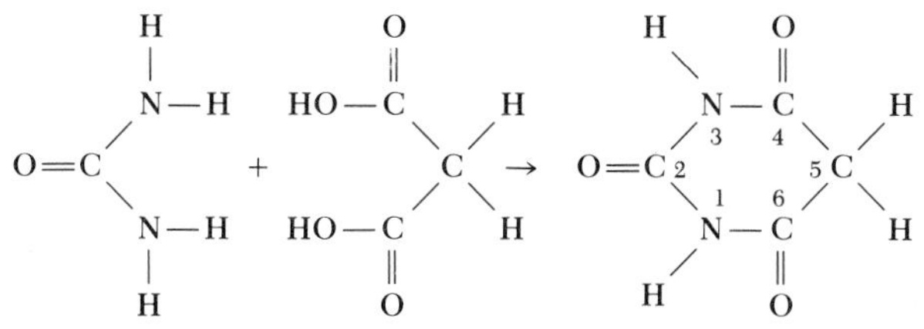

In 1904 Fischer and von Mering prepared diethyl barbituric acid* and determined that it possessed hypnotic activity. Most clinically useful barbiturates are prepared by substituting appropriate groups for the hydrogens on carbon atom number 5 of the barbituric acid molecule. The most significant substitution other than those on carbon-5 is to replace the carbon-2 oxygen with sulfur. This produces the thiobarbiturates, which are used as intravenous general anesthetics. Table 6-1 shows the substitutions on the barbiturate nucleus to form commonly used barbiturates.

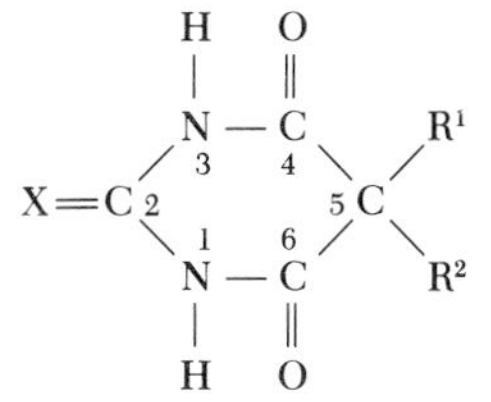

Barbiturate nucleus

In the free acid form the barbiturates are colorless, odorless, crystalline solids that are relatively insoluble in water. The free acids are converted to their sodium salts for the preparation of parenteral solutions. Both the free acid and sodium salts can be used orally.

Body handling

The barbiturates are well absorbed orally, rectally, and intramuscularly. The high alkalinity of parenteral solutions prohibits their use subcutaneously and limits the thiobarbiturates to the intravenous route.

The more lipophilic barbiturates, such as the thiobarbiturates, become quickly concentrated in the brain. These drugs then redistribute from the brain, first to muscle and then to fat. It is this redistribution that is responsible for the ultrashort duration of action of methohexital and the thiobarbiturates. The less lipophilic barbiturates reach brain tissues more slowly and become rather

---

*Ethyl groups substituted for hydrogens on C_5.

| Urea | Malonic acid | Barbituric acid |

Table 6-1. Trade names and substitutions of commonly used barbiturates

Barbiturate	Trade name	R^1	R^2	X
Amobarbital	Amytal	ethyl	isoamyl	0
Aprobarbital	Alurate	allyl	isopropyl	0
Barbital	Veronal	ethyl	ethyl	0
Butabarbital	Butisol	ethyl	1-methylpropyl	0
Methohexital*	Brevital	allyl	1-methyl-2-pentenyl	0
Pentobarbital	Nembutal	ethyl	1-methylbutyl	0
Phenobarbital	Luminal	ethyl	phenyl	0
Secobarbital	Seconal	allyl	1-methylbutyl	0
Thiamylal*	Surital	allyl	1-methylbutyl	S
Thiopental*	Pentothal	ethyl	1-methylbutyl	S

*General anesthetics.

Table 6-2. Classification, route of administration, and dosages of commonly used barbiturates

Barbiturate	Route of administration	Oral adult dosage (in mg)*	
		Sedative	Hypnotic
Ultrashort acting (immediate onset)			
Methohexital sodium	IV		
Thiamylal sodium	IV		
Thiopental sodium	IV		
Short acting (oral onset about 30 minutes; duration up to 3 hours)			
Pentobarbital	O, R, IM, IV	100	100-200
Secobarbital	O, R, IM, IV	100	100-200
Intermediate acting (oral onset 40 to 60 minutes; duration 3 to 6 hours)			
Amobarbital	O, R, IM, IV	100	100-300
Aprobarbital	O	100	120
Butabarbital	O	15-30	50-100
Long acting (oral onset 2 to 3 hours; duration over 6 hours)			
Phenobarbital	O	15-30	30-60

O, Oral; *R*, rectal; *IM*, intramuscular; *IV*, intravenous.
*Children's dosages should be calculated or obtained from manufacturers' recommendations (PDR).

uniformly distributed throughout the body. They cross the placenta and also appear in a nursing mother's milk.

The thiobarbiturates are slowly metabolized by the liver. The short- and intermediate-acting barbiturates are more rapidly and almost completely metabolized by the liver. Consequently, patients with liver damage may exhibit exaggerated responses to these drugs. The long-acting barbiturates, such as phenobarbital and barbital, are excreted to a great extent (30% to 40%) as free drug in the urine. As a result of this, renal impairment will lead to cumulation and an exaggerated response.

Classification, administration, and dosage

The most practical clinical classification of the barbiturates is by duration of action. This classification of commonly used barbiturates, their routes of administration, and sedative and hypnotic dosages are shown in Table 6-2.

The distinction between a sedative and hypnotic dose is not distinct. Responses to barbiturates vary among different people. Additionally, the presence or absence of food in the stomach and the environment in which the drug is taken (dark, quiet room as opposed to the deck of a sinking ship) influence the sedative effects obtained. Greater sedation will follow a barbiturate taken on an empty stomach by a small person than if it is taken on a full stomach by a large individual. A sedative dose taken at bedtime by a tired person in a relaxed atmosphere may produce sleep. Consequently, you should not accept stated doses as being absolute; they must be individualized.

Pharmacologic effects

The principal effects of the barbiturates are on the central nervous system. Sedative and hypnotic doses are believed to act mainly at the level of the thalamus and ascending reticular activating system to depress the transmission of impulses to the cortex.[3] Higher doses appear to act at all levels of the central nervous system. Thus sufficiently high doses may depress cortical centers, motor functions, and medullary centers. The basic mechanism of action is unclear. Following is the progression of effects with increasing doses of barbiturates:

Sedation
↓
Hypnosis
↓
General anesthesia
(with progressive respiratory and cardiovascular depression)
↓
Respiratory arrest

Sedative doses do not ordinarily produce clinically significant degrees of respiratory depression, but hypnotic doses may cause minor depression. Respiratory and cardiovascular depression, which is progressive during general anesthesia, prohibits the use of barbiturate anesthesia for other than short procedures. Cardiovascular depression may include both a reduction of cardiac output and peripheral vasodilation.

Barbiturate sedation impairs mental and physical skills to some degree. Therefore a patient taking barbiturates should be warned against driving a car or operating dangerous equipment or machinery. He should be accompanied to and from the dental office by a responsible individual.[4]

Except at extremely high doses, the barbiturates have no significant analgesic effects. Even doses that produce general anesthesia do not preclude reflex responses to pain. Patients in pain may become agitated and even

delirious if barbiturates are administered without analgesics.[5] Consequently, barbiturates should not be prescribed for patients in pain unless an analgesic is also prescribed. When a barbiturate is prescribed with an analgesic, the patient's relaxation that is obtained may potentiate the effect of the analgesic. If an analgesic that produces sedation is used, the practitioner should remember that this sedation will be additive to that produced by the barbiturate.

The barbiturates have anticonvulsant effects. The short-acting drugs are generally effective to terminate convulsions, and the long-acting agents such as phenobarbital have had great use in preventing the convulsions of epilepsy.

In addition to previously mentioned pharmacologic effects, high doses of barbiturates may reversibly depress liver and kidney function, reduce gastrointestinal motility, and reduce body temperature.[6]

Adverse reactions

Sedative and hypnotic doses of the barbiturates are relatively safe. However, one should be aware of the fact that central nervous system depression may be exaggerated in elderly and debilitated patients and those with impaired liver or kidney function. It is also important to remember that the sedative effects of these drugs are additive to sedation produced by alcohol and other central nervous system depressants. In some people, particularly the elderly, the barbiturates may cause an idiosyncratic excitement rather than sedation. Rashes and nausea may occur. Serious allergic reactions are rare.

Anesthetic doses of the barbiturates result in blood concentrations that are close to the lethal blood level. Consequently, great care must be exercised to avoid compromising respiratory and cardiovascular function. As previously noted, this becomes impossible except for short durations of anesthesia. Coughing and/or laryngospasm are also rather frequently seen during the intravenous use of the barbiturates.

Acute poisoning represents a serious concern relative to the use of barbiturates. Many deaths occur each year from intentional and unintentional acute overdoses of barbiturates. In 1967, 506 accidental deaths and 1694 suicides caused by barbiturates were reported in the United States.[7] Some unintentional poisonings result from automatism.* Although a lethal dose can only be approximated, moderately severe poisoning will follow the ingestion of five to ten times the hypnotic dose, and life is seriously threatened if over fifteen times the hypnotic dose is consumed.[8] However, if the individual is not discovered early, eight to ten times the hypnotic dose may be fatal.[9] Consequently, the practitioner should not prescribe over five or six hypnotic doses of a barbiturate at one time. The cause of death when overdose occurs is respiratory depression, although circulatory failure may exist concurrently.

Some considerations in the treatment of overdose as reported by Meyers and colleagues[9] include (1) continuous observation; (2) support of respiration; (3) prevention or treatment of shock (blood or plasma substitutes, possibly vasopressors); (4) maintenance of renal function (adequate fluid intake, possibly 5% glucose); and (5) increasing rate of excretion of drug (osmotic and alkaline diuresis; peritoneal dialysis or hemodialysis may be necessary in profound depression). The following should *not* be used:[9] (1) Gastric lavage which adds the risk of aspiration, cardiac arrhythmias, and respiratory arrest; (2) convulsant stimulants and analeptics such as pentylenetetrazol (Metrazol) and picrotoxin, the benefits of which are believed doubtful and additional hazards are imposed (convulsions and hyperpyrexia); and (3) narcotic antagonists, which do not counteract barbiturate depression but, in fact, will add to it.

Long-term use of barbiturates can lead to psychic and physical dependence. Some people become euphoric with barbiturates, but long-term use leads to a state similar to alcohol intoxication. A particularly unfortunate aspect of barbiturate addiction is that whereas the narcotic addict who continues to receive a narcotic can function relatively normally, the barbiturate addict becomes progressively depressed and is unable to function. Tolerance that develops to the barbiturates is much less than that seen with narcotics, and no tolerance is apparent relative to the lethal dose. There is cross-tolerance between different barbiturates but none between barbiturates and narcotics.

*Automatism is a sedative-induced state of confusion wherein a patient forgets that he has taken previous doses and repeats doses until poisoning ensues.

Other precautions and contraindications related to the use of barbiturates are the following:

1. The practitioner must be continuously alert to the fact that barbiturate depression is additive to that produced by antihistamines, alcohol, and other central nervous system depressants and is potentiated by phenothiazine tranquilizers and monoamine oxidase inhibitors.
2. Solutions of barbiturates for intravenous use, such as 2.5% thiopental sodium, are highly alkaline. Consequently, they may cause considerable tissue damage if injected perivascularly or intra-arterially.
3. The practitioner must be alert to possible allergies to these agents.
4. They are absolutely contraindicated in patients with intermittent porphyria.

Drug interactions

Barbiturates are potent stimulators of liver microsomal enzyme production (enzyme induction). These enzymes are involved with the metabolism of a number of other drugs; therefore, when the enzymatic activity is increased, the rate of metabolism will be increased effectively reducing the usual response. Enzyme induction has been reported to occur after 7 days of continuous therapy with barbiturates, with a return to normal in about 1 month. Some of the drugs whose effectiveness is believed to be reduced by this mechanism include warfarin, chlorpromazine, and the anti-inflammatory steroids.

Phenobarbital has been shown to reduce the clinical effectiveness of the antifungal drug griseofulvin, perhaps through a reduction of absorption.[10]

Uses and preparations

The barbiturates are used to provide sedation for anxiety and essential hypertension and hyperthyroidism. They are used to induce sleep in cases of insomnia. The ultra-short-acting barbiturates are important intravenous general anesthetics. The long-acting members, notably phenobarbital, are of value as antiepileptics.

The principal use of the barbiturates in the practice of dentistry is in preoperative medication to reduce anxiety. The short-acting members are most appropriate here. A 100 to 200 mg oral dose of pentobarbital or secobarbital 1 hour before an appointment will generally provide effective sedation in adults. The quality of this type of sedation can be improved with a similar dose at bedtime on the evening before the appointment. The usual oral dose for preoperative sedation in children is 1 mg/lb of body weight. Available preparations are the following:

Pentobarbital
  Oral elixir—20 mg/5 ml
Pentobarbital sodium
  Capsules—30, 50, and 100 mg
  Rectal suppositories—30, 60, 120, and 200 mg
  Parenteral solution—50 mg/ml
Secobarbital
  Oral elixir—22 mg/5 ml
Secobarbital sodium
  Capsules—30, 50, and 100 mg
  Rectal suppositories—30, 60, 120, and 200 mg
  Parenteral solution—50 mg/ml

NONBARBITURATE SEDATIVE HYPNOTICS

During the latter half of the nineteenth century, the bromides and chloral hydrate (synthesized in 1862) began to replace opium, alcohol, and belladonna as drugs for the production of sedation. Paraldehyde was introduced in 1882 and the barbiturates in 1904. As previously noted, the barbiturates became and until recently remained the principal sedative-hypnotic drugs in dental and medical practice. Numerous nonbarbiturate sedatives of varying chemical structures have been produced over the last 20 years.

The nonbarbiturate sedative-hypnotic drugs have essentially the same undesirable features as the barbiturates and in some cases are known to have additional disadvantages. Although the use of huge quantities of barbiturates over many years has rather completely elucidated their adverse potentialities, the nonbarbiturate drugs are less well known. The nonbarbiturate drugs are generally weaker than the barbiturates and offer no particular advantage. Preoperative sedation in dental practice can usually be adequately obtained with a properly selected dose of a tranquilizer or a barbiturate. Except for those few patients in whom other sedatives are contraindicated, no clear-cut indications exist for the use of the following drugs.

A number of sedative-hypnotic mixtures are available. Their value over equivalent doses of a single drug is highly questionable. For this reason they are not discussed. Certain antihistamines and tranquilizers have been used for preoperative sedation in dentistry and will be considered in their separate chapters.

Several sedative-analgesic mixtures that fulfill the special purpose of providing both sedation and relief from pain are available. Since pain and anxiety are often associated, some of these mixtures will be discussed.

Bromides

The bromide ion produces mild sedation by directly depressing the sensory and motor cortex. Some antiepileptic effect is also obtained. The prolonged use of bromides produces bromide intoxication (bromism). The kidney does not differentiate between chloride and bromide ions. Consequently, after long-term use of high dosages of bromides (usually as the sodium or potassium salts), the blood and tissue chloride/bromide ratio decreases and bromism results. Signs and symptoms include a rash resembling acne; bullous erythema multiforme[11]; increased oral, nasal, and lacrimal secretions; and in extreme cases, toxic psychoses.

The bromides are still found in some proprietary mixtures (Bromo-Seltzer, Miles-Nervine) but have been largely replaced by more effective drugs with less adverse potentialities.

Chloral hydrate

Chloral hydrate $(CCl_3—CH(OH)_2)$ is an inexpensive, orally effective sedative-hypnotic drug with a rapid onset (20 to 30 minutes) and fairly short duration of action (about 4 hours). It is a relatively safe drug. It is too irritating to be used parenterally. Therapeutic doses do not produce pronounced respiratory or cardiovascular depression,[3] but an exaggeration of effects is seen in patients with advanced liver or kidney disease. Large doses or long-term use may produce peripheral vasodilation and hypotension with some degree of myocardial depression.[11] Gastric irritation with nausea and vomiting is not uncommon; consequently, it should not be used in patients with ulcers or gastroenteritis. Gastric irritation can be minimized by taking chloral hydrate in dilute solutions and with milk. The highly irritating effect of this drug on mucosa is illustrated by a report of laryngospasm in a child that was believed to be caused by the aspiration of chloral hydrate.[12] Some liver and kidney damage has been observed. Psychological or physical dependence may follow the prolonged use of chloral hydrate.

Although chloral hydrate is an excellent sedative, its use declined significantly after the introduction of the barbiturates. It appears to have regained popularity in some institutions. The principal use of chloral hydrate today is as a single oral dose hypnotic at bedtime. It has been used rectally in status epilepticus in children and for eclamptic seizures. It has been used successfully for the preoperative sedation of children in dentistry[13] and can be used as an effective substitute for barbiturates in adults. An effective oral dose for preoperative sedation in adults is about 1 Gm (0.5 to 2 Gm) given 30 minutes before the appointment. The oral or rectal sedative dose for children must be highly individualized, but the following guideline dosages have been recommended[14]:

Age	Approximate weight (lb)	Dose (mg)
6 months	15	100
1 year	20	150
3 years	30	200
5 years	40	300
7 years	50	400

The disagreeable odor and taste of chloral hydrate are masked in a flavored syrup containing 500 mg/5 ml. It is also available in 250 and 500 mg capsules and 500 mg suppositories.

Chloral betaine

Chloral betaine (Beta-Chlor) was introduced in 1963 as a chemical complex of chloral hydrate and betaine. It has essentially the same effectiveness and undesirable effects as chloral hydrate but is more expensive. It is available as an 870 mg tablet, which is equivalent to 500 mg of chloral hydrate. The usual oral dose for preoperative sedation in adults and children over 12 years of age is 870 mg. Chloral betaine has a slower onset than chloral hydrate and should be given 1 hour preoperatively.

Paraldehyde

Paraldehyde (polymer of acetaldehyde) is an inexpensive, orally effective sedative hypnotic. It has a rapid onset but a longer duration of action than chloral hydrate. Paraldehyde is a safe drug, but as little as 30 ml has been fatal. Paraldehyde has a very disagreeable taste and odor. Since approximately 25% of the drug is exhaled, an extremely offensive breath has limited patient acceptance. In view of the degree to which paraldehyde is eliminated by the respiratory route, its use in patients with bronchopulmonary disease is questionable. The drug not exhaled is metabolized by the liver; consequently, severe liver damage may exaggerate its effects. Since gastric irritation occurs, its use is best avoided in patients with ulcers or gastroenteritis. Psychological and physical dependence with paraldehyde may follow long-term use. The use of paraldehyde is greatly limited by patient acceptance, and it has little to offer in dental practice.

Ethinamate

Ethinamate (Valmid) is a weak sedative hypnotic with a fast onset and short duration of action. Since its introduction in 1954, adverse reactions to ethinamate have been minimal. Excitement is occasionally seen in children, and gastrointestinal upset and skin rashes are sometimes observed. Thrombocytopenic purpura has been reported but is rare. Psychological and physical dependence may follow long-term use. Teratogenic studies are insufficient to recommend its use in pregnant or nursing women. Ethinamate's short duration of action precludes its use as a daytime sedative.

Its rapid onset and short duration of action has led to some use as a preoperative sedative in dentistry. The usual oral dose of ethinamate for preoperative sedation in adults is 500 mg to 1 Gm given 30 minutes before the procedure. It is available in 500 mg tablets.

Ethchlorvynol

Ethchlorvynol (Placidyl) was introduced in 1954. It is a weak sedative hypnotic with a fairly rapid onset and a duration of 6 to 8 hours. Ethchlorvynol is a relatively safe drug, but its use has been associated with hypotension, gastric upset, aftertaste, dizziness, blurring of vision, facial numbness, urticaria, and mild excitation. High doses have caused mental confusion and hallucinations. Syncope, prolonged hypnosis, and profound muscular weakness have been reported but are rare. Ethchlorvynol is contraindicated in patients with porphyria. Physical or psychological dependence may follow prolonged use. Teratogenic studies are insufficient to recommend its use during pregnancy. Ethchlorvynol is used as a daytime sedative and as a mild hypnotic, but it has no particular indication in dental practice.

Glutethimide

Glutethimide (Doriden) was introduced in 1955. It is a weak sedative hypnotic with a rapid onset and a duration of 6 to 8 hours. Glutethimide is a fairly safe drug, but its use has been associated with gastrointestinal distress, rash, urticaria, excitation, blurring of vision, acute allergic reactions, porphyria, and blood dyscrasias, including aplastic anemia. Physical or psychological dependence may follow prolonged use. Glutethimide is contraindicated in patients with porphyria, and teratogenic studies are insufficient to recommend its use during pregnancy. Information is insufficient to recommend its use in children. Glutethimide is used as a daytime sedative and as a mild hypnotic. Although it has been used for preoperative sedation, it has no particular importance in dental practice.

Other nonbarbiturate sedative hypnotics

The following are nonbarbiturate sedative hypnotics that have no particular indication in dentistry but may be administered by physicians to patients whom the dentist may see. As with all sedative hypnotics, the special considerations that are listed afterward pertain to these drugs.

Bromisovalum (Bromural)
Chloral hydrate derivatives
Chlorhexidol (Lora)
Petrichloral (Periclor)
Methaqualone (Quaalude, Sopor)
Methylparafynol (Dormison)
Methyprylon (Noludar)
Tybamate (Tybatran)

SEDATIVE-ANALGESIC COMBINATIONS

Provision for concomitant sedation and analgesia is rational for three reasons: (1) Sedation and pain relief are frequently required together, (2) sedatives potentiate analgesics, and (3) sedatives may induce excitement in patients experiencing uncontrolled pain. Both sedation and analgesia can be obtained from the narcotic drugs used singly. Meperidine is particularly effective in this regard. However, it is not desirable to use a narcotic to add sedation to analgesia unless the analgesic potency of the narcotic is required. When analgesia can be adequately obtained with a nonnarcotic such as aspirin or acetaminophen, these drugs and a sedative can be prescribed separately. Some fixed-dosage combinations of mild analgesics with depressant drugs, such as Fiorinal and Equagesic, have been mentioned in Chapter 10. When more complete pain relief is required with sedation, a narcotic can be considered. Some clinicians believe that more dependable sedation-analgesia is obtained with certain fixed-dosage combinations such as the meperidine-promethazine mixtures.

Meperidine-promethazine (Mepergan, Mepergan Fortis)

Meperidine (Demerol) is discussed in Chapter 10, and promethazine (Phenergan) is discussed in Chapter 15. Some studies have shown that the addition of promethazine allows the reduction of the required analgesic dose of meperidine by about one half. The smaller required dose of meperidine should reduce the narcotic side effects. Additionally, the sedation produced by promethazine adds to that provided by the meperidine. Although there is little doubt that significant analgesia and sedation can be obtained with this combination, definite evidence of advantages over higher doses of meperidine is lacking.

Adverse effects that might be expected with either constituent singly should be considered as untoward potentialities of the combination. The most common possibilities are drowsiness, dizziness, xerostomia, and blurring of vision. The discussions of meperidine and promethazine should be consulted for other possible adverse effects.

The combination of meperidine and promethazine has been reported as useful for preoperative sedation in dentistry.[15] The adult oral dosage is 50 mg meperidine with either 12.5 or 25 mg promethazine every 4 to 6 hours. The adult intramuscular dosage is 25 to 50 mg of each drug. The recommended intramuscular dosage for children up to the age of 12 years is 0.5 mg of each constituent per pound of body weight.

The following meperidine-promethazine preparations are available: Mepergan Fortis capsules, comprising 50 mg meperidine HCl and 25 mg promethazine HCl; and Mepergan injection, comprising 25 mg meperidine HCl and 25 mg promethazine HCl per milliliter.

SPECIAL CONSIDERATIONS

Certain generalizations should always be kept in mind relative to the use of sedative-hypnotic drugs.[4]

1. The practitioner should not rely exclusively on drugs to provide a calm and cooperative patient. The dentist's confident but relaxed manner and a pleasant, soothing office atmosphere are of great importance in relaxing an anxious patient. Drugs should not be substituted for patient education or for the proper psychological approach to patient care.

2. When a sedative hypnotic is required, the selection of the specific drug should be based on a knowledge of the advantages and disadvantages of the agents available and an understanding of the needs and contraindications that relate to the case at hand. In most instances a barbiturate should be the drug of choice.

3. Regardless of the sedative hypnotic selected, the following precautions pertain:

   a. Patients with immature or impaired elimination may experience exaggerated effects of medication. These individuals include the young, the elderly, the debilitated, and those with liver or kidney disease.

   b. Depression caused by all sedative hypnotics will add to depression caused by other depressants that the patient may be taking. The patient should be made aware of this, particularly in regard to alcohol; over-the-counter sleep aids may also be a potential source of hazard.

   c. The patient should understand that the drug which the practitioner is prescribing may make it unsafe for him to perform acts requiring full alertness and muscular coordination, such as driving a car. This is particularly important if the patient has not taken the drug previously and his response to it is consequently less predictable.

   d. Psychic and physical dependence have been observed with almost all sedative-hypnotic drugs. The dentist should consider all sedative-hypnotic drugs to have a potential for abuse and should limit their use accordingly. This is particularly important in regard to psychologically unstable individuals because of their greater potentiality for addiction.

   e. Suicide is commonly accomplished with depressant drugs. Consequently, the amount of the drug prescribed should be limited to that absolutely required to accomplish the therapeutic objective.

   f. Newer drugs of this or any other group should not be administered to women of childbearing age if potential maternal of fetal dangers are not known. An exception here would include a situation in which the clinical demands outweigh the risks.

   g. Sedatives do not provide analgesia. In fact, the use of a sedative without adequate pain control may cause the patient to become highly excited and act irrationally. However, sedatives may potentiate the effect of an analgesic taken concomitantly.

REFERENCES

1. McCarthy, F.: Sudden, unexpected death in the dental office, J.A.D.A. 83:1091, 1971.
2. Jastak, J. T., and Paravecchio, R.: An analysis of 1,331 sedations using inhalation, intravenous, or other techniques, J.A.D.A. 83:1242-1249, 1975.
3. Cutting, W. C.: Handbook of pharmacology, ed. 4, New York, 1969, Appleton-Century-Crofts.
4. Pharmacotherapeutics in dental practice (NAVPERS 10486), Washington, D.C., 1969, U.S. Bureau of Naval Personnel.
5. Goth, A.: Medical pharmacology: principles and concepts, ed. 7, St. Louis, 1974, The C. V. Mosby Co.

6. Sutherland, V. C.: A synopsis of pharmacology, ed. 2, Philadelphia, 1970, W. B. Saunders Co.

7. U.S. Department of Health, Education, and Welfare, Public Health Service, National Center for Health Statistics: Vital statistics of the U.S., Part A—Mortality, Washington, D.C., 1967, U.S. Government Printing Office, Vol. 2.

8. DiPalma, J. R., editor: Basic pharmacology in medicine, New York, 1976, McGraw-Hill Book Co.

9. Meyers, F. H., Jawetz, E., and Goldfien, A.: Review of medical pharmacology, ed. 3, Los Altos, Calif., 1972, Lange Medical Publications.

10. Evaluations of drug interactions, ed. 2, Washington, D.C., 1976, American Pharmaceutical Association.

11. American Medical Association Council on Drugs: AMA drug evaluations—1973, Chicago, 1973, American Medical Association.

12. Granoff, D. M., McDaniel, D. B., and Borkowf, S. P.: Cardiorespiratory arrest following aspiration of chloral hydrate, Am. J. Dis. Child. **122:**170, 1971.

13. Robbins, M. B.: Chloral hydrate and promethazine as premedicants for the apprehensive child, J. Dent. Child. **34:**327, 1967.

14. Finn, S. B., et al.: Clinical pedodontics, ed. 3, Philadelphia, 1967, W. B. Saunders Co.

15. Small, E. W.: Preoperative sedation in dentistry, Dent. Clin. North Am. **14:**769, Oct., 1970.

7

Psychotherapeutic drugs

BARBARA F. ROTH-SCHECHTER

Many drugs are known to have psychotropic activity; that is, they can affect mental activity. This chapter, however, deals exclusively with those agents that are presently employed in the management of major psychiatric disorders. The pharmacology of minor psychiatric disorders and various anxiety states is presented in Chapter 8. For information on psychotogenic drugs (drugs that *induce* psychosis-like behavior) the reader is referred to Chapter 30. The psychotherapeutic drugs will be presented according to their predominant clinical use. For this reason a brief description of the psychiatric illnesses treated with the drugs to be discussed is appropriate.

PSYCHIATRIC DISORDERS

Psychiatric disorders can be classified according to their known or suspected cause of origin and as such are one of two types: organic or functional.

Organic illnesses are defined as (1) those caused by or associated with acquired injuries or diseases that have damaged the brain (for example, tumor, trauma), and (2) those caused by congenital defects (for example, phenylketonuria). In contrast, functional psychiatric disorders by definition are at least partially of psychogenic origin and do not exhibit any clearly defined structural or biochemical abnormality in the brain. The four major classes of functional psychiatric illnesses are the psychoses, neuroses, psychophysiologic (somatic) disorders, and personality disorders.

Within the framework of this discussion, the psychoses and neuroses are of primary interest. During the past two decades major advances have been achieved in the pharmacologic treatment of these two classes of psychiatric disorders.

Psychoses can be termed the most violent type of psychiatric disorders. The two main types of psychoses are the schizophrenias and the affective disorders. A great variety of conditions exist under the heading of schizophrenia, and it is far beyond the scope of this discussion to describe the various forms of this disease. Suffice it to say that schizophrenia is a long-term psychosis characterized by extensive disturbance of the individual's personality function with an obvious loss of the perception of reality.

Affective disorders include the various types of depression, that is, the endogenous (involutional) and exogenous (reactive) depression, as well as the syndrome of manic depression. Endogenous depression is generally considered to be the more severe type of depression and is characterized by an onset apparently unrelated to external events and a high suicidal risk. Exogenous depression appears to be a psychotic reaction to a specific external event and seldom exhibits the severity of the endogenous type. Manic-depressive illness is a cyclic affective disorder characterized by alternating periods of mania (elation) and depression.

Neuroses, or psychoneurotic disorders, are the second major category of psychiatric disorders responsive to psychopharmacologic agents. Although less severe than psychosis, neurosis is a distinct psychiatric entity. It includes various forms of anxiety, phobia, and compulsiveness.

In summary, it must be emphasized that the classifications and definitions given in this introduction are oversimplified, but it is believed that the generally reported specific responses to different psychotherapeutic agents justify this approach. Furthermore, it is intended to aid the reader in the understanding and appreciation of the use of psychopharmacologic drugs. These agents will be presented under two main categories. The first group will include those drugs used in the treatment of psychoses, often referred to as major tranquilizers. The second group will deal with those drugs used to treat affective disorders. The discussion of minor tranquilizers in the management of various neuroses is discussed in Chapter 8.

DRUGS USED IN THE TREATMENT OF PSYCHOSES

Prior to the introduction of drugs into the management of psychiatric disorders, many physical treatment methods were discovered empirically. Some of these are still being used, alone or in combination with drug therapy, such as electroconvulsive therapy; others have been abandoned after a relatively short period of extensive use, such as physical shock treatment like sudden ducking and submersion of the mentally ill patient. Psychosurgery deserves mention because it appears to enjoy renewed interest. Although initially introduced as prefrontal lobotomy (section of the white matter in the plane of the coronal suture), it now has been refined into a highly specific surgical ablation of presumably behavior-controlling central structures. Undoubtedly, however, the introduction of specific psychopharmacologic drugs—not merely sedatives—has superseded many other types of treatment.

The first two psychopharmacologic drugs to be introduced into psychiatry, the phenothiazines and the *Rauwolfia* alkaloids, appeared almost simultaneously in Western medicine. Although extracts of *Rauwolfia serpentina* had been used extensively in Hindu medicine for a variety of diseases, including hypertension and insanity, it was not until 1954 that reserpine was reportedly used in Western medicine for the treatment of psychotic and hypertensive patients, respectively.[1,2] It soon became apparent that the phenothiazines were more effective and easier to control than the *Rauwolfia* compounds. For these reasons *Rauwolfia* alkaloids and their derivatives (reserpine, deserpidine, rescinnamine) are only occasionally used currently for the treatment of psychoses. The use of these drugs in the treatment of hypertension is discussed in Chapter 19.

By far the most widely used group of antipsychotic agents are the phenothiazines,

followed by the butyrophenones and the thioxanthines, the latter being chemically closely related to the phenothiazines. Recently, dihydroindolone has been introduced as an antipsychotic unrelated chemically to any other antipsychotic drug.[3] These four types of antipsychotic agents will be discussed separately.

The phenothiazines

Phenothiazine itself was used as early as 1934 as a urinary antiseptic and anthelminthic. Subsequently, many derivatives were synthesized, and the first important discovery was promethazine, which was found to be a powerful antihistamine with additional sedative effects. It was the sedative effect of promethazine that initiated attempts to improve on this central effect of phenothiazine derivatives, resulting in the synthesis of chlorpromazine (CPZ). The French psychiatrist Laborit first observed the unique psychopharmacologic action of CPZ: "There is no loss in consciousness, not any change in the patient's mentality but a slight tendency to sleep and above all disinterest for all that goes on around him."[4] Those psychiatrists who first used phenothiazine derivatives immediately noted that these effects were far superior to those of any drugs previously used in the treatment of schizophrenic disorders. The use of CPZ quickly spread throughout the world, and its use paralleled a steady decrease in the number of hospitalized psychiatric patients.

Chemistry. Phenothiazine is void of any antipsychotic activity. Substitutions of pharmacologic significance are in positions $10(R^1)$ and $2(R^2)$. Substitutions at position 10 provide the basis for subclassification of the various antipsychotic phenothiazines. Chlorpromazine is the representative example of those phenothiazines that have an *aliphatic side chain (A)* substituted at the nitrogen in position 10. Members of this group are characterized by moderate extrapyramidal effects and an apparently higher rate of agranulocytosis than are members of the other groups of derivatives. The most potent phenothiazine derivatives are provided by members of the *piperazine side-chain substitutions (B)* (for example, trifluoperazine). These phenothiazines have a higher incidence of extrapyramidal side effects but have less sedative properties. An increase in anti-

Table 7-1. Phenothiazine derivatives with antipsychotic activity

Substitution at R^1	Commonly available drugs of that group	Usual oral anti-psychotic dose range (mg/24 hr)	Side effects		
			Frequent	Occasional	Rare
A—Aliphatic side chain	Chlorpromazine (Thorazine)	300-800	Oversedation Orthostatic hypotension Atropine-like effects*	Cholestatic jaundice Parkinsonism Akathisia Menstrual changes Dystonic reactions	Lenticular pigmentation ECG abnormalities Blood dyscrasias Photosensitivity
	Promazine (Sparine)	500-1000			
	Triflupromazine (Vesprin)	100-300			
B—Piperazine side chain	Acetophenazine (Tindal)	30-120	Parkinsonism Akathisia Atropine-like effects* Dystonic reactions	Photosensitivity Orthostatic hypotension Menstrual changes	Jaundice Blood dyscrasias Decreased libido Allergic reactions Sedation
	Fluphenazine HCl (Prolixin)	4-15			
	Trifluoperazine (Stelazine)	3-15			
C—Piperidine side chain	Mesoridazine (Serentil)	150-400	Oversedation Atropine-like effects* Orthostatic hypotension Weight gain	Parkinsonism Akathisia Photosensitivity Menstrual changes	Jaundice Blood dyscrasias Pigmentary retinopathy Dystonic reactions
	Piperacetazine (Quide)	25-150			
	Thioridazine (Mellaril)	100-500			

*Atropine-like (anticholinergic) effects include dry mouth, mydriasis, cycloplegia, urinary retention, tachycardia, decreased gastrointestinal motility.

emetic potency is generally obtained by the additional substitution by a halogen at position 2. The less toxic phenothiazines result from substitution by a piperidine side chain (C) whose members afford intermediate antipsychotic activity (Table 7-1). Generally, substitution in position 2 of the ring results in increased antipsychotic activity. Depending on the type of substitution, this increased antipsychotic activity may or may not be accompanied by a simultaneous increase in antiemetic or side effects, or both. It is worthwhile to note that all antipsychotic phenothiazines have a 3-carbon bridge between ring and side chain nitrogen, whereas phenothiazines with predominantly antihistamine action have only 2 carbons in this position. (Antihistamines are described in Chapter 15.)

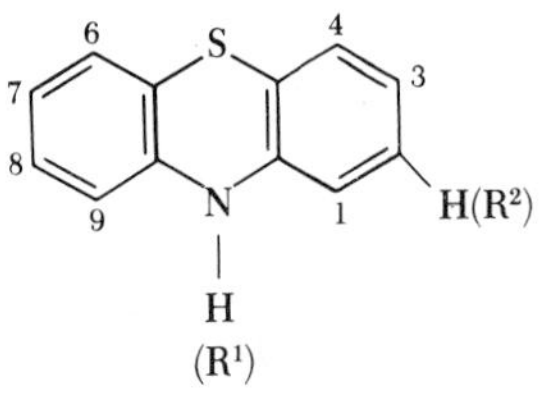

Phenothiazine

Phenothiazine derivatives

A, Aliphatic side chain (for example, chlorpromazine)

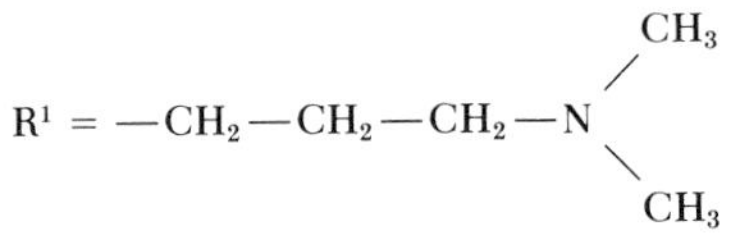

$$R^1 = -CH_2-CH_2-CH_2-N\begin{smallmatrix}CH_3\\ \\CH_3\end{smallmatrix}$$

B, Piperazine side chain (for example, trifluoperazine)

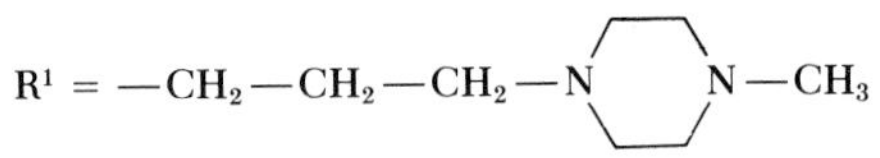

$$R^1 = -CH_2-CH_2-CH_2-N\bigcirc N-CH_3$$

C, Piperidine side chain (for example, thioridazine)

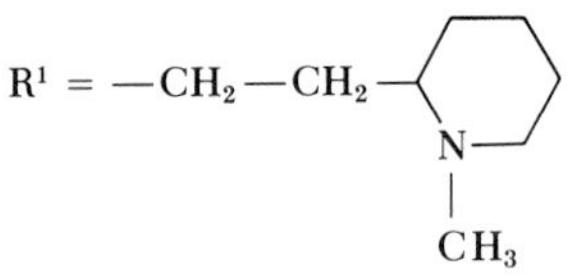

$$R^1 = -CH_2-CH_2-\bigcirc N-CH_3$$

Absorption, metabolism, and excretion. All phenothiazines are well absorbed after oral as well as parenteral administration. Particularly after oral administration, a considerable proportion of the dose is removed into active enterohepatic circulation and is only slowly released into the general circulation. This is considered to be responsible for the long half-life of phenothiazines. For that reason sustained-release preparations of phenothiazines are of no advantage.

There is no specific and pharmacologically significant preferential tissue distribution of the phenothiazines. Hydroxylation followed by conjugation with glucuronic acid represents the major pathway of metabolism. In addition, numerous other metabolites have been postulated and some isolated. These are excreted in about equal proportions by way of the urine and feces. The important fact to appreciate, however, is that the ultimate half-life of a chronically administered phenothiazine is very long. For months after discontinuation of the drug, metabolites as well as free unchanged drug can be identified in the urine.

Addiction and tolerance. Although the phenothiazines are not addicting as defined in Chapter 30, rare and mild cases of physical dependence have been reported. Apparently, there is no development of central tolerance to their antipsychotic effect; however, some degree of tolerance to several of their side effects does occur. Psychological dependence has not been observed with even long-term use, probably because of the lack of any euphoriant action of the phenothiazines.

Pharmacologic effects. The pharmacologic spectrum of phenothiazines is exceptionally wide and diverse.

Central effects of phenothiazines

1. The phenothiazines' main pharmacologic action is their antipsychotic effect that induces the "neuroleptic syndrome." This syndrome consists of a slowing of psychomotor activity in the agitated and disturbed patient, an emotional quieting with suppression of hallucinations and delusions and loss of affect without loss of intellectual function.

2. Various degrees of sedation and drowsiness are effected by different phenothiazine derivatives. They are, however, to be differentiated from other sedatives in that phenothiazines will not induce anesthesia, even with large doses, and although drowsy, the patient can always be easily aroused under the influence of the drug. As mentioned earlier, there is no tolerance developed to the antipsychotic effect, but tolerance to the sedative action occurs within 1 to 2 weeks, the same time period necessary for the full antipsychotic effect to become mani-

fested. Thus the combination of sedative and antipsychotic action of phenothiazines provides maximal initial benefit for the agitated and disturbed psychotic patient. The mechanism of action of the phenothiazines in producing their major pharmacologic effect is not understood. Together with the extrapyramidal stimulation observed (see later), the antipsychotic action could be explained by a blockade of dopamine receptors, which by a negative feedback mechanism leads to enhanced dopamine turnover. Specifically, it has been suggested that activation of a limbic (antipsychotic) and caudate (extrapyramidal) adenylate cyclase by dopamine is blocked by antipsychotic drugs.[5]

All other effects of the phenothiazines are either minor therapeutic or strictly side effects. Among the many phenothiazines marketed, no single phenothiazine is clearly superior to any other in its antipsychotic action. There are advantages and disadvantages with respect to side effects of each individual compound, and the consideration of the differential risk of all side effects remains a matter of clinical judgment. Chlorpromazine will be discussed here as the typical and most widely used phenothiazine.

3. The third, although minor, pharmacologic effect of therapeutic significance of CPZ is an antiemetic action. This stems from specific depression of the chemotherapeutic trigger zone. Chlorpromazine is particularly potent in producing this effect at nonsedative doses. The antiemetic effect of phenothiazines has been found useful in controlling nausea and vomiting occurring during uremia, gastroenteritis, carcinomatosis, and drug-induced emesis. But since CPZ acts by depressing the chemotherapeutic trigger zone, it is ineffective in controlling motion sickness or any other nausea from vestibular stimulation.

4. The hypothalamus is another central structure that is apparently uniformly depressed by CPZ. This action manifests itself in a number of mostly undesirable side effects.

   a. The vasomotor center is depressed at relatively low doses; specifically, sympathetic outflow from the hypothalamus appears to be suppressed. Together with peripheral autonomic effects (see later), this action manifests itself as orthostatic hypotension.

b. Temperature-regulating systems are disrupted, and a tendency toward poikilothermy can be observed. In case of environmental hypothermia this effect combined with peripheral vasodilation can become detrimental.

c. Release of pituitary gonadotropins is suppressed by CPZ, which may cause delay in ovulation and menstruation in female patients, sometimes even induction of pseudopregnancy. A certain degree of tolerance has been observed to develop to this effect.

d. Secretion of growth hormone, oxytocin, and adrenocorticotropic hormone is suppressed by CPZ, but it remains to be unequivocally established whether adrenocortical secretion and thyroid activity are also reduced.

5. The medullary respiratory center is depressed only slightly at low doses of CPZ, but this central depressive action has to be kept in mind when a sedative or other central nervous system depressant is administered to a patient who is receiving long-term phenothiazine therapy or at toxic doses of CPZ.

6. Central motor effects can be either inhibitory or stimulatory.

a. Skeletal muscular relaxation, which contributes to the neuroleptic syndrome, can be produced in other spastic conditions as well. It appears to be of central origin, possibly caused by depression of cerebral gamma motor systems.

b. Chlorpromazine and other phenothiazines stimulate the extrapyramidal system, giving rise to the most common and most disagreeable series of side effects. There is considerable variation in individual susceptibility to the extrapyramidal syndrome. Side effects may occur early during therapy, but the incidence increases with long-term administration, with some of the effects being directly related to the cumulative dose.[6] Extrapyramidal stimulation manifests itself in dyskinesia (bizarre movements of tongue, face, and neck), the well-known Parkinson's disease (resting tremor, rigidity, akinesia), and various forms of akathisia (extensive motor restlessness). Only some of these side effects are responsive to anti-Par-

kinson therapy, and there have been reports of rare cases of persistence of the effects long after discontinuation of the phenothiazine medication.[7]

In dyskinetic patients, spasms of the muscles of mastication may be a phenothiazine-induced complication. The typical symptom is sudden and severe intermittent pain in the region of the temporomandibular joint. In an acute attack it becomes difficult to open or close the jaw, and unilateral or bilateral dislocation of the mandible may occur. Without any treatment the spasm will generally subside within several hours. Intravenous administration of amobarbital sodium or diphenhydramine hydrochloride, as well as oral administration of phenobarbital and methocarbamol, have been successful in relieving the acute spasm.

Peripheral effects of phenothiazines

1. Phenothiazine derivatives have extensive autonomic effects. Adrenergic receptors appear to be blocked by CPZ, which augments the central sympatholytic effect mentioned earlier. The observable clinical manifestation is orthostatic hypotension with a compensatory tachycardia. Tolerance usually develops during the first weeks of medication.

There are mild anticholinergic side effects of CPZ, primarily of the antimuscarinic type, that is, blurred vision, xerostomia, and constipation. Alone, the anticholinergic actions of phenothiazines are weak, but they can become of major significance when other anticholinergic medication is administered together with phenothiazines.

2. Chlorpromazine can induce local anesthesia when injected proximally to a nerve, being twice as effective as meperidine, but this action is of no clinical value by itself.

3. Chlorpromazine is known to have a diuretic effect, which is thought to be due to a decreased release of antidiuretic hormone, a direct action of CPZ on the renal tubule, or a combination of both actions.

4. Phenothiazines have a direct negative inotropic effect on the heart. The main manifestation of CPZ on the heart, however, is tachycardia, which is partially compensatory to the hypotensive action and partially caused by its atropine-like action.

5. Several other peripheral actions of CPZ have been observed; they are believed to be either allergic and hypersensitivity reactions

or long-term effects of unknown origin. Blood dyscrasias are known to occur, the most serious of which is agranulocytosis, which usually occurs within the first 6 to 8 weeks of medication. Although the occurrence is rare, the mortality is high (30%). Chlorpromazine-induced cholestatic jaundice is considered an allergic reaction, with most cases being benign and a return to normal liver function occurring on discontinuation of the drug. A variety of skin eruptions has been associated with CPZ medication, including urticarial, petechial, and edematous types. Photosensitivity reactions resembling severe sunburn as well as blue-gray metallic discoloration of skin and eyes are known to occur.

Drug interactions and overdose toxicity. In view of the actions of phenothiazines, it is not surprising that they interact in an additive or even potentiating fashion with all central nervous system depressants, such as barbiturates, alcohol, general anesthetics, and opiates. Chlorpromazine greatly enhances the respiratory depression produced by meperidine. For additive psychotherapeutic benefit phenothiazines are often successfully combined with the tricyclic antidepressants. With this combination, however, the antihypertensive effect of guanethidine may be blocked. On the other hand, with all other antihypertensive drugs phenothiazines may act in an additive fashion, probably by their blockade of dopamine receptors. The same mechanism is thought to be responsible for the interaction of phenothiazines with levodopa, which results in a decreased anti-Parkinson effect. To control excessive extrapyramidal stimulation, phenothiazine therapy often has to be combined with anti-Parkinson medication of anticholinergic type. This combination is bound to exacerbate antimuscarinic peripheral effects, like xerostomia, urinary retention, bowel paralysis, and inhibition of sweating. Lastly, it should be emphasized that epinephrine should never be used for vasomotor collapse in a patient receiving phenothiazine medication because of the alpha-adrenergic blocking action of these drugs.

Acute overdose toxicity results from a combination of central and peripheral effects. It usually includes respiratory failure, convulsions or excessive extrapyramidal symptoms, cardiovascular collapse, and hypothermia. Chronic overdose toxicity generally manifests itself in exacerbation and intensification of most of the side effects described. A specific oral syndrome—primarily attributable to excessive anticholinergic action—can be described as dry mouth, diffuse redness of mucous membranes, loosened dentures, denture stomatitis, and black or white hairy tongue, all of which disappear on discontinuation of medication.

In general, the treatment of acute overdose toxicity is of a supportive and symptomatic nature to provide adequate respiration and circulation and to maintain body temperature. The treatment of chronic overdose toxicity consists of gradual withdrawal of the phenothiazine.

Therapeutic uses. Despite their wide spectrum of side effects, phenothiazines are relatively safe drugs. They have revolutionized mental hospitals and are the first line of defense against schizophrenia.[8] They also have been used, although with variable results, in the management of various neuroses and some character disorders. Treatment with phenothiazines is strictly on an individual basis. It should be appreciated that long-acting injectable phenothiazines are available with a duration of action of up to 4 to 6 weeks, thus allowing the effective control of chronic schizophrenia in patients who fail to take their oral medication regularly. Phenothiazines have been tried in the treatment of acute withdrawal from many abused central nervous system drugs. Although they seem of little use in the management of withdrawal from narcotics, they are being used successfully in the management of alcoholic hallucinosis. A second, minor therapeutic indication of chlorpromazine and other phenothiazines is as antiemetics, particularly in the control of vomiting of gastroenteritis, uremia, carcinomatosis, and drug-induced vomiting. Lastly, chlorpromazine has been used successfully in the control of intractable hiccoughs. For obvious reasons of additive interactions, phenothiazines are contraindicated in patients with myasthenia gravis, brain damage and epileptic disorders, cardiac disease, and hepatitis and in patients receiving antihypertensive therapy.

The butyrophenones

History. The first butyrophenone to be introduced for the treatment of psychoses was haloperidol. It was synthesized by Janssen[9] after an extensive synthetic program following the successful introduction of the analgesic meperidine. Haloperidol was made available for therapeutic use in 1960.

Chemistry. In contrast to other antipsychotic drugs, which tend to constitute more or less successful modifications of the basic phenothiazine structure, butyrophenones are chemically entirely different psychotherapeutic agents. The chemical formula of haloperidol is as follows:

Despite the structural dissimilarity, the butyrophenones resemble closely in their actions the piperazine phenothiazines. They also block the effects of dopamine and increase its turnover rate, which is believed to be their mechanism of action. The two members available in the United States are haloperidol and droperidol. This discussion will focus on the former, since it is by far the most widely used butyrophenone in the United States.

Absorption, metabolism, and excretion. At present, haloperidol is available for oral and parenteral administration. In human beings it has a long biologic half-life with persistence of the drug for several weeks after a single dose. Haloperidol concentrates in the liver; however, its primary pathway of excretion is by way of the kidney. Haloperidol has not been found to be addictive, or does it exhibit the phenomenon of central tolerance.

Pharmacologic effects. The main pharmacologic action of haloperidol is its highly potent antipsychotic effect combined with a sedative and general central nervous system depressive action. This depression manifests itself in tiredness, lowering of blood pressure (apparently only of central origin), and a fall in body temperature. Both the sedative and the hypotensive effects of haloperidol are less severe than those of the phenothiazines. Furthermore, autonomic side effects are also less pronounced than those of the phenothiazines. Within low to medium therapeutic dose range side effects

of butyrophenones are restricted to extrapyramidal manifestations like parkinsonism and dystonic reactions. In high therapeutic dose ranges side effects consist of blood dyscrasias, hypotension, and depression, all of which respond to a reduction in dosage. Hypersensitivity and allergic reactions have been observed only rarely. Like the phenothiazines, haloperidol on occasion has been found to induce tardive dyskinesia that may be irreversible.

Drug interactions. Butyrophenones potentiate the sedative effect of other central nervous system depressants like barbiturates, general anesthetics, and analgesics. In high doses butyrophenones decrease the anticoagulant action of phenindione by stimulating its metabolism. They are contraindicated in any type of depressive state because of their potential to induce depression themselves.

Therapeutic uses. Butyrophenones are highly effective antipsychotic drugs, not only in the various forms of schizophrenia but also in the management of the manic phase of manic-depressive illness. In addition, they have been found to be effective in the treatment of Gilles de la Tourette's syndrome. Butyrophenones are preferred for use in patients with coronary or cerebrovascular disease because they produce less hypotension.

The thioxanthines

Thioxanthines are a less potent group of antipsychotic drugs when compared with the phenothiazines or butyrophenones. They are closely related chemically to the phenothiazines. Thioxanthines have a lower incidence of adverse reactions than do the other antipsychotic drugs, consisting primarily of oversedation, but they are also considerably weaker antipsychotics. They have almost the same but weaker pharmacologic and toxicologic spectrum as the phenothiazines. Nevertheless, thioxanthines have a definite place in the antipsychotic armamentarium for the management of certain schizoaffective disorders. In addition to chlorprothixene, thiothixene and clopenthixol are available. Their entire therapeutic spectrum remains to be established.

The dihydroindolones

The only dihydroindolone presently available is molindone, which is chemically unrelated to any other antipsychotic drug. When compared with a representative phenothiazine (triphenoperazine), it was found to be equally effective in patients with acute or chronic schizophrenia. Its adverse reactions are similar to those of the phenothiazines, including extrapyramidal symptoms, postural hypotension, and tachycardia. Molindone has not been used long enough for an appreciation of its full potential or full range and severity of side effects.

DRUGS USED IN THE TREATMENT OF DEPRESSION

Until the late 1950s, there was no widely accepted pharmacologic treatment for depression. Forms of mild depression were treated with psychotherapy, and severe depression was treated with electroconvulsive therapy (ECT). Although several drugs are now available for the treatment of depression, all of them share the same drawback: an onset of at least 1 to 2 weeks. Therefore in severe suicidal depression ECT still remains superior to any drug treatment presently available.

The dibenzazepines (tricyclic antidepressants)

Although the dibenzazepines were not the first antidepressive drugs developed, they now constitute the most widely used and are considered by many to be the most effective compounds. Many dibenzazepines had been synthesized as early as 1889, but they were not clinically investigated until the late 1950s. This can most probably be attributed to their close chemical and to some extent pharmacologic similarity to the phenothiazines, which resulted in overlooking them for their specific antidepressant action.

Chemistry. The close structural similarity between the tricyclic antidepressants and the phenothiazines can be appreciated by consideration of the illustrations at the top of the next column:

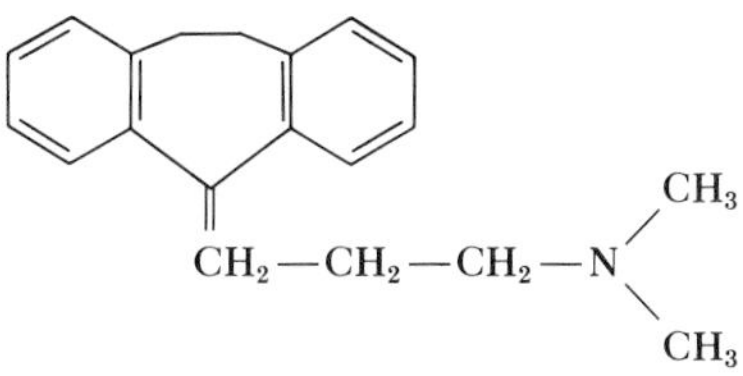

The replacement of the sulfur atom of chlorpromazine *(A)* by a CH_2-CH_2 bridge pharmacologically results in a change from an antipsychotic to an antidepressant agent, and pharmacokinetically prevents conjugation of this ring. Two different series of tricyclics are derived, depending on whether a nitrogen or carbon is in position 10 *(A-C)*. The two types of derivatives are the (1) iminodibenzyl compounds with imipramine (Presamine, Tofranil) *(B)* and (2) dibenzocyclo-

A, Chlorpromazine

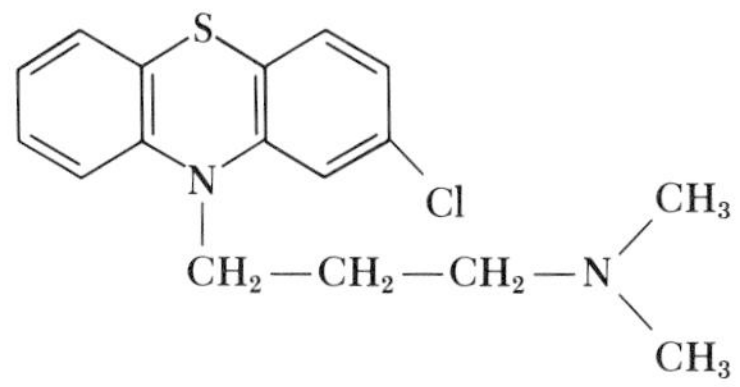

B, Imipramine

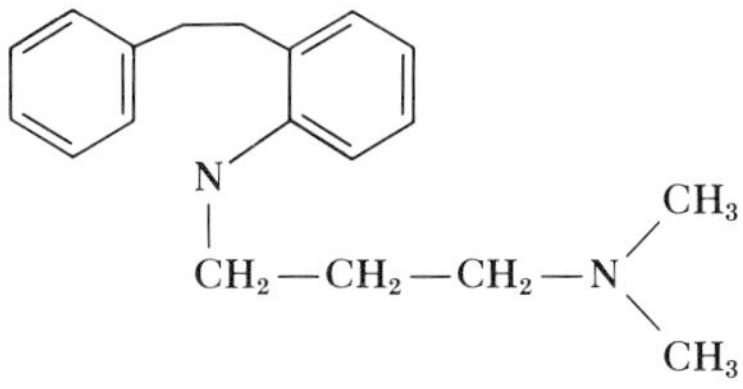

C, Amitriptyline

heptenes with amitriptyline (Elavil, Triavil) *(C)* as their representative example. Their actions and side effects are sufficiently similar so that a discussion of the subtle differences of the two types of tricyclic antidepressants is not warranted. Suffice it to point out that the latter tricyclic derivatives exhibit sedative side effects more frequently than do the others. For convenience, pharmacodynamics and pharmacology of the dibenzazepines will be discussed in terms of imipramine, and differences will be emphasized only when necessary.

Absorption, metabolism, and excretion. Imipramine is rapidly and well absorbed into the general circulation, independent of the route of administration. The biologic half-life is surprisingly short in comparison with the long latency of onset of action of the drug (see later). Dibenzazepines are predominantly metabolized by hepatic ring hydroxylation, glucuronide conjugation, and demethylation. Metabolites and unchanged drug are excreted by way of the kidneys, amounting to a total of 70% of administered dose within the first 72 hours.

Pharmacologic effects. The therapeutically important action of imipramine is on the central nervous system and differs between normal and depressed individuals. Many of its central actions resemble those of the pheno-thiazines. Particularly in normal persons, imipramine produces mild sedation and fatigue accompanied by strong antimuscarinic (atropine-like) side effects as well as reduction of psychomotor activity, potentiation of central nervous system depressants, and hypothermia. In contrast, depressed patients respond to imipramine therapy with an elevation of mood and a feeling of well-being but without any euphoriant action. However, the onset of these actions in depressed patients is between 1 and 3 weeks. Tricyclic antidepressants should be given for 4 weeks before they are considered to be ineffective in the treatment of depression. Furthermore, depressed patients respond to imipramine therapy with increased mental and physical activity, together with a reduction in their morbid preoccupation with suicide. The primary effect of tricyclic antidepressants in depressed individuals has been described as a "dulling of depressive ideation,"[10] but it may be accompanied by initial difficulty in concentration and thinking. The mechanism of the central nervous system effects of imipramine is not understood. The most plausible hypothesis at present relates changes in the metabolism of central biogenic amines to its antidepressant effect.

The medullary respiratory center is unaffected by therapeutic doses of imipramine, but respiratory depression has been observed after poisoning with imipramine and amitriptyline.

Adverse effects and drug interactions. Some tricyclic antidepressants have tremorigenic activity of central origin. It apparently is not attributable to extrapyramidal stimulation, and it therefore does not respond to anti-Parkinson medication. It consists of a fine tremor in the upper extremities and occurs in at least 10% of patients treated with the drug.

Primary peripheral effects of imipramine are on the autonomic nervous system. It has distinct anticholinergic effects, resulting in dry mouth, blurred vision, tachycardia, constipation, and urinary retention. Tolerance to these atropine-like effects tends to develop with continued use. Similarly to the phenothiazines, imipramine initially produces orthostatic hypotension, and tolerance is acquired to this effect also.

The most serious peripheral side effect is from imipramine's cardiac toxicity. Myocardial infarction and precipitation of congestive heart failure during the course of treatment have occurred. Various arrhythmias and episodes of tachycardia have been attributed to imipramine's antimuscarinic effects.

Hypersensitivity reactions like skin rashes, blood dyscrasias, and obstructive jaundice have rarely been observed with the use of tricyclic antidepressants.

Unlike the phenothiazines, tricyclic antidepressants potentiate the behavioral actions of amphetamines and other central nervous system stimulants. Simultaneous administration of imipramine and monoamine oxidase inhibitors has resulted in severe reactions consisting of signs and symptoms of severe atropine toxicity. It is generally agreed that at least a 1-week interval should be observed after the discontinuation of one drug and the initiation of the other type of drug. Similar precautions should be kept in mind when treating a patient who is receiving imipramine therapy with any anticholinergic drug. Imipramine-like compounds will potentiate the pressor effects of injected norepinephrine, apparently because of an interference with uptake mechanism of this amine. Probably for the same reason, tricyclics block the antihypertensive action of guanethidine.

The combination of phenothiazines and tricyclics has been employed successfully and safely in the treatment of severely anxious and agitated depressed individuals. Tricyclic antidepressants can also be well combined with electroconvulsive therapy; this may be of greatest advantage during the initial phase of drug therapy, in severe suicidal risks, since the onset of action of imipramine may be as long as several weeks. Because of the cardiac and autonomic side effects, tricyclic antidepressants are to be used cautiously in cardiac patients, and epileptics, as well as patients with glaucoma or prostatic hypertrophy.

Accidental poisoning with tricyclics has become more common, and such overdose can be lethal. Acute overdose toxicity consists of severe hypertension, cardiac arrhythmias, hyperpyrexia, convulsions, coma, and respiratory failure. Survivors may have permanent myocardial damage. Treatment is symptomatic and should be conservative in view of the known interactions with other central nervous system vasopressor agents. Physostigmine has been reported to be effective in treating severe poisoning by tricyclic antidepressants.[11]

Tricyclic antidepressants have very rarely been found to produce psychic or physical dependence and certainly not the entire syndrome of addiction with central tolerance and the necessary increase in dose for an adequate antidepressant action. Slight withdrawal effects after abrupt discontinuation of the drug have been reported. Tolerance to many side effects, central as well as peripheral, develops with different time courses.

Therapeutic uses. Tricyclic antidepressants can be considered the initial pharmacologic approach to depression. This evaluation is based on a consideration of both the efficacy and the toxicity of all drugs used in the management of depression. The eventual effectiveness of the tricyclic agents approaches that of electroconvulsive therapy but has the additional advantage of preventing relapses and thus provides long-term control of this psychiatric disorder. Imipramine-like agents have been used with moderate success in the control of nocturnal enuresis in children.

The monoamine oxidase inhibitors (MAOIs)

The heading of monoamine oxidase inhibitors includes a variety of drugs all of which share in the ability to inhibit monoamine oxidase (MAO) and thus to block oxidative deamination of naturally occurring amines. With a few exceptions these drugs inhibit MAO noncompetitively and irreversibly; that is, recovery from their action can occur only by synthesis of new enzyme, which is a matter of weeks. Long-term inhibition of MAO has been shown to result in the accumulation of norepinephrine, epinephrine, serotonin, dopamine, tyramine, or tryptamine in various tissues. The relationship between MAO inhibition, the accumulation of these biogenic amines, and the therapeutic usefulness of these drugs in psychiatry remains to be established. Furthermore, one should keep in mind that MAOIs also inhibit many other enzyme systems such as dopamine-β-oxidase, several decarboxylases, and hepatic oxidative enzymes, as well as having numerous effects unrelated to enzyme inhibition.

Presently used MAOIs are isocarboxazid (Marplan) and nialamide (Niamid), both of which are hydrazides; phenelzine (Nardil), which is a hydrazine derivative; tranylcypromine (Parnate); and pargyline (Eutonyl). Although chemically heterogeneous, MAOIs can be discussed as an entity as far as pharmacodynamics, their pharmacologic effects, and their uses are concerned.

Absorption, metabolism, and excretion. All currently available MAOIs are readily absorbed with either oral or parenteral administration. The metabolism of hydrazides and hydrazines apparently consists of cleavage resulting in inactivation. Tranylcypromine is partially metabolized to benzoic acid. Other unidentified metabolites and unchanged drugs are excreted primarily in the urine with a half-life of approximately 1 or 2 days.

Pharmacologic effects. The most useful psychopharmacologic action of certain MAOIs is their ability to elevate the mood of depressed patients. (For a discussion of antihypertensive MAOIs, see Chapter 19.) This antidepressive action of MAOIs is described as euphoric stimulation and occurs in normal as well as depressed subjects. The onset of antidepressive action is slow, and usually several weeks are required for full benefit to become evident.

Adverse reactions and drug interactions. Frequent side effect of MAOIs consist of restlessness and insomnia, which in rare cases may lead to manic reactions and even hallucinations. The peripheral side effects of MAOIs are hypotension (Chapter 19), dry mouth, nausea, constipation, and anorexia. Rare side effects may include paresthesia, skin rashes, and muscle spasms.

Knowing the many enzyme systems affected by MAOIs, one is not surprised that the actions of many different drugs are being modified by the presence of a MAOI. Since MAO metabolizes endogenous as well as exogenous amines, the action of any sympathomimetic amine administered is potentiated. In addition, since MAO is an intraneuronal enzyme, it is understandable that indirectly acting amines (tyramine, amphetamine) are potentiated to a greater extent than directly acting amines (norepinephrine, epinephrine). Many foods and beverages contain high levels of tyramine (cheeses, fish, beer). For this reason ingestion of such food poses the danger of precipitation of a hypertensive crisis in a patient receiving long-term MAOI therapy. In several cases intracranial bleeding, excessive fever, and death occurred because of this interaction.

Because of their general enzyme-inhibiting properties, mentioned earlier, MAOIs interfere with the detoxifying mechanism of many drugs. They are known to potentiate the central nervous system–depressing action of barbiturates, alcohol, and analgesics. The MAOIs also prolong and intensify the effect of tricyclic antidepressants as well as anticholinergic agents used in the treatment of parkinsonism.

Acute toxicity from overdosages is characterized by hallucinations, hyperreflexia, convulsions, hyperpyrexia, and hypertensive crisis more often than hypotensive collapse. Treatment has to be conservative and aimed at the maintenance of body temperature, respiration, blood pressure, and electrolyte balance. Treatment of choice of the hypertensive crisis is the administration of a short-acting alpha-adrenergic blocking agent like phentolamine.

Therapeutic uses. It has been stated repeatedly that MAOIs are more successful in the treatment of exogenous rather than endogenous depression. However, the former is also known to respond much better to psychotherapy, and it appears that many successes attributed to MAOI therapy were primarily caused by an increased responsiveness to psychotherapy in the presence of the MAOI. On the other hand, MAOIs undoubtedly have euphoriant and antidepressive action, with tranylcypromine being the most effective and nialamide the least effective of the group. With their great potential for dietary and drug interactions as well as their own toxicity, combined with the availability of the tricyclic antidepressants, MAOIs are being used much less in recent years for the treatment of depression. They are being reserved mainly for patients whose condition is refractory to any other form of treatment and for patients who are reliable enough to be trusted with a potentially highly toxic drug.

Lithium salts

As outlined earlier, manic depressive illness constitutes one major segment of the affective disorders. It is characterized by the cyclic recurrence of mania alternating with depression. Lithium carbonate has been used intermittently to treat the manic phase for more than 20 years, but only recently has it been approved by the FDA in the United States, both as maintenance therapy and as adjunctive or primary therapy for acute episodes.[12]

Chemically, lithium is a monovalent cation and belongs in the group of alkali metals. It is used as lithium carbonate (Li_2CO_3) and is administered orally only.

After ingestion lithium is readily absorbed, with peak plasma levels being reached between 2 and 4 hours after administration. Lithium is apparently rather uniformly distributed throughout the body, since it has been identified in both cerebrospinal fluid and milk of lactating mothers. The main route of excretion is through the kidneys, and there it apparently is handled like sodium, since under conditions of lowered sodium intake lithium excretion is reduced, and thus the potential of lithium toxicity rises under those circumstances. No tolerance of any origin has been detected during the use of lithium in the treatment of psychiatric disorders.

The mechanism of action of lithium in unknown. It appears to act rather specifically, since it does not have any psychoactivity in normal individuals. Because 3 to 10 days of therapy are needed for lithium to become effective, a severely manic patient should be hospitalized and should receive phenothiazines together with the lithium in the first few days. All experts agree that to assure safety and effectiveness lithium serum concentrations should be monitored weekly and maintained below 1.5 mEq/L to avoid serious toxicity.

Side effects consist of polyuria, fine hand tremor, and mild thirst; in more severe cases they may extend to slurred speech, ataxia, nausea, vomiting, and diarrhea. Overdose toxicity is primarily manifested by central nervous system symptomatology. Muscular ridigity, hyperactive deep reflexes, excessive tremor, and muscle fasciculations are observed, together with loss of consciousness and coma. Immediate cessation of medication is the treatment of choice. In severe cases intravenous administration of urea or mannitol may be used to enhance lithium excretion by osmotic diuresis. The drug is obviously contraindicated in patients with impaired renal function and should not be given to patients taking a restricted salt diet or diuretic therapy.

PSYCHOTHERAPEUTIC AGENTS IN PEDIATRICS AND GERIATRICS

Before this chapter is closed, a brief discussion of differences in response to and problems with the use of psychotherapeutic agents in the very young patient and in the elderly is considered to be mandatory.

Use in pediatrics

Although the use of psychotherapeutic drugs is widespread in children, few well-controlled studies are available in pediatric psychopharmacology. This appears to stem from a combination of many factors. There is an increased difficulty in differentiating drug-induced changes from maturational changes. Also, children are more suggestible and dependent on their surroundings than are adults, thereby increasing possible placebo reactions. Nevertheless, most of the psychotherapeutic agents used in the adult are employed in children, although not always for the same purpose.

The phenothiazines, possibly because of their relatively long existence, are the most widely used drugs for the treatment of emotional disorders in children, not however, to treat mild or moderate neurotic behavior. In general, the phenothiazines are less potent in children than in adults. Similarly, side effects like drowsiness, constipation, and skin reaction occur less frequently. With the exception of extrapyramidal dystonic reactions and seizure occurrence, children can tolerate a higher milligram of drug per kilogram of body weight than adults can.

The tricyclic antidepressants have been claimed to be of additional value for children with a large number of disturbances, such as hyperactivity, stammering, behavior problems, or poor learning, but at present only nocturnal enuresis has been established as a condition that is effectively treated by imipramine-like drugs. The most common side effects of imipramine in enuretic children are nervousness, sleep disorders, and mild gastrointestinal disturbances. Furthermore, adverse reactions rarely seen in adults include cardiac arrhythmias and agranulocytosis. Thus, although imipramine appears to be effective in the treatment of enuresis in some children, it should be administered with the utmost care.[13]

The use of sedatives in children for the control of emotional disorders seems to be unjustified. Since they have no antipsychotic or antidepressant effect, they have been found to be inferior to placebo therapy.

Use in geriatrics

The use and effectiveness of any drug, and particularly the psychotherapeutic drugs in the geriatric patient is largely limited by his physical state. Also, the degree of variability found among individuals in their response to drugs is much larger in an older population. Changes in the rates of absorption, metabolism, and excretion as a function of pathophysiologic changes are the most obvious factors determining such variability. Generally, adverse effects of a given dose increase, whereas the primary effect remains the same or decreases. In any case the therapeutic index decreases. For this reason lower initial doses of psychotherapeutic drugs should be used in the older patient compared with doses in a young adult. The use of phenothiazines in geriatric psychopharmacology is primarily limited by two sets of side effects. Tardive dyskinesia has a considerably higher incidence in the elderly, and the autonomic side effects are of more problematic consequences. Hypotensive reactions and parasympatholytic effects on the gastrointestinal tract, the genitourinary system, and the eye are more severe than in young adult patients.

For the treatment of depression the use of tricyclic antidepressants in geriatrics has the same limitation as that of the phenothiazines: The toxic effects occur at a relatively lower dosage and with a higher incidence. Some authorities believe that, in the elderly, electroconvulsive therapy is to be preferred. There is uniform agreement that MAOI antidepressant therapy is to be used as a last resort only, since elderly individuals usually have to take other medication more frequently and are susceptible to dietary complications. Thus the potential of adverse drug interactions is greatly increased and does not justify the use of these drugs until all other possibilities have been explored.

In conclusion, use of psychotherapeutic agents in pediatric and geriatric patients should be guided by a more careful approach with anticipation of possible paradoxical reactions on the one hand and increased toxicity and complications on the other.

REFERENCES

1. Kline, N. S.: Use of *Rauwolfia serpentina Benth* in neuropsychiatric conditions, Ann. N.Y. Acad. Sci. **59:**107-132, 1954.
2. Wilkins, R. W.: Clinical usage of *Rauwolfia* alkaloids, including reserpine (Serpasil), Ann. N.Y. Acad. Sci. **59:**36-44, 1954.
3. Molindone—a new antipsychotic drug, The Medical Letter **17:**59-60, 1975.
4. Hordern, A.: Psychopharmacology: some historical considerations. In Joyce, C. R. B., editor: Psychopharmacology, London, 1968, Tavistock Publications.
5. Clement-Cormier, Y. C., Kebabian, J. W., Petzold, G. L., and Greengard, P.: Dopamine-sensitive adenylate cyclase in mammalian brain: a possible site of action of antipsychotic drugs, Proc. Natl. Acad. Sci. U.S.A. **71:**1113-1117, 1974.
6. Simpson, G. M., and Angus, G. W. S.: Drug-induced extra-pyramidal disorders, Acta Psychiatr. Scand. **212:**7-58, 1970.
7. Crane, G. E.: Dyskinesias and neuroleptics, Arch. Gen. Psychiatry **19:**700-703, 1968.
8. Davis, J. M.: Overview: maintenance therapy in psychiatry. I. Schizophrenia, Am. J. Psychiatry **132:**1239-1245, 1975.
9. Janssen, P. A. J.: The pharmacology of haloperidol, Int. J. Neuropsychiatry **3:**S10-S18, 1967.
10. Cole, J. O.: Therapeutic efficacy of antidepressant drugs, J.A.M.A. **190:**448-455, 1964.
11. Burks, J. S., Walker, J. E., Rumack, B. H., and Ott, J. E.: Tricyclic antidepressant poisoning J.A.M.A. **230:**1405-1407, 1974.
12. Johnson, F. N., editor: Lithium research and therapy, New York, 1975, Academic Press, Inc.
13. Imipramine for enuresis, The Medical Letter **16:**21-24, 1974.

8

Minor tranquilizers and centrally acting muscle relaxants

RICHARD L. WYNN
BARBARA F. ROTH-SCHECTER

Drugs described in this chapter have the ability to relieve anxieties (minor tranquilizers) and to diminish skeletal muscle tone and involuntary movement by actions on the central nervous system (centrally acting muscle relaxants). Since many of the minor tranquilizers exert muscle relaxant actions in themselves, it is convenient to discuss the pharmacology of these two drug classes in a single chapter.

Both groups of drugs constitute a major portion of pharmaceuticals that are consumed by the public. In addition, the minor tranquilizers play an important therapeutic role as premedications for the anxious dental patient. Thus the drugs in this chapter will be discussed in terms of their use by the general public and in the practice of dentistry.

MINOR TRANQUILIZERS

Anxiety constitutes a major psychoneurotic disorder. Although less severe than psychosis, it is believed to have fundamental psychological causes, but undoubtedly there are organic factors along with the functional ones. Anxiety is expressed by means of psychophysiologic mechanisms and thus manifests itself by a diverse group of signs and symptoms. There is a feeling of apprehension, panic, and fear coupled with and positively reinforced by muscular tension, restlessness, choking, palpitation, and excessive sweating and in the chronic form developing into irritability, fatigue, and insomnia.

In the practice of dentistry many forms of anxiety can be observed, ranging from a short episode of anxiety preceding a dental operative procedure to a full-blown neurosis. The symptomatology is usually the same as that just described and differs in severity only.

Antianxiety agents in general are ineffective against psychotic episodes but appear to have a definite antianxiety component. In addition, they usually have a wide spectrum of peripheral effects that contribute to and reinforce their antianxiety action. It must be appreciated that antianxiety agents constitute strictly symptomatic treatment; their use may alleviate the syndrome of anxiety temporarily but not cure the underlying psychopathologic defect. In dentistry these drugs have been employed for their ability to reduce tension and anxiety in the preoperative situation. Furthermore, they have recently been introduced as sedatives (intravenously) during dental procedures and thus promise to remain an important group of drugs in the hands of the dentist.

The three major chemical groups of antianxiety drugs or minor tranquilizers and their representatives are as follows:

Propanediols (propyl alcohol derivatives)
  Emylcamate (Listica)
  Ethinamate (Valmid)*
  Meprobamate (Equanil, Miltown)
  Phenaglycodol (Ultran)
  Tybamate (Solacen)
Benzodiazepine derivatives
  Chlordiazepoxide (Libritabs, Librium)
  Clorazepate dipotassium (Tranxene)
  Diazepam (Valium)
  Flurazepam (Dalmane)
  Oxazepam (Serax)
Diphenylmethanes
  Benactyzine (Deprol)
  Buclizine (Softran)
  Diphenhydramine (Benadryl)†
  Hydroxyzine (Atarax, Vistaril)

---

* Discussed as a nonbarbiturate sedative in Chapter 6.
† Discussed as an antihistamine in Chapter 15.

The propanediols

Meprobamate and phenaglycodol are discussed as representatives of the propanediols.

Meprobamate

Meprobamate (Miltown, Equanil) is the most popular propanediol. It was developed to prolong the central muscle–relaxing action of mephenesin. Its assumed potential to relieve anxiety, together with a sedative component, furthered its rapid acceptance. The structural formula of meprobamate is as follows:

$$H_2N-\overset{\overset{O}{\|}}{C}-OCH_2-\overset{\overset{C_3H_7}{|}}{\underset{\underset{CH_3}{|}}{C}}-CH_2O-\overset{\overset{O}{\|}}{C}-NH_2$$

Absorption, metabolism, and excretion. When administered orally, meprobamate is readily absorbed from the gastrointestinal tract and becomes uniformly distributed throughout the body. It is metabolized by oxidation, hydroxylation, and glucuronide conjugation. Excretion of unchanged and metabolized drug is by way of the urine. Prolonged use of meprobamate will result in the occurrence of central tolerance, compulsive use, and physical dependence. The last two characteristics are demonstrated by a withdrawal syndrome after abrupt discontinuation of the drug. Withdrawal resembles that observed after barbiturate withdrawal and consists of convulsions, psychotic behavior, and coma.

Pharmacologic effects. The difficulty is now appreciated of differentiating pharmacologically between meprobamate and the sedative barbiturates. Meprobamate clearly has sedative properties and anticonvulsant action, but with increasing dosage, relief of anxiety appears to be a more prominent effect rather than simple sedation. This relief of anxiety is accompanied by an increased reaction time and definite slowing of learning.

Meprobamate, like its predecessor mephenesin, has muscle-relaxing properties. The origin of this effect (central as opposed to peripheral) has not been established. Undoubtedly, the overall effect is beneficial for the anxious individual, since increased muscle tension always appears to be associated with anxiety.

Adverse reactions and drug interactions. In therapeutic doses meprobamate has a rather limited spectrum of side effects and is a relatively safe drug. However, it has occasionally been associated with the development of aplastic anemia and other hematologic disorders. Allergic reactions of a dermatologic nature have been reported. An unexplained hypotensive effect has been observed primarily in elderly patients.

Acute overdose toxicity from meprobamate is caused by excessive central nervous system depression and results in loss of consciousness, cardiovascular collapse, respiratory depression, and death. The treatment of choice is similar to that for barbiturate overdose, that is, primarily supportive and symptomatic.

The concomitant use of meprobamate with other central nervous system depressants must be carried out with caution. Interaction of meprobamate with them is determined by the duration of use of meprobamate, that is, whether central as well as pharmacodynamic tolerance has been induced. In the acute and subacute situation other sedatives and hypnotics are potentiated by the simultaneous presence of meprobamate. In the chronic, tolerant situation meprobamate could be expected to exhibit cross-tolerance with most of the nonopiate central nervous system depressants, including alcohol.

Uses, preparation, and dosages. Meprobamate is widely used in a great variety of anxiety states and as a daytime sedative or nighttime hypnotic. It is used in combination therapy with other muscle-relaxing medication and has been used in dentistry as an antianxiety agent. Meprobamate has been found to be particularly useful in conditioning the dental patient for the acceptance of a new prosthetic appliance.[1] The dosage in this study was 400 mg four times every 24 hours. Other studies have shown that meprobamate was effective in the management of the apprehensive dental patient with a dose schedule of 400 mg given the night before operative procedures.[2,3] A review of the use of meprobamate in dentistry for children is available to the reader.[4] In view of its wider margin of safety or favorable therapeutic index, it has been suggested that the use of meprobamate may be preferable to that of barbiturates in patients who are considered to be suicidal risks (New Drugs [AMA], 1967). It has also been used to relieve muscle spasm, but the question remaining is whether this effect is primarily attributable to direct muscle relaxation or the sedative effect. Meprobamate has also been used for the control of petit mal epilepsy. It is available in 200 and 400 mg tablets and as a 200 mg/5 ml suspension. The usual adult dose for anxiety is 400 mg every 6 to 8 hours.

Phenaglycodol

The pharmacologic properties and effectiveness of phenaglycodol are similar to those of meprobamate. There have been few reports of significant adverse side effects and neither physical nor psychological dependence has been reported. Drowsiness may occur after large doses.

Phenaglycodol is available in 300 mg capsules and 200 mg tablets. The usual adult dose for mild anxiety is 300 mg every 6 to 8 hours.

The benzodiazepines

The benzodiazepines are among the most widely used drugs in medicine. In 1974 over 80 million prescriptions for these minor tranquilizers were filled in United States retail pharmacies, with 59.3 million filled for diazepam (Valium), 19.5 million for chlordiazepoxide (Librium), and the remainder for flurazepam (Dalmane). The gross dollar yield to the manufacturers, wholesale, for diazepam and chlordiazepoxide was $313 billion in 1974 and represented 81% of the total market for all tranquilizers in the United States.[5] These drugs are also popular for use in hospitalized patients. In 1973, 30% of all medical inpatients in two Boston teaching hospitals received diazepam and 32% received flurazepam.[6]

Chemistry. The benzodiazepines are so called because they are derivatives of the 1,4-benzodiazepine nucleus shown in Fig. 7. Chlordiazepoxide was the first of the deriva-

tives synthesized by chemist Leo H. Sternbach and his associates at Roche Laboratories in 1955. The structures of chlordiazepoxide and the popular diazepam are shown in Fig. 8. Other derivatives that are currently available for use in the United States include oxazepam (Serax), flurazepam (Dalmane), and clorazepate dipotassium (Tranxene). Chlordiazepoxide was shown in 1957 to elicit sedative, hypnotic, and anticonvulsant activity similar to that of meprobamate in animals. Trials in humans have since confirmed this compound to be a clinically useful antianxiety and anticonvulsant agent.

Because of the success of chlordiazepoxide, thousands of other benzodiazepine derivatives were screened for psychopharmacologic activity, as a result of which, diazepam (Valium) was synthesized in 1959 and marketed in 1963. Although having similar actions as chlordiazepoxide, it was shown to be a more potent muscle relaxant and anticonvulsant in animals. Oxazepam (Serax) was found to be a pharmacologically active, hydroxylated and demethylated end product of the metabolism of diazepam and was marketed in 1965. Substitution of a halogen at the ortho position (R^2) in the 5-phenyl ring of the benzodiazepine nucleus (Fig. 7) was shown to enhance

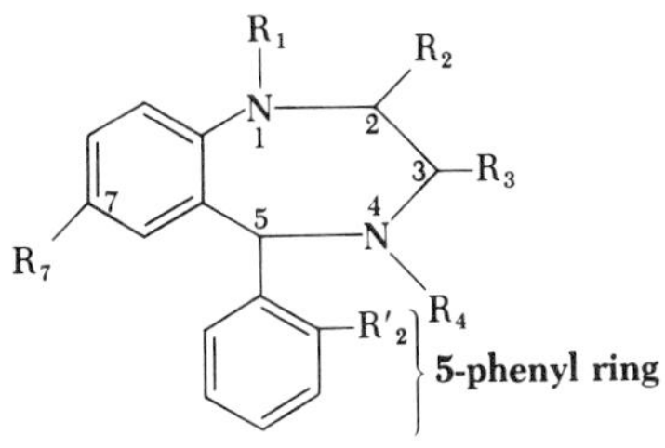

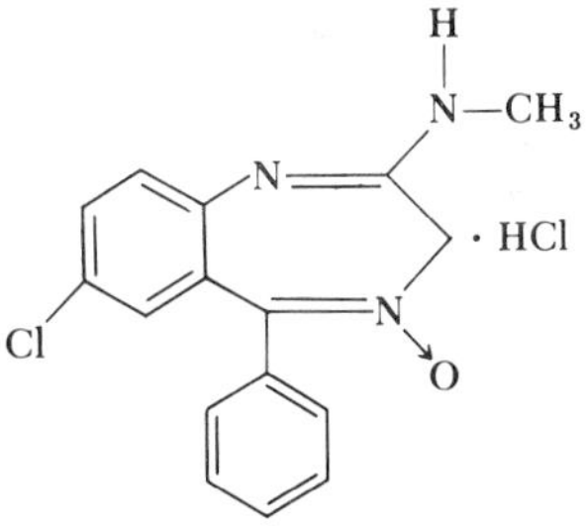

Chlordiazepoxide hydrochloride

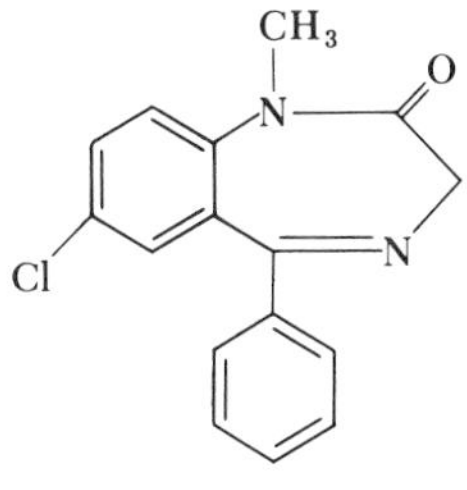

Diazepam

Fig. 8. Chemical structures of chlordiazepoxide and diazepam.

Fig. 7. 1,4-Benzodiazepine nucleus.

the activity of these compounds.[7] Flurazepam (Dalmane) is such a derivative. This drug is used as a hypnotic agent and was marketed in 1970. Clorazepate dipotassium (Tranxene) is the newest member of the benzodiazepines marketed in the United States (1972).

Some benzodiazepine derivatives include a nitro ($-NO_2$) group at position R^7. Nitrazepam (Mogadon) is one such derivative that is a useful hypnotic in most other areas of the world. Finally, the chlorine substitution of oxazepam led to the discovery of lorazepam, which was found to be one of the most potent benzodiazepine derivatives available.[8] Nitrazepam and lorazepam are presently *not available* in the United States.

Body handling. Chlordiazepoxide is available for clinical use as the water-soluble hydrochloride salt. It is well absorbed after oral administration. Parenterally, it is effective after intravenous administration but is absorbed slowly and erratically after intramuscular administration. The oral or intravenous routes should be used to achieve reliable sedative effects. Peak blood concentra-

tions are reached 4 hours after oral dosing, and the biologic half-life varies considerably, that is, between 6 and 30 hours.[9] Biotransformation occurs in the liver, consisting of initial demethylation to form desmethylchlordiazepoxide, oxidative deamination to form demoxepam, and subsequent conjugation with glucuronic acid.[10] Both desmethylchlordiazepoxide and demoxepam are psychopharmacologically active, and repeated dosage of chlordiazepoxide produces cumulative clinical effects because of the accumulation of these two metabolites.

Diazepam is water insoluble and relatively lipid soluble and is administered both orally and parenterally. Absorption is rapid and complete after oral administration, with peak blood levels occurring 2 hours after treatment.[11] Intramuscular absorption is slow and erratic and associated with a high incidence of pain.[12,13] Oral or intravenous routes are used to achieve reliable sedative effects. After a single oral or intravenous dose, diazepam rapidly distributes to all tissues, after which biotransformation occurs slowly, and it has a biologic half-life of 20 to 40 hours. Me-

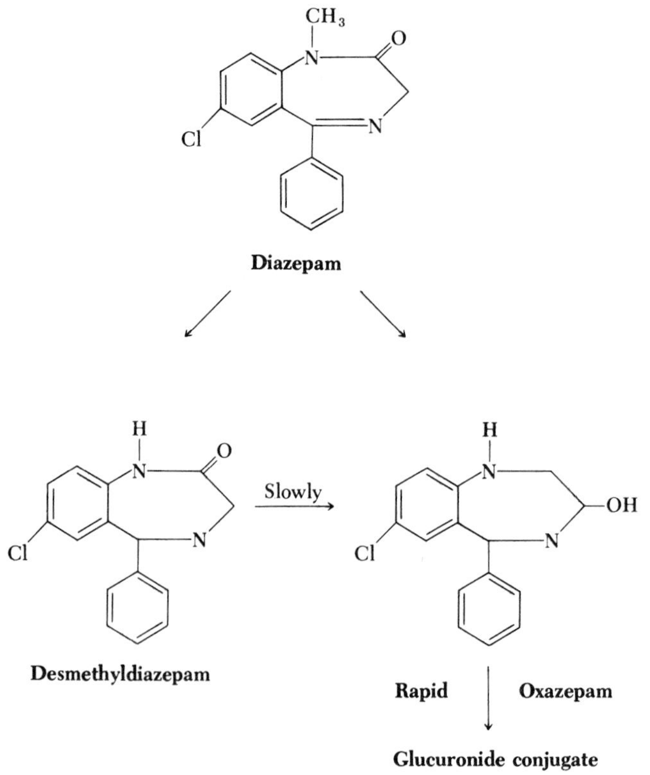

Fig. 9. Biotransformation of diazepam.

tabolism occurs in the liver with the formation of two active metabolites. Desmethyldiazepam is initially formed by removal of the N-l methyl group, whereas the hydroxylation at the number 3 position of diazepam and removal of the N-l methyl group yield oxazepam. The desmethyldiazepam is subsequently biotransformed extremely slowly, but the oxazepam is rapidly glucuronidated and excreted in the urine as the major urinary metabolite of diazepam (Fig. 9). Repeated administration of diazepam leads to accumulation of diazepam and desmethyldiazepam in the blood, and after termination of long-term administration one or both compounds may be detected in the blood for a week or more.[11]

Oxazepam is available only as an oral preparation, and the completeness of oral absorption has not been determined. The biologic half-life of the drug is 3 to 21 hours, with no cumulative effects reported.[14] As mentioned earlier, oxazepam is rapidly metabolized to an inactive glucuronide conjugate with no metabolic intermediates identified to date. Flurazepam is available as a water-soluble dihydrochloride salt for oral administration only. It is rapidly metabolized to a psychopharmacologically active metabolite by removal of the N-l side chain. This metabolite undergoes slow biotransformation and has a biologic half-life of 50 to 100 hours.[15] Since this metabolite can accumulate in the blood, repeated dosage of flurazepam produces cumulative effects as well as residual effects after termination of therapy. Clorazepate may be rapidly hydrolyzed to the N-l demethylated analog of diazepam, desmethyldiazepam.[6] Desmethyldiazepam is slowly biotransformed, and long-lasting and cumulative effects can be anticipated during treatment with clorazepate. Clorazepate is supplied as an oral preparation of the water-soluble dipotassium salt.

Pharmacologic effects. Pharmacologic effects of the benzodiazepines are mediated through the central nervous system. The various derivatives have qualitatively similar actions but vary in potency. These agents affect behavior, have anticonvulsant actions, and elicit relaxation of skeletal musculature.

Effects on behavior have been determined mainly through animal studies and may differ greatly from actual effects in humans. Behavioral effects in animals with appropriate doses of these drugs include a suppression of behavior motivated by punishment, a restoration of behavior suppressed by lack of reward, and an alteration of behavior accompanying stress and frustration. These animal effects are thought to be analogous to their clinical antianxiety effects. At high doses in animals the benzodiazepines will produce ataxia and other symptoms of nonspecific central nervous system depressions, which are considered to be side effects of these agents. These drugs also have the ability to reduce aggression and hostility in animals. In general, clinical effects on behavior by these drugs parallel their effects on animals, that is, anxiety reduction at low doses and drowsiness and other nonspecific central nervous system depression at higher doses. The mechanism of behavioral effects probably involves a selective depression of the limbic system activity at doses that do not depress the rest of the brain. More specifically, these agents probably depress electrical activity arising from the amygdaloid nuclei within the limbic system.

Benzodiazepines, particularly diazepam, have strong anticonvulsant actions in animals and humans. They prevent or arrest generalized seizure activity produced by electric shock or analeptic agents. Recently, diazepam has been shown to be an effective anticonvulsant for the prevention of local anesthetic–induced seizures.[16] The mechanism for anticonvulsant activity of these tranquilizers has not been established but may be similar to that for phenytoin. When an anatomic seizure focus exists, the benzodiazepines prevent propagation of seizures in surrounding tissue but have little effect on discharges at the focus itself. Diazepam and phenytoin have similar molecular conformation and might interact with similar receptor sites. Diazepam may be the drug of choice for protection against lidocaine-induced convulsions. DeJong and Heavner[16] reported that 0.25 mg/kg diazepam given intramuscularly increased the tolerance to intravenously administered lidocaine by two thirds in nonhuman primates and that 0.1 mg/kg given intravenously completely arrested lidocaine convulsions in these same species.

Chlordiazepoxide and diazepam can produce relaxation of skeletal musculature. Although the mechanism of this effect is unknown, it does occur within the central nervous system. Animal studies have shown that muscular relaxation by these drugs appears to require an intact spinal cord.[17] There probably is more than one site of action within the central nervous system, however, since diazepam can depress motor nerve and muscle function in healthy persons[18] and relax spastic musculature in patients with spinal cord transection.[19]

Therapeutic doses of benzodiazepines have no adverse effect on the circulation and respiration, and very large doses of diazepam produce only minor degrees of cardiovascular and respiratory depression.[20] Transient episodes of bradycardia, hypotension, or apnea have occurred occasionally after rapid intravenous injection of diazepam. A recent study suggested that intravenously administered diazepam can dilate coronary blood vessels and enhance coronary blood flow.[21]

Use in general medicine. The benzodiazepines are useful in treating anxiety, insomnia, certain seizures, alcohol withdrawal, and some neuromuscular diseases. They also enjoy selected uses in anesthesia and surgery.

Neurotic anxiety is the most common indication for the use of benzodiazepines in general medicine. Anxiety is a major psychoneurotic disorder and describes a psychophysiologic response resembling fear. Manifestations of anxiety have been discussed earlier. The clinical efficacy of the benzodiazepines in treating neurotic anxiety is difficult to demonstrate. Most well-controlled clinical trials have compared the antianxiety effect of the benzodiazepines with those of placebo, barbiturates, and meprobamate. Benzodiazepines were definitely more effective than placebo in most studies and also more effective than barbiturates in that they produced less drowsiness with less frequency. It is questionable, however, whether these agents are superior to meprobamate.

If insomnia is a manifestation of anxiety, sleep will usually improve when chlordiazepoxide or diazepam is administered at bedtime with an antianxiety drug. Flurazepam is specifically indicated as a hypnotic, and 30 mg of the drug improves insomnia as effectively as the barbiturate hypnotics.[6] The benzodiazepines have two distinct advantages over the barbiturates as hypnotic agents. First, true addiction is rare, and second, the danger of serious poisoning after intentional overdosage is less.

Diazepam is effective when given intravenously in the treatment of grand mal, petit mal, and psychomotor and myoclonic seizures when intractable, repetitive seizures require parenteral therapy. The drug is usually administered through a large peripheral vein at 5 to 10 mg/min until seizure activity is controlled or until a total dose of approximately 0.5 mg/kg is reached. Orally administered diazepam is of little value as a prophylactic or maintenance anticonvulsant in the preceding seizure disorders.

Chlordiazepoxide has become a mainstay in the treatment for the alcohol-withdrawal syndrome.[22] Diazepam and oxazepam appear to be equally effective, but oxazepam cannot be given parenterally. In severe mainfestations of withdrawal, 50 to 100 mg chlordiazepoxide or 5 to 20 mg diazepam is given orally and repeated hourly until adequate sedation is achieved. In the early stages of withdrawal intravenous therapy is preferable.

Benzodiazepines are used to control muscle spasticity that accompanies cerebral palsy, multiple sclerosis, parkinsonism, and cerebrovascular accidents. Diazepam is specifically utilized for relief of pain and spasm caused by back strain and disk lesions. Studies have suggested that diazepam is superior to other muscle relaxants such as methocarbamol, carisoprodol, and chlormezanone in this regard.[6]

Benzodiazepines enjoy a variety of uses in anesthesia and surgery. As premedicant sedatives administered before surgical procedures using general anesthesia, diazepam (10 mg orally) and chlordiazepoxide (100 mg orally) have been shown to be effective. Diazepam given intravenously at a dose of 10 to 20 mg effectively produces sedation and anterograde amnesia before cardioversion procedures. Similar doses of diazepam are also used to facilitate gastroscopy, sigmoidoscopy, and cystoscopy. Finally, parenterally administered diazepam and chlordiazepoxide are suitable adjuncts to local and systemic analgesics given during labor.

Dental use. In dentistry the benzodiazepines, particularly diazepam, have been employed for their ability to reduce preoperative tension and anxiety. Also, diazepam is popular as an intravenously administered sedative and amnesiac during dental procedures (Chapter 26). A double-blind trial of orally administered diazepam has shown the drug to be more effective than placebo in allaying apprehension in patients undergoing restorative procedures.[23] This study also concluded that an initial treatment with the assistance of diazepam will increase the likelihood of subsequent successful treatment without it. The dose of diazepam used in this study was one 5 mg tablet on retiring, one tablet on arising, and one tablet 2 hours before the dental appointment. Another study reported the use of diazepam in children undergoing ear, nose, or throat surgery.[24] A dose of 0.2 mg/kg was orally administered to 101 children 2 to 9 years of age 2 hours before general anesthesia. The results showed 47 children asleep after 2 hours, 35 drowsy or calm, 7 apprehensive, 10 tearful, and 2 noisy. A combination of diazepam (0.2 to 0.3 mg/lb) and scopolamine (0.25 mg/lb) has been used successfully as an oral premedication sedative in children who fear injections.[25] Chlordiazepoxide was found to be an effective premedicant for 2 adult patients who underwent extensive restorative dental procedures.[26] During the course of the treatment, 10 mg capsules were prescribed four times every 24 hours.

Clorazepate dipotassium is a potentially good candidate for use as a sedative in dentistry. Two recent studies showed the drug to be superior to diazepam in the management of chronic anxiety. In the first study a dose of 22.5 to 37.5 mg/24 hr gave excellent overall responses in 25 out of 32 adult patients, whereas diazepam produced excellent responses in only 2 out of 31 patients.[27] In the second study clorazepate produced better effects than diazepam in the management of anxiety and the feeling of muscular tension.[28] A third study has confirmed that a long-term dose of 22.5 to 45 mg/24 hr clorazepate was as effective in relieving anxiety as a 15 to 30 mg/24 hr dose of diazepam.[29]

Adverse effects. The most common side effect attributed to benzodiazepines is central nervous sytem depression manifested as fatigue, drowsiness, muscle weakness, and ataxia. This side effect is more likely to occur in elderly persons and less likely to occur in heavy cigarette smokers.[30] Diazepam causes local pain in many patients receiving it intravenously or intramuscularly. Phlebitis also results in a few patients after intravenous diazepam administration. One study reported an incidence of phlebitis of 3.5% in patients receiving the drug by the intravenous route.[31] Pain on injection may be caused by precipitated particles of drug or by the propylene glycol vehicle. Diazepam also has been shown to decrease salivary secretions in humans—a response that can be considered a side effect. Basal and stimulated salivary secretion was inhibited 30 minutes after the oral administration of 10 mg diazepam and lasted up to 4 hours.[31]

The benzodiazepines can be abused, and they produce physiologic addiction if large doses are taken over a long period of time. Their abuse and addiction potential is less, however, than that of the other sedative-hypnotic agents such as barbiturates, glutethimide, methaqualone, and meprobamate. One of the great advantages of benzodiazepines over the barbiturates is their wide range of "safe" dosage. Overdose poisoning with these drugs has been rare and appears to be difficult to achieve. Excessively large doses have to be ingested to achieve respiratory and central vasomotor depression.

Like all other antianxiety agents, benzodiazepines interact in additive fashion with other central nervous system depressants, notably alcohol, barbiturates, and phenothiazines. As pointed out before, prolonged intake of large doses of chlordiazepoxide will result in central tolerance. There exists cross-tolerance between chlordiazepoxide and other central nervous system depressants. This is believed to be the underlying mechanism for the fact that chlordiazepoxide can substitute for ethyl alcohol, as indicated by its ability to relieve the symptoms of delirium tremens precipitated by acute alcohol withdrawal.

Preparations and dosage. Chlordiazepoxide hydrochloride (Librium) is supplied as capsules (5, 10, and 25 mg) and tablets (5, 10, and 25 mg). A parenteral solution is also available. The usual oral dose for mild to moderate anxiety is 5 to 10 mg every 6 to 8 hours. Diazepam (Valium) is supplied as 2, 5, and 10 mg tablets and as an injectable preparation. The usual oral dose for the symptomatic relief of tension and anxiety states is 2 to 10 mg, two to four times every 24 hours. Oxazepam (Serax) is supplied as 10, 15, and 30 mg capsules and 15 mg tablets. The usual dose to treat mild to moderate anxiety is 10 to 15 mg three or four times every 24 hours. Flurazepam hydrochloride (Dalmane) is available in 15 and 30 mg capsules. The usual hypnotic dose is 30 mg before retiring. Clorazepate dipotassium (Tranxene) is supplied as 3.75, 7.5, and 15 mg capsules and as a 22.5 mg tablet. The usual dose to treat mild to moderate anxiety is 30 mg/24 hr in divided doses.

The diphenylmethanes

The commonly used compounds of the diphenylmethane group are hydroxyzine (Atarax), benactyzine (Deprol), buclizine (Softran), and diphenhydramine (Benadryl). These compounds are clearly of minor effectiveness as antianxiety drugs, and their limited use does not justify extensive discussion here. Pharmacologically, these drugs are primarily antispasmodics and antihistamines. Hydroxyzine has had some use in dental practice and is discussed as a representative of the group.

Hydroxyzine (Atarax, Vistaril) has sedative, antihistaminic, antispasmodic, and antiemetic actions. It has been used clinically as a minor tranquilizer and in the management of anxiety-related allergies. It has been used in the treatment or prevention of nausea and vomiting, excluding that of pregnancy. Hydroxyzine has been used to allay anxiety, control nausea and vomiting, and reduce the narcotic requirement in preoperative and postoperative sedation. Since the intravenous route is no longer recommended, hydroxyzine should only be used orally or intramuscularly for preoperative sedation. The effect of therapy with hydroxyzine in controlling the behavior of 76 apprehensive and fearful pedodontic patients has been studied. The administration of 50 mg hydroxyzine 1 hour prior to the scheduled appointment was found to reduce significantly the behavioral difficulties exhibited by these patients.[32]

The most common side effect of hydroxyzine is drowsiness. Its overall toxicity appears to be low, and blood dyscrasias and adverse effects on the liver have not been reported.

Neither psychological nor physical dependence has been attributed to hydroxyzine. However, caution should be exerted in prolonged administration to patients believed to be particularly susceptible to drug dependence. Fetal abnormalities have been caused by hydroxyzine in experimental animals, and clinical data are inadequate to establish that the drug is safe for humans during pregnancy. Consequently, its use during pregnancy is contraindicated. Hydroxyzine potentiates the effect of phenothiazines, opiates, barbiturates, and other central nervous system depressants.

Hydroxyzine hydrochloride is available in 10, 25, 50, and 100 mg tablets and also in 10 mg/5 ml syrup and in parenteral solutions. Hydroxyzine pamoate is available in 25, 50, and 100 mg capsules and as a 25 mg/5 ml oral suspension. The usual adult oral dose of hydroxyzine for mild to moderate anxiety must be individualized and may vary from 25 to 100 mg every 6 to 8 hours.

CENTRALLY ACTING MUSCLE RELAXANTS

Drugs classified as centrally acting muscle relaxants exert effects on the central nervous system to cause skeletal muscle relaxation. A distinction between these agents and the curare-like neuromuscular blocking agents should be made. Neuromuscular blocking agents exert their effects on peripheral neuromuscular junctions, whereas the centrally acting agents depress spinal polysynaptic reflexes in the central nervous system. This group of drugs does not affect the neuromuscular junctions, the motor cortex, or the reticular formation like other drugs known to alter skeletal muscle function.

The list of indications for these drugs is long and includes skeletal muscle disorders such as muscle spasms, tetanus, sprains, spasms accompanying bursitis, slipped disk, multiple sclerosis, brain tumor, cerebrovascular accidents, and cerebral palsy. A sedative effect is exhibited to some degree by all the central muscle relaxants. Clinical testing indicates that for some of these drugs, sedative effects may predominate over selective muscle relaxant activity. In normal animals these agents can cause a decrease in skeletal muscle tone and in large doses cause transient flaccid paralysis and death from respiratory depression.

The side effects associated with these drugs are drowsiness, dizziness, headache, blurred vision, weakness, and ataxia. Nausea and vomiting are also observed after large oral doses.

Centrally acting muscle relaxants, when administered intravenously, have shown usefulness in treating acute muscle spasms and in producing muscle relaxation for certain orthopedic procedures. Orally administered muscle relaxants do not produce the flaccidity obtainable in humans with intravenous ad-

Table 8-1. Centrally acting skeletal muscle relaxants

Generic name	Trade name	Oral dose (mg 24 hr)	NAS–NRC evaluation*
Carisoprodol	Rela, Soma	1000-1400	Possibly effective
Chlormezanone	Trancopal	300-400	No rating
Chlorphenesin	Maolate	1600-2400	No rating
Chlorzoxazone	Paraflex	1500-3000	Possibly effective
Mephenesin	Tolserol	3000-12,000	Possibly effective
Metaxalone	Skelaxin	2400-3200	Ineffective
Methocarbamol	Robaxin	4000-9000	Possibly effective
Orphenadrine	Disipal	150-300	Possibly effective
Styramate	Sinaxar	600-1200	No rating

*From National Academy of Sciences–National Research Council: Drug efficacy study, Washington, D.C., 1969, National Academy of Sciences.

ministration, and this is thought not to occur with clinically used oral doses. Thus, until definitive studies show otherwise, it is reasonable to ascribe the beneficial effects of these drugs to their sedative actions.

A recent review of these drugs by the National Academy of Sciences–National Research Council (NAS–NRC) led to a rating of ineffective, effective, or possibly effective for each agent in treating skeletal muscle disorders.[33] This classification is adequate until further documentation is made for effectiveness. Table 8-1 provides this information on the individual products.

In conclusion, none of these drugs is effective in reducing spasticity in neurologic disease or spinal cord injury, and their effectiveness in reducing muscle spasms under other conditions after oral dosage is questionable. Their limited effectiveness is probably a result of sedation or placebo effects.

REFERENCES

1. Wilson, H. D., and Parker, E. B.: Tranquilizing drugs as an aid to patient acceptance of dental prostheses, Dent. Surv. **34:**171-174, 1958.
2. Lefkowitz, W.: Use of meprobamate before operative procedures: a preliminary report, Ohio Dent. J. **32:**27-30, 1958.
3. Lund, L., and Anholm, J. M.: Clinical observations on the use of meprobamate in dental procedures, Oral Surg. **10:**1281-1286, 1957.
4. Kopel, H. M.: The use of ataraxics in dentistry for children, J. Dent. Child. **26:**14-24, 1959.
5. Cant, G.: Valiumania, N.Y. Times Magazine, Feb. 1, 1967.
6. Greenblatt, D. J., and Shader, R. I.: Drug therapy —benzodiazepines, N. Engl. J. Med. **291:**1011-1015, 1974.
7. Sternback, L. H., Randal, L. O., Banziger, R., and Lehr, H.: Structure activity relationships of the 1,4-benzodiazepine series. In Burger A., editor: Drugs affecting the central nervous system, New York, 1968, Marcel Dekker, Inc., Vol. 2.
8. Gluckman, M. L.: Pharmacology of 7-chloro-5-(o-chlorophenyl)-1,3-dihydro-3-hydroxy-2H-1,4-benzodiazepine-2-one (lorazepam: Wy 4036), Arzneim. Forsch. **21:**1049-1055, 1971.
9. Schwarts, M. A., Postma, E., and Gaut, Z.: Biological half-life of chlordiazepoxide and its metabolite, demoxepam, in man, J. Pharm. Sci. **60:**1500-1503, 1971.
10. Schwarts, M. A., and Postma, E.: Metabolic N-demethylation of chlordiazepoxide, J. Pharm. Sci. **55:**1358-1362, 1966.
11. Kaplan, S. A., Jack, M. L., and Alexander, K.: Pharmacokinetic profile of diazepam in man following single intravenous and oral and chronic oral administrations, J. Pharm. Sci. **62:**1789-1796, 1973.
12. Baird, E. S., and Hailey, D. M.: Plasma levels of diazepam and its major metabolite following intramuscular administration, Br. J. Anaesth. **45:**546-548, 1972.
13. Assaf, R. A. E., Dundee, J. W., and Gamble, J. A. S.: The influence of the route of administration on the clinical action of diazepam, Anaesthesia **30:**152-158, 1975.
14. Knowles, J. A., and Ruelius, H. W.: Absorption and excretion of oxazepam in humans: determination of the drug by gas-liquid chromatography with electron capture detection, Arzneim. Forsch. **22:**687-692, 1972.
15. Kaplan, S. A., DeSilva, J. A. F., and Jack, M. L.: Blood level profile in man following chronic oral administration of flurazepam hydrochloride, J. Pharm. Sci. **62:**1932-1935, 1973.
16. deJong, R. H., and Heavner, D. V. M.: Diazepam prevents and aborts lidocaine convulsions in monkeys, Anesthesiology **41:**226-230, 1974.
17. Przybyla, A. C., and Wang, S. C.: Locus of central depressant action of diazepam, J. Pharmacol. Exp. Ther. **163:**439-447, 1968.
18. Hopf, H. C., and Billman, F.: The effect of diazepam on motor nerves and skeletal muscle, Z. Neurol. **204:**255-262, 1973.
19. Cook, J. B., and Nathan, P. W.: On the site of action of diazepam in spasticity in man, J. Neurol. Sci. **5:**33-37, 1967.
20. Rao, S., Sherbaniuk, R. W., and Prasad, K.: Cardiopulmonary effects of diazepam, Clin. Pharmacol. Ther. **14:**182-189, 1973.

21. Ikram, H., Rubin, A. P., and Jewkes, R. F.: Effect of diazepam on mycoardial blood flow of patients with and without coronary artery diasease, Br. Heart J. **35:**626-630, 1973.

22. Greenblatt, D. J., and Greenblatt, M.: Which drug for alcohol withdrawal? J. Clin. Pharmacol. **12:**429-431, 1972.

23. Baird, E. S., and Curson, I.: Orally administered diazepam in conservative dentistry: a double blind trial, Br. Dent. J. **128:**25-27, 1970.

24. Boyd, J. D., and Manford, M. L. M.: Premedication in children, Br. J. Anaesth. **45:**501-506, 1973.

25. Root, B., and Loveland, J. P.: Pediatric premedication with diazepam or hydroxyzine: oral versus intramuscular route, Anesth. Analg. **52:**717-723, 1973.

26. Ahlin, J. H., and Steinberg, A. I.: Chlordiazepoxide HCl (Librium) as a premedicant for dental patients: a preliminary report, J. Dent. Med. **24:**39-41, 1969.

27. Feurst, S. I.: Clorazepate dipotassium, diazepam and placebo in chronic anxiety, Curr. Ther. Res. **15:**449-459, 1973.

28. Norman, B.: Clinical and experimental comparison of diazepam, clorazepate and placebo, Psychopharmacologia **40:**279-284, 1975.

29. Ricca, J. J.: Clorazepate dipotassium in anxiety: a clinical trial with diazepam and placebo controls, J. Clin. Pharmacol. **12:**286-290, 1972.

30. Boston Collaborative Drug Surveillance Program: Clinical depression of the central nervous system due to diazepam and chlordiazepoxide in relation to cigarette smoking and age, N. Engl. J. Med. **288:**277-280, 1973.

31. Steiner, J. E., Birnbaum, D., Karmelli, F., and Cohen, S.: Effect of diazepam on human salivary secretion, Digestion **3:**262-268, 1970.

32. Lang, L. L.: An elevation of the efficacy of hydroxyzine (Atarax, Vistaril) in controlling the behavior of child patients, J. Dent. Child. **32:**253-258, 1965.

33. National Academy of Sciences–National Research Council: Drug efficacy study, Washington, D.C., 1969, National Academy of Sciences.

9

Nonnarcotic analgesics

SAM. V. HOLROYD
J. MAX GOODSON

Pain and dentistry have always been uniquely related. It is often pain that brings the patient to the dentist. Conversely, fear of pain can be the factor that keeps the patient from seeking dental care at the appropriate time. Thus the dentist often works on the inflamed, hypersensitive tissues of a patient who suffers from mental fatigue after long endurance of pain.

> . . . Pain is perfect misery, the worst of evils, and excessive, overturns all patience.
>
> JOHN MILTON, *Paradise Lost*

Skillful use of drugs for the control of pain is therefore of major importance to the dentist and the patient.

PAIN AND ANALGESIC THERAPY

The sensation of pain is the means by which the body is made urgently aware of the presence of tissue damage.[1] For the person experiencing pain, it represents a protective reflex for self-preservation. Just as the hand is quickly removed from a hot object, a painful dental abscess brings the subject to seek professional assistance for its resolution. For the dentist, pain represents a diagnostic symptom of underlying pathology. Although the relief of pain is an immediate objective, only treatment of the underlying cause is its ultimate resolution.

The treatment of pain differs from other types of therapy in the major contribution of an emotional component. Although individuals are surprisingly uniform in their *percep-*

tion of pain, they differ greatly in their *reaction* to it.[2] Predisposition toward a greater reaction to pain has been associated with emotional instability, fatigue, youth, women, fear, and apprehension.[3] As a result, analgesic therapy must be selected for the individual. A level of discomfort that may not require drug treatment in one individual may require extreme therapy in another. Although approximately 15% of patients undergoing routine exodontia require no postoperative medication,[4,5] it is commonly reported that even the strongest analgesics will not completely control postoperative extraction pain in some individuals. For the same reason the effectiveness of placebo treatment of dental pain cannot be ignored.[6] As much as 80% of the effectiveness of any analgesic drug may be attributed to its placebo effect.[7] Thus, to obtain maximum analgesic effectiveness, the practitioner should relate confidence in the drug. The confidence that the patient has in his dentist will then be conveyed to the analgesic.

Pharmacologic relief from pain is accomplished by the use of *anesthetics*, which eliminate all modalities of sensibility, or by *analgesics*, which eliminate or reduce specifically only pain sensations. In this section and the next the properties of analgesic drugs and their use in dental therapy will be considered.

GENERAL CHARACTERISTICS OF NONNARCOTIC ANALGESICS

Nonnarcotic analgesics relieve pain without altering consciousness. Although they are ineffective for severe discomfort, most pain of dental origin can be controlled by these drugs. This is particularly important because the nonnarcotic analgesics are safer than

□ The opinions or assertions contained herein are the private ones of the writers and are not to be construed as official or as reflecting the views of the Navy Department or the naval service at large.

narcotics, produce fewer side effects, and are not addicting.

A principal difference between nonnarcotic and narcotic analgesics is their site of action. Nonnarcotic analgesics act principally at the peripheral nerve endings, whereas the action of narcotic analgesics is within the central nervous system.[8] Nonnarcotic analgesics inhibit the synthesis of prostaglandins that occurs at sites of tissue inflammation.[9] Since the prostaglandins sensitize pain receptors to endogenous pain producing substances such as bradykinin, a reduction in prostaglandin tissue levels is accompanied by a decrease in pain perception.

As a result of the mechanism by which this group of drugs acts, two corollaries useful in clinical therapy emerge. First, nonnarcotic analgesics are most effective when given *before* prostaglandin synthesis due to inflammation that has occurred. Second, these analgesics are never *completely* effective because they do not affect the formation of the primary pain mediators such as bradykinin. Since dental disease is usually accompanied by inflammation, the common use of these drugs in dental therapy is well justified.

Nonnarcotic analgesics have the advantage that long-term use does not produce addiction or tolerance. Furthermore, the toxicity of these agents is much lower than that of the narcotic analgesics. In general, however, nonnarcotic analgesics are only effective in the treatment of mild to moderate pain. The use of narcotic analgesics is necessary to relieve severe pain of dental origin. Since it is clear that narcotic and nonnarcotic analgesics act at completely different sites by totally different mechanisms, their combination in analgesic therapy may produce more complete relief.

Nonnarcotic analgesics are all organic acids that are excreted by the kidney either unchanged or after partial biotransformation. The most common undesirable side effect of many of these drugs is gastric upset and bleeding, and long-term use in high doses can produce kidney damage.

The principal pharmacologic actions of therapeutic utility exhibited to a greater or lesser degree by agents of this drug group include (1) analgesia, (2) antipyresis, and (3) anti-inflammatory action.

THE SALICYLATES

Extracts of willow bark containing the bitter glycoside salicin have been used since antiquity to reduce fever. The recognition and medical use of this natural product for its analgesic properties occurred in 1763.[10] After the isolation and identification of the active component, salicylic acid, acetylsalicylic acid (aspirin) was introduced into medical therapy in 1899. Since that time, numerous agents have been introduced with similar properties, yet none has achieved the widespread general use of aspirin. Salicylates other than aspirin are either too toxic for internal use (salicylic acid and methyl salicylate) or less effective than aspirin (sodium salicylate and salicylamide). The chemical structure of aspirin is as follows:

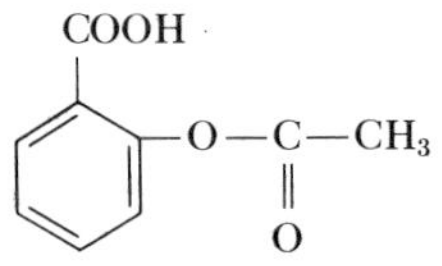

Aspirin

Therapeutically useful salicylates and their importance are as follows:

Salicylic acid—parent compound, toxic internally, topical fungicide, keratolytic agent

Sodium salicylate—internal use as an analgesic, less effective than aspirin

Methyl salicylate (oil of wintergreen)—external use as a counterirritant, flavoring in cooking

Salicylamide—internal use as an analgesic, less effective than aspirin, possibly less gastrointestinal irritation

Acetylsalicylic acid—widespread use as an analgesic, antipyretic, and antirheumatic

The pharmacologic effects of the salicylates are qualitatively similar. Since aspirin is probably the most widely employed drug in medical and dental practice, it will be discussed as being representative of the salicylates.

Acetylsalicylic acid (aspirin)

Pharmacologic effects and mechanism of action. A common mechanism by which aspirin and other nonsteroidal anti-inflammatory drugs may exert their action has been elucidated. The observations that have led to clarification of the mechanism of pharmacologic action of this group of drugs has resulted from a clearer definition of the role of the prostaglandins in the inflammatory response. Prostaglandins are lipids that are synthesized locally by inflammatory stimuli and exert biologic activity at the site of their production. The precursors for prostaglandin synthesis are the essential fatty acids such as arachidonic acid, which are found in all cell membranes in the phospholipid lecithin. The inflammatory stimulus activates or releases a phospholipase, which cleaves the essential fatty acid from membrane lecithin, thereby making it available for prostaglandin synthesis by the membrane-bound enzyme complex, prostaglandin synthetase. Aspirin-like drugs inhibit the prostaglandin synthetase reaction. This sequence of events is illustrated below.

The *analgesic* action of aspirin-like drugs is explained by synergism between prostaglandins and pain-producing substances such as bradykinin that are produced or released locally by the inflammatory process. In the presence of prostaglandin, which by itself is not a pain-producing substance, a subthreshold concentration of bradykinin becomes painful. Thus the inhibition of prostaglandin synthesis by aspirin-like drugs leads to analgesia by decreasing the sensitivity of pain fibers to the presence of pain-producing substances.

The *antipyretic* action of aspirin-like drugs results from inhibition of prostaglandin synthesis in the hypothalamus. Hypothalamic prostaglandin synthesis is caused by elevated blood levels of leukocyte pyrogens induced by inflammation. Increased hypothalamic prostaglandin levels produce an increased body temperature. Therefore the inhibition of hypothalamic prostaglandin synthesis results in a return to more normal body temperature, even though infection and pyrogens may still be present. Although aspirin-like drugs may reduce an elevated temperature, they have no effect on normal body temperature.

The *anti-inflammatory* effects of aspirin-like drugs are also derived from their ability to inhibit prostaglandin synthesis. The prostaglandins are potent vasodilator agents that also increase capillary permeability. Therefore aspirin therapy will lead to decreased redness and swelling of the inflamed area. Patients with rheumatic fever and other kinds of arthritis are often given large doses of aspirin (5 to 8 Gm/24 hr) to provide symptomatic relief of joint pain associated with these inflammatory diseases.

It is undoubtedly an oversimplification to attribute all effects of aspirin-like drugs to their ability to inhibit prostaglandin synthesis. As more information is obtained on their biochemical effects, subtle pharmacologic differences that are seen between the various agents will be more accurately defined. However, all drugs considered in this chapter possess the ability to inhibit prostaglandin synthesis, a property that offers an explanation for their principal actions.

The anti-inflammatory effect of aspirin-like drugs is different from that of the anti-inflammatory steroids. The steroids apparently act either to reduce local production of lymphocyte-derived products, the lymphokines, or to decrease release of lysosomal enzymes from polymorphonuclear leukocytes. In general, the anti-inflammatory activity of aspirin is weaker than that of the steroids, but it is associated with fewer undesirable side effects.

Aspirin has been used in therapy for certain conditions, causing several effects that are poorly understood, including the following[11]:

1. *Antidiabetic effect.* Aspirin increases peripheral utilization of glucose and reduces blood glucose levels in diabetics.

2. *Thyroid-stimulating effect.* Long-term aspirin consumption will produce an elevated free thryoid hormone level in the blood, apparently by competitive displacement of the thyroid hormones from their blood protein binding sites.

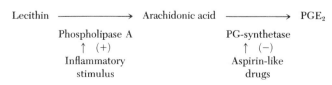

3. *Uricosuric effect.* Large doses of aspirin (over 5 Gm/24 hr) increase uric acid secretion and decrease plasma urate concentration. However, even small doses of aspirin will annul the uricosuric effect of agents such as probenecid that are used to treat gout. Aspirin therefore should not be given to patients being treated for gout.

4. *Antithrombotic effect.* At usual therapeutic doses aspirin will decrease blood platelet adhesiveness and prolong bleeding time. Even with normal patients this effect will last from 4 to 7 days after taking one or two aspirin tablets. The therapeutic utility of this effect for the prophylaxis of patients concerned with coronary or cerebral thrombosis is being actively investigated.

Adverse effects. Although aspirin is an extremely safe drug, troublesome and sometimes serious and fatal reactions occur. The most frequently observed adverse effect is gastrointestinal upset, which can generally be avoided if aspirin is taken with food or with a full glass of milk or water. Gastrointestinal discomfort may be limited to simple dyspepsia ("heartburn"), nausea, and vomiting or may include gastrointestinal bleeding. For some time the adverse gastrointestinal effects of aspirin were considered to be strictly the result of direct irritation of the gastric mucosa. However, since intravenously administered salicylates cause similar gastrointestinal problems, a systemic effect is apparently operative.[12]

The administration of aspirin causes a degree of increased gastric bleeding tendency in almost all individuals. Salicylate-induced gastric bleeding is painless and in most cases does not significantly affect the patient's health. However, in patients with upper gastrointestinal tract disease such as ulcers, gastritis, or hiatus hernia, it is wise to avoid aspirin altogether. Conditions that predispose to nausea, vomiting, dyspepsia, or gastric ulceration should receive careful consideration before aspirin is prescribed. In the amounts present in most buffered aspirin preparations, the buffering agent does not produce a meaningful decrease in gastric acidity,[13] or can it be relied on to reduce gastrointestinal upset.[14] Timed-release and enteric-coated aspirin offer no specific benefits and can contribute to erratic absorption.[13,15] The gastric erosive effects of aspirin are considerably lessened when taken with

plenty of water.[16] For the majority of patients aspirin is unlikely to have injurious gastric effects to the extent that its use would be contraindicated.

A less frequently observed untoward effect of aspirin therapy, but one with a more dangerous potentiality, is that of allergy. Many individuals, perhaps as many as 2 per 1000,[17] are allergic to salicylates. Allergic reactions to aspirin are frequently serious, and deaths have occurred. This reaction may be characterized by asthmatic symptoms, urticaria, angioneurotic edema, and anaphylactic shock. Many patients who exhibit allergic reactions to aspirin have a history of allergic disease, especially asthma. The dentist should therefore observe caution in prescribing aspirin for patients with asthma and should ensure that a patient's medical history does not include indication of allergic reaction to salicylates. In avoiding aspirin, the dentist should be aware that most multiple-entity analgesic preparations include aspirin or other salicylates.

When the toxic blood level for salicylate is exceeded, either by cumulation or by overdose, a wide variety of signs and symptoms ensue. A mild toxic reaction is termed *salicylism* and is characterized by tinnitus, headache, nausea, vomiting, dizziness, and dimness of vision. In more severe cases of salicylism, psychological, circulatory, and respiratory changes may occur. The symptoms of salicylism usually disappear when the drug is withdrawn.

If the blood level of salicylate is sufficiently high, the individual proceeds quickly through the signs and symptoms of salicylism and is faced with a serious toxic crisis. A concise and excellent description of the sequence of events in serious salicylate poisoning has been presented by Koch-Weser.[18] Briefly, this is the sequence: Hyperventilation causes a loss of blood carbon dioxide, with a consequent increase in blood pH. The renal excretion of bicarbonate, sodium, and potassium in an attempt to bring pH back toward normal (compensatory alkalosis) decreases the buffering capacity of the extracellular fluid. The system is then predisposed to respiratory and metabolic acidosis, which results from (1) depression of the respiratory center (carbon dioxide accumulation); (2) renal impairment from dehydration and hypotension (inorganic and metabolic acids ac-

Table 9-1. Poisonings by analgesics in the United States (1965 and 1967)

Drug	Fatalities 1965[19]		Fatalities 1967[20]	
	Accidental	Suicide	Accidental	Suicide
Aspirin and salicylates	175	80	153	87
Morphine and derivatives	69	6	176	6
Other analgesics and soporific drugs	345	608	744	716

cumulate); and (3) impaired carbohydrate metabolism which increases the production of metabolic acids, which the kidney, depressed by dehydration and hypotension, cannot adequately excrete. Severe acidosis and electrolyte imbalance place the situation in extremis and are usually the causes of death.

These emergency situations generally occur as accidental poisonings in children, suicide attempts in adults, and therapeutically administered overdose in infants, children, and severely debilitated adults. These reactions usually involve aspirin, but methyl salicylate liquid, which is commonly found in household flavorings, is often the agent in accidental poisonings in children. Fatalities resulting from the accidental and intentional overdose of analgesics for 1965 and 1967, as reported to the National Center for Health Statistics, are presented in Table 9-1.

It is not realistic to believe that the statistics presented in Table 9-1 are complete, or that they reflect fatalities from therapeutically administered overdose. However, they do illustrate the dangerous potential in salicylate poisoning. The lethal adult dose of aspirin is between 10 and 30 Gm (30 to 100 of the 5-grain tablets).

The young child is highly susceptible to salicylate poisoning. An important clinical consideration in aspirin use is the fact that children, particularly debilitated children or those under 3 years of age, are highly susceptible to "therapeutic overdose." Craig and co-workers have stated that "in the preschool child more aspirin deaths are caused by faulty therapeutics than by accident."[21] They state that the child who is likely to be given aspirin is also more likely to have a less than desirable fluid intake and may be constipated, both of which conditions encourage the accumulation of salicylate.[21] When the dentist prescribes aspirin for a

child, he should ensure that (1) the dosage is accurately determined, (2) good fluid intake is maintained, and (3) the parent is cognizant of the dangers of salicylate poisoning. The latter is of special importance because many parents consider aspirin to be almost completely innocuous.

The treatment of severe toxic reactions to salicylate requires immediate hospitalization and the use of intravenous fluids to correct acidosis and electrolyte imbalance. Since the degree of the severity of the reaction may be difficult to assess early, one should overestimate rather than underestimate the potential for severity. The responsibility of the dentist is to (1) be aware of the toxic potentiality of salicylates, particularly in regard to young patients, (2) counsel parents whose children are taking salicylates, (3) recognize a toxic reaction to salicylate early, (4) induce emesis, and (5) obtain immediate medical treatment, particularly in regard to instituting intravenous therapy.

Although hypoprothrombinemia occurs as a result of salicylate overdose, its importance is secondary to acidosis and electrolyte imbalance. However, hypoprothrombinemia can result from doses well below the toxic level, particularly after long-term use. Aspirin is known to prolong prothrombin time and inhibit platelet function.[22,23] In fact, Mielke and Britten[23] have reported that one therapeutic dose of aspirin can prolong the bleeding time for about 5 days. However, this is not likely to be clinically important except in patients with hemorrhagic diseases or those with peptic ulcers.

One should anticipate possible prothrombin deficiency in patients who have been taking aspirin over a relatively long period of time, such as in patients with arthritis or rheumatic fever. Aspirin should also be expected to increase bleeding tendencies when taken with anticoagulants. When surgery is anticipated, prothrombin time and coagulation time measurements should be performed on these patients, particularly if petechiae are observed. Since aspirin interferes with the hepatic production of prothrombin by blocking the utilization of vitamin K, an acceptable prothrombin and coagulation time can usually be restored by one of the following regimens (adult dosages): (1) 2 mg menadione sodium bisulfite or vitamin K_1 subcutaneously, which should provide a 20% improvement in prothrombin time in 12 hours; or (2) 5 mg/24 hr menadione sodium bisulfite orally for 4 to 7 days prior to surgery.[24]

The adjustment of prothrombin levels by the use of menadione or vitamin K should be carried out in collaboration with the patient's physician.

Several drug interactions with aspirin can be related to its ability to displace other drugs from plasma protein binding sites and thereby increase their free level in the blood, thus amplifying their toxic effects. The most commonly encountered condition in which this effect may be seen is in the patient receiving anticoagulant therapy. Drug levels in patients taking dicumarol or related anticoagulants are carefully titrated to obtain a lowered prothrombin level. In these patients, prothrombin time is approximately twice that of normal individuals. The administration of salicylates to these patients can dramatically increase prothrombin time and at the same time promote gastrointestinal bleeding. For these reasons aspirin should not be given to patients receiving anticoagulant therapy.

A second example of drug interaction with aspirin is with cancer treatment. Chemotherapeutic agents given for the treatment of cancer are extremely toxic, and the administration of aspirin to a patient taking an anticancer drug such as methotrexate can produce fatal blood levels by displacement from plasma protein binding sites.

Glucose-6-phosphate dehydrogenase (G-6-PD) deficiency is a relatively common inborn error of metabolism that can lead to hemolysis after the administration of several drugs, including aspirin. The incidence of G-6-PD deficiency has been estimated to be 13% in American black males[25] and is also common in Orientals and patients of Mediterranean

origin. This enzyme (G-6-PD) is essential for the maintenance of adequate levels of reduced glutathione in the red blood cell. Inadequate glutathione levels labilizes the erythrocyte to oxidative destruction and hemolysis. The administration of aspirin to these patients rarely causes hemolysis except in high doses. Symptoms include abdominal or back pain, anemia, jaundice, and hemoglobinuria.

The use of aspirin in the pregnant woman is not contraindicated, since there is no evidence that therapeutic doses of aspirin produce fetal damage.[11] However, the administration of large doses of aspirin should be avoided. Effects reported include lengthening of gestation, increasing frequency of postmaturity, prolonged spontaneous labor, and possible incomplete closure of the ductus arteriosus.

Although aspirin is by no means a dangerous drug, long experience in its use has clearly defined those situations in which a hazard may be associated with its administration. A summary of these conditions appears in Table 9-2. The adverse effects of newer drugs discussed later in this chapter are less well known than those of aspirin. Consequently, one should not conclude from the less detailed consideration of their adverse effects that they are intrinsically safer than aspirin.

Administration, absorption, and metabolism. Aspirin is almost always administered orally. It is absorbed rapidly from the stomach and small intestine. A 600 mg oral dose (two 5-grain tablets) normally produces a peak blood level in about 30 minutes.[26] Despite the fact that it is the nonionized form of aspirin which is absorbed, buffered aspirin has been shown to produce higher blood levels more quickly than unbuffered aspirin.[26] However, a double-blind clinical comparative study of five proprietary analgesic compounds was unable to show any important differences between buffered and unbuffered aspirin in regard to speed of onset or degree or duration of analgesia.[14] Absorption of aspirin in the mouth is poor, and effects obtained are the result of that which is swallowed in the saliva. Topical application to the oral mucosa is of no analgesic value, and painful ulceration is produced. Although rectal absorption is slower than that obtained

Table 9-2. Precautions and contraindications for the administration of aspirin

Disease/condition	Drug taken	Reasons for precaution or contraindication (*)
Peptic ulcer*		Gastric irritant effect
Hemophilia*		Gastric bleeding
Gout	Probenecid*	Antagonizes uricosuric effect
Myocardial infarct	Dicumarol* ⎫	Displaces drug from protein-binding site,
Cancer	Methotrexate* ⎭	increasing its toxicity
Asthma		High incidence of hypersensitivity reactions
Hypoprothrombinemia ⎫ Vitamin K deficiency ⎭		Weak inhibition of prothrombin synthesis
Glucose-6-phosphate dehydrogenase deficiency		Hemolysis
Rheumatic fever		May be taking large quantities already
Pregnancy		Possible alteration of gestation period and labor

orally, aspirin may be administered rectally in solution or suppositories where emesis precludes retention of oral medication.

Once absorbed, aspirin is rapidly hydrolyzed in the plasma to salicylic acid, which becomes unevenly distributed throughout the body. Relatively high concentrations are found in the lungs, liver, and kidney; lower levels are obtained in muscle and brain. Salicylate crosses the placental barrier and also appears in the milk of lactating mothers.

Products of salicylate conjugation and oxidation, formed principally in the liver, are excreted by the kidney. Renal excretion, particularly that of free salicylate, is increased by alkalinization of the urine (as by administration of sodium bicarbonate) and by diuresis.[11] Very little salicylate is excreted in the feces.

Uses. Aspirin is used primarily as an analgesic for mild to moderate pain. It also has important uses in the control of fever (antipyretic effect), in the treatment of rheumatic fever and arthritis (anti-inflammatory–antirheumatic effects), and in the treatment of gout (uricosuric effect). The hypoglycemic effect of aspirin has been used in the control of diabetes. The use of aspirin to prevent arterial thrombosis has also been suggested.

Dosage and preparations. The adult dosage of aspirin for pain and fever is 600 mg (two 5-grain tablets) every 4 hours. The analgesic-antipyretic dosage for children is 65 mg/kg/24 hr (maximum 3.6 Gm/24 hr) divided into four to six doses.[27] Dosage for children should never exceed 60 mg (1 grain)

per year of age, five times a day, and administration to infants should never go beyond 2 days.[21]

Single entity forms of aspirin include the commonly used 300 mg (5-grain) tablets and 75 mg (1¼-grain) children's tablets. Aspirin is available in a wide variety of multiple-entity preparations.

Drugs found in combination with aspirin include the following:

1. *Other analgesics* (numerous preparations). The combination of aspirin with narcotic analgesics is a common practice that may produce greater analgesic effectiveness.[11] The antipyretic and anti-inflammatory effects of the aspirin may enhance the analgesic effectiveness of the narcotic.

2. *Antacids* (Ascriptin, Cope, Bufferin). The amount of antacid included in most analgesic preparations is insufficient to substantially affect gastric acidity and does not dependably reduce gastric irritation.

3. *Sedatives* (Fiorinal, Darvo-Tran, Equagesic). Under certain conditions concurrent administration of a sedative with aspirin may be of value. In most cases, however, this may be accomplished in a more controlled manner by prescription of a sedative agent as a separate entity. The administration of a fixed combination of aspirin with a sedative has the potential risk of either overdose of aspirin to obtain the desired level of sedation or inadequate sedation at the recommended aspirin dosage. Furthermore, sedation throughout the period that analgesia is required may not be desirable.

4. *Antihistamines* (Synalgos and Synalgos-D.C.). The primary purpose of concurrent administration of an antihistamine and aspirin is for the sedative side effects obtained. Although the antihistaminic effects could be of value in the treatment of certain allergic conditions, the combination for this purpose with aspirin has no rational basis in therapy.

5. *Caffeine.* There is no rational inclusion of caffeine in analgesic preparations. The original stated purpose was a belief that it increased analgesic effectiveness, had a unique effect on relief of headache, or created a favorable effect on mood. None of these beliefs has been substantiated by clinical experimentation.

6. *Anticholinergics.* Several analgesics include anticholinergic agents such as hyoscyamine for the stated purpose of reducing gastric distress. The effectiveness of their presence in analgesic mixtures has not been demonstrated.

The para-aminophenols

The parent of the para-aminophenol group of drugs is acetanilid, which was introduced into medical practice in 1886 and was rapidly shown to be excessively toxic. Although acetanilid is not a para-aminophenol, it was found that a substantial fraction of it was converted to para-aminophenol derivatives. Subsequently, acetaminophen (paracetamol) and phenacetin (acetophenetidin) were introduced into therapy and found to be relatively devoid of the principal toxicity of acetanilid. Acetaminophen has become the accepted alternative to aspirin in its analgesic and antipyretic uses.[11] Phenacetin is less favored for reasons that will be discussed and is found only in drug mixtures. The chemical structures of these drugs are as follows:

Phenacetin   **Acetaminophen**

Administration, absorption, and metabolism. The para-aminophenols are absorbed rapidly and completely from the gastrointestinal tract to achieve therapeutic levels in 30 to 60 minutes. Acetaminophen is 20% to 50% bound to plasma proteins and excreted with a half-life of 1 to 3 hours. Acetaminophen is metabolized by the liver microsomal system principally to a glucuronate conjugate (80%), which is excreted in the urine. Phenacetin is rapidly converted by the body to acetaminophen[28] but also undergoes unique conversion to para-phenetidin. The various hydroxylated metabolites of this group of drugs are responsible for the principal toxicity of methemoglobinemia, hepatotoxicity, and renal toxicity. Patients with a genetically deficient ability to metabolize para-aminophenols will convert a greater percentage to toxic metabolites. Patients with kidney disease have higher plasma levels of conjugated forms but little difference in the levels of free drug.

Pharmacologic effects. The analgesic and antipyretic effects of acetaminophen and phenacetin are approximately those of aspirin. However, the anti-inflammatory activity of these drugs is less than that of aspirin[16] and does not appear to be clinically significant. For this reason para-aminophenols are not used to treat arthritis. The ability of acetaminophen to inhibit prostaglandin synthesis in the brain is greater than its ability to inhibit prostaglandin synthesis in peripheral tissues.[9]

Therapeutic doses of acetaminophen or phenacetin have no effect on the cardiovascular or respiratory system. These drugs do not produce gastric bleeding, do not affect platelet adhesion,[29] and do not affect uric acid excretion. Acetaminophen enhances water transport in the kidney and has been used with some success in the treatment of diabetes insipidus.[30] Phenacetin given in 2 Gm doses has been reported to produce a sedative effect equivalent to 150 mg pentobarbital.[31]

Adverse effects. The principal toxic effects of the para-aminophenols are (1) methemoglobinemia, (2) hemolytic anemia, (3) hepatic necrosis (large doses), and (4) nephrotoxicity (long-term usage).

Methemoglobinemia is a condition that results from conversion of the iron in hemoglobin to an oxidized state (ferric) that cannot effectively carry oxygen.[32] The condition may occur spontaneously as a disease or from the effect of certain drugs. Therapeutic doses of phenacetin convert 1% to 3% of the total hemoglobin to methemoglobin, and acetaminophen produces even less methemo-globin. Levels produced by these drugs are seldom of clinical significance. However, in the presence of preexisting methemoglobine-mia, congenital deficiency of the ability to metabolize para-aminophenols, or in the presence of other drugs such as prilocaine (Citanest) that cause methemoglobinemia, the combined effect can be significant. The clinical signs of methemoglobinemia are cya-nosis, dyspnea on exertion, and functional anemia. Over 30% of the blood hemoglobin must be converted before these signs appear.

Hemolytic anemia that occurs with para-aminophenols is most often associated with *long-term* ingestion. Hemolysis is caused by minor metabolites that oxidize glutathione in the red blood cell and thereby labilize the erythrocyte membrane to oxidative destruc-tion. *Acute* hemolytic anemia may occur in patients with glucose-6-phosphate dehydro-genase deficiency.[25] A similar reaction can occur in patients who are allergic to the para-aminophenols. In this case antigen-antibody complexes to the drug absorb onto the sur-face of the erythrocyte and lead to activation of complement and cell destruction. Allergy to aspirin does not confer allergy to the para-aminophenols.[33] Large doses of phenacetin have been reported to produce hemolytic anemia.[34] Clinical signs and symptoms of hemolytic anemia are abdominal or lower back pain, jaundice, hemoglobinuria, and anemia.

Hepatic necrosis may occur in adults after the ingestion of a single dose of 10 to 15 Gm acetaminophen[35]; 25 Gm or more is po-tentially fatal. Symptoms during the first 2 days after intoxication are minor. Nausea, vomiting, anorexia, and abdominal pain may occur. Liver injury becomes manifest on the second day, with alterations in plasma en-zyme levels (elevated transaminase and lactic hydrogenase), elevated bilirubin levels, and prolongation of prothrombin time. Hepato-toxicity may progress to encephalopathy, coma, and death. There are no known anti-dotes to acetaminophen toxicity. In nonfatal cases the condition is reversible over a period of weeks to months.

Nephrotoxicity has been associated with *long-term* consumption. The primary lesion appears to be a papillary necrosis with sec-ondary interstitial nephritis. Although no single agent in the numerous preparations available can be identified as being specifi-cally toxic, it is apparent that prolonged con-sumption of analgesics can lead to kidney dis-ease.[36] It is important that patients be con-vinced that daily intake of analgesics for long periods must be avoided. Since the use of analgesics in dental practice is rarely on other than a short-term basis, the possibility of nephrotoxicity does not present a significant problem in dental therapy.

Uses. Phenacetin and acetaminophen are employed as analgesics and antipyretics. Phenacetin is generally used in combination with other drugs such as aspirin and has had its greatest use as the *P* in APC (aspirin, phenacetin, and caffeine). Any advantage in reducing the aspirin content of a preparation to add phenacetin has not been demon-strated. The use of phenacetin in modern medicine is questionable. It is inferior to as-pirin and perhaps to acetaminophen in its analgesic and antipyretic properties, and it causes more methemoglobinemia and hemo-lytic anemia. Furthermore, phenacetin in combination analgesics contributes additively rather than synergistically so that there is little reason for its occurrence in multiple entity products.

Acetaminophen has gained popularity as an aspirin substitute. It is specifically valu-able in patients who are allergic to aspirin or in whom aspirin-induced gastric irritation would present a special problem. Although this point is not well established, there is some indication that acetaminophen causes less alteration in acid-base balance than aspi-rin and consequently may present a reduced toxic potential in young children. It is not known to what degree the long-term use of acetaminophen might produce the renal le-sions that have been attributed to its struc-tural congener phenacetin.

Dosage and preparations. Acetaminophen is available in many combinations and elixirs

Table 9-3. Dosage of acetaminophen for children

Age	Weight (mg)	Elixir (120 mg/5 ml)	Drops (60 mg/0.6 ml)
Under 1 year	60	½ tsp	0.6 ml
1-3 years	60-120	½-1 tsp	0.6-1.2 ml
3-6 years	120	1 tsp	1.2 ml
Over 6 years	240	2 tsp	

(Datril, Nebs, Tempra, Tylenol). The usual adult dose is one or two tablets (325 to 650 mg) three or four times every 24 hours. Various exilirs that are convenient for administration to children are available, and they most commonly have a concentration of 120 mg/5 ml (1 teaspoonful). The usual dosage for children are given in Table 9-3.

Single oral doses of 1000 mg acetaminophen have been reported to produce superior analgesia when compared with regular doses.[37] However, the potential toxicity of this dosage level has not been adequately investigated to determine if treatment with acetaminophen is sufficiently free of adverse effects to be routinely used at this higher dose.

OTHER ANTI-INFLAMMATORY ANALGESICS

A continued search for agents that possess analgesic activity without the undesirable side effects of aspirin has resulted in the synthesis and testing of thousands of compounds, a few of which have shown some promise in clinical trials. Although many of the drugs thus far tested claim a lower incidence of gastric irritant effects when compared with aspirin, none is devoid of that characteristic. Furthermore, as clinical experience with the use of these drugs is gained, undesirable effects unique to the agents tested have become apparent (mefenamic acid). In some cases relatively new analgesics, either those representing new chemical types (naproxen and ibuprofen) or newly evaluated congeners of chemicals long known as analgesic compounds (phenylbutazone and oxyphenylbutazone), have found greater usefulness and a more rational application as analgesics against inflammatory disease rather than as simple analgesics. Although several promising new drugs have been introduced, their use for the treatment of dental pain is, as present, speculative.

Mefenamic acid

Mefenamic acid (Ponstel) was introduced in 1963 for clinical testing as an analgesic. its chemical structure is as follows:

Mefenamic acid

Mefenamic acid possesses analgesic effectiveness approximately equal to that of aspirin.[11] It is a fairly potent inhibitor of prostaglandin synthesis[38] and is both anti-inflammatory and antipyretic.

Troublesome and sometimes serious adverse reactions have occurred after its use, the most common of which are gastrointestinal effects and include severe diarrhea, constipation, nausea, vomiting, abdominal pain, and gastrointestinal bleeding. Drowsiness, dizziness, vertigo, and headache have been seen. Hemolytic anemia, agranulocytosis and thrombocytopenia purpura have been reported to be associated with the use of mefenamic acid. As with any new drug, the potential for damage to the renal, hepatic, and hematopoietic systems must be considered, and appropriate function tests should be performed in all but short-term use.

Mefenamic acid should be used with caution in asthmatic patients because acute exacerbations have been reported. This drug is contraindicated with inflammatory diseases of the gastrointestinal tract and in patients with renal impairment. The safety of using mefenamic acid during pregnancy and for children under 14 years of age is not established and should not be so prescribed.

Intestinal absorption of mefenamic acid is relatively slow, with a maximum blood level being obtained in 2 to 4 hours. For this reason it should be started 2 to 4 hours prior to surgical procedures where the need for postoperative analgesia is anticipated. It is excreted principally in the urine as free drug and products of oxidation.

Mefenamic acid has been used orally against mild to moderate pain. Documentation of its use in dentistry is completely lacking. It is available in 250 mg capsules. The recommended dosage for adults and children over 14 years of age is 500 mg initially, followed by 250 mg every 6 hours. Since mefenamic acid is not superior to better known analgesics and can cause serious toxicity, it is difficult to justify its use in dental practice. If it is used, administration should not extend beyond 7 days. If severe diarrhea occurs, it should be discontinued and not used again in that patient.

Naproxen

Naproxen (Naprosyn) was introduced for clinical testing soon after the report of its anti-inflammatory properties in 1970. It has analgesic, antipyretic, and anti-inflammatory properties and is used in the symptomatic treatment of rheumatoid arthritis. Its chemical structure is as follows:

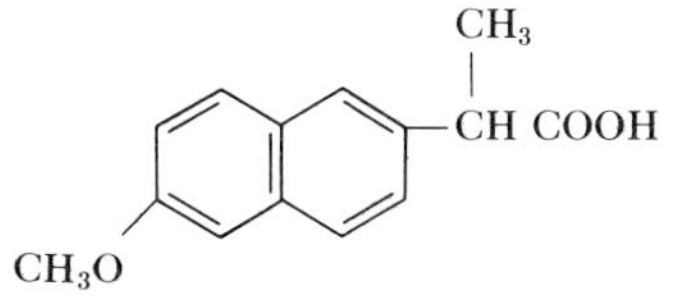

Naproxen

Initial reports suggest that the analgesic effectiveness of naproxen is superior to that of aspirin-codeine[39] and orally administered meperidine,[40] with a lower incidence of adverse gastric effects than aspirin.[41] Coadministration of aspirin and naproxen has been reported to produce greater analgesic effectiveness, even though aspirin appeared to accelerate the renal clearance of naproxen.

Naproxen is completely absorbed after oral administration and peak plasma levels are obtained 2 to 4 hours after administration. Naproxen is almost completely bound to plasma protein and may therefore affect the toxicity of concomitantly administered drugs such as dicumarol.

Because of the relative lack of experience in treating patients with naproxen, it is not recommended for women during pregnancy or lactation or for children. Naproxen has been associated with a high incidence of adverse reactions, and 1 patient in 7 has reported gastrointestinal problems such as abdominal pain, nausea, vomiting, diarrhea, stomatitis, and gastrointestinal bleeding. Consequently, it should be given with caution if at all to patients susceptible to upper gastrointestinal tract disease. Like aspirin, naproxen decreases platelet adhesiveness and prolongs bleeding time. Other relatively frequent reactions include headache, drowsiness, dizziness, vertigo, visual disturbances, edema, skin eruptions, and palpitation.

Naproxen is primarily marketed for the treatment of arthritis. The recommended adult dose is 250 mg twice every 24 hours.

Ibuprofen

Ibuprofen (Motrin was introduced for clinical testing in 1969. It has analgesic, antipyretic, and anti-inflammatory properties and has been used in the treatment of rheumatoid arthritis and osteoarthritis. Compared with aspirin, ibuprofen causes less occult bleeding, and there are fewer complaints of gastric upset. The chemical formula of ibuprofen is as follows:

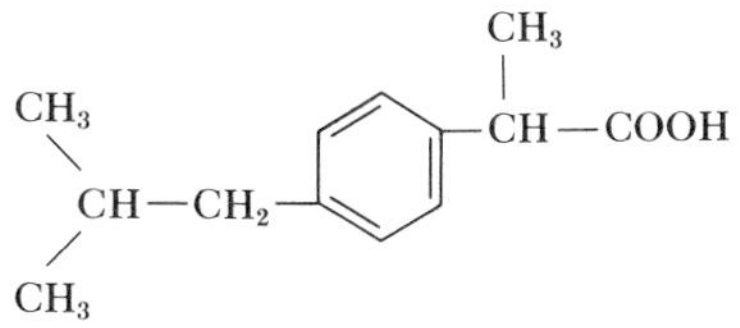

Ibuprofen

Clinical testing of the analgesic effectiveness of ibuprofen indicates that it is superior to placebo[44] and comparable to aspirin[43,44] with less gastrointestinal upset. Reported side effects include gastrointestinal distress, dizziness, headache, visual field defects, and alteration of hepatic function.

Ibuprofen is primarily marketed for treatment of arthritic conditions, for which it has been used in doses of 300 to 400 mg or 3 or 4 times every 24 hours.

THE PYRAZOLONES

Prior to 1935 two pyrazolone derivatives, antipyrine and aminopyrine, were used extensively as antipyretic and antirheumatic analgesics. Although they continue to be used to some extent in Europe, the realization by 1931 to 1933 that these drugs caused agranulocytosis has led to their almost complete elimination from use in the United States. The seriousness of this adverse effect and the fact that they are no more effective than aspirin contraindicate their use as analgesics.

A third pyrazolone, dipyrone (Narove, Pyrilgin) is available in several trade and generic preparations. Its relative potency as an analgesic and antipyretic has not been established. Dipyrone is a highly toxic drug and may produce fatal agranulocytosis even after short-term use. Hemolytic anemia and numerous other untoward effects have occurred after its use. Since dipyrone provides no therapeutic advantage over less toxic drugs, it should not be used in dental practice. Its use in medical practice may be justified as a parenteral antipyretic in life-threatening febrile conditions in children when other measures and drugs have failed.

Another pyrazolone, phenylbutazone (Butazolidin) has a greater anti-inflammatory effect than other pyrazolones and the salicylates. It has been used in various arthritic and inflammatory conditions. It has a uricosuric action and has been employed in gout. Phenylbutazone is a relatively toxic drug, particularly with prolonged use. It has caused gastrointestinal distress, edema, hepatitis, agranulocytosis, thrombocytopenia, and leukemic changes. Xerostomia and salivary gland enlargement have also been reported, even after short-term use.[45] Phenylbutazone is recommended only for short-term use against gout and inflammatory conditions for which less toxic agents are not effective. It should not be used as an analgesic in dental practice. Although reports on the use of oxyphenbutazone (Tandearil), a chemical relative of phenylbutazone, have been favorable after surgery for impactions,[46] evidence is too limited at the present time to justify its general use in dentistry.

SUMMARY

The drug of choice for mild to moderate pain is aspirin. Special caution must be exercised in regard to overdosage in children and in patients allergic to aspirin or susceptible to gastrointestinal distress. In cases where aspirin is contraindicated or undesirable, acetaminophen is usually a good substitute. If aspirin or acetaminophen is inadequate for the relief of pain, increased effects may be obtained by using these drugs in combination with the narcotic analgesics, which will be discussed in the next chapter.

REFERENCES

1. Merskey, H., and Spear, F. G.: The concept of pain, J. Psychosom. Res. **11:**59-67, 1967.
2. Guyton, A. C.: Textbook of medical physiology, ed. 3, Philadelphia, 1966, W. B. Saunders Co.
3. Monheim, L. M.: Local anesthesia and pain control in dental practice, ed. 4, St. Louis, 1969, The C. V. Mosby Co.
4. Chilton, N. W., Lewandowski, A., and Cameroy, J. R.: Double-blind evaluation of a new analgesic agent in postextraction pain, Am. J. Med. Sci. **342:**704, 1961.
5. Popkes, D. L., and Folsom, T. C.: Comparative study of three analgesic agents used in oral surgical procedures, J. Oral Surg. **27:**950-954, 1969.
6. Beecher, H. K.: The powerful placebo, J.A.M.A. **159:**1602-1606, 1955.
7. Wagner, W. A., and Hubbell, A. O.: Pain control with a mixture containing dextropropoxyphene hydrochloride, a mixture containing codeine phosphate and a placebo, J. Oral Surg. Anesth. Hosp. Dent. Serv. **17:**14, 1959.
8. Lim, R. K. S.: Salicylate analgesia. In Smith,

M. J. H., and Smith, P. K., editors: The salicylates: a critical bibliographic review, New York, 1966, John Wiley & Sons, Inc.
9. Ferreira, S. H., and Vane, J. R.: New aspects of the mode of action of nonsteroid anti-inflammatory drugs, Annu. Rev. Pharmacol. **14:**57-73, 1974.
10. Cutting, W. C.: Handbook of pharmacology, ed. 5, New York, 1972, Appleton-Century-Crofts.
11. Goodman, L. S., and Gilman, A.: The pharmacological basis of therapeutics, ed. 5, New York, 1975, The Macmillan Co.
12. Grossman, M. I., Matsumoto, K. K., and Lichter, R. J.: Fecal blood loss produced by oral and intravenous administration of various salicylates, Gastroenterology **40:**383, 1961.
13. Is all aspirin alike? Med. Lett. Drugs Ther. **16:**57-59, 1974.
14. DeKornfeld, T. J., Lasagna, L., and Frazier, T. M.: A comparative study of 5 proprietary analgesic compounds, J.A.M.A. **182:**1315, 1962.
15. Gastrointestinal disturbances with aspirin, Med. Lett. Drugs Ther. **7:**76, 1965.
16. Acetaminophen, Valadol, and analgesic renal injury, Med. Lett. Drugs Ther. **13:**74-76, 1971.
17. DiPalma, J. R., editor: Basic pharmacology in medicine, New York, 1976, McGraw-Hill Book Co.
18. Koch-Weser, J.: Harrison's principles of internal medicine, ed. 6, New York, 1970, McGraw-Hill Book Co.
19. U.S. Department of Health, Education, and Welfare, Public Health Service, National Center for Health Statistics: Excerpt from Vital Statistics of the U.S., vol. II—Mortality, Washington, D.C., 1965, U.S. Government Printing Office.
20. U.S. Department of Health, Education, and Welfare, Public Health Service, National Center for Health Statistics: Excerpt from Vital Statistics of the U.S., vol. II—Mortality, Washington, D.C., 1967, U.S. Government Printing Office.
21. Craig, J. O., Ferguson, I. C., and Syme, J.: Infants, toddlers, and aspirin, Br. Med. J. **5490:**757-761, 1966.
22. O'Brien, J. R.: Effect of salicylates on human platelets, Lancet **1:**1431, 1968.
23. Mielke, C. H., Jr., and Britten, A. F. H.: Aspirin: a new nightmare for blood bankers, N. Engl. J. Med. **286:**268-269, 1972.
24. McFarland, W.: Drugs for hematologic disorders. In Modell, W., editor: Drugs of choice 1976-1977, St. Louis, 1976, The C. V. Mosby Co.
25. Glucose-6-phosphate dehydrogenase deficiency, Med. Lett. Drugs Ther. **17:**3-4, 1975.
26. Truitt, E. B., Jr., and Morgan, A. M.: A comparison of the gastrointestinal absorption rates of plain and buffered acetylsalicylic acid, Arch. Int. Pharmacodyn. Ther. **135:**105, 1962.
27. Hughes, J. G.: Synopsis of pediatrics, ed. 4, St. Louis, 1975, The C. V. Mosby Co.
28. Brodie, B. B., and Axelrod, J.: Fate of acetophenetidin (phenacetin) in man and methods for estimation of acetophenetidin and its metabolites in biological material, J. Pharmacol. Exp. Ther. **97:**58, 1949.
29. Mielke, C. H., Jr., and Britten, A. F. H.: Use of aspirin or acetaminophen in hemophilia, N. Engl. J. Med. **282:**1270, 1970.
30. Nusynowitz, M. L., and Forsham, P. H.: The anti-

diuretic action of acetaminophen, Am. J. Med. Sci. **252:**429-435, 1966.

31. Eade, N. R., and Lasagna, L.: A comparison of acetophenetidin and acetaminophen. II. Subjective effects in healthy volunteers, J. Pharmacol. Exp. Ther. **155:**301-308, 1967.
32. Bodansky, O.: Methemoglobinemia and methemoglobin-producing compounds, Pharmacol. Rev. **3:** 144-196, 1951.
33. Fein, B. T.: Aspirin shock associated with asthma and nasal polyps, Ann. Allergy **29:**598-601, 1971.
34. Hutchison, H. E., Jackson, J. M., and Cassidy, P.: Phenacetin-induced hemolytic anemia, Lancet **2:** 1022, 1962.
35. Boyer, T. D., and Rouff, S. L.: Acetaminophen-induced hepatic necrosis and renal failure, J.A.M.A. **218:**440-441, 1971.
36. Phenacetin, Med. Lett. Drugs Ther. **6:**79, 1964.
37. Hopkinson, J. H., et al.: Acetaminophen (500 mg) versus acetaminophen (325 mg) for the relief of pain in episiotomy patients, Curr. Ther. Res. **16:**194-200, 1974.
38. Scherrer, R. A., and Whitehouse, M. W., editors: Antiinflammatory agents: chemistry and pharmacology, New York, 1974, Academic Press, Inc., Vol. I.
39. Ruedy, J.: A comparison of the analgesic efficacy of naproxen and acetylsalicylic acid–codeine in patients with pain after dental surgery, Scand. J. Rheumatol. **2**(supp.):60-63, 1973.

40. Stetson, J. B., Robinson, K., Wardell, W. M., and Lasagna, L.: Analgesic activity of oral naproxen in patients with postoperative pain, Scand. J. Rheumatol. **2**(supp.):50-55, 1973.
41. Halvorsen, L., Dotevall, G., and Sevelius, H.: Comparative effects of aspirin and naproxen on gastric mucosa, Scand. J. Rheumatol. **2**(supp.):43-47, 1973.
42. Lopken, P., Olsen, I., Bruaset, I., and Norman-Pedersen, K.: Bilateral surgical removal of impacted lower third molar teeth as a model for drug evaluation: a test with ibuprofen, Eur. J. Clin. Pharmacol. **8:**209-216, 1975.
43. Bloomfield, S. S., Barden, T. P., and Mitchell, J.: Comparative efficacy of ibuprofen and aspirin in episiotomy pain, Clin. Pharmacol. Ther. **15:**565-570, 1974.
44. Needle, S. E., and Cooper, S. A.: Evaluation of the analgesic activity of ibuprofen, J. Dent. Res. **55:** B327 (abs. 1062), 1976.
45. Cohen, L., and Banks, P.: Salivary gland enlargement and phenylbutazone, Br. Med. J. **1:**1420, 1966.
46. van Geel, C. J.: Erfahrungen mit landeril in der Kieferchirurgie, Schweiz. Monatsscher. Zahnheilk. **78:**257, 1968.

10

Narcotics

SAM V. HOLROYD

Narcotics are drugs that produce narcosis (stupor). Except for potency, rate of onset, and duration of action, the differences among the narcotic analgesics are not great. Clinically important similarities among narcotic agents are that they all produce (1) potent analgesia, (2) addiction, (3) respiratory depression, (4) sedation, (5) emesis, and (6) constipation. Tolerance readily develops to the narcotics, and cross-tolerance as well as cross-addiction exist. Another common characteristic is that they are all antagonized by specific narcotic antagonists.

The narcotics are important in dental practice for pain that cannot be controlled by the less potent nonnarcotic drugs. Reynolds has recently said, "In order to control moderately severe pain, the use of narcotics is imperative. It is hard to understand how many dentists can practice without a federal narcotics license."[1]

Because of their addicting liabilities, the narcotics are subject to control under the Controlled Substance Act of 1970. They can be prescribed only by practitioners who register annually with the Drug Enforcement Administration (DEA), as described in Chapter 4.

CLASSIFICATION

The narcotic analgesics can be categorized as follows:

Opium alkaloids
  Morphine
  Codeine
Semisynthetic derivatives of morphine
  Heroin
  Dihydromorphinone or hydromorphone (Dilaudid, Hymorphan)

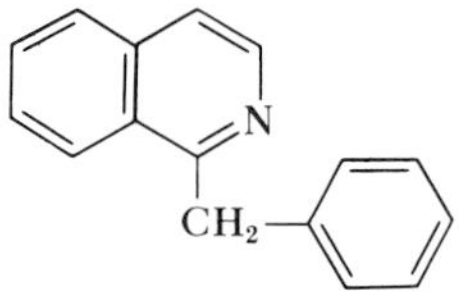

☐ The opinions or assertions contained herein are the private ones of the writer and are not to be construed as official or as reflecting the views of the Navy Department or the naval service at large.

Dihydrocodeinone (Dicodeine, Dicodid)
Oxymorphone
Oxycodone
Synthetic narcotics
  Meperidine (Demerol)
  Ethoheptazine (Zactane)
  Alphaprodine (Nisentil)
  Anileridine (Leritine)
  Piminodine (Alvodine)
  Methadone (Dolophine)
  Propoxyphene (Darvon)
  Levorphanol (Levo-Dromoran)
  Pentazocine (Talwin)

OPIUM ALKALOIDS

Opium is the dried juice obtained from the unripe seed capsules of the poppy plant *Papaver somniferum*. Approximately 25% of opium consists of alkaloids: 10% morphine, 0.5% codeine, 0.2% thebaine, 6% narcotine, 1% papaverine, and others. These alkaloids are either phenanthrene derivatives or benzylisoquinoline derivatives. The basic chemical structure, principal properties, and members of each group are as follows. Only morphine and codeine are of great clinical importance.

Phenanthrene: Analgesic and addicting (morphine, codeine, thebaine)

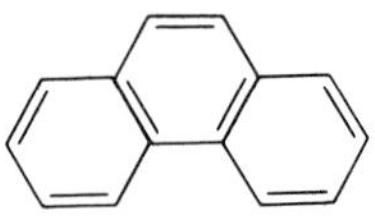

Benzylisoquinoline: Depressor of smooth muscle, nonanalgesic, nonaddicting (narcotine, papaverine)

Morphine

Morphine was isolated in pure form from opium by Serturner in 1803. Although synthesized in 1952 by Gates and Tschudi, it is still commercially obtained from the natural source. The structure of morphine is as follows:

Pharmacologic effects (therapeutic and adverse)

Unlike many drugs, the significant adverse effects of morphine do not relate to a direct damaging effect on hepatic, renal, or hematologic tissues. The principal adverse effects of morphine result from undesirable alterations of the function of several organ systems. Consequently, in this chapter, the discussions on adverse effects and pharmacologic effects are considered together. Allergic reactions occur but are infrequent and usually mild and dermatologic in nature. Anaphylaxis has occurred but is rare.

Analgesia and sedation. Morphine provides effective analgesia against severe pain. The greater potency over nonnarcotic analgesics is related to the fact that in addition to raising the pain threshold, the narcotics also affect the cerebral cortex to depress the reaction to pain. Analgesic doses also produce sedation, which undoubtedly potentiates the analgesic effect. Euphoria is produced by analgesic doses in some people. Tolerance develops to the analgesic, sedative, and euphoric effects.

Respiratory depression. Morphine sharply depresses the respiratory center in the medulla. Respiratory depression parallels the analgesic potency[2] and is associated with a reduced sensitivity to carbon dioxide.[3] Tolerance develops to this effect. Respiratory depression is the cause of death in overdose and represents an extremely important clinical consideration. Although the usual adult doses of morphine have minimal effects on respiration in healthy patients, even therapeutic doses may dangerously decrease pulmonary ventilation in elderly or debilitated patients and those with severe pulmonary

diseases.[4] Morphine and other narcotics have been said to be contraindicated in cases of myxedema, Addison's disease, and cirrhosis of the liver because small doses may cause respiratory failure.[5] Special care is also indicated in patients with other respiratory limitations such as those in shock or those suffering from severe asthma or chronic lung disease. The use of narcotics in pregnant women should be avoided when possible to preclude possible anoxia to the fetus. The practitioner should reduce the dosage of morphine for patients who are taking other drugs that also depress respiration, such as the barbiturates.

Emesis and nausea. Analgesic doses of morphine tend to cause nausea and vomiting in many people. This is attributable to direct stimulation of the trigger zone for emesis, which is located in the medulla.[6] This trigger zone is distinct from the vomiting center, which is depressed by morphine.

Cough suppression. Although morphine depresses the cough center, antitussive effects are generally obtained therapeutically by less addicting drugs.

Gastrointestinal effects. Analgesic doses of morphine cause constipation by reducing gastrointestinal secretions and motility. No tolerance develops to these effects. Although the constipating effect may be useful in diarrhea, morphine is not normally used for this single purpose.

Renal effects. Morphine may cause urine retention by increasing the smooth muscle tone of the urinary tract. It also produces an antidiuretic effect by stimulating the release of the antidiuretic hormone of the pituitary. Although analgesic doses do not pose a threat to the healthy patient, they may cause acute urinary retention in patients with prostatic hypertrophy or stricture of the urethra.[4]

Increased intracranial pressure. Morphine causes cerebral vasodilation, which appears to be secondary to respiratory depression. This results in an increase in intracranial and spinal fluid pressure. Consequently, morphine should not be used in patients with head injuries or where intracranial pressure may already be present. It should also be noted at this point that since the presence of depression and nausea are important in determining the extensiveness of head injuries, the imposition of these factors by a drug cannot help but complicate the diagnosis.

Central nervous system stimulation. Very high doses of morphine and its chemical relatives have produced convulsions by direct action on the cerebral cortex. Although relatively low doses of morphine may produce excitation in some animals (cats, lions, tigers, horses, cows, sheep, and goats), this generally does not present a therapeutic problem in humans.

Cardiovascular effects. Morphine depresses the vasomotor center and stimulates the vagus. These effects would generally not be clinically significant at the usual dosage levels, but higher doses may cause hypotension and bradycardia.

Miosis. Morphine constricts the pupils. There is no tolerance to this effect, and it serves as an important diagnostic sign in morphine overdose.

Bronchiolar constriction. Morphine causes bronchiolar constriction. The effect is usually minor but may present a serious problem if combined with asthmatic respiratory depression.

Hepatic effects. Although liver damage does not occur, high doses in some people may sufficiently constrict the biliary duct to cause biliary colic.

Addiction

Morphine is highly addicting—a fact that represents an important limitation to its therapeutic use. Although patients with personality problems are more susceptible to addiction, others are also highly susceptible. This is a greater problem in medicine than in dentistry because the dental use of morphine is almost always of short duration. Despite this, the dentist should not minimize the importance of this potentiality. Every effort should be made to control pain with nonnarcotic analgesics or narcotics with less addicting liability, such as codeine, before resorting to the use of morphine.

The morphine addict may appear completely normal except for constipation and miosis, to which tolerance does not develop. A "withdrawal syndrome" results if the addict does not continue to receive morphine. This syndrome can be brought on almost immediately by the narcotic antagonists, which are discussed later. Symptoms of withdrawal range from depression to delirium and include lacrimation, perspiration, rhinorrhea, yawning, and progression to a restless sleep, which is followed by dilated pupils, gooseflesh, anorexia, irritability, tremor, nausea, vomiting, intestinal spasm, abdominal cramps, chills, tachycardia, and increased blood pressure.[6]

Overdose

As noted earlier, the principal danger in morphine overdose is respiratory depression. The diagnostic triad of overdose consists of coma, depressed respiration, and pinpoint pupils.

The treatment of choice is the use of specific narcotic antagonists, naloxone (Narcan), levallorphan (Lorfan), or nalorphine (Nalline), which will bring prompt recovery. One must be aware that although adequate respiration will be quickly restored, this recovery will be associated with varying degrees of withdrawal symptoms. The latter in some cases may present greater hazards than does the pretreatment respiratory depression. Therefore the use of narcotic antagonists should not be taken lightly.

Administration and body handling

Although the opiates are absorbed orally, morphine is not very effective by this route, probably because of slow absorption. Consequently, morphine is usually administered subcutaneously and is sometimes used intramuscularly or intravenously.

The rate of absorption from subcutaneous or muscle tissues may vary considerably because of differences in tissue circulation, but ordinarily peak activity is seen in 45 to 90 minutes.[7]

Once absorbed, morphine is rapidly distributed to the tissues, particularly the kidney, lung, liver, and spleen. It is metabolized by the liver, principally by conjugation with glucuronic acid. Conjugates and some free drug are excreted in the urine.

Use, dosage, and preparations

Morphine, as the sulfate salt, is used parenterally for severe pain. The usual adult dose of 10 to 15 mg subcutaneously should cover severe pain of dental origin for about 6 hours. For children the dose is 0.1 to 0.2 mg/kg/dose, with the maximal dose being 15 mg.[4] Close observation should follow the use of morphine in a child. Parenteral solutions of morphine sulfate that contain 8, 10, 15, and 30 mg/ml are available.

Codeine

Codeine is produced by methylation of morphine. It is the most frequently used narcotic in dental practice and has the same pharmacologic actions as morphine but to different degrees. Tolerance and addiction to codeine develop more slowly than to morphine.

Therapeutic comparison to morphine

Whereas morphine is only used parenterally, codeine is effective orally. Codeine has less than one sixth the analgesic potency of morphine and a shorter duration of action, and consequently it is not effective for severe or moderately severe pain. Codeine equals morphine as an antitussive.

Toxicity comparison to morphine

Just as codeine has the same therapeutic actions as morphine, its adverse effects are qualitatively similar although quantitatively different. Doses of codeine between 60 and 120 mg are likely to cause about as many troublesome effects as 10 mg morphine.[7] Although most patients will be sedated to some degree by 30 to 60 mg codeine, euphoria is not likely to be seen at these doses. Little or no respiratory depression should follow the usual analgesic doses of codeine (about 60 mg). However, 120 mg is believed to produce respiratory depression that is approximately equal to that produced by 10 mg morphine.[6]

Emesis, nausea, and constipation may be seen with analgesic doses of codeine but will be less than that seen with morphine. Increased intracranial pressure is not likely to present a problem, unless doses are used that would significantly depress respiration. Miosis and adverse renal, hepatic, cardiovascular, and bronchial effects are not likely to be seen with therapeutic doses of codeine. The excitatory effects of codeine may be greater than those of morphine, and convulsions have been seen in children.

Addiction comparison to morphine

Although codeine is addicting, the liability is much less than that associated with morphine. The short-term use of codeine, as would be employed in dental practice, does not present a particularly great problem.

Administration and body handling

Codeine is absorbed well orally and is usually administered by this route. It is sometimes used subcutaneously. Wide tissue distribution is obtained. Codeine is metabolized in the liver to morphine and norcodeine, which are sequentially conjugated and excreted in urine. The analgesic and other effects of codeine may be attributable to the morphine and norcodeine that are formed.

Use, dosage, and preparations

Codeine is used for mild to moderate pain. It is employed in dental practice for pain that cannot be controlled by nonnarcotic analgesics but that does not require the use of the more potent narcotics. It has additional use in medicine as an antitussive. It is almost always used orally, and the usual adult analgesic dosages are 15 to 60 mg (¼ to 1 grain) every 4 to 6 hours. Unless a patient has developed tolerance to narcotics, a maximal analgesic potency is generally obtained with 60 mg. This dosage will not equal that of 10 mg morphine. Increasing the dosage beyond 60 mg will prolong the duration, but for greater analgesic depth the practitioner must go to a more potent analgesic. A somewhat greater analgesic effect may be obtained by giving the drug subcutaneously.

Codeine sulfate and codeine phosphate are available as 15, 30, and 60 mg tablets and as 15, 30, and 60 mg/ml parenteral solutions. Codeine is also available in various preparations with aspirin (Ascodeen 30, Empirin Compound with codeine, etc.) and acetaminophen (Codalan, Dialog with codeine, Percogesic-C, Phenaphen, etc.), which add analgesic and antipyretic effects. To estimate the value of the analgesic additive effect, one may assume that 30 mg codeine equals approximately 600 mg (10 grains) aspirin or acetaminophen. The particular advantage of using codeine with aspirin or acetaminophen is that one can obtain the additional analgesic effect with lower doses of codeine, thereby avoiding the side effects of codeine that might occur at higher doses. As a general rule, it is less expensive to prescribe codeine and aspirin or acetaminophen separately rather than to prescribe the combination products.

Aside from what has already been said, it is unnecessary to comment individually on the large number of analgesic combination products. By knowing the therapeutic and adverse effects of each constituent, one may estimate the advantages and disadvantages of a particular commercial preparation.

SEMISYNTHETIC DERIVATIVES OF MORPHINE
Heroin

Heroin is produced by the acetylation of morphine. It is a highly euphoric and addicting drug. Although it has analgesic properties, its enormous addicting liability has precluded its therapeutic usefulness. It cannot be legally manufactured or imported into the United States.

Dihydromorphinone or hydromorphone

Dihydromorphinone (Demorphone, Dilaudid, Hymorphan) is a more potent analgesic than morphine, and its tendency to produce adverse side effects is correspondingly high. The analgesic effects and the occurrence of typical narcotic side effects, including respiratory depression, of 2 mg dihydromorphinone approximately equals that of 10 mg morphine. Its addicting liability equals that of morphine. Because of its rapid onset and short duration of action, its principal use is for acute pain of short duration. The usual adult dose is 2 to 5 mg orally or 1 or 2 mg subcutaneously.

Dihydrocodeinone or hydrocodone

Dihydrocodeinone (Dicodeine, Dicodid, Mercodinone) has approximately the same analgesic potency as codeine but a greater antitussive effect. Analgesic doses may depress respiration noticeably.[3] Its addiction liability equals that of morphine. Its principal use today is as an antitussive.

Oxymorphone

Oxymorphone (Numorphan) is similar to dihydromorphinone in that although it is more potent than morphine (eight to ten times), its undesirable effects are correspondingly high. It is extremely addicting and a potent respiratory depressant. The usual adult dose is 1 mg subcutaneously.

Oxycodone

Chemically, oxycodone is to codeine what oxymorphone is to morphine. Oxycodone is more potent and more addicting than codeine and produces similar side effects. It is used in antitussive preparations and is available as an analgesic only in the multiple entity product Percodan. This preparation contains 4.5 mg oxycodone hydrochloride, 0.38 mg oxycodone terephthalate, 0.38 mg homatropine terephthalate, 224 mg aspirin, 160 mg phenacetin, and 32 mg caffeine. Percodan-Demi contains one half of the preceding quantities of oxycodone and homatropine. The inclusion of homatropine contraindicates its use in patients with glaucoma.

Although there is little doubt that this product will alleviate most mild to moderate pain of dental origin, any advantage over single-entity preparations or simpler mixtures is not established.

SYNTHETIC NARCOTICS

Meperidine, alphaprodine, anileridine, piminodine, and ethoheptazine are all piperidine derivatives and consequently are closely related chemically. Although they are related pharmacologically to the opiates, they are chemically different. All have the following structural nucleus and differ mainly by the group at R.[*]

Piperidine nucleus

Meperidine

Meperidine (Demerol) is probably the most used narcotic in dental practice except for codeine. Although not as potent as morphine, it provides effective analgesia against moderately severe pain. Associated effects are similar to but less potent than those of morphine; these include sedation, respiratory depression, and stimulation of gastrointestinal and biliary muscle. It produces less euphoria, bronchoconstriction, and constipation than morphine. Meperidine is addicting and tolerance develops. Its effects are counteracted by narcotic antagonists.

The most frequently observed side effects

---

[*]Ethoheptazine is identical chemically to meperidine (both have CH_3 at R), except that the nitrogen-containing ring in ethoheptazine is seven membered (contains an additional carbon).

of meperidine are dizziness, nausea, vomiting, postural hypotension, sweating, and xerostomia. Reactions to overdose include tachycardia, excitement, disorientation, delirium, hallucinations, and convulsions. All precautions observed for morphine should be exercised with meperidine.

Meperidine is absorbed well orally, but analgesic effects are produced best parenterally. It is metabolized principally by the liver. Metabolites and some free drug are excreted in the urine.

The usual adult doses of meperidine (50 to 100 mg orally, subcutaneously, or intramuscularly) will be effective against moderate to severe pain of dental origin. It will be particularly valuable when used parenterally to obtain rapid analgesia and sedation. The 100 mg dose approaches the analgesic potency of 10 mg morphine.

Meperidine HCl is available in 50 and 100 mg tablets, an oral elixir containing 50 mg/5 ml, and solutions for injection containing 25, 50, 75, and 100 mg/ml. Meperidine HCl is available in combination with acetaminophen (Demerol-APAP: tablets containing 50 mg meperidine HCl and 300 mg acetaminophen). It may be prescribed in this way or taken separately with acetaminophen or aspirin. The use of meperidine with aspirin or acetaminophen increases the analgesic effect provided by meperidine and provides antipyresis. Meperidine HCl is available with promethazine HCl as Mepergan Fortis capsules: 50 mg meperidine HCl and 25 mg promethazine HCl. It is not completely determined as to how much the analgesic effect of meperidine is enhanced by the antihistamine promethazine. The sedating effects of these drugs are additive, perhaps even potentiating. Consequently, this combination may be useful when sedation is particularly important. However, one must be cautioned that promethazine and other phenothiazines can exaggerate the respiratory depression caused by meperidine and other narcotics.

Ethoheptazine

Ethoheptazine was introduced in 1958 and marketed as ethoheptazine citrate (Zactane citrate). It is prepared synthetically and has a chemical structure similar to that of the narcotic meperidine.

The only therapeutic effect of ethoheptazine is that of analgesia, but its relative analgesic potency is difficult to assess. When used alone, its potency is inferior to that of aspirin.[8] In fact, a recent study showed it to be less effective than a placebo.[9]

Adverse effects of therapeutic dosages of ethoheptazine are mild and similar to those associated with propoxyphene, principally dizziness and gastrointestinal disturbances. Addiction to ethoheptazine has not been reported, and the number of cases of severe overdosage are inadequate to allow a complete evaluation of the problem. Cumulative toxicity may develop after large doses over several days and lead to dizziness, nervousness, and syncope.

Ethoheptazine is adequately absorbed orally and is administered only by this route. The distribution of ethoheptazine in the tissues and its metabolic alterations have not been established.

Ethoheptazine citrate has been used for mild to moderate pain, almost always in combination with aspirin and phenacetin. The usual adult oral dose is 75 to 150 mg every 6 to 8 hours. The following preparations are available as tablets:

75 mg ethoheptazine citrate (Zactane)
75 mg with 325 mg aspirin (Zactirin)
100 mg with APC* (Zactirin Compound-100)
75 mg with 250 mg aspirin and 150 mg meprobamate (Equagesic)†

Alphaprodine

Alphaprodine (Nisentil) is similar to meperidine. In equivalent doses (40 to 60 mg) it provides analgesia and adverse effects that are qualitatively and quantitatively the same as those of meperidine. Alphaprodine has a shorter duration of action, which may be advantageous in some situations. It is only used parenterally.

Anileridine

In equivalent doses there are no distinctive differences between anileridine (Leritine) and meperidine. The usual adult dose is 25 to 50 mg every 6 hours orally, intramuscularly, or subcutaneously. It is available as the hydrochloride in 25 mg tablets and as the phosphate in solutions containing 25 mg/ml.

---

*227 mg aspirin, 162 mg phenacetin, and 32.4 mg caffeine.
† Minor tranquilizer.

Piminodine

Piminodine (Alvodine) has essentially the same therapeutic and adverse effects as meperidine. The usual adult dosage for moderately severe pain is 25 to 50 mg orally every 4 to 6 hours or 10 to 20 mg intramuscularly or subcutaneously every 4 hours. Piminodine esylate is available in 50 mg tablets and a parenteral solution containing 20 mg/ml.

Methadone

Methadone (Dolophine) is chemically distinct from both the opiates and the meperidine type of synthetics.

Methadone

Methadone was synthesized in Germany during World War II and was shown to produce the effects of morphine: potent analgesia, respiratory depression, sedation, addiction, smooth muscle spasm, and miosis. Although methadone can be used to relieve severe pain, the fact that it prevents and alleviates the opiate withdrawal syndrome has led to its wide use as a narcotic substitute. Withdrawal from methadone appears to be accomplished more easily than from morphine.

Patients taking methadone exhibit the usual opiate side effects of constipation, nausea, vomiting, dizziness, xerostomia, and mental depression.

Methadone is well absorbed orally and may also be used parenterally. It is metabolized chiefly by the liver, and metabolic products are eliminated in the feces and urine.

The usual adult analgesic dose of methadone for severe pain is 10 mg. This equals the analgesia provided by 10 mg morphine and produces less sedation and euphoria. Methadone hydrochloride is available in 5 and 10 mg tablets, in a syrup containing 10 mg/30 ml, and in a parenteral solution containing 10 mg/ml.

Propoxyphene

Propoxyphene was introduced in 1957 and marketed as propoxyphene hydrochloride (Darvon). It is produced synthetically and has a chemical structure similar to that of the narcotic methadone.

Propoxyphene

The only therapeutic effect of propoxyphene is that of analgesia. Although it is sometimes said to equal codeine in analgesic potency or to have analgesic effects similar to those of codeine,[10] dental studies have found it to be slightly inferior to codeine with fewer side effects,[11] statistically less effective than codeine,[12] significantly inferior to aspirin,[13] equal to a placebo,[13,14] and inferior to a placebo.[15] Beaver[16] has stated that propoxyphene is superior to a placebo in doses of 65 mg or more but is of questionable efficacy in doses lower than 65 mg. He further states that propoxyphene is "certainly no more, and probably less, effective than the usually used doses of aspirin or APC." A study by Moertel and co-workers[9] found propoxyphene to be no more effective than a placebo. Apparently the psychological effect of propoxyphene administration is of great importance in determining the degree of its analgesic effect. Since propoxyphene does not produce sedation, its site of action is probably subcortical.

Adverse effects of therapeutic dosages of propoxyphene are mild and consist primarily of nausea, vomiting, abdominal pain, dizziness, headache, insomnia, and skin rashes. Although some cases of euphoria, tolerance, and psychological and physical dependence have been reported, the addictive liability of propoxyphene is low. Despite this, drug abuse with propoxyphene appears to have obtained significant proportions, and a number of overdose deaths have been reported.

Severe overdosage may produce symptoms of inebriation, convulsions, respiratory depression, cyanosis, coma, circulatory failure, and death. Overdosage can be counteracted by narcotic antagonists such as nalorphine or levallorphan. Central nervous system stimulants such as amphetamine or caffeine should not be used because fatal convulsions may be induced. The safety of using propoxyphene in pregnant women and children has not been established.

Propoxyphene is adequately absorbed orally and is given only by this route. It cannot be used parenterally because of local irritation. The tissue distribution of propoxyphene has not been determined. It is metabolized primarily in the liver; metabolites and some active drug are excreted in the urine.

Propoxyphene hydrochloride is used against mild to moderate pain. The usual adult dosage is 32 to 65 mg every 6 to 8 hours. Propoxyphene is frequently administered with aspirin and phenacetin to provide an antipyretic effect and increase its analgesic potency. The following preparations are available as capsules:

> 32 or 65 mg propoxyphene HCl (Darvon)
> 32 mg with APC* (Darvon Compound)
> 65 mg with APC* (Darvon Compound-65)
> 65 mg with 325 mg aspirin (Darvon with aspirin)
> 32 mg with 325 mg aspirin and 150 mg phenaglycodol† (Darvo-Tran)

Problems that were encountered with the instability of propoxyphene hydrochloride when in close contact with aspirin required additional manufacturing steps.[17] Consequently, other propoxyphene salts were evaluated. Two napsylate salt preparations have been made available commercially. The pharmacologic effects of the napsylate salt are apparently similar to those of the hydrochloride.[18] The usual adult oral doses of the napsylate salts are 100 mg three or four times every 24 hours. Available preparations are listed as follows:

> 100 mg tablets propoxyphene napsylate (Darvon-N)
> 100 mg tablets with 325 mg aspirin (Darvon-N with Aspirin)
> 50 mg/5 ml suspension of propoxyphene napsylate (Darvon-N suspension)

Levorphanol

Levorphanol (Levo-Dromoran) is a phenanthrene synthetic that is closely related chemically and pharmacologically to morphine. It is a more potent analgesic than morphine, but adverse effects are equivalent. Consequently, it provides no advantage over morphine.

---

*227 mg aspirin, 162 mg phenacetin, and 32.4 mg caffeine.
†Minor tranquilizer.

Pentazocine

Pentazocine (Talwin) is a relatively new, potent, synthetic analgesic that was introduced in 1967. It is related chemically to the opiates and has quickly become a potent analgesic of importance in dental practice. Pentazocine has the following chemical structure:

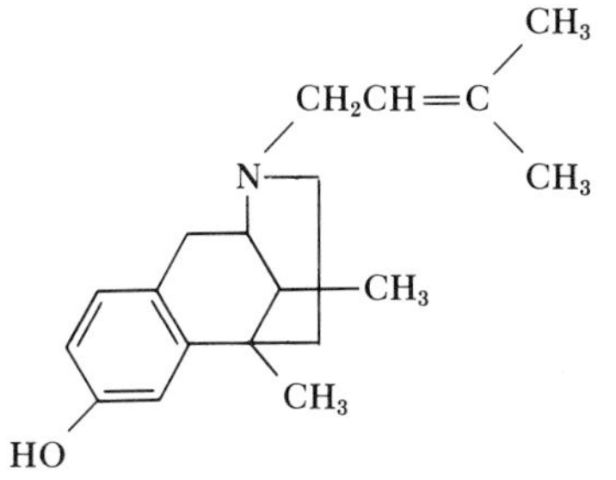

Maximal parenteral dosages of this drug appear to provide analgesia equal to that obtainable with meperidine and morphine.[19-21] This is to say that when all three drugs are administered parenterally, 30 mg pentazocine equals 10 mg morphine or 50 to 100 mg meperidine. Onset and duration are similar. Orally administered pentazocine has been observed to be one third as potent as the parenteral form.[22] Other studies of oral analgesic potency have shown 50 mg pentazocine to equal 60 mg codeine with a slightly faster onset.[23,24] Pentazocine at a 50 mg dosage has also been said to equal 100 mg meperidine given intramuscularly.[25] Onset of analgesia with orally administered pentazocine occurs in 15 to 30 minutes, and the duration is about 3 hours. Analgesic doses produce sedation but do not have antipyretic or anti-inflammatory properties. Information on tissue distribution and metabolism of pentazocine are lacking.

Pentazocine is addicting, is the subject of abuse,[26,27] and should be prescribed with the same care and concern as are applied to the prescribing of other narcotics. Adverse effects after the use of pentazocine are qualitatively and quantitatively similar to those produced by morphine and other narcotics. Sedation, dizziness, vertigo, nausea, vomiting, euphoria, and headache are most frequently seen. Less frequently, a wide variety of adverse effects occur, including hallucinations, respiratory depression, constipation, sweating, abdominal distress, diarrhea, anorexia, delusions, dermatitis, visual disturbances, vertigo, tightness of the chest, tachycardia, and changes in blood pressure. Although reproductive studies in animals have not reported developmental defects resulting from pentazocine, it is too early to recommend the use of this drug in pregnant women. Clinical experience is inadequate to recommend its use in children under 12 years of age.

Pentazocine should be useful for dental pain when codeine and nonnarcotic analgesics are ineffective. It is available as the lactate for parenteral use (30 mg/ml) and as the hydrochloride for oral use (50 mg tablets). The usual recommended adult dose is 30 mg intramuscularly, subcutaneously, or intravenously, or 50 mg orally every 3 to 4 hours. An oral dose of 100 mg can be used.

NARCOTIC ANTAGONISTS

Nalorphine, levallorphan, and naloxone prevent, reduce, or abolish the depressant effects of morphine and all other narcotics. However, they do not antagonize respiratory depression caused by nonnarcotic depressants such as the barbiturates. Their chemical structures are closely related to that of morphine.

Nalorphine

Nalorphine (Nalline) is a semisynthetic derivative of morphine, and when administered to a patient not taking a narcotic, it produces the effects of a weak morphine. It will depress respiration except in those cases where it relieves narcotic-induced respiratory depression. Consequently, nonnarcotic induced respiratory depression will be deepened by nalorphine. The usual adult dose of nalorphine is 5 to 10 mg intravenously. The effects of narcotic overdose are promptly relieved, and as noted earlier, withdrawal symptoms are precipitated in the addict. Since the duration of action of nalorphine (1½ hours) may be less than that of the narcotic, the dose may need to be repeated if respiration again becomes depressed.

Levallorphan

Levallorphan (Lorfan) is a new synthetic narcotic antagonist. Except for greater potency, its pharmacologic effects are essentially the same as those of nalorphine. The adult intravenous dose of 0.5 to 1 mg has a duration of action of about 2 hours.

Naloxone

Naloxone (Narcan) is a synthetic congener of oxymorphone. Unlike nalorphine and levallorphan, it does not produce morphine-like effects in addition to its action as a narcotic antagonist. The only pharmacologic activity of naloxone appears to be the reversal of narcotic-induced depression and the precipitation of withdrawal symptoms in narcotic addicts. Also, unlike nalorphine and levallorphan, naloxone is effective in reversing depression caused by pentazocine. The usual initial adult dose of naloxone is 0.4 mg intravenously, intramuscularly, or subcutaneously. Effects should be observed within 2 minutes; doses may be repeated at 2- to 3-minute intervals. If significant improvement is not obtained after two or three doses, the practitioner should suspect that the depression is not narcotic induced. As with the other narcotic antagonists, the duration of action may be less than that of the narcotic causing the depression, and the dosage may need to be repeated if respiration again becomes depressed.

BENZYLISOQUINOLINE OPIATES

As previously noted, these opium alkaloids depress smooth muscle, do not produce analgesia, and are not addicting. Like the phenanthrene alkaloids they have some antitussive effects.

Narcotine (Nectadon) has had some use as a cough suppressant, and papaverine (Cerespan, Lutag) has been used as a peripheral vasodilator. Neither drug is particularly important clinically.

REFERENCES

1. Reynolds, D. C.: Pain control in the dental office, Dent. Clin. North Am. **15:**319, April, 1971.
2. Cutting, W. C.: Handbook of pharmacology, ed. 5, New York, 1972, Appleton-Century-Crofts.
3. Sutherland, V. C.: A synopsis of pharmacology, ed. 2, Philadelphia, 1970, W. B. Saunders Co.
4. American Medical Association Council on Drugs: AMA drug evaluations—1971, Chicago, 1971, American Medical Association.
5. American Medical Association Council on Drugs: New drugs 1967, Chicago, 1967, American Medical Association.
6. Goodman, L. S., and Gilman, A.: The pharmacological basis of therapeutics, ed. 5, New York, 1975, The Macmillan Co.
7. Modell, W., editor: Drugs of choice—1974-1975, St. Louis, 1974, The C. V. Mosby Co.
8. Non-narcotic analgesics, Med. Lett. Drugs. Ther. **8:**8, 1966.
9. Moertel, C. G., Ahmann, D. L., and Taylor, W. F.:

A comparative evaluation of marketed analgesic drugs, N. Engl. J. Med. **286:**813, 1972.

10. Gruber, C. M., Jr., Codeine phosphate, propoxyphene HCl, and placebo, J.A.M.A. **164:**966, 1957.

11. Koslin, A. J.: A single-blind comparison of codeine PO_4 and dextropropoxyphene HCl, Oral Surg. **12:** 1203, 1959.

12. Chilton, N. W., Lewandowski, A., and Cameron, J. R.: Double blind evaluation of a new analgesic agent in post-extraction pain, Am. J. Med. Sci. **242:**702, 1961.

13. Ahlström, U., and Lantz, B.: A comparison between dextropropoxyphene hydrochloride and acetyl salicylic acid as analgesics after oral surgery, Odontol. Revy **19:**55, 1968.

14. Berdon, J. K., Strahan, J. D., Meriza, K. B., and Wade, A. B.: The effectiveness of dextropropoxyphene HCl in the control of pain after periodontal surgery, J. Periodontol. **35:**106, 1964.

15. Scopp, I. W., Morgan, F. H., Gillette, W. B., Fredrics, H. J., Peskin, M. J., and Kleinman, D.: A double blind clinical study of Dialog, Darvon and a placebo in the management of postoperative dental pain, J. Oral. Ther. **4:**123, 1967.

16. Beaver, W. T.: Mild analgesics: a review of their clinical pharmacology, Am. J. Med. Sci. **250:**577, 1965.

17. Gruber, C. M., Stevens, V. C., and Terrill, P. M.: Propoxyphene napsylate: chemistry and experimental design, Toxicol. Appl. Pharmacol. **19:**423, 1971.

18. Darvon and Darvon-N, Med. Lett. Drugs Ther. **14:**27, 1972.

19. Sadov, M. S., and Balagot, R. C.: Pentazocine—a new nonaddicting analgesic, J.A.M.A. **193:**887, 1965.

20. Gaines, H. R.: Preoperative and postoperative use of pentazocine, Ill. Med. J. **131:**320, 1967.

21. Stoelting, V. K.: Analgesic action of pentazocine compared with morphine in postoperative pain, Anesth. Analg. **44:**769, 1965.

22. Beaver, W. T., Wallenstein, S. L., Houde, R. W., and Rogers, A.: A clinical comparison of the effect of oral and intramuscular administration of analgesics, Clin. Pharmacol. Ther. **9:**582, 1968.

23. Kontos, T. G., Sunshine, A., Loska, E., Meisner, M., and Hopper, M.: Oral analgesic studies, Clin. Pharmacol. Ther. **7:**447, 1966.

24. Nasits, B. J.: Analgesia following dental surgery, Ariz. Dent. J. **13:**11, 1967.

25. Marks, M. M.: Talwin (pentazocine), new nonnarcotic analgesic in rectal surgery: a three year evaluation, Int. Surg. **48:**519, 1967.

26. Pentazocine (Talwin), Med. Lett. Drugs Ther. vol. 11, May 16, 1969.

27. American Medical Association Council on Drugs: The misuse of pentazocine: its dependence-producing potential, J.A.M.A. **209:**1518, 1969.

11

Central nervous system stimulants

RICHARD L. WYNN

The central nervous system stimulants consist of a heterogeneous group of compounds that produce various degrees of stimulation, depending on the compound, the dose, and the occasion of its use. Agents such as pentylenetetrazol, picrotoxin, nikethamide, and bemegride act mainly to stimulate respiration and to oppose the respiratory depressant actions of barbiturates. Because of their ability to overcome drug-induced respiratory depression and hypnosis, these drugs are termed *analeptics*. Other stimulants such as strychnine have selective stimulant actions on the spinal cord. In contrast, caffeine, amphetamines, and methylphenidate exert their primary actions on the cerebral cortex. In addition, the actions of some of these stimulants are not restricted to the central nervous system. For example, caffeine and two of its congeners, theophylline and theobromine, elicit various effects on other organ systems that have important therapeutic implications. The central nervous system effects and other miscellaneous effects of these stimulant drugs will be discussed in this chapter.

As a general rule, dentists do not prescribe central nervous system stimulants. However, the increasing abuse of amphetamines and methylphenidate and the ingestion of large quantities of caffeine by the public cause an increase in the number of dental patients under the influence of these drugs. Also, since the effects of these drugs are not restricted to the nervous system, this raises the possibility of many drug interactions with these agents and their resulting change in the activity of other organs.

In the past, most of the central nervous system stimulants were widely used therapeutically, but only a limited few have any therapeutic usefulness today.

ANALEPTICS AND RESPIRATORY STIMULANTS
Pentylenetetrazol (Metrazol)

Pentylenetetrazol is a stimulant to the respiratory and cardiovascular systems and a central nervous system convulsant. The chemical structure of pentylenetetrazol is shown in Fig. 10. The drug causes increases in respiration and blood pressure by the direct stimulation of the medullary respiratory and vasomotor centers. Convulsant activity occurs with higher doses because of activation of both the cerebrum and brain stem. The drug probably acts by stimulating excitatory cerebral neurons that are unopposed by inhibitory pathways. The drug also causes a decrease in the recovery time of these excitatory neurons.

Pentylenetetrazol enjoys limited use as a diagnostic aid to activate epileptogenic foci in epilepsy to characterize this cerebral disorder. As a convulsant in laboratory animals, it is used as a laboratory tool in the evaluation of potential anticonvulsant drugs. It has previously been used as a convulsant for shock therapy in involutional depression—a use superseded by electroconvulsive therapy (ECT). The drug has also been used in the past to elevate the mood in chronically depressed patients and to relieve confusion and memory loss in geriatric patients. Any real benefit in this regard is questionable, however.

Pentylenetetrazol is not useful as an analeptic in drug-induced respiratory depression. The stimulant effect of the drug is brief and may be followed by a subsequent depression. Also, a narrow dose margin exists between respiratory stimulation of drug-depressed respiration and convulsions. The drug is available as 100 mg tablets and as a 10% aqueous solution.

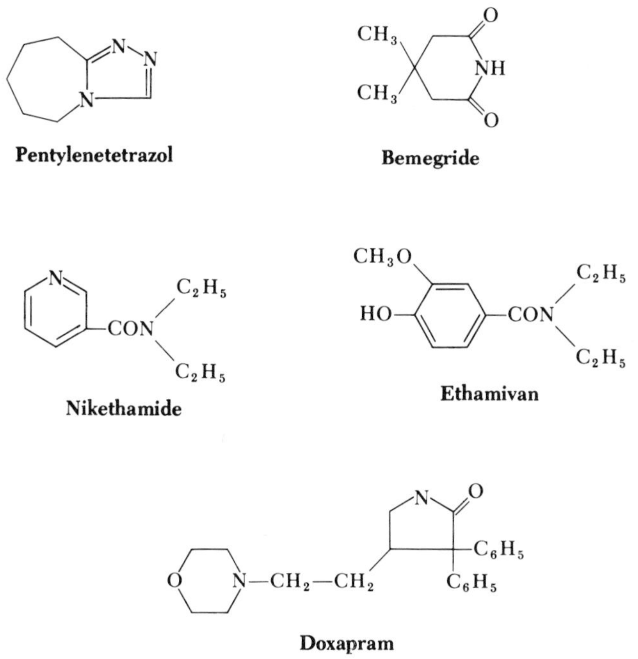

Fig. 10. Structural formulas of some central nervous system stimulants.

Bemegride (Megimide)

Bemegride is structurally similar to the barbiturates (Fig. 10) and was originally used as a specific antagonist to the depressant effects of these drugs. Bemegride has been shown to exert its effects equally as well against nonbarbiturate depressants. Bemegride resembles pentylenetetrazol in action and has been used as an analeptic, respiratory stimulant, and diagnostic aid in epilepsy. It has not been shown to be superior to pentylenetetrazol, however. Bemegride is administered by intravenous injection when used as a respiratory stimulant.

Nikethamide (Coramine)

Nikethamide is the diethyl derivative of the vitamin nicotinamide. Its chemical structure is shown in Fig. 10. The drug stimulates respiration at nonconvulsive doses and has been shown to stimulate morphine-induced respiratory depression effectively. Larger doses produce convulsions that are indistinguishable from those produced by pentylenetetrazol. Nikethamide also exerts a central depressive action after its stimulant effect—an action that renders it useless as an analeptic agent. The drug has little effect on the cardiovascular system.

Clinically, nikethamide has been used as a respiratory stimulant to counter the effects of central depressant drugs. An intravenous dose of 1 to 3 ml of a 25% solution is usually sufficient for this purpose. Nikethamide has been recommended for use as a respiratory stimulant in lung disease.[1]

Ethamivan (Emivan)

Ethamivan chemically resembles nikethamide but is more potent in its central nervous system stimulant action. It stimulates all levels of the cerebrospinal axis and stimulates the medullary respiratory centers in doses below those that cause convulsions. Like nikethamide it is recommended therapeutically as a respiratory stimulant, and its use in drug-induced respiratory depression has the same disadvantages that the other compounds have in such a situation. Ethamivan has been shown to be useful as a respiratory stimulant in hypoventilatory states.[2]

Doxapram (Dopram)

Doxapram is an effective respiratory stimulant and analeptic used to hasten arousal and the return of protective pharyngeal and laryngeal reflexes in the postanesthetic period after general anesthesia. The chemical structure of doxapram is shown in Fig. 10. The drug produces a significant increase in tidal volume and respiratory rate, and is of very short duration (2 to 5 minutes). Doxapram can also produce generalized central nervous system convulsions. Its margin of safety is sufficient, since the dose required to improve respiration is considerably below the dose needed to induce convulsions. Serious adverse effects have been produced by doxapram, including hypertension, tachycardia, arrhythmias, muscle rigidity, and vomiting.[3] Doxapram's short duration of action precludes its usefulness as a respiratory stimulant in drug-induced depression. Its untoward cardiovascular effects may be greatly increased in patients receiving sympathomimetic drugs or monoamine oxidase inhibitors.

Picrotoxin

Picrotoxin is a natural substance occurring in the seeds of the plant *Anamirta cocculus.* These seeds have been used for poisoning fish, hence the name "fish berries." Picrotoxin has been assigned the empirical formula $C_{30}H_{34}O_{13}$, and when dissolved in water, it splits into equal parts of *picrotin* and *picrotoxinin.*

Picrotoxin is a powerful stimulant to the central nervous system. The target cells are probably in the medulla, since convulsions produced by the drug persist after the removal of the cerebral hemispheres in laboratory animals. Tonic-clonic seizures occur with the drug, and respiratory volume is stimulated in the presence of drug-induced depression. Medullary stimulation of the respiratory and vasomotor centers accounts for the respiratory stimulation, hypertension, salivation, nausea, and vomiting that accompany the drug's use. The mechanism of convulsive activity is suggested to be a blockade of presynaptic inhibition[4] as opposed to pentylenetetrazol, which stimulates excitatory cerebral neurons.

The use of picrotoxin in the past has been limited to analepsis in drug-induced respiratory depression, particularly barbiturate overdosage. However, as has been stated before, the use of such an agent in this circumstance is controversial.

STRYCHNINE

Strychnine is a central nervous system convulsive agent of primarily toxicologic interest with no established therapeutic use. Strychnine is the alkaloidal component of nux vomica seeds of a tree native to India, *Strychnos nuxvomica.* This agent acts at all levels of the cerebrospinal axis, resulting in restlessness, increased respiration, muscle twitching, and convulsions. Opisthotonos and the initiation of tetanic convulsions by even the slightest sensory stimulus are the classic manifestations of its poisoning. The mechanism of strychnine is well known. The drug blocks postsynaptic inhibitory reflexes within the central nervous system, particularly in the spinal cord, allowing for the propagation of excitatory impulses throughout the complex interconnections in the cerebrospinal axis.[5] This mechanism explains why the stronger extensor muscles acting unopposed produce the characteristic posture of opisthotonos and why a variety of sensory stimuli elicit the characteristic seizures.

Strychnine was used for many years as a tonic—the tonic effect comprised the bitter taste, stimulation of the gastrointestinal tract, and an increase in tone of voluntary muscle. The latter two effects are difficult to achieve with therapeutic doses, however, and there remains no rational basis for the use of this drug in medicine.

Death from strychnine is usually due to asphyxia from respiratory arrest during tetanic convulsions. Treatment is generally aimed at blocking convulsions with intravenously administered barbiturates, an inhalant anesthetic, or a muscle relaxant, by the use of artificial respiration and oxygenation, and by minimizing sensory stimuli from the environment. Diazepam is superior to the intravenously administered barbiturates and today is considered the drug of choice to treat strychnine poisoning. Prompt control of convulsions by diazepam with little accompanying sedation affords distinct advantages over the more depressant barbiturates. Convulsions are terminated by 10 mg diazepam administered intravenously.[6] The minimum lethal oral dose of strychnine is approximately 100 mg. There exists no official preparation of strychnine.

XANTHINES

Caffeine, theophylline, and theobromine are members of a class of compounds known as xanthines.

Caffeine

Caffeine is the 1,3,7-trimethylxanthine and is the most widely ingested central nervous system stimulant by the public, since it is so readily accessible as a component in caffeinated beverages. The structures of the basic xanthine nucleus and caffeine are as follows:

Xanthine   1,3,7,-Trimethylxanthine
(caffeine)

The pharmacologic effects of caffeine that are of therapeutic interest are those acting on the central nervous system. The drug increases mental alertness, decreases drowsiness, and provides for a clear flow of ideas. Respiration may be quickened because of stimulation of the medulla. Effects other than on the central nervous system include bronchodilation, diuresis, increased gastric secretions, and cardiovascular effects. The drug increases the force of contraction of the myocardium to cause an increase in the cardiac output. There are mixed effects on blood pressure with a decrease occurring because of peripheral dilation and an increase due to the myocardial stimulation. The resulting blood pressure is determined by the balance of these two effects.

Caffeine is used therapeutically to treat common headache in combination with analgesics such as aspirin and phenacetin (APC tablets) and to treat migraine headache in combination with the ergot alkaloid ergotamine. The rationale for the use of caffeine in headache remedies is the increase in cerebral vascular resistance that results from its ability to constrict the cerebral blood vessels. Caffeine is not an effective analeptic in severe drug-induced depression.

Side effects to the use of caffeine are nervousness, irritability, tremors, insomnia, and epigastric distress. Large doses (150 mg intramuscularly) will cause the respiratory stimulation mentioned earlier. Acute toxicity by caffeine is manifested as central nervous system effects of restlessness, irritability, and generalized convulsions and as cardiovascular effects of tachycardia, hypertension, and circulatory failure. An excess of 10 Gm is required to induce convulsions, but no fatalities have been reported after its use. Habituation to caffeine is a well-known phenomenon, and tolerance develops to the insomniac and alerting effects of the drug.[7] Withdrawal symptoms to caffeine have been difficult to establish.

Caffeine is contraindicated in patients with a history of gastric ulcers. Caffeine should be used with caution in patients with coronary thrombosis, since it does increase cardiac work by stimulating the myocardium. In combination with nicotine (heavy smoking) and fatigue, caffeine has been known to cause paroxysmal atrial tachycardias. Caffeine has also been shown to cause chromosomal breakage in humans.[8] The ingestion of caffeinated beverages does not increase the mutation rate above the natural rate, however, and does not seem to present a toxic hazard in humans.

Caffeine is present in percolated or drip coffee at a concentration of 100 to 150 mg/cup, instant coffee 50 to 65 mg/cup, decaffeinated coffee 13 to 35 mg/cup, tea 43 to 110 mg/cup, and cola beverages 35 to 55 mg/12 oz. Caffeine citrate tablets are available in strengths of 60, 100, and 250 mg, and caffeine sodium benzoate is available as an intramuscular injection in ampules containing 0.25 Gm/2 ml.

Theophylline and theobromine

Theophylline and theobromine are the 1,3-dimethylxanthine and 3,7-dimethylxanthine respectively. Their chemical structures are as follows:

1,3-dimethylxanthine   3,7-dimethylxanthine
(theophylline)   (theobromine)

Theophylline and theobromine are weaker central nervous system stimulants than caffeine but have other useful properties that warrant discussion. The xanthine derivatives interfere with sodium reabsorption in the proximal renal tubules, resulting in a diuretic effect. Theophylline is the most potent and caffeine the least potent in this regard. The xanthines are also smooth muscle relaxants, with theophylline the most potent and caffeine the least potent. This action is direct and not mediated by autonomic mechanisms. As a result of smooth muscle relaxation, a therapeutically beneficial bronchodilating action is demonstrable in asthmatic patients, resulting in a concomitant decrease in airway resistance and respiratory effort.

Theophylline is the most potent and caffeine the least potent cardiac agent. A direct myocardial stimulating action of theophylline occurs, resulting in increased heart rate and force of contraction. This effect of theophylline is occasionally useful in treating acute congestive heart failure.

The mechanism of action of the xanthines is unknown. However, it may be related to the fact that methylxanthines, particularly theophylline, are competitive inhibitors of cyclic nucleotide phosphodiesterase, the enzyme that catalyzes the conversion of cyclic adenosine monophosphate (AMP) to 5'-AMP.[9] Concentrations of cyclic AMP are thus increased in certain tissues after exposure to methylxanthines. It has also been postulated that the xanthines act by reducing the binding of calcium in muscle cell membranes, thereby affecting muscle contraction.[10]

Theophylline is available as the free base but is generally used in combination with ethylene diamine and known as aminophylline. Aminophylline is available as tablets for oral administration, as a parenteral preparation, and as rectal suppositories. Aminophylline is useful in the treatment of severe attacks of asthma—particularly status asthmaticus. It is also given over prolonged periods by mouth to reduce the number and severity of asthma attacks. A single dose of 0.25 Gm is given three or four times every 24 hours. Theobromine is available as the free alkaloid and also as a variety of complexes such as theobromine calcium salicylate (Theocalcin), theobromine sodium acetate, and theobromine salicylate.

AMPHETAMINES

The amphetamines include methamphetamine (Methedrine, Desoxyn), dextrorotatory amphetamine sulfate (Dexedrine), racemic amphetamine sulfate (Benzedrine), and levoamphetamine (Levonor). The central nervous system effects of the amphetamines are manifested as a general alerting action—an increased alertness, attentiveness, wakefulness, and decreased sense of fatigue. These effects are accompanied by an elevation of mood resembling elation or euphoria. The euphoric effects predispose these compounds to misuse and abuse. The amphetamines also exhibit anorexiant and analeptic effects, cause an increase in psychomotor activity, and provide sympathomimetic effects on the autonomic nervous system. They cause a release of catecholamines, an action that may partly account for their sympathomimetic activity. The anorexiant activity of these compounds may result in weight loss primarily from appetite suppression. Tolerance continues to this effect, however, and continued weight loss requires dietary restrictions. Analeptic activity is noticed only with high doses. Systolic and diastolic blood pressure and pulse pressure are usually increased, and reflex bradycardia becomes predominant with the continued use of these drugs.

Acute toxicity from overdosage of the amphetamines includes dizziness, mental confusion, hallucinations, and convulsions. Cardiovascular toxicities occur as hypertension, palpitations, and arrhythmias. Chronic toxicity from the long-term use of these drugs is characterized by physical exhaustion and collapse, weight loss, insomnia, dermatitis, and psychotic episodes. Psychic dependence is well known for the amphetamines, but physical dependence is less completely established. Withdrawal reactions associated with a so-called physical dependence have been documented as rebound exhaustion, mental depression, and an increase in the rhomboencephalic phase of the electroencephalographic pattern during sleep.

Therapeutic use of the amphetamines depends on their central effects rather than their sympathomimetic actions. They are used in patients with obesity, narcolepsy, parkinsonism, and mild depressions. Their use as analeptics has been unsuccessful. The amphetamines should be used with caution in the presence of hypertension, cardiac and cerebrovascular disease, and hyperthyroidism and in emotionally unstable individuals predisposed to drug abuse.

MISCELLANEOUS AGENTS
Methylphenidate (Ritalin)

Methylphenidate is structurally related to the amphetamines, and its pharmacology is essentially similar to these drugs. Methylphenidate produces mild central nervous system stimulation, but large doses can produce generalized central nervous system excitement leading to convulsions. Methylphenidate also shares the abuse potential of the amphetamines.

The effectiveness of methylphenidate to treat overdosage of depressant drugs and to relieve lassitude from various causes is not well established. It probably enjoys its greatest use as an adjunct in the therapy of hyperkinetic syndromes in children characterized as having minimal brain dysfunction (MBD).[11] The drug improves both behavior and learning ability in these children. Methylphenidate also has been used in the treatment of narcolepsy.

Flurothyl (Indoklon)

Krantz and co-workers,[12] while screening for potential fluorinated anesthetics, showed that bis (2,2,2-trifluoroethyl) ether (flurothyl) produced convulsions in laboratory animals when the vapor was inhaled or the liquid administered systemically. Subsequent clinical trials indicated that the compound was useful as a convulsive agent for therapy of mental disorders. In clinical use flurothyl has been substituted for electroconvulsive therapy in treating schizoaffective reactions associated with depression and in acute schizophrenic reactions associated with excitement or withdrawal from reality.

REFERENCES

1. Feinsilver, O.: The role of nikethamide as a respiratory stimulant in the management of pulmonary insufficiency, Curr. Ther. Res. 4:165-177, 1962.
2. Rodman, T., Fennelly, J. F., Kraft, A. J., and Close, H. P.: Effect of ethamivan on alveolar ventilation in patients with chronic lung disease, N. Engl. J. Med. 267:1279, 1962.
3. Wolfson, B., Siker, E. S., and Ciccarelli, H. E.: A double blind comparison of doxapram, ethamivan and methylphenidate, Am. J. Med. Sci. 249:391-398, 1965.
4. Eccles, J. C., Schmidt, R., and Willes, W. D.: Pharmacological studies on presynaptic inhibition, J. Physiol. (Lond.) 168:500-530, 1963.
5. Bradley, K., Easton, D. W., and Eccles, J. C.: An investigation of primary or direct inhibition, J. Physiol. (Lond.) 122:474-488, 1953.
6. Jackson, G., Ng, S. H., Diggle, G. E., and Bourke, I. G.: Strychnine poisoning treated successfully with diazepam, Br. Med. J. 3:519-520, 1971.
7. Colton, T., Gosselin, R. E., and Smith, R. P.: The tolerance of coffee drinkers to caffeine, Clin. Pharmacol. Ther. 9:31-39, 1968.
8. Ostertag, W., Duisberg, E., and Sturmann, M.: The mutagenic activity of caffeine in man, Mutat. Res. 2:293-296, 1965.
9. Butcher, R. W., and Sutherland, E. W.: Adenosine 3',5'-phosphate in biological materials, J. Biol. Chem. 237:1244-1250, 1962.
10. Gubareff, T. de, and Sleaton, W., Jr.: Effects of caffeine on mammalian atrial muscle and its interaction with calcium, J. Pharmacol. Exp. Ther. 148:202-214, 1965.
11. Millichap, J. G.: Drugs in the management of minimal brain dysfunction, Ann. N.Y. Acad. Sci. 205:321-334, 1973.
12. Krantz, J. C., Jr., Truitt, E. B., Jr., Ling, A. S. C., and Speers, L.: Anesthesia IV. The pharmacological response to hexafluorodiethyl ether, J. Pharmacol. Exp. Ther. 121:362-308, 1957.

12

Anticonvulsant drugs

SEBASTIAN G. CIANCIO

Although all convulsions are not epileptic per se, the most common convulsive disorder treated with anticonvulsant drugs is epilepsy. It is estimated that approximately 1 in every 200 persons is afflicted with some form of epilepsy. In view of the incidence of this disorder, dentists will often encounter epileptics in their daily practice. Since some anticonvulsant drugs cause gingival hyperplasia and other clinically important side effects, they are of special interest to dentistry.

TYPES OF EPILEPSY

Epilepsy can result from trauma, metabolic diseases, developmental defects, tumors, or brain disease. However, the etiology is unknown in most cases and is therefore classified as idiopathic.

Epileptic seizures can be classified as grand mal, petit mal, psychomotor, or Jacksonian. Grand mal seizures are characterized by the following:

1. A sensation, usually visual or auditory, which generally precedes a seizure (aura)
2. Loss of consciousness
3. Muscle contractions (duration 1 to 5 minutes)
4. Amnesia during the convulsion

Petit mal seizures are characterized by the following:

1. No aura
2. Minor erratic head, eye, or extremity movements (duration 5 to 30 seconds)
3. Manifestations that in some seizures may only be detectable by an examination of brain wave patterns
4. Amnesia

Psychomotor seizures are characterized by the following:

1. Preceded by an aura
2. Impairment of consciousness

3. Patterned attacks of confused behavior (duration, 30 seconds).

These seizures have also been referred to as temporal lobe seizures, since abnormal brain wave activity associated with them is centered on the anterior temporal lobe of the brain.

Jacksonian seizures are characterized as follows:

1. May or may not be preceded by an aura
2. No effect on consciousness
3. Convulsions confined to a single limb or muscle group
4. May progress to grand mal seizure

Based on the description of these seizures, grand mal and petit mal seizures are representative of generalized seizures, and psychomotor and Jacksonian ones are representative of partial seizures. A more detailed discussion of epilepsy can be found in various textbooks and journal reports.[1,2]

PHARMACOLOGIC MANAGEMENT

The antiepileptic drugs are central nervous system depressants with sufficient specificity to prevent epileptic seizures without causing excessive drowsiness. Although the mechanism of action of these drugs as anticonvulsants is not completely known, it is believed that their primary effect is to prevent the spread of abnormal cerebral electrical discharges.

The choice of an anticonvulsant drug is based on the type of seizure rather than on the cause of the seizure. However, since convulsive episodes may be diagnostic for certain serious brain disorders, the physician utilizes this information in reaching a final diagnosis, and although he uses an anticonvulsant drug to treat symptoms, the overall objective is to determine the cause of the convulsion and treat the etiologic factor whenever possible.

The appropriate dosage of any drug or combination of drugs depends on the age, size, and condition of the patient, his response to treatment, and the possible synergistic or antagonistic effect of other drugs given in conjunction with the anticonvulsant drug. The dosage of anticonvulsants for children is usually somewhat larger on a weight basis than that for adults. Except for control of an acute convulsion, patients are generally started on a small or moderate dose, which is increased slowly until the convulsions are controlled or minor signs and symptoms of toxicity are manifested. If toxic signs develop before control is obtained, another drug is usually prescribed. At times, when control cannot be achieved with a single drug, combination with another drug results in good control and minimal toxicity.

Most drugs useful in the treatment of epilepsy can be categorized as follows. The main areas of usefulness are also indicated.

Barbiturates (grand mal and psychomotor)
    Mephobarbital (Mebaral)
    Metharbital (Gemonil)
    Phenobarbital (Luminal)
Primidone (Mysoline) (grand mal and psychomotor)
Hydantoins (grand mal and psychomotor)
    Ethotoin (Peganone)
    Mephenytoin (Mesantoin)
    Phenytoin or diphenylhydantoin (Dilantin)
Oxazolidones (petit mal)
    Paramethadione (Paradione)
    Trimethadione (Tridione)
Succinimides (petit mal)
    Ethosuximide (Zarotin)
    Methsuximide (Celontin)
    Phensuximide (Milontin)
Miscellaneous anticonvulsants
    Acetazolamide (Diamox) (grand mal and petit mal)
    Phenacemide (Phenurone) (psychomotor)

Barbiturates

The three most commonly used barbiturates in the treatment of epilepsy are mephobarbital (Mebaral), metharbital (Gemonil) and phenobarbital (Luminal). Although a low incidence of gingival hyperplasia has been reported with the use of these drugs, the degree of hyperplasia is seldom clinically significant.[3] Metharbital and mephobarbital are somewhat less potent than phenobarbital but are useful in some cases where phenobarbital has not been effective. Phenobarbital was first introduced as an anticonvulsant in 1912. It is long acting and is still the most widely used anticonvulsant. The reader is referred to Chapter 6 for a discussion of barbiturates as sedatives.

Phenobarbital is given alone or in conjunction with phenytoin for the control of epilepsy. It is sometimes the initial drug of choice because it controls multiple types of seizures and is relatively safe. In general, the drugs that are effective in grand mal epilepsy are usually not effective in petit mal epilepsy and vice versa. Phenobarbital is an exception to this rule in that it is used to control both types of seizures. However, it is most effective in controlling seizures of the grand mal and psychomotor type.

Since phenobarbital is a sedative, drowsiness, which is usually transient, is the most common adverse effect. However, some children exhibit an opposite effect and become hyperactive. It is thought that when this drug elicits excitation, underlying minimal brain dysfunction may be present. With time, tolerance to the sedative effects occurs but not to the anticonvulsant effects. Although long-term treatment with barbiturates results in physical and psychic dependence, the doses given for epilepsy seldom present a problem of addiction.

Although the barbiturates are respiratory depressants, this usually becomes a clinical problem only when overdose occurs. If an epileptic patient being treated with a barbiturate presents with breathing difficulties, a possible barbiturate overdosage must be suspected and the patient's physician should be contacted. Also, in these patients inhalation anesthetics such as nitrous oxide should not be administered, since a respiratory problem is probably present.

When phenobarbital is administered in the management of epilepsy, 2 weeks of therapy may be necessary before a determination can be made of its effectiveness in controlling convulsions.

Phenobarbital is prepared as the sodium salt for injection intramuscularly or intravenously in the control of severe, continuous convulsions classified as status epilepticus. However, the current trend is to use diazepam (Valium) for this purpose.

Primidone (Mysoline)

Primidone is chemically similar to the barbiturates and is partially metabolized to phenobarbital. Its principal use is as a substitute for barbiturates in patients not responding to other drug therapy. When used for this reason, larger doses are needed than with phenobarbital. As with the barbiturates, sedation diminishes with continued administration. In contrast to the barbiturates, skin eruptions and anemia have been reported in conjunction with its use. Other side effects include dizziness, nausea, vomiting, diplopia, and nystagmus. Patients taking this drug for long periods of time have complained of vague gingival pains.[4] The etiology of this complaint is not clear.

Hydantoins

A number of drugs are classified as hydantoins and include phenytoin (Dilantin), ethotoin (Peganone), and mephenytoin (Mesantoin). Periodic blood studies are indicated in patients taking these medications, since anemia (megaloblastic type) has been associated with their use. Lymphadenopathies simulating malignant lymphomas have been related to therapy with these drugs, particularly with the use of mephenytoin. Usually this is reversible with cessation of therapy. On occasion liver disorders have been related to therapy with the hydantoins. Gingival hyperplasia has been associated with two of the drugs in this group, for example, phenytoin and to a lesser extent mephenytoin.

Ethotoin (Peganone)

Ethotoin is a hydantoin derivative that is less effective and less toxic than phenytoin but has not been associated with gingival hyperplasia. Therefore it may be an excellent alternative drug for the hyperplasia susceptible patient.

Mephenytoin (Mesantoin)

Mephenytoin is as effective as phenytoin for many major convulsive disorders but is more toxic.

Mephenytoin has a sedative effect that is usually absent with phenytoin. On the other hand, it has a lower incidence of gingival hyperplasia, hirsutism, and gastric distress but is more toxic than phenytoin. Serious side effects associated with its usage include skin eruptions, blood dyscrasias, hepatitis, systemic lupus erythematosus, and lymphadenopathy simulating malignant lymphomas.

When mephenytoin is used, it is generally given concurrently with other agents, in the lowest dose possible, and only in patients who fail to respond to or do not tolerate safer agents. Because of its sedative effects, it is more often employed concurrently with phenytoin than with phenobarbital or primidone.

Phenytoin (Dilantin)

Phenytoin, also referred to as diphenylhydantoin is the most useful drug for the treatment of grand mal type of convulsion, and it is used by itself or in combination with phenobarbital or primidone. It has also been used with some success to relieve the pain of trigeminal neuralgia. The mechanism of action of phenytoin is thought to be related to its stabilizing effect on cell membranes and its alteration of synaptic transmission. These events are probably related to the alteration of movement of ions across cell membranes. However, all the aspects of its mechanism of action have not been elucidated.

An advantage of phenytoin over the barbiturates is that it does not produce sedation in normal therapeutic doses. Although not absorbed from the gastrointestinal tract as rapidly as the barbiturates, it is absorbed well enough to warrant oral administration. Once it is ingested, absorption is variable with peak plasma concentrations occurring between 3 and 12 hours after ingestion. Once in plasma, the drug is highly bound to protein (70% to 95%).

A number of toxic effects of phenytoin have been reported. These include skin eruptions, gastric distress, peripheral neuropathy, gingival hyperplasia, hirsutism, hepatitis, bone marrow depression, systemic lupus erythematosis, Stevens-Johnson syndrome, and lymphadenopathy resembling malignant lymphomas. Dental personnel should be aware of these toxicities and be prepared to alert the patient if any of them is detected at the patient's dental visit.

Various investigators have reported that the incidence of hyperplasia of the gingival tissue in children receiving phenytoin ranges between 3% and 62%, with a mean of 50%. These epidemiologic studies have used populations whose members have been taking phenytoin for varying periods. A number of investigators have suggested that gingival hyperplasia can be prevented with good oral hygiene.[5-7]

Table 12-1. Miscellaneous anticonvulsants

Generic name	Trade name	Side effects
Acetazolamide	Diamox	Drowsiness, facial and extremity paresthesia, fatigue, renal disorders, gastrointestinal disturbances
Carbamazepine	Tegretol	Mood elevation, increased alertness, abnormal involuntary movements, neurologic disturbances, peripheral neuritis, paresthesia, blood dyscrasias, dermatologic disorders, adverse effects on cardiovascular, hepatic, and genitourinary systems
Ethosuximide	Zarontin	Gastrointestinal disturbances, drowsiness, headache, euphoria, rash, hiccough, behavioral changes, blood dyscrasias
Methsuximide	Celontin	Gastrointestinal disturbances, drowsiness, headache, severe mental depression
Paramethadione	Paradione	Similar to trimethadione but less severe
Phenacemide	Phenurone	Hepatitis, blood dyscrasias, toxic psychosis, depression, nephropathy, rash, gastrointestinal disturbances
Phensuximide	Milontin	Nausea, drowsiness, rash, reversible nephropathy
Trimethadione	Tridione	Severe dermatologic disorders, nephropathy, hepatitis, blood dyscrasias, hair loss, congenital defects

When gingival hyperplasia occurs, it is usually more severe if the patient receives the medication at 15 years of age of younger. Adults who are receiving phenytoin seldom show a high incidence or severity of gingival hyperplasia. The hyperplasia first manifests itself as an enlargement of the interproximal papillae and progresses from this point. In some cases the gingival enlargement is merely seen as nodular papillae. In other cases it has been noted to extend over the occlusal surfaces of the teeth and thus interfere with chewing. The hyperplasia is more severe in the anterior portion of the oral cavity and sometimes creates severe esthetic and psychological problems for the patient.

When the gingival hyperplasia interferes with plaque control, esthetics, or mastication, periodontal surgery is indicated. If plaque control is excellent after periodontal surgery, the degree and speed of recurrence can be minimized.

Some investigators have reported a successful reduction in gingival hyperplasia after the use of pressure devices on gingival tissues.[8] However, these findings are contradicted by other reports. Consequently, the value of using pressure devices to reduce hyperplasia is not clear at present.

The mechanism by which phenytoin produces gingival hyperplasia is not clear. It appears that this drug can stimulate collagen production by fibroblasts and thus result in clinical signs of hyperplasia.[9] There is also some evidence that phenytoin indirectly affects soft tissue metabolism through an alteration in the activity of the adrenal gland.[10]

Miscellaneous anticonvulsants

A number of other drugs are occasionally used for the treatment of convulsions. These drugs are generally less effective than those previously described and therefore are not used as often. The side effects of these less frequently used drugs are summarized in Table 12-1.

DENTAL CONSIDERATIONS

Although it is not the intent of this chapter to discuss the dental care of the epileptic patient, certain pharmacologic considerations should be noted.

Except for emergency care, the epileptic should not undergo dental treatment until the proper medical control of his seizures has been obtained. The patient's physician should be consulted to obtain a status report on the patient and ascertain any contraindications or special considerations relative to the specific patient. Even "controlled" epileptics may experience a convulsion in the dental office. Some seizures may be evoked by fear and excitement. Consequently, a calm approach to treatment is imperative, and preoperative sedation should be considered. The dentist should also be aware that excitement which may occur during induction with nitrous oxide may dispose to seizures.

If a convulsion does occur in the dental office, the following points should be kept in mind:

1. A bite-block or appropriate substitute should be available to protect the tongue and teeth during a convulsion.
2. The patient should be protected from injury but not heavily restrained.
3. Although adequate oxygenation generally does not present a problem, the patient should be observed for signs of anoxia.

Most antiepileptic drugs cause various symptoms related to central nervous system depression. This should be considered in developing a treatment plan for plaque control in these patients. They will require a slower approach with fewer initial demands placed on them and patience on the part of the practitioner.

Facial paresthesia has been reported with two anticonvulsant drugs, namely carbamazepine and acetazolamide. Therefore complaints of numbness in the head and neck area may be related directly to these drugs and not to a severe dental problem. It should be noted that carbamazepine is sometimes used by patients with trigeminal neuralgia.[11]

Since blood dyscrasias have been reported after the long-term use of many anticonvulsants, an adequate blood workup should be done for patients on long-term therapy prior to surgical procedures. If a blood dyscrasia is present, it could result in poor wound healing and postoperative infection.

The dentist should be aware of the other adverse effects and drug interactions associated with the anticonvulsant drugs and be alert to their recognition. Drug interactions of anticonvulsant drugs are considered in Chapter 12.

REFERENCES

1. Gastaut, H.: Clinical and electroencephalographical classification of epileptic seizures, Epilepsia 11:102, 1970.
2. Aird, R. B., and Woodbury, D. M.: Management of epilepsy, Springfield, Ill., 1974, Charles C Thomas, Publisher.
3. Panuska, H. J., Gorlin, R. J., Bearman, J. E., and Mitchell, D. F.: The effect of anticonvulsant drugs upon the gingiva: a series of 1048 patients, II, J. Periodontol. 32:15, 1961.
4. Anticonvulsants. In American Dental Association–Council on Dental Therapeutics: Accepted dental therapeutics, ed. 36, Chicago, 1975, American Dental Association.
5. Ziskin, D. E., Stowe, L. R., and Zegarelli, E. V.: Dilantin hyperplastic gingivitis, Am. J. Orthod. 27:350, 1941.
6. Hall, W. B.: Prevention of dilantin hyperplasia: a preliminary report, Bull. Acad. Gen. Dent. 20: June, 1969.
7. Ciancio, S. G., Yaffee, S. J., and Catz, C. C.: Gingival hyperplasia and diphenylhydantoin, J. Periodontol. 43:411, 1972.
8. Aiman, R.: The use of positive pressure mouthpiece as a new therapy for dilantin gingival hyperplasia, Chron. Omaha Dent. Soc. 131:244, 1968.
9. Shafer, W. G.: Effect of dilantin sodium on various cell lines in tissue culture, Proc. Soc. Exp. Biol. Med. 108:694, 1961.
10. Werk, E. E., Thrasher, K., Shilton, L. J., Olinger, C., and Young, C.: Cortisol production in epileptic patients treated with diphenylhydantoin, Clin. Pharmacol. Ther. 12:698, 1971.
11. Miscellaneous drugs: AMA drug evaluations, ed. 2, Acton, Mass., 1973, Publishing Sciences Group, Inc.

13
Autonomic drugs

TOMMY W. GAGE

Drugs affecting the autonomic nervous system play an important role in clinical dental therapeutics. The practical application of vasoconstrictors in local anesthetics and of agents that reduce salivary flow are perhaps the best known examples of autonomic drugs used in dentistry. Drugs that have effects on other body systems may also influence autonomic function. Indeed, many drug responses such as change in heart rate, blood pressure, and intestinal motility result from secondary effects on the autonomic nervous system. Therefore it is important for dentists to have a working knowledge of autonomic drugs for use in dental therapy and to be able to predict possible patient responses resulting from medical treatment with drugs having either a direct or indirect effect on autonomic function.

ORGANIZATION OF THE AUTONOMIC NERVOUS SYSTEM
Anatomic organization

The autonomic nervous system is divided into two divisions, the sympathetic and parasympathetic, as distinguished by the location of their originating nerve cell bodies. Even though these cell bodies are located within the central nervous system and receive considerable input centrally, they must be regarded as peripheral in modes of action and drug reactions.[1]

Cell bodies giving rise to the sympathetic division are located in the intermediolateral horn of the spinal cord beginning at the first thoracic through second or third lumbar vertebrae. Projections from these cell bodies, termed *preganglionic fibers*, pass out of the spinal column with the segmental spinal nerves. The preganglionic fibers leave the spinal nerves almost immediately on exiting from the cord and enter the sympathetic chain located along each side of the spinal column. Once a part of the sympathetic chain, preganglionic fibers may synapse with other cell bodies at the same segmental level or they may project up or down the sympathetic chain to synapse with cell bodies of different spinal segments. Some preganglionic fibers pass through the sympathetic chain without synapsing and enter into collateral ganglia. Preganglionic fibers synapse with those cell bodies which give origin to the postganglionic fibers. The postganglionic fibers then terminate at the effector organ or tissue site.[2]

A single sympathetic preganglionic fiber may form multiple synaptic junctions with numerous postganglionic neurons. The high ratio of synaptic connections between preganglionic and postganglionic fibers allows for a diffuse response from the sympathetic division. The adrenal medulla also receives innervation from sympathetic preganglionic fibers. It functions much like a large sympathetic ganglion, with the glandular tissues of the medulla representing the postganglionic component. Discharge of the sympathetic division causes release of epinephrine and norepinephrine from the adrenal medulla into the circulation, accounting for an even more complete and diffuse response.[3]

Cell bodies giving rise to the preganglionic fibers of the parasympathetic division have their origin in the nuclei of the third, seventh, ninth, and tenth cranial nerves, as well as second through fourth sacral segments. Parasympathetic ganglia are located on or in proximity to the effector organ rather than in a paravertebral chain as in the case of the sympathetic division. There is, with certain exceptions, a much lower ratio of synaptic connections between preganglionic and postganglionic neurons; thus the response to parasympathetic discharge is not as pronounced or diffuse as that of the sympathetic division.[4]

Functional organization

The autonomic nervous system is concerned with the maintenance of a constant internal environment providing for optimal cellular function and survival. This includes such things as reflex vasodilation, where shifting the blood supply helps to regulate body temperature. Blood glucose level, cardiac rate, water balance, and metabolism may be regulated through autonomic mechanisms. The sympathetic division is designed to cope with sudden emergencies such as that described by the fright and flight phenomenon. On the other hand, the parasympathetic division is concerned with the conservation of bodily processes. Reflex slowing of the heart rate is an example of parasympathetic activity.[5]

The autonomic nervous system innervates almost all body tissues, with many organs receiving innervation from both the sympathetic and parasympathetic divisions. When this occurs, the functional capacity of the tissue is equal to the algebraic sum of the excitatory and inhibitory influences of the two divisions. Table 13-1 summarizes the response of the major tissue and organ systems to the autonomic nervous system.

Neurotransmitters

In order to comprehend the manner in which drugs influence the response of the autonomic nervous system, one needs to understand the concept of chemical neurotransmitters and synaptic relay. Nerves transmit signals along their length by self-propagated electrical signals termed *action potentials or impulses*. These signals are carried across synapses, that is, from nerve to nerve or nerve to effector organs and tissues, by chemical mediators called *neurotransmitters*. These neurotransmitters cross the synaptic space and stimulate the postsynaptic nerve or effector tissue.[6]

Neural tissues synthesize and store the neurotransmitter. After the transmitter has interacted with the postsynaptic tissues, its effect may be terminated by (1) enzymatic inactivation, (2) dilution by body fluids, or (3) a reuptake mechanism in the presynaptic endings.[7] Therefore drugs may affect the autonomic nervous system by altering the synthesis, storage, release, or disposition of the neurotransmitter or its action at the receptor site.

The chemical mediators of the autonomic nervous system are now well known. Acetylcholine is the specific chemical mediator at all parasympathetic synapses and at sympathetic preganglionic synapses.[9] It is also the mediator at neuromuscular junctions in skeletal muscle. In the special case of the sweat glands, acetylcholine also mediates sympathetic postganglionic responses. The principal chemical mediators of the sympathetic postganglionic fibers are norepinephrine and epinephrine. Whereas norepinephrine is the major chemical mediator

Table 13-1. Response of major tissue and organ systems to autonomic nervous system

Organs or tissues (effector)	Parasympathetic division	Sympathetic division
Salivary	Vasodilation	Vasoconstriction
	Secretion (thin, high water content)	Secretion (viscid, low water content)
Heart	Cardiac slowing	Cardiac acceleration
	Coronary constriction (?)	Increase in force of contraction
		Coronary dilation (?)
Bronchial smooth muscle	Constriction	Relaxation
Iris of eye	Constriction	Dilation
	Accommodation, for near vision	Accommodation for distant vision
Adrenal medulla	—	Secretion of neurohumoral agents
Vessels of skeletal muscles	Dilation, if any	Dilation
Vessels of skin	Dilation, if any	Constriction
Intestines	Increase in peristalsis and secretions	Decrease in peristalsis and secretions
	Sphincters relax	Sphincter constriction
Liver	—	Glycogenolysis
Spleen capsule	—	Constriction

released at the postsynaptic endings, epinephrine is the major mediator released by the adrenal medulla. It has been traditional to classify the response produced by nerves on the basis of the chemical transmitter released at the synapse. Thus nerves that release acetylcholine are termed *cholinergic* and those releasing norepinephrine are termed *adrenergic*, presumably after the adrenal gland.[8]

PHARMACOLOGY OF THE PARASYMPATHETIC DIVISION
Acetylcholine

Acetylcholine has been identified as the principal mediator of the parasympathetic division as well as the ganglia of the sympathetic division. It is a quaternary ammonium compound that is synthesized in the neural tissues[10] and stored in vesicles located in the presynaptic terminals of the nerves.

An action potential traveling along the neuron causes the release of stored acetylcholine from the synaptic storage vesicles. A sufficient quantity of acetylcholine must be released to cross the synaptic cleft and initiate a response in the postsynaptic tissue. If the postsynaptic tissue is a postganglionic nerve, the usual consequence is depolarization with generation of an action potential in that neuron. In the case of the postganglionic parasympathetic fibers, the postsynaptic tissue is an effector organ and the response will be that of the effector.

The fact that some postsynaptic tissues respond to acetylcholine and not other mediators implies that acetylcholine must possess certain characteristics acceptable to the responding tissues. Therefore it must fit physically and chemically a specifically structured postsynaptic tissue component (the receptor) to be an effective mediator. It can be demonstrated that usual doses of atropine can block the action of acetylcholine at postganglionic endings but not at the neuromuscular junction. Other drugs have been used to illustrate similar stimulating or blocking effects at the various sites of action of acetylcholine. This information implies that different types of receptors may be located at the synapses where acetylcholine has been identified as the mediator. Some of these receptors may be affected by one drug but not another. As an example, curare blocks the response of skeletal muscle to acetylcholine but does not block its effect on the salivary glands. Other

factors, such as the quantity of acetylcholine released, the size of the synaptic cleft, and the tissue penetrability of drugs, may also account for differences in receptor response to drugs at acetylcholine-mediated junctions.[11]

For acetylcholine to function as a physiologic neurotransmitter, its action must be reversible and terminate rapidly. The actions of acetylcholine are reversible, since it is inactivated rapidly by the enzyme, acetylcholine esterase. This enzyme is found associated with the synaptic tissues and can hydrolyze acetylcholine more rapidly than do other nonspecific plasma choline esterases. The molecule is enzymatically hydrolyzed to inactive choline and acetic acid.[12]

Mechanism of action

The action of many drugs may now be predicted and explained on the basis of the information presented about acetylcholine neurotransmission. Drugs can be synthesized that resemble acetylcholine in structure and can imitate its effects when administered. Such drugs are referred to as *cholinergic* or *parasympathomimetic*, and they have the physical and chemical characteristics necessary to fit the acetylcholine receptor. In addition, side chains or radicals may be added so that their rate of enzymatic hydrolysis is reduced, thereby changing their duration of action and route of administration. Drugs are also available that selectively affect certain acetylcholine-mediated synapses but not others. It is possible to prolong the effects of acetylcholine with the use of drugs that are specific inhibitors of the enzymatic action of acetylcholine esterase. Finally, the action of acetylcholine may be blocked by the use of drugs that prevent its union with the receptor. Such drugs are termed *anticholinergic* or *parasympatholytic*.

Cholinergic drugs
Choline esters

The natural prototype of the choline esters is acetylcholine. However, acetylcholine is not useful as a therapeutic agent because of its rapid destruction by plasma esterases and its lack of a selective action. Since acetylcholine has a powerful parasympathetic stimulant action, efforts have been made to synthesize drugs of a similar chemical structure to that of acetylcholine but with a longer and more selective action. These efforts have met

Table 13-2. Drugs of choline ester structure and their uses

Drug name	Medical use
Acetylcholine chloride	Not useful
Methacholine chloride (Mecholyl chloride)	Infrequent use in heart block
Bethanechol chloride (Urecholine chloride)	Postoperative abdominal distension and urinary retention
Carbachol	Ophthalmology (glaucoma)
Furtrethonium iodide (Furamon, Furanol)	Overcome urinary retention

with limited success. Drugs in this category, all having the basic choline ester structure, and their uses are shown in Table 13-2. As one can observe from the table, these drugs have their greatest usefulness in medicine.

The pharmacology of the choline esters reflects the actions of acetylcholine. The most noticeable effects being a fall in blood pressure attributable to generalized vasodilation, flushing of the skin, a slowing of the heart rate, and increased tone and activity of both the gastrointestinal and urinary tract. Topical application of the drugs to the eye causes miosis (constriction of the pupil) and a decrease in intraocular pressure. Central nervous system effects are not observed with the usual therapeutic doses. Other manifestations of parasympathetic activity are observed in varying degrees depending on the dose employed and individual patient sensitivity to the drug.

The side effects and toxic reactions associated with the use of the choline esters resemble those of a general stimulation of parasympathetic activity. Included in these reactions are excessive salivation, flushed skin, abdominal cramps with diarrhea, bradycardia, and a decrease in blood pressure. A cholinergic sympathetic response is associated with an increase in sweating. Larger doses may provoke serious cardiovascular problems resulting in shock.

The choline esters have limited application in dental therapeutics, if any. Attempts to use some of these drugs to promote salivation have been unsuccessful because of their widespread effect on various body systems. In case there should arise a situation whereby a dentist would utilize these drugs, the contraindications to their use should be noted, as follows: (1) bronchial asthma, (2) hyperthyroidism, (3) mechanical obstruction of the gastrointestinal or urinary tract, (4) severe cardiac disease, and (5) in patients receiv-

ing neostigmine for myasthenia gravis therapy.[13]

Alkaloids

In addition to the synthetic choline esters, there are three naturally occurring alkaloids that can stimulate the peripheral postsynaptic acetylcholine receptor. These drugs are muscarine, pilocarpine, and arecoline. The latter two can also stimulate the ganglia. Muscarine is useful as a research tool, and the action of acetylcholine at postganglionic parasympathetic sites is often referred to as a muscarinic response. Pilocarpine is the most useful of the alkaloids in medicine being employed as a miotic. It has been used, with varying degrees of success, to increase salivary flow. The usual adult dose is 5 mg given orally or by subcutaneous injection. If used this way, the patient should be cautioned about the possibility of other parasympathetic effects such as sweating and visual disturbances. It should be pointed out that treatment of dry mouth may present a special management problem in that the lack of salivary flow may reflect a systemic disease which requires special care.[14,15]

Cholinesterase inhibitors

Prolongation of the effects of acetylcholine may be achieved by the use of drugs that inhibit the enzyme, acetylcholine esterase. This may be accomplished with a rather large and heterogeneous group of agents, each with varying degrees of application in medicine. Table 13-3 lists drugs with anticholinesterase activity and their usual therapeutic indication.

The anticholinesterase drugs may be divided into three categories based on the reversibility of their reaction with the esterase enzyme. Physostigmine and neostigmine are slowly reversible, whereas adrophonium is rapidly reversible. The chemical warfare agents and insecticides are essentially non-

Table 13-3. Drugs with anticholinesterase activity and their usefulness

Anticholinesterase agent	Major usefulness
Alkaloids	
Physostigmine salicylate (Eserine)	Miotic, anticurare action
Synthetic agents	
Neostigmine (Prostigmin)	Anticurare agent, miotic, myasthenia gravis
Pyridostigmine bromide (Mestinon)	Myasthenia gravis
Ambenonium chloride (Mytelase)	Myasthenia gravis
Demecarium bromide (Humorsol)	Glaucoma
Echothiophate iodide (Phospholine)	Glaucoma
Edrophonium chloride (Tensilon)	Diagnosis of myasthenia gravis, anticurare agent
Chemical agents	
Malathion	Insecticide
Parathion	Insecticide
Sarin (GB)	Chemical warfare agent
Tabun	Chemical warfare agent

reversible and hence have a long duration of action. Most of the useful drugs are employed in ophthalmology to treat glaucoma or in the treatment of myasthenia gravis.[16]

More recently a new use has been suggested for physostigmine. An occasional side effect of delirium has occurred with the use of some of the benzodiazepine class of drugs, that is, diazepam and lorazepam. Small doses of physostigmine given by injection have been reported to terminate the apparent hallucinogenic component of this side effect effectively. It can be suggested that the synthetic anticholinesterase drugs would not produce a similar effect because they are quaternary compounds and will not cross the blood-brain barrier.

The side effects and toxic reactions associated with the use of anticholinesterase agents can be observed as a prolonged effect of acetylcholine. Such reactions include defecation, contracted pupils, sweating, excessive salivation, bronchial constriction, and skeletal muscle fasciculation. Undue exposure to the insecticides leads to reactions that may extend over a longer period of time, progressing to tremor, ataxia, hallucinations, respiratory paralysis, and death. Treatment requires the support of vital signs, artificial respiration, and atropine sulfate.[17]

It is important to note on the dental records if a patient is taking one of these anticholinesterase agents, particularly neostigmine. There is the danger that use of atropine to reduce salivary flow could interfere with the cholinergic action of the drug. Since the choline esters and the anticholinesterase agents have little use in dentistry, doses of these drugs were omitted.

Anticholinergic drugs

The parasympatholytics or anticholinergic drugs consist of a large group of natural and synthetic drugs that prevent the action of acetylcholine at postganglionic parasympathetic endings. Acetylcholine release is not prevented, but its interaction with the receptor is blocked. Thus the anticholinergic drugs effectively block the action of acetylcholine on smooth muscle, glandular tissues, and the heart. In the therapeutic dosage used by dentists, little or no effect will be observed at the ganglia and neuromuscular junction.

The principal drugs in this category are the naturally occurring belladonna alkaloids atropine and scopolamine, which are useful in dentistry as agents to control salivary secretion and as preanesthetic medication. Most of the synthetically prepared anticholinergic drugs have been designed to provide a longer duration of action and have a greater selectivity for action on the smooth muscle of the intestines.

Many are combined with a barbiturate or a tranquilizer to reduce either the patient's underlying psychic influence on gastrointestinal secretions or the central nervous system's influence on parasympathetic activity. The rationale for such therapy is still under investigation.[18]

The pharmacologic actions of atropine and scopolamine are similar in many respects as might be expected, since they differ from one another by only an oxygen atom. Atropine in the usual dose employed in dentistry does not show a central nervous system response, although in larger doses stimulation may occur. Scopolamine, however, has a depressant effect on the central nervous system that accounts for its usefulness as a preanesthetic agent and perhaps its use in motion sickness in several over-the-counter preparations. Both drugs will reduce salivary flow and, in larger doses, block the cardiac slowing effect of the vagus nerve with a resultant tachycardia. This latter effect is useful in preventing cardiac slowing during general anesthesia.[19]

Atropine, scopolamine, and the synthetic derivatives are also extremely useful in therapy and examination of the eye. These drugs produce dilation (mydriasis) and paralysis of accommodation for distant vision and light (cycloplegia). Such effects are generally long lasting and can also be manifested by larger systemic doses of the drugs.

The use of atropine and scopolamine in dentistry is limited to preanesthetic medication and reduction of salivary flow. Atropine sulfate may be used either orally or by injection to reduce salivation. Doses for adults range from 0.3 to 1 mg and should be given at least 1 or 2 hours prior to the dental procedure. It should be noted that careful dosage adjustment is required in children because they are more responsive to the effects of these drugs.[20] After the use of atropine to reduce salivation, the patient should be warned that he will feel a dryness and burning of the throat that will persist for a few hours. Additionally, vasodilation of the skin with flushing may occur, along with blurred vision. Nursing mothers excrete atropine in their milk; therefore one must consider the real need for reduction of salivation in these patients to prevent a drug response in the infant. Scopolamine hydrobromide may also be used, but it is more useful in premedication for general anesthesia in doses of 0.3 to 0.6 mg for adults when given by injection.[21]

There are at least fifty-four different synthetic anticholinergic drugs designed to be an aid to peptic ulcer therapy and related disorders. Many of these agents have the side effect of reducing salivary flow; thus dentists have utilized this side effect to their advantage. Since so many of these agents exist, an example of only one will be used to illustrate how the antispasmodic drugs may be utilized. *Accepted Dental Therapeutics*[22] lists propantheline bromide (Pro-Banthine) as a possible selection. Methantheline (Banthine) has also been used, but propantheline may cause fewer side effects. It should be given orally at least 30 to 45 minutes preoperatively. The usual dose for an adult is 7.5 to 15 mg, and occasionally 30 mg may be required. Since only single doses are employed, the incidence of side effects associated with more frequent use of such drugs may be avoided. However, even with a 15 mg oral dose, one patient was observed to have tachycardia. The practitioner must constantly keep in mind that each patient is an individual who is subject to varying responses to the usual dose of a drug. Note on the patient's chart the dose used and the response so that future side effects and greater therapeutic response may be attained by dosage adjustments at subsequent appointments.

Specific contraindications to the use of the anticholinergic agents include glaucoma, prostate hypertrophy (may cause urinary retention), and intestinal obstruction. Since these drugs affect the cardiovascular system, caution should be observed when using them in patients with severe cardiovascular problems.

Side effects are common with the anticholinergic drugs and include blurring of vision, tachycardia, urinary retention, constipation, decreased salivation, sweating, and dry skin. Some of the effects can last several hours. Toxic reactions are most often associated with overdose or accidental poisoning and can include delirium, hallucinations, convulsions, and respiratory depression. Dry skin and elevation of body temperature also occur. Treatment is largely symptomatic to control vital signs, with sponge baths to lower body temperature.

The chief medical use of the atropine substitutes and belladonna preparations includes functional gastrointestinal disorders and peptic ulcer. In addition, these agents have been used to control secretions of the common cold and in some cases of asthma. Drugs with anticholinergic effects are also used in treating parkinsonism and motion sickness. A good medical history will usually provide the information concerning which drug the patient is receiving. Additional anticholinergic drugs in these individuals may not be required for control of salivary flow.

Interaction with other medically useful drugs

Drugs in the cholinergic and anticholinergic categories have limited usefulness in dentistry. These drugs are more important to dentists because of the possible interactions with other categories of drugs that also have autonomic effects. The cholinergic and anticholinergic drugs are widely used in medicine and affect so many body systems that it is important to be able to recognize or anticipate synergistic and antagonistic drug reactions. Some of these reactions are clinically important and some may not be so clinically significant. Be that as it may, it is good practice to note these reactions so that patients achieve the intended therapeutic benefits of a drug.

The choline esters and anticholinesterases, when given together, potentiate cholinergic responses. Adrenergic drugs and atropine can antagonize the miotic effects of the cholinergics. Antihistamines are reported to reduce the activity of cholinesterase inhibitors and also produce dryness of the mouth similar to that of the anticholinergics.[23]

Anticholinergic drugs react with a wide assortment of other agents to produce a variety of responses. Those agents that can be considered to potentiate anticholinergic drugs include adrenergics, alphaprodine, meperidine, antihistamines, tricyclic antidepressants, corticosteroids, monoamine oxidase inhibitors, methylphenidate, the nitrates, tranquilizers, and urinary alkalinizers. Drugs that antagonize or inhibit anticholinergic actions include achlorhydria agents, urinary acidifiers, anticholinesterases, guanethidine, and reserpine. Levodopa, the latest drug developed for treatment of parkinsonism, may be potentiated by the anticholinergics. This list is far from exhaustive but should include most of the drugs commonly encountered in a day-to-day practice.[24]

PHARMACOLOGY OF THE SYMPATHETIC DIVISION
Epinephrine and norepinephrine

It has been well established that epinephrine and norepinephrine are the neurotransmitters of the sympathetic division. Norepinephrine is the major transmitter released at the nerve ending, since epinephrine appears to be released only in small quantities. Just the opposite occurs in the adrenal medulla, where epinephrine is the major neurohumoral agent released and norepinephrine is discharged in smaller quantities. The neurotransmitters released by the adrenal medulla are distributed by the circulatory system, reaching almost every part of the body.

As was the case with acetylcholine, both epinephrine and norepinephrine are synthesized in the neural tissues and stored in synaptic vesicles. The synthesis of the adrenergic mediators is more complex than that for acetylcholine because a number of steps and different enzymes are required. It is important to list these steps, since drugs are now being used in therapy that exert their effects by influencing the synthesis pathway. The synthesis steps are as follows[25]:

1. Tyrosine $\xrightarrow[\text{Hydroxylase}]{\text{Tyrosine}}$ Levodihydroxyphenyl-alanine (levodopa)

2. Levodopa $\xrightarrow[\text{Decarboxylase}]{\text{Levodopa}}$ Dopamine

3. Dopamine $\xrightarrow[\text{Beta-hydroxylase}]{\text{Dopamine}}$ Norepinephrine

4. Norepinephrine $\xrightarrow[\text{N-methyltransferase}]{\text{Phenylethanolamine}}$ Epinephrine

The structures of epinephrine and norepinephrine are shown later in this chapter.

Adrenergic receptors

In 1948 Ahlquist[26] proposed the existence of two types of adrenergic receptors and suggested they be termed *alpha* and *beta.* This concept presented the proposition that the "activation" of alpha receptors by an adrenergic drug caused one type of response and the "activation" of beta receptors caused a different response. The excitation of alpha receptors causes the contraction of smooth muscle (vasoconstriction), whereas the excitation of beta receptors causes the relaxation of smooth muscle (vasodilation) and cardiac stimulation (increased heart rate and strength of contraction).

Epinephrine has a potent effect on both alpha and beta receptors, with beta receptors showing the greater response to lower doses. Norepinephrine has its main action on alpha receptors. In addition, the alpha receptor is more responsive to epinephrine than norepinephrine. Isoproterenol acts principally on beta receptors, and phenylephrine almost exclusively activates alpha receptors. It is extremely important to separate the actions of adrenergic drugs on the receptors, since their entire pharmacology is based upon this concept.

Most tissues have both alpha and beta receptors with one type predominant. The response of the tissue to a specific adrenergic drug will depend principally on the majority of the receptor type present. The vessels of the skin, mucosa, and kidney contain alpha receptors that respond to both norepinephrine and epinephrine with vasoconstriction. Vessels located in skeletal muscles contain a majority of beta receptors; therefore epinephrine is most effective and causes vasodilation. If norepinephrine were put into these vessels, vasoconstriction would occur because norepinephrine does not stimulate the beta response.

Epinephrine and norepinephrine are metabolized by at least two identifiable enzymes, monoamine oxidase (MAO) and catechol-O-methyl transferase (COMT). COMT appears to be specific for a characteristic group referred to as the *catecholamines*. This term is given to those adrenergic drugs containing two hydroxyl groups attached to the aromatic ring. Thus the catecholamine drugs include dopa, dopamine, norepinephrine, epinephrine, and isoproterenol. Monoamine oxidase is found within the mitochondria, whereas COMT is concerned with metabolism of the circulating amines. The end products of metabolism are excreted in the urine where they can be readily measured.[27]

The inactivation of norepinephrine and epinephrine is not entirely dependent on enzymatic action as was the case with acetylcholine. The factor most responsible for the termination of their activity is a reuptake mechanism associated with the nerve ending. This accounts for the longer duration of action of the biogenic amines and acts also to conserve the transmitter substance.

Mechanism of action

The complex synthesis and the difference in mediators released at various sites, as well as receptor specificity, allows for a rather large group of drugs that can influence the sympathetic division. Drugs may be used to inhibit the enzymes at the various steps of synthesis and thus inhibit sympathetic responses, or different substrates for the enzymes may be given in the form of drugs in place of epinephrine or norepinephrine so that "false transmitters" are produced. Drugs may be prepared synthetically that can either block or imitate the action of the adrenergic mediators at the receptor. Unlike those drugs encountered in the parasympathetic division, certain adrenergic drugs not only stimulate adrenergic receptors but also cause release of the sympathetic transmitters from their storage vesicles. Some drugs may act by preventing the reuptake process and therefore inhibit sympathetic activity. Thus the number of drugs that can influence the sympathetic division is larger and more complex when compared with the parasympathetic division.

Adrenergic drugs
Epinephrine hydrochloride (Adrenalin)

The most useful and perhaps the best example of a drug that imitates the activity of sympathetic discharge is epinephrine. Its major effects are on the myocardium and smooth muscles of the blood vessels and lung. Therefore epinephrine acts as a direct cardiac stimulant. Both small and large doses of epinephrine cause an increase in strength of contraction, cardiac rate, cardiac output, and oxygen utilization.

The receptors located in the vessels of the skin, mucous membranes, and kidney are predominantly alpha so that epinephrine will cause vasoconstriction. Receptors in those vessels located in skeletal muscle are, for the most part, beta with some alpha. Therefore epinephrine will cause vasodilation in skeletal muscles. These two responses are extremely important in the regulation of blood pressure. Slow intravenous infusion of low doses of epinephrine will cause an increase in cardiac activity associated with a rise in systolic pressure but with a decrease in diastolic pressure because of the vasodilation occurring in skeletal muscles. Larger doses produce a rise in both systolic and diastolic pressures because the cutaneous alpha response predominates. Since the alpha response is of a shorter duration than the beta, a fall in pressure will be observed after the initial increase. The smooth muscles of the bronchi contain beta receptors and hence are relaxed by epinephrine. Alpha receptors located in the vascular smooth muscle of pulmonary arterioles respond with vasoconstriction to epinephrine. The net result is a reduction in resistance to air flow, which provides relief during asthmatic attacks.

The central nervous system effects of epinephrine are more prominent when accidental intravenous injections occur or when excessive doses are used. These effects are manifested by anxiety, apprehension, restlessness, weakness, and occasionally tremor.[14] Epinephrine also stimulates metabolism.

Epinephrine hydrochloride is available for use in the commercial form of Adrenalin. It is supplied in ampules of a 1:1000 aqueous solution for injection either subcutaneously, intramuscularly, or for extreme emergencies, intravenously. The most often used route of administration is the subcutaneous route, which allows the drug to be absorbed over a longer period of time with less central nervous system stimulation. If given intravenously, 1 ml should be diluted to 10 ml with sterile water for injection and then given very slowly. Do not confuse the 1:100 dilution used for inhalation or topical application with the injectable form because disastrous results might occur. A topical solution, 1:1000, is also available for use as a hemostatic agent on bleeding gingival or pulpal tissues. Small quantities of the solution should be placed in a clean dappen dish for this purpose; cotton pledgets should not be saturated directly from the original container. Contaminants may cause premature deterioration of the epinephrine solution. All epinephrine should be stored in the original dark containers because light will also decompose the solution. The presence of a brownish color indicates an epinephrine solution that has lost its potency and should be discarded.[22]

Epinephrine is the drug of choice for acute asthmatic and allergic reactions. It may be injected subcutaneously, intramuscularly, or intravenously in doses of 0.2 to 0.5 ml of the 1:1000 aqueous solution. The drug is employed as a vasoconstrictor in local anesthetics. It is also employed as a cardiac stimulant in patients with cardiac arrest where fibrillation is absent. Because the drug is a direct cardiac stimulant, it could cause ventricular fibrillation in certain cardiac emergencies. For this reason its use in patients with hemorrhagic, traumatic, or cardiogenic shock is not recommended. Epinephrine is contraindicated for use in certain types of glaucoma (congestive narrow angle) and for use with cyclopropane and halogenated hydrocarbon anesthetics. It should be used with caution in elderly people and in those with cardiovascular disease, hypertension, and hyperthyroidism. As with any drug, every situation must be evaluated on its own merits as to the safety and possible interaction with other drugs or disease processes.

Norepinephrine bitartrate

The principal neurohumoral agent released from sympathetic neurons is norepinephrine. It is primarily an alpha stimulator and causes vasoconstriction in the cutaneous vessels, which leads to an increase in peripheral resistance and increase in both systolic and diastolic blood pressure. Baroreceptors are stimulated by the elevated pressure and cause a reflex firing of the vagus nerve, resulting in bradycardia. It does not relax bronchial smooth muscle, since this is a beta response. Alpha constriction of arterioles in the lungs will not provide sufficient reduction in airway resistance to be useful in asthma. The metabolic effects seen with epinephrine apparently do not occur with norepinephrine.

Norepinephrine bitartrate is available as the commercial product Levophed. It is intended to be used only in certain cases of hypotension associated with shock. It should not be part of the dental emergency kit because other adrenergic drugs are more suitable. It produces severe vasoconstriction in cutaneous vessels so that necrosis and tissue slough can occur. Therefore there can be little justification for its use in local anesthetics.[21]

Toxic and side effects associated with the use of norepinephrine resemble those seen with epinephrine. Hypertension caused by norepinephrine is likely to be more severe, especially in the hyperthyroid patient. Contraindications to the use of norepinephrine are also similar to those for epinephrine.

Isoproterenol or isopropylnorepinephrine

Isoproterenol is a synthetic adrenergic derivative of epinephrine with action limited to the beta receptors. When injected, it acts as a direct cardiac stimulant, increasing both the rate and strength of cardiac contraction.

Since it stimulates only the beta receptor, a decrease in diastolic pressure is observed. It also decreases bronchial spasm by relaxation of the bronchial smooth muscle. Vasoconstriction of pulmonary vessels does not occur, since this represents an alpha response.

Isoproterenol hydrochloride is available commercially as Isuprel. Its primary use is in the treatment of bronchial asthma and heart block. Preparations include an inhalation product in a concentration of 1:400. Sublingual tablets are supplied in 10 and 15 mg dosage forms, and a 1:5000 (1 ml) ampule for injection is also available. Its side effects are similar to those of epinephrine, and like epinephrine and norepinephrine, it is not effective orally.

Ephedrine

Ephedrine is a naturally occurring sympathomimetic agent that can stimulate the adrenergic receptor and also cause release of the adrenergic transmitters from their neuronal storage sites. Unlike the previously mentioned drugs, it is effective when given orally and is used in numerous oral preparations intended for use in patients with bronchial asthma. Solutions of the drug have been used in ophthalmology to cause pupillary dilation (mydriasis). Since it has both alpha- and beta-stimulating effects, it is used in intranasal solutions to produce vasoconstriction for a localized decongestive effect. An isomer of ephedrine, pseudoephedrine, is also used effectively in the treatment of asthmatic and allergic disorders.

Synthetic adrenergic drugs

Competition among pharmaceutical manufacturers has prompted the development of a large number of drugs having adrenergic properties. Each of these agents possesses the basic characteristic of vasoconstriction. Some are intended as nasal decongestants only; others are effective agents in combating hypotension. The use of one over the other is largely a matter of personal preference and familiarity.

Phenylephrine hydrochloride (Neo-Synephrine). Phenylephrine has vasoconstrictive properties that make it useful in the treatment of hypotension. It has also been employed as a vasoconstrictor in local anesthetics. Phenylephrine is not as potent as norepinephrine and can be used to elevate pressure

without the danger of direct cardiac stimulation. It may be administered by injection or by mouth. Ophthalmic preparations provide excellent mydriasis.

Metaraminol bitartrate (Aramine). Metaraminol is a highly potent adrenergic agent used almost exclusively to treat severe hypotension. It also has cardiac-stimulant properties. Metaraminol is reported to be taken up by sympathetic nerve terminals in a manner similar to norepinephrine. In this way it becomes a "false mediator," being released by sympathetic discharge. Its duration of action is longer than that of norepinephrine. As with all vasoconstrictors, one must exercise care when giving potent agents.

Mephentermine sulfate (Wyamine). Mephentermine is used as a vasoconstrictor to treat hypotension. It has also been employed as a nasal decongestant, but this is somewhat less popular. Dentists could select this agent either to place in their emergency drug kit for their use or to have on hand for use by medical personnel. It reportedly does not produce central nervous system stimulation as observed with other vasoconstrictors. The route of administration is either subcutaneous or intramuscular in a dosage range of 15 to 30 mg for adults.[28]

Miscellaneous drugs

Nasal decongestants. There appears to be an almost endless variety of adrenergic drugs that can be utilized for vasoconstriction. Symptomatic relief by the use of nasal decongestants reduces the swelling by vasoconstriction of vessels in the mucous membranes. Within a short time the congestion returns and the vasoconstrictor must be used again. If the recommended dosage schedules are not followed, a condition referred to as "congestion rebound" occurs. Vasodilation and congestion is then complicated by irritation and local tissue edema. Repeated use of stronger solutions, closely spaced dosages, and systemic absorption could provoke greater problems than congestion rebound. It should be emphasized that these agents provide only symptomatic relief. The following is a list of adrenergic drugs used as nasal decongestants: naphazoline HCl (Privine), tetrahydrozoline HCl (Tyzine), tuaminoheptane sulfate (Tuamine), oxymetazoline HCl (Afrin), xylometazoline HCl (Otrivin), phenylephrine HCl (Neo-Synephrine), cyclopentamine HCl (Clopane), and phenylpropan-olamine HCl (Propadrine). The list is incomplete and is intended to be illustrative only.[18]

Amphetamines. The amphetamines are a group of drugs that have indirect adrenergic stimulant effects manifested by increases in blood pressure and reflex cardiac slowing. However, they are potent central nervous system stimulants. The more prominent members of this category of drugs include amphetamine sulfate (Benzedrine), dextroamphetamine sulfate (Dexedrine), and methamphetamine HCl (Desoxyn, Methedrine, or "speed"). The abuse potential associated with the use of this category of drugs has prompted their inclusion as controlled substances under the recent federal drug laws. Therefore prescriptions for these drugs must meet all the requirements for Schedule II agents, that is, the same as the potent narcotic analgesics.[29]

The use of these agents is limited in both medicine and dentistry. Medical uses have included treatment of mental depression, hyperkinesis, appetite control, and narcolepsy. The action of these agents in reducing appetite is still a matter of conjecture, since after a few days these drugs seem to loose their appetite-suppressant effects.

Prolonged use of these drugs may lead to such side effects as physical dependence, apprehension, wakefulness, and mental depression and may evoke suicidal tendencies. Toxic reactions associated with overdosage may result in cardiac irregularities, cardiovascular collapse, coma, and death.[30]

Vasoconstrictors and their use in local anesthetics

A general discussion of the use of vasoconstrictors in local anesthetic solutions is presented in Chapter 14. Further consideration of specific agents is given here.

Extracts from the adrenal medullas of animals once constituted the major source of epinephrine; as such, it usually contained quantities of norepinephrine. Fortunately, epinephrine may now be prepared synthetically, thereby eliminating other isomeric contaminants. All of the commonly used vasoconstrictors in local anesthetics are of synthetic origin.

The following chemical structures depict the subtle molecular changes that occur among the most commonly employed agents.

Although the changes in structure may seem small, the pharmacologic differences occurring as a result of the change are of extreme importance.[10]

Epinephrine

Norepinephrine

Phenylephrine

Levonordefrin

Pharmacologic activity

Epinephrine. Although the basic pharmacology of epinephrine has been discussed, its effect on cutaneous blood vessels should be mentioned again. Mucous membrane contains, for the most part, alpha receptors. The response to alpha stimulation is vasoconstriction; hence, epinephrine can be used in concentrations smaller than those of other vasoconstrictors to give satisfactory results. Accidental intravascular injection may cause pronounced central nervous system and cardiac responses.

Norepinephrine. Norepinephrine has been discussed as having only indirect cardiac effects. It is such a potent vasoconstrictor that it can cause necrosis and slough of tissues when injected locally. Excessively high blood pressures and cardiac slowing may be seen with accidental intravascular injections. Its use as a vasoconstrictor in local anesthetics should be discouraged because its disadvantages are too great.

Phenylephrine. Phenylephrine is another vasoconstrictor with alpha receptor–stimulating properties that has been used in local anesthetics. As might be surmised from the type of receptor involved, there is little, if any, myocardial stimulation. However, the quality of vasoconstriction does not appear any better, and a larger dose of the drug is required to produce vasoconstriction. Cardiac slowing could occur because of reflex vagal inhibition.

Levonordefrin. Levonordefrin appears to be an effective vasoconstrictor. Claims made for the drug include less central nervous system excitation and less cardiac stimulation. Its effects resemble those of alpha receptor stimulation. Levonordefrin is stated to be less potent than epinephrine, but potency is used only to distinguish between the relative doses of drugs to produce a similar effect. The dose of levonordefrin is less than that for phenylephrine but greater than for epinephrine.

Mechanism of action. The action of the vasoconstrictors is a matter of stimulation of the proper receptor located in the vascular smooth muscle. The duration and degree of activity varies with each agent and probably to some degree with the amount of vasodilation inherent in the local anesthetic. Using concentrations in excess of the optimum amount does not offer any appreciable advantage.[31]

Absorption and excretion. All the vasoconstrictors utilized are absorbed systemically from the site of injection and are carried throughout all the body tissues. Accidental intravenous injection could result in alarming or hazardous consequences. Since the enzyme systems responsible for the metabolism of these drugs are similar, their rates of metabolism will be similar and the metabolites appear in the urine.

Commonly used concentrations

Vasoconstrictors are used in the following concentrations:

Epinephrine HCl	1:50,000 to 1:250,000; optimum—1:100,000
Norepinephrine bitartrate	1:30,000 to 1:50,000
Phenylephrine HCl	1:2000 to 1:2500
Levonordefrin HCl	1:20,000 to 1:30,000

Side effects and toxicity. Epinephrine hydrochloride, being the most commonly employed vasoconstrictor and the classic representative of the sympathetic nervous system, is perhaps the drug of choice when describing side effects and toxic reactions to adrenergic vasoconstrictors. It should be noted that vasoconstrictors behave as desired except when excessive dosages are employed and accidental intravascular injections are made.[32]

Patients may demonstrate many sympathetic and central nervous system reactions to epinephrine. These sympathetic reactions may appear as side effects characterized by palpitation, tachycardia, hypertension, and headache. If the central nervous system is also stimulated, the patient may show anxiety, restlessness, and weakness, may appear pale, and complain of dizziness. Many times these reactions may be wrongfully assigned to the local anesthetic, thereby creating future problems for the patient when more dental work is scheduled. Toxic reactions to vasoconstrictors are most often associated with dosages higher than those usually employed in dental local anesthtic solutions.[33]

Precautions in use. Over the years, many controversies have arisen concerning the use of epinephrine or other vasoconstrictors in patients with hypertension, hyperthyroidism, and cardiovascular diseases. It is not uncommon for dentists to hear a word of caution from the patient's physician in regard to vasoconstrictors. All too often this is a problem in communication that could be resolved by the dentist's explaining to the physician about the strength and amount of vasoconstrictor employed.

In 1964, the *Journal of the American Dental Association*[34] carried a report of a joint conference by the American Dental Association and the American Heart Association on problems with the patient who had cardiovascular disease and required dental treatment. The conference urged the careful cooperation of the physician and dentist in evaluating the use of both local anesthetics and vasoconstrictors. Vasoconstrictors are not contraindicated for the patient whose condition is diagnosed and controlled when they are used with careful aspiration and in optimal dosages. Premedication is suggested to help alleviate apprehension in these patients. Most information presented in the past years suggests the inclusion rather than the omission of vasoconstrictors so that a more profound and longer lasting anesthesia is possible. Fear, apprehension, and pain may be responsible for the patient elaborating more endogenous vasoconstrictor than the dentist would think about injecting.

There are a number of specific incidences where the vasoconstrictor should not be employed, such as in the hypertensive and hyperthyroid patient whose condition is uncontrolled. Epinephrine should be avoided in patients undergoing general anesthesia with cyclopropane or the halogenated hydrocarbons. These general anesthetic agents are capable of sensitizing the myocardium to epinephrine in such a way that cardiac arrhythmias and even fibrillation can occur.

Use for gingival retraction. There are numerous commercial preparations consisting of some type of string or cord impregnated with epinephrine or a racemic mixture of epinephrine isomers. Regardless of claims made by one over the other, these agents depend on the vasoconstrictive action of epinephrine on gingival blood vessels to bring about a retraction of tissue or hemorrhage control. The dentist should be aware that the concentrations of epinephrine in these preparations are relatively high and that systemic absorption does occur. Therefore these preparations may represent a potential source of danger in the cardiovascular and hyperthyroid patient. This also applies to the use of epinephrine-impregnated cords during general anesthesia with cyclopropane and the halogenated hydrocarbons. Wetting the gingival retraction cord with saliva in the floor of the mouth allows the epinephrine to be absorbed rapidly from this site for a systemic effect and could account for some arrhythmias or tachycardia observed in patients during general anesthesia.[35]

Medically useful drugs modifying sympathetic responses

There is a large group of drugs that have the capability of reducing or blocking sympathetic activity. Contrary to what might be expected, the development of drugs with the property of blocking alpha or beta adrenergic receptors confirmed that the two receptors were plausible. Most of these agents are used in the treatment of peripheral vascular disease, hypertension, and specific cardiac problems. Except for extremely rare instances, they are not suitable therapeutic agents for dentistry but are important in medical practice. Because epinephrine and related catecholamines have been identified in the central nervous system, drugs are available that can also modify the psychic response in patients by means of interference

with the metabolic inactivation of the catecholamines. These drugs also affect, to some degree, peripheral autonomic mechanisms and will be briefly mentioned.

Adrenergic blocking agents prevent the response of the receptor to both the endogenous and exogenous adrenergic agents. The alpha blocking agents were the first to be developed, and they are used in the treatment of peripheral vascular diseases (Raynaud's and Buerger's disease) and in the control of an adrenal medullary tumor, pheochromocytoma. The drugs included in this category are phenoxybenzamine (Dibenzyline), phentolamine (Regitine), azaptine (Ilidar), and tolazoline (Priscoline). The ergot alkaloids also have alpha blocking properties, but their usefulness is in the area of migraine headache rather than the control of hypertension. As with all drugs that block alpha responses, the use of therapeutic doses of epinephrine may produce a lowering rather than an increase in blood pressure. The phenothiazine tranquilizers, such as chlorpromazine, also possess the ability to block alpha receptors.

There are several agents capable of causing beta blockage, but only one, propranolol (Inderal), has proved therapeutic usefulness. Other drugs with beta blocking activity are currently under investigation. Beta blocking agents have been used to treat angina pectoris, cardiac arrhythmias, thyrotoxicosis, and pheochromocytoma. Some research currently involves its use in alcoholics. Since this drug blocks beta receptors, it is contraindicated in asthmatics.

The adrenergic neuronal blockers are distinguished from the adrenergic blocking agents in that the neuronal blockers prevent the discharge of stored transmitter. Circulating amines and those injected are not blocked. The principal drug employed for this purpose is guanethidine (Ismelin), the main use of which is in the treatment of hypertension. It is important to note the long-lasting effects of this drug even when therapy has been discontinued. Hypotension and weakness may accompany its use. Reserpine and its related alkaloids are also used to treat hypertension by a mechanism involving the depletion and blockage of catecholamine storage. Alpha methyldopa has been used to treat hypertension by blocking the action of the dopa decarboxylase enzyme and interfering with the synthesis of both epinephrine and norepinephrine.

Those drugs that have either a blocking or stimulating effect on the autonomic ganglia have a limited usefulness in medicine. Nicotine, the alkaloid obtained from tobacco, is an interesting agent in that it can both stimulate and block the ganglia, depending on the doses used. Some of the sympathetic responses that a person feels after having stopped smoking and then beginning again are examples of its stimulating effects. The *ganglionic blocking agents* are used in the treatment of hypertension. These drugs include mecamylamine (Inversine), trimethaphan (Arfonad), and pentolinium (Ansolysen). Both divisions of the autonomic nervous system show a peripheral response to the ganglionic blockers. One of the side effects associated with these drugs is dryness of the mouth.[18]

Interactions with other drugs

The sympathetic-related drugs react in many ways with an exceptionally large number of other drugs. This is not only a reflection of the diffuse activity of the sympathetic amines but also that of so many other drugs having an indirect autonomic response.

The drugs that potentiate the activity of adrenergic stimulators include alcohol, antihistamines, cocaine, doxapram, ergot drugs, ganglionic blockers, and the xanthine group. Of course, adrenergic drugs are used together at times to potentiate decongestant effects. The halogenated anesthetics and cyclopropane increase the hazard of cardiac arrhythmias and should be avoided in combination with the adrenergic drugs. Digitalis is also associated with a predisposition to cardiac arrhythmias.

Two groups of drugs, the tricyclic antidepressants and the monoamine oxidase inhibitors, may present special difficulties in treating patients with sympathomimetic drugs. These relationships are discussed in Chapters 7 and 29.

The list of drugs that can interact with the adrenergic blocking agents is extensive. Dentists would be wise to consult where these drugs are used. They should be alert to the antagonism of propranolol for antihistamines and anti-inflammatory agents (salicylates) and its potentiation of general anesthetics, hexobarbital, and morphine. The thiazide diuretics have the capability of lowering blood pressure by a peripheral action on arterioles and hence can potentiate alpha blocking agents and ganglionic blocking drugs producing a hypotensive state.[23,24]

REFERENCES

1. Patton, H. D.: Higher control of autonomic outflows: the hypothalamus. In Ruch, T. D., and Patton, H. D., editor: Neurophysiology, Philadelphia, 1965, W. B. Saunders Co.
2. Truex, R. C., and Carpenter, M. S.: Strong and Elwyn's human neuroanatomy, Baltimore, 1964, The Williams & Wilkins Co.
3. Carisson, A., and Hillarp, N. A.: On the state of catecholamines of the adrenal medullary granules, Acta Physiol. Scand. **44**:163, 1958.
4. Koelle, G. B.: Neurohumoral transmission and the autonomic nervous system. In Goodman, L. S., and Gilman, A. Z., editors: The pharmacological basis of therapeutics, ed. 5, New York, 1975, The Macmillan Co.
5. Brody, M. J.: Neurohumoral mediation of active reflex vasodilation, Fed. Proc. **25**:1583, 1966.
6. Hodgkin, A. L.: The conduction of the nerve impulse, Springfield, Ill., 1964, Charles C Thomas, Publisher.
7. Glowinski, J.: Some new facts about synthesis, storage and release processes of monoamines in the central nervous system. In Snyder, S. H., editor: Perspectives in neuropharmacology, London, 1972, The Oxford University Press.
8. Eccles, J. C.: The physiology of synapses, Berlin, 1964, Springer-Verlag.
9. Loewi, O., and Navratil, E.: Über humorale Übertragbarkeit der Herznervenwirkung; über das Schicksal des Vagusstoffs, Pflueger's Arch. Ges. Physiol. **214**:678, 1926.
10. Wilson, C. O., Gisvald, O., and Doerge, R. F.: Textbook of organic medicinal and pharmaceutical chemistry, Philadelphia, 1966, J. B. Lippincott Co.
11. Paton, W. D. M.: Receptors as defined by their pharmacological properties. In Porter, R., and O'Conner, M., editors: Molecular properties of drug receptors, A Ciba Symposium, London, 1970, J. & A. Churchill, Ltd.
12. Davis, R., and Koelle, G. B.: Electron microscopic localization of acetylcholine esterase and nonspecific cholinesterases at the neuromuscular junction by the gold-thiocholine and gold-thioacetate acid methods, J. Cell. Biol. **34**:157, 1967.
13. Volle, R. L.: Cholinomimetic drugs. In DiPalma, J. R., editor: Drill's pharmacology in medicine, New York, 1971, McGraw-Hill Book Co.
14. Goth, A.: Medical pharmacology: principles and concepts, ed. 8, St. Louis, 1976, The C. V. Mosby Co.
15. Waser, P. G.: Chemistry and pharmacology of muscarine, muscarone and some related compounds, Pharmacol. Rev. **13**:465, 1961.
16. Schwab, R. C.: The pharmacologic basis of the treatment of myasthenia gravis, Clin. Pharmacol. Ther. **1**:319, 1960.
17. Polson, C. J., and Tattersall, R. N.: Clinical toxicology, ed. 2, Philadelphia, 1969, J. B. Lippincott Co.

18. Melmon, K. L., and Morelli, H. F., editors: Clinical pharmacology, New York, 1972, The Macmillan Co.
19. Eger, E. I.: Atropine, scopolamine and related compounds, Anesthesiology 23:365, 1962.
20. Kutscher, A. H., Zegarelli, E. V., and Hymon, G. A.: Pharmacotherapeutics of oral disease, New York, 1964, McGraw-Hill Book Co.
21. Jorgensen, N. B., and Hayden, J.: Premedication, local and general anesthesia in dentistry, Philadelphia, 1967, Lea & Febiger.
22. Accepted dental therapeutics, ed. 36, Chicago, 1975, American Dental Association.
23. Gage, T. W., and Radman, W. P.: Drug interactions—a professional responsibility, J.A.D.A. **84:** 848, 1972.
24. Martin, E. W., editor: Hazards of medication, Philadelphia, 1971, J. B. Lippincott Co.
25. Axelrod, J.: Enzymatic formation of adrenaline and other catecholamines from monophenols, Science **140:**499, 1963.
26. Ahlquist, R. P.: A study of the adrenotropic receptors, Am. J. Physiol. **153:**586, 1948.
27. Axelrod, J.: The metabolism, storage and release of catecholamines, Recent Progr. Horm. Res. **21:** 597, 1965.
28. DiPalma, J. R., editor: Basic pharmacology in medicine, New York, 1976, McGraw-Hill Book Co.
29. Department of Justice, Bureau of Narcotics and Dangerous Drugs: Regulations implementing the Comprehensive Drug Abuse Prevention and Control Act of 1970, Fed. Reg. **36:**7776, 1971.
30. Ray, O. S.: Drugs, society and human behavior, St. Louis, 1972, The C. V. Mosby Co.
31. Bishop, J. G., Dorman, H. L., and Matthews, J. L.: Vasoconstrictors in local anesthetics, Dent. Clin. North Am., p. 279, July, 1971.
32. Special Committee of the New York Heart Association: Use of epinephrine in connection with procaine in dental procedures, J.A.D.A. **50:**108, 1955.
33. Holroyd, S. V., Watts, D. T., and Welch, J. T.: The use of epinephrine in local anesthetics for dental patients with cardiovascular diseases: a review of the literature, J. Oral Surg. **18:**492, 1960.
34. Conference report: Management of dental problems in patients with cardiovascular disease, J.A.D.A. **68:**333, 1964.
35. Woycheshin, F. F.: An evaluation of the drugs used for gingival retraction, J. Prosth. Dent. **14:** 769, 1964.

14

Local anesthetics

SAM V. HOLROYD

No drugs are employed more frequently in dental practice than are the local anesthetics. Their use can become so routine that one loses sight of the fact that these are drugs which have important systemic as well as local potentialities. It behooves the dentist to know the local anesthetic drugs well. Clinically related pharmacology should particularly be reviewed at frequent intervals. The dentist should also exert leadership in giving direction to research and evolving a philosophy of use relative to local anesthetic agents.

HISTORY

Discovery. Although primitive man undoubtedly observed the local anesthetic effect of chewing certain plants or leaves, clinical local anesthesia was established by three events: (1) the isolation of cocaine from the leaves of the coca plant (Niemann, 1860), (2) the topical use of cocaine in surgery of the eye (Köller, 1884), and (3) the use of cocaine for nerve block in surgery (Halsted, 1885).

The recognition that cocaine was toxic and addicting led to a search for local anesthetic agents of equal efficacy but greater safety. The synthesis of procaine by Einhorn in 1905 initiated a new era in local anesthesia.

Trends in local anesthesia for dentistry. Sometimes it helps to look back to see where we are going. If the first volume of *Accepted Dental Remedies** (1934) is examined, the reader will find that 2% procaine (Novocain)

with epinephrine is considered to be the most effective local anesthetic for conduction anesthesia and 1% to 2% is considered most effective for infiltration anesthesia. ADR does not reflect any significant changes in dental local anesthesia over the next several years. Butethamine (Monocaine) was added in the 1941 edition. The 1945 ADR indicated that procaine-epinephrine solutions continue to be the predominant local anesthetic in dentistry. The commercially available procaine solutions were 2%, except for a 2.2% solution with nordefrin (Cobefrin), 1:9000.

During the late 1940s there was a growing concern over the routine use of 4% procaine and mixtures of procaine and more powerful anesthetics such as tetracaine (Pontocaine), which had appeared commercially.[1] The combination of 2% procaine, 0.15% tetracaine, and 1:10,000 nordefrin was not accepted by ADR in 1945; however, it was accepted in 1950. Also in 1950 tetracaine was added to the listings, and commercial dental solutions of 4% procaine increased in number.

In 1952 lidocaine (Xylocaine) and another tetracaine combination, 2% procaine, 0.15% tetracaine, and 1:2500 phenylephrine, were added to ADR. By 1954 another tetracaine combination, 2% procaine, 0.15% tetracaine, and 1:30,000 levarterenol (Levophed), was accepted. Propoxycaine (Ravocaine) entered ADR in 1957. Since its potency is similar to that of tetracaine, a combination with 2% procaine followed, and the combination of 0.4% propoxycaine and 2% procaine with 1:10,000 nordefrin was added to ADR and in a second solution with 1:30,000 levarterenol. In 1958 metabutethamine (Unacaine), meprylcaine (Oracaine), and metabutoxycaine (Primacaine) were added, with a view

---

□ The opinions or assertions contained herein are the private ones of the writer and are not to be construed as official or as reflecting the views of the Navy Department or the naval service at large.

*Later renamed *Accepted Dental Therapeutics.*

toward shorter duration anesthesia. Levo-nordefrin (Neo-Cobefrin) was added in 1:20,000 concentration in 1959 as the vasoconstrictor in a 2% procaine–0.15% tetracaine combination. In 1961 chloroprocaine (Nesacaine), mepivacaine (Carbocaine), and isobucaine (Kincaine) were added to ADR. In 1962 chloroprocaine was removed and there were no additions. From 1962 to the present there have been additions of pyrocaine (Dynacaine) in 1964, dyclonine (Dyclone) in 1966, and prilocaine (Citanest) in 1967. Since 1967, metabutoxycaine (Primacaine), naepaine (Amylsine), meprylcaine (Oracaine), butethamine (Monocaine), and metabutethamine (Unocaine) have been deleted.

Over the last 15 years we have seen the almost complete replacement of procaine by more potent local anesthetics. More recently, "short duration anesthesia," accomplished by increasing concentrations from 2% to 3% or 4% and eliminating the vasoconstrictor, has been promoted.

SAFETY OF DENTAL LOCAL ANESTHESIA

The history of local anesthetic safety can be considered as occurring in three eras, the first being the era of cocaine; the second, the era of procaine; and the third and present, the era of increased potency. The addicting properties and high toxicity of cocaine are well documented in the medical and dental literature for the years when this anesthetic was in great use. The synthesis of procaine in 1905 led to the replacement of cocaine in dentistry by this nonaddicting and less toxic drug. The *Index to Dental Literature* reflects the early investigations of procaine (1906-1910), the enthusiasm for procaine (1911-1915), the taking over by procaine (1916-1920), and the obvious predominance of procaine anesthesia in dentistry by 1921. The movement toward more potent local anesthesia in dentistry was making itself felt by 1950. This brief introduction to the consideration of local anesthetic safety was necessary because the statistics on fatalities for any particular period reflect the dangers of the predominant anesthetics of the period. For instance, statistical studies conducted from 1930 to 1950 may provide significant data relative to procaine toxicity but do not provide a basis for the security or lack of security in using lidocaine, mepiva-caine, prilocaine, and other subsequently developed local anesthetic agents.

The American Medical Association became concerned with deaths from local anesthesia in 1924 and appointed a committee to survey related fatalities. This committee reported 43 deaths from local anesthesia.[2] In 1928, 14 more deaths were reported.[3] A committee appointed by the Philadelphia Medical Society found 29 local anesthetic deaths in the Philadelphia area from 1935 to 1946,[4] and Dealy[5] reported 5 local anesthetic deaths at Queens General Hospital in New York from 1936 to 1941. It is difficult to assess the overall dangers in local anesthesia from such scattered reports; however, the lethal potential of local anesthetics is well illustrated. Adriani and Campbell have stated, "Accurate statistics on the frequency of untoward reactions and fatalities due to local anesthetics are not available, because few such mishaps are reported."[6] They indicated that 10 unreported deaths and numerous other nonfatal reactions have occurred at their hospital in a 15-year period. The 10 deaths reported by Adriani and Campbell occurred from the topical application of tetracaine. On the other hand, tetracaine was used 20,000 times in spinal anesthesia at this hospital during the same time period without a death. Other mortality reports attributable to topical application of local anesthetics seem to illustrate further the importance of the method of administration.[7-9] One may therefore conclude that medical statistics probably do not reflect the dangers or lack of dangers in using local anesthetics in dentistry. However, fatal allergic reactions, such as those reported by Criep and Ribeiro[10] could occur as easily from dental use as from medical use.

Fortunately, five studies that provide a limited assessment of the dangers of local anesthesia in dentistry have been conducted. Seldin and Recant[11] surveyed the mortality files of the City of New York for the period 1943 to 1952. They found 2 deaths attributed to dental local anesthesia during the 10-year period, in which they estimate 90,000,000 local anesthesias (mostly procaine) must have been administered for dental purposes. Seldin[12] made a nationwide survey of anesthetic mortality for 1950 to 1956 in oral surgery. A questionnaire was sent to each member of the American Society of Oral Surgeons. The 406 answers indicated that approximately

Table 14-1. Local anesthetic deaths

Dates of survey	Total number of cases	Procedure	Mortality rate
1905-1950[7]	30,000	ENT (C)*	1:10,000
Before 1950[8]	39,299	ENT (C and T)	1.8:10,000
1948-1952[9]	58,700	Spinals (T)	3.7:10,000
	152,000	Regional and topical (P and C)	1.3:10,000
1943-1952[11]	90,000,000	Dental (P)	1:45,000,000
1950-1956[12]	4,316,027	Oral surgery (P)	1:1,438,000
During 1962[13]	71,874,000	Dental (L)	1:36,000,000
During 1965[14]	1,493,000	Oral Surgery (L)	1:1,493,000
During 1972[15]	1,853,750	Oral Surgery (L)	1:1,853,000

*Primary anesthetic: C, cocaine; L, lidocaine; P, procaine; T, tetracaine.

4,316,027 local anesthetics were administered and 3 deaths occurred as a result of the anesthetic.

In the American Dental Association's *The 1962 Survey of Dental Practice*, an extrapolation of survey data from general practice found a death rate attributed to local anesthesia of 1:36,000,000.[13] Questionnaire surveys of oral surgical practices for 1965 by Driscoll[14] and for 1972 by the American Society of Oral Surgeons[15] found death rates of 1:1,493,000 and 1:1,853,000, respectively. Table 14-1 illustrates these statistics. Data concerning local anesthetic fatalities in medicine are shown for comparison.

Although anesthetic morbidity figures are highly subject to error, it would seem that dental local anesthesia is relatively safer than medical local anesthesia. This is logical in view of the fact that, in dentistry, less anesthetic is generally used and the patient is usually in better overall health. Dental surgery is also less of a complicating factor than most medical surgery.

It would also appear that local anesthetic mortality figures for general dentistry (approximately 1:40,000,000) are more favorable than for oral surgery (approximately 1:1,500,000). This probably results from the same factors that make the combined dental data more favorable than the medical data.

Although local anesthetic morbidity data are limited, it appears that dental local anesthesia is an extremely safe procedure. The dentist's commendable measures of aspiration, minimizing dosage, and attention to the patient's medical history have been highly successful. Some will say that, "One death is one too many." I certainly agree but

must relate a germane case history. A dental patient went into anaphylactic shock 3 minutes after the injection of lidocaine. The dentist injected 0.5 ml 1:1000 epinephrine intramuscularly and administered oxygen. The patient quickly responded and survived without residual effects. This survival allowed a determination that the patient was *not* allergic to lidocaine but to a type of grass that was being mowed outside the dentist's office as the patient entered. If this patient had died, the death would have been a lidocaine statistic. The point I wish to make is that *even if practitioners injected water, they would never obtain a zero morbidity figure.*

In spite of an excellent record of safety in dental local anesthesia, dentists must be aware of the potential dangers and not lessen their precautionary measures of *aspiration, minimizing dosage, and attention to the patient's medical history.* Lidocaine appears to have an excellent safety record, yet even with a good record serious and fatal reactions have occurred in dentistry[16-18] and medicine.[19-21] The toxicity and allergenicity of mepivacaine are approximately the same as those of lidocaine. Overall, dental local anesthesia can be considered to be remarkably safe.[22]

DESIRABLE QUALITIES OF A LOCAL ANESTHETIC

A large number of chemical agents are capable of producing local anesthesia. However, not all are clinically acceptable. The basis of clinical acceptability is safety to the patient and adequacy of the anesthesia produced. Ideally, a local anesthetic would do the following.[23]

1. Provide potent and reversible local anesthesia with a minimum of adverse local or systemic reactions
2. Have a rapid onset of action and provide a satisfactory duration of action
3. Have tissue-penetrating properties
4. Be inexpensive, stable in solution, and capable of being sterilized by heat

The degree to which a particular agent approaches the ideal varies with the drug itself and also with the needs of a particular case.

CHEMISTRY

Most clinically acceptable local anesthetics consist of an aromatic nucleus (R^1) connected by an ester or amide linkage to an aliphatic chain containing a secondary or tertiary amino group.

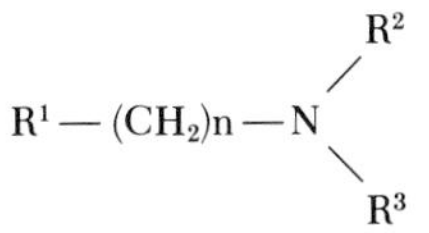

$$R^1-(CH_2)n-N\begin{smallmatrix}R^2\\\\R^3\end{smallmatrix}$$

With the exception of cocaine, the local anesthetics are synthetic and are formed by the attachment of various chemical groups to the aromatic nucleus, the aliphatic chain, or the amino group. The drugs thus formed are, almost without exception, white, generally odorless, viscid liquids or amorphous solids that are fat soluble but relatively insoluble in water. All are bases and form water-soluble and stable salts with acids.

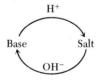

Base	Salt
1. Viscid liquids or amorphous solids	1. Crystalline
2. Fat soluble	2. Water soluble
3. Unstable	3. Stable
4. Alkaline	4. Acidic

The first local anesthetics were esters of benzoic acid (cocaine) or para-aminobenzoic acid (procaine). Subsequently, more diverse chemical structures have evolved. A chemical classification of local anesthetics with an example of each is as follows:

Esters of benzoic acid: cocaine

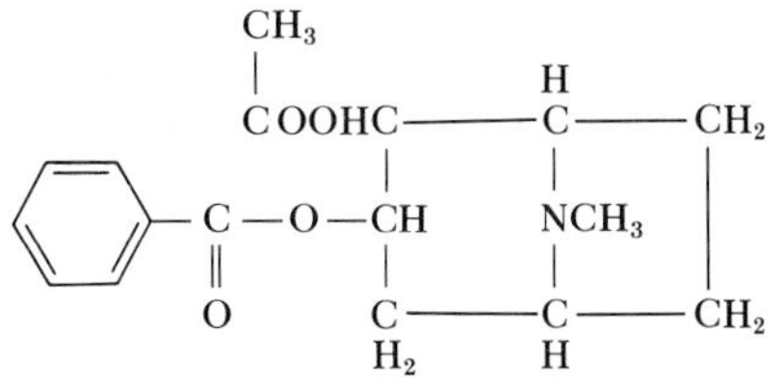

Esters of para-aminobenzoic acid: procaine

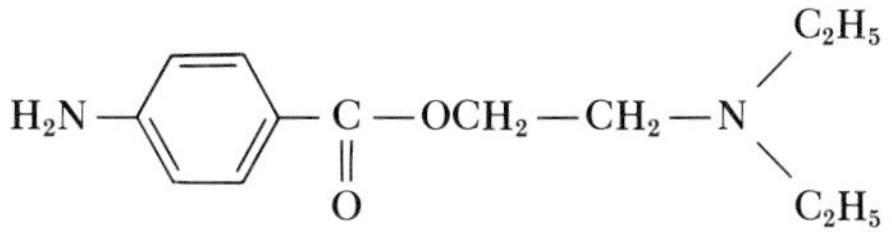

Esters of meta-aminobenzoic acid: metabutethamine

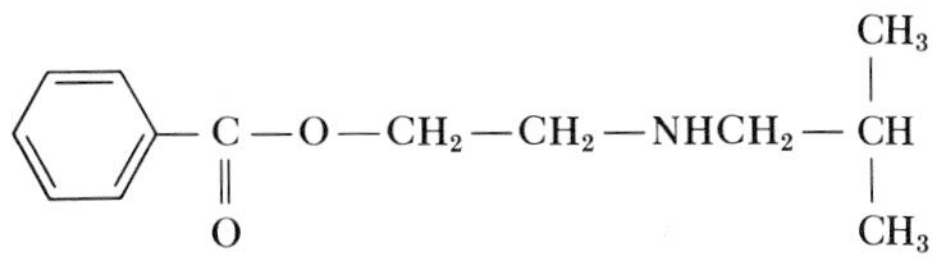

Amide derivatives of xylidine

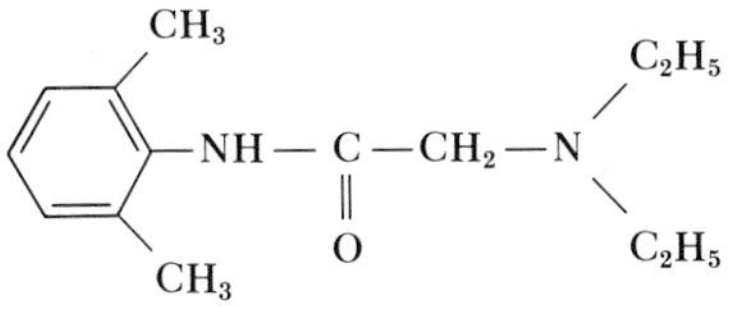

Lidocaine

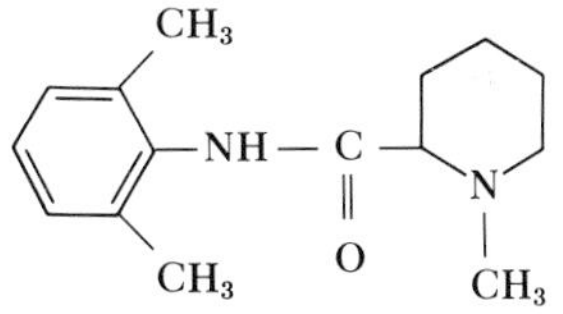

Mepivacaine

Amide derivatives of toluidine: prilocaine

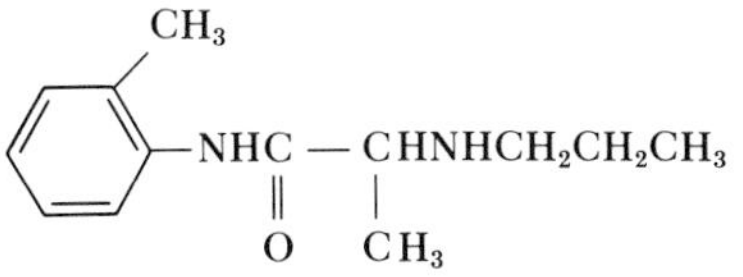

DRUGS AVAILABLE

A large number of local anesthetics are available. Some have little or no dental use. These include benoxinate HCl (Dorsacaine), phenocaine HCl (Holocaine HCl) and proparacaine HCl (Ophthaine), which are used for surface anesthesia in ophthalmology, and cyclomethycaine (Surfacaine), diperodon HCl (Disthane HCl), and pramoxine HCl

(Tronothane HCl), which provide surface anesthesia of damaged skin and mucosa. Dimethisoquin HCl (Quotane HCl) and diperodon HCl (Diothane HCl) are used for surface anesthesia. Dibucaine HCl (Nupercaine HCl), which is the most potent, toxic, and long-acting local anesthetic in current use,[24] is used for spinal and surface anesthesia. Bupivacaine HCl (Marcaine HCl) is a relatively new amide that is chemically related to mepivacaine. It is a potent and toxic drug with a long duration of action. It has been used for infiltration, block, and peridural anesthesia. Although piperocaine HCl (Metycaine HCl), chloroprocaine HCl (Nesacaine) and hexylcaine HCl (Cylcaine HCl) are all useful for infiltration and block anesthesia, they are seldom used in dentistry. Piperocaine and hexylcaine are also used topically, and the latter has additional use in spinal anesthesia. To emphasize agents of particular use in dentistry, I will not discuss the preceding local anesthetics further. The following drugs of historic or current importance in dental practice are shown in their respective chemical categories. These drugs will be described in individual monographs after the general discussion of local anesthetics. Drugs indicated by an asterisk are used only topically.

Esters of benzoic acid
  Cocaine*
  Meprylcaine (Oracaine)
Esters of para-aminobenzoic acid (PABA)
  Benzocaine*
  Butacaine (Butyn)*
  Butethamine (Monocaine)
  Procaine (Novocain)
  Propoxycaine (Ravocaine)
  Tetracaine (Pontocaine)
Esters of meta-aminobenzoic acid (MABA)
  Metabutethamine (Unacaine)
Amide derivatives of xylidine
  Lidocaine (Xylocaine)
  Mepivacaine (Carbocaine)
  Pyrrocaine (Dynacaine)
Amide derivatives of toluidine
  Prilocaine (Citanest)
Miscellaneous
  Chlorobutanol*
  Dyclonine (Dyclone)*

PHARMACOLOGIC EFFECTS

Peripheral nerve conduction. Reversible blockade of peripheral nerve conduction is the principal clinical function of local anesthetics. They inhibit the propagation of nerve impulses along fibers, at sensory endings, at myoneural junctions, and at synapses.[25] They do not penetrate the myelin sheath and therefore affect myelinated fibers only at the nodes of Ranvier. Local anesthetics affect small, unmyelinated, or thinly myelinated fibers first and large or heavily myelinated fibers last. Consequently, the losses in the usual order obtained are autonomics, sense of cold, warmth, pain, touch, pressure, vibration, proprioception, and motor.[26]

Central nervous system effects. If the systemic blood level of a local anesthetic reaches a certain concentration, effects on the central nervous system are observed. These effects represent the toxic reaction to local anesthesia and are discussed under the subject of adverse effects.

Myocardial effects. The myocardium is depressed by high systemic doses of local anesthetics. Electrical excitability, conduction rate, and cardiac output are reduced. This is the basis for the use of procaine amide and lidocaine as antiarrhythmic agents.

Effects on smooth muscle. Smooth muscle is relaxed, possibly by the depression of sensory receptors.[27] This allows arteriolar dilation and a spasmolytic effect on intestinal and bronchial smooth muscle. Although vasodilation with procaine requires the use of a vasoconstrictor for adequate dental local anesthesia, little or no vasodilation is seen with lidocaine, mepivacaine, and prilocaine.

ABSORPTION AND METABOLISM

As soon as a local anesthetic is injected or absorbed topically, it begins to (1) establish anesthesia, (2) distribute through the tissues, and (3) enter systemic circulation. Aside from the chemistry of the drug itself, the rate at which it leaves the site of administration and enters the circulation depends principally on the vascularity of the tissues injected and the presence or absence of a vasoconstrictor in the solution.

Greater vascularity, the absence of a vasoconstrictor, the application of heat or massage, and the presence of a spreading agent such as hyaluronidase increase absorption. Less vascularity, the presence of a vasoconstrictor, and vasoconstriction induced by the application of cold decrease absorption.

The systemic blood concentration that is ultimately obtained depends on the amount of drug that enters the circulation per unit of time (total dose and rate of entry), the volume of distribution, and the rate at which the drug is broken down and eliminated. One should note at this point that the absorption of some drugs from topical application may be rapid. Investigators have shown that in dogs the blood level obtained from the application of tetracaine to mucous membrane closely simulates that of rapid intravenous injection.[6,28] This is of particular significance in view of the fact that tetracaine is one of the more toxic local anesthetics and is found in 2% concentration in topical sprays that are used in dentistry.

Once in systemic circulation, local anesthetics permeate most tissues, particularly the liver, kidney, brain, heart, and lungs. They also cross the placenta. In humans the ester type of local anesthetics, particularly procaine and chloroprocaine, are hydrolyzed by both plasma and liver esterases. Most procaine is degraded to para-aminobenzoic acid (PABA) and diethylaminoethanol in plasma. Lidocaine and probably most other local anesthetics of the amide type are metabolized principally in the liver. Metabolites of both ester and amide anesthetics and some free drug are excreted in urine. The practitioner should be cautioned that severe liver disease will allow the systemic accumulation of local anesthetics, particularly the amides.

MECHANISM OF ACTION

Ionization factors. As previously noted, the local anesthetic free bases are fat-soluble (lipophilic) drugs. They are converted to their water-soluble (hydrophilic) hydrochloride salts to allow the preparation of solutions for injection. These solutions are stable and have a pH of 4.5 to 6.0. In solution an equilibrium is established between the ionized and nonionized forms of the local anesthetic drug. The proportion of the drug in ionized form depends, of course, on the pKa of the drug and the pH of the solution. At the usual solution pH of 6.0 or lower, most local anesthetics are almost completely in ionized form. The clinical importance of this fact is that only the nonionized free base form of the drug can readily penetrate tissue membranes. Consequently, local anesthesia can be obtained only if sufficient free base is available. The lower the pKa of the

drug, and the higher the pH of the solution or injected tissues, the more free base will be available.

Once the local anesthetic is injected, the buffering capacity and pH of the tissues (pH 7.4) tip the equilibrium in favor of free base formation. This conversion to free base allows greater tissue penetration of the local anesthetic. At physiologic tissue pH (7.4), 20% of lidocaine (pKa 7.86) is in free base form, whereas only 2% of procaine (pKa 8.92) exists as the free base. The presence of infection or inflammation in an injection area may lower the local tissue pH to the point where there is a significant inhibition of liberation of free base. Consequently, the depth of anesthesia is reduced.

The free base form of the local anesthetic is necessary for penetrating the nerve membrane. However, once the anesthetic has gained access to the interior of the axon, it is the ionized form of the anesthetic that is the active form of the drug. The site of action of the local anesthetic is on the inside surface of the neuronal membrane.

Action on the nerve fiber. Physiologically, a proportionally large number of negative ions (anions) accumulate on the inside of nerve fiber membranes, and a proportionally large number of positive ions (cations) accumulate on the outside of the membrane. Thus the resting nerve fiber is electronegative on the inside and electropositive on the outside (Fig. 11, *A*). A nerve impulse (nerve action potential) is a transient reversal of this polarity, which is propagated down the fiber like a wave. This reversal of polarity, or depolarization, results from an increase in the permeability of an area of the fiber membrane to sodium ions. Since a much greater concentration of sodium exists on the outside of the membrane, a large influx of sodium ions enters the fiber to reverse the polarity (Fig. 11, *B*). This local depolarization then transits the fiber as a nerve impulse. The fiber behind the traveling impulse is repolarized by the efflux of potassium ions and the active transport of sodium ions back out of the fiber (Fig. 11, *C*). The latter mechanism is the classic sodium "pump."

Local anesthetics block nerve conduction by decreasing the membrane permeability to sodium, thus interfering with the influx of sodium, which is essential for the depolarization of the fiber. The exact mechanism by

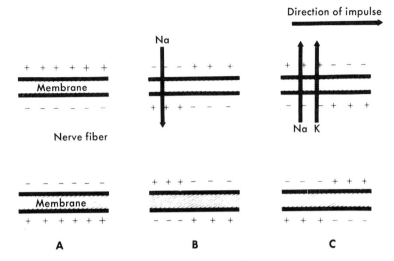

Fig. 11. The nerve impulse. **A,** Resting nerve fiber. **B,** Generation of a nerve impulse—a reversal of polarity resulting from an influx of sodium. **C,** Repolarization behind the impulse resulting from an efflux of potassium and sodium.

which local anesthetics decrease membrane permeability to sodium is not known.

ANTIHISTAMINES AS LOCAL ANESTHETICS

Antihistamines have weak local anesthetic properties. The only clinical significance of this fact is that they may be useful when a patient is allergic to several types of local anesthetics, or in emergency cases where the patient recalls a severe allergic reaction to an unknown local anesthetic.

One percent tripelennamine (Pyribenzamine) and 1% diphenhydramine hydrochloride (Benadryl) have been injected as local anesthetics.[29] Both were found to provide satisfactory local anesthesia for tooth extraction. The average volume injected was 3 ml, and the maximal dose was 5 ml. The average duration of local anesthesia obtained with the antihistamines was about one half that obtained with 2% lidocaine with epinephrine 1:100,000. Another study compared 2% lidocaine and 1% diphenhydramine, both with 1:100,000 epinephrine.[30] The diphenhydramine solution had a slower onset, about one half the duration of action, and produced profound anesthesia in fewer patients. However, diphenhydramine provided profound or satisfactory anesthesia for the removal of 22 out of 25 partially embedded, carious, and malposed third molars without postanesthetic complications. The maximal dose of diphenhydramine used was 4 ml (40 mg).

COMPOSITION OF ANESTHETIC SOLUTIONS

In addition to the anesthetic drug, local anesthetic solutions usually contain a vasoconstrictor (epinephrine, levonordefrin) and an antioxidant to preserve the vasoconstrictor (sodium bisulfite or sodium pyrosulfite). Antiseptics such as methylparaben are added to multiple-dose vials and sometimes to cartridges. Experimentally, antibiotics, meperidine, alkalinizing agents, and hyaluronidase have been added to local anesthetic solutions.

VASOCONSTRICTORS IN LOCAL ANESTHETICS

Vasoconstrictors are included in local anesthetic solutions to (1) prolong and increase the depth of anesthesia by retaining the anesthetic in the area injected, (2) reduce the toxic effect of the drug by delaying its absorption into the general circulation, and (3) render the area of injection less hemorrhagic. A pharmacologic comparison of the various vasoconstrictors is presented in Chapter 13.

Eliminating the vasoconstrictor. Whenever a local anesthetic solution does not contain a vasoconstrictor, the anesthetic drug will be removed from the injection site and into systemic circulation faster than if the solution did contain a vasoconstrictor. This will provide a shorter duration of action and allow a more rapid buildup of a systemic blood level of the anesthetic. Any advantage gained by eliminating the vasoconstrictor (shorter duration?) must be weighed against the adverse potentialities. The latter will be determined by the nature, toxicity, and concentration of the anesthetic drug, the volume of drug required, and the size, age, and general health of the patient involved.

Concentration of the vasoconstrictor. How much vasoconstrictor is needed in a local anesthetic solution? A sufficient concentration should be present to allow anesthesia of adequate depth, duration, and safety. How much is this? On the point of safety, dentists have established an excellent safety record using 1:50,000 and 1:100,000 epinephrine or equivalent concentration of levonordefrin with 2% procaine, lidocaine, and mepivacaine. The question then becomes: If adequate safety is obtained with 1:100,000 epinephrine, does one need the 1:50,000 concentration?

In 1963 Keesling and Hinds[31] carried out a double-blind study of various concentrations of epinephrine with 2% lidocaine in 119 subjects. They found that 2% lidocaine with 1:250,000 epinephrine was as effective in increasing the depth and duration of anesthesia as the solutions containing 1:50,000 or 1:100,000 epinephrine. Reeve stated in 1970, "There is no need at any time to use a concentration of epinephrine greater than 1:100,000 for dental anesthesia."[32] In spite of the fact that for years the dental profession used epinephrine in local anesthetic solutions at a concentration of 1:50,000, the use of 1:100,000 concentrations will provide an adequate prolongation of anesthesia and protection against rapid absorption.

I do not believe there is justification for the use of epinephrine in a concentration greater than 1:100,000 except in those infrequent cases where 1:50,000 is necessary to provide hemostasis.

Vasoconstrictors in patients with cardiovascular disease. During the 1930s and 1940s, statements were frequently made in the literature that vasoconstrictors should not be used in dental local anesthetics for patients with cardiovascular disease. The fear was that the vasoconstrictor might cause a rise in blood pressure which could not be tolerated by a patient with cardiovascular disease. Although these early fears were associated with a certain amount of logic, the effect of vasoconstrictors on the cardiovascu-

lar system in the quantities used in dental practice had not been adequately studied at that time. Additionally, physicians were accustomed then, as they are now, to think of epinephrine in terms of greater concentrations than are used in dentistry.

During the 1950s, a number of studies demonstrated that the small amount of vasoconstrictor contained in dental local anesthetics had no effect on blood pressure. Notable here were the studies by McCarthy,[33] Wallace and co-workers,[34] Tainter and Winter,[35] Follmar and associates,[36] Salman and Schwartz,[37] Cheraskin and Prasertsuntarasai,[38-41] and Costich.[42] During the same period, Dick,[43] Follmar and associates,[36] and Mead[44] had indicated that discomfort after inadequate anesthesia would produce more endogenous epinephrine than that introduced in a local anesthetic solution. It is interesting to note that the *resting* adrenal medulla of a 70 kg man produces approximately 0.014 mg per minute epinephrine.[45] This equals the amount of epinephrine in 1.4 ml of a 1:100,000 solution.

The current status of vasoconstrictors in patients with cardiovascular disease is as follows:

1. A Working Conference of the American Dental Associations and American Heart Association has said, "The concentration of vasoconstrictor normally used in dental local anesthetic solutions is not contraindicated in patients with cardiovascular disease when administered carefully and with preliminary aspiration. The following concentrations can be used: epinephrine, 1:50,000–1:250,000; levarterenol, 1:30,000; levonordefrin, 1:20,000; and phenylephrine 1:2,500."[46]

2. The New York Heart Association has stated, "The dentist should have information from the physician about the nature and severity of the heart disease in the patient. He should also have knowledge of medication the patient is receiving, particularly such medication as might increase the activity of epinephrine. This knowledge is important because ordinary dental procedures may produce some emotional stress and cause cardiac disturbances which might be wrongly attributed to epinephrine."[47] As a guideline, the New York Heart Association recommends that for any one session no more than 0.2 mg epinephrine be administered. This is the amount of epinephrine

in 10 ml of a 1:50,000 solution or 20 ml of a 1:100,000 solution.

ADVERSE EFFECTS

Despite the enviable record of safety in dental local anesthesia, the practitioner must be aware of the adverse potentialities. Adriani has said, "Few potentially hazardous drugs are used as thoughtlessly, as indiscriminately and with less knowledge of their pharmacology as are the local anesthetics."[48] One must not consider local anesthesia as being without danger. A lack of caution will result in needless serious and fatal reactions. The treatment of adverse effects is discussed in Chapter 24.

Adverse reactions to local anesthetics can be local or systemic. Although these drugs can damage tissues locally,[49,50] this does not appear to present a significant clinical problem in dentistry. Adverse systemic effects include toxic reactions, allergic reactions, and effects of the vasoconstrictor.

Toxic effects. As with any drug, toxic reactions to local anesthetics occur when a certain tolerable blood-tissue concentration (toxic level) is exceeded. The particular concentration of a drug that causes a toxic reaction depends basically on the toxicity of the specific drug. Table 14-2 shows the relative toxicities of some local anesthetics of importance in dentistry. One should remember that the blood level that will cause a toxic response is likely to vary somewhat among individuals and may also vary with time in the same individual. Children and elderly and debilitated patients may show toxic reactions at blood levels lower than those that are adverse in young healthy adults. One should note that the severity of toxic effects are proportioned to the toxicity of the drug and the blood level that exists.

Although the factors that determine the height of a particular blood level obtained after the injection of a local anesthetic have been mentioned earlier, a more detailed consideration relative to toxicity should be made at this point.

1. *Nature of drug.* The rates at which currently used local anesthetics enter the circulation after submucosal injection are not significantly different. Although the ester type of drugs cause more vasodilation than do the amides, the clinical effects of vasodilation are usually counteracted by the inclusion of greater concentration of a vasoconstrictor. However, drugs such as tetracaine enter the circulation after topical application much more rapidly than does lidocaine.

2. *Concentration of drug.* Obviously, the higher the concentration of drug used the greater will be the amount of drug per unit of injected volume that will enter the systemic circulation.

3. *Route of injection.* The inadvertent intravenous injection of a local anesthetic is probably the most frequent reason for high systemic blood levels obtained in dental practice. This points up the importance of aspiration prior to injection.

4. *Vascularity of site.* Greater innate vascularity of an area or the presence of hyperemia as produced by inflammation or the application of heat will increase the rate of drug entry into systemic circulation. Vasoconstriction as produced by the application of cold will reduce systemic absorption.

5. *Presence of a vasoconstrictor.* The vasoconstrictor reduces systemic absorption. Adequate reduction in systemic absorption of the currently available local anesthetics is accomplished with 1:100,000 epinephrine.

6. *Volume of distribution.* A dose of a local anesthetic administered to a 50-pound child will obtain higher blood-tissue concentration than if administered to a 150-pound adult.

Table 14-2. Relative toxicities and maximum recommended doses

Drug	Relative toxicity	Maximum recommended dose (Monheim[51])*	Milliliters of a 2% solution
Procaine	1	400 mg	20
Lidocaine	2	300 mg	15
Mepivacaine	2	300 mg	15
Prilocaine	1.5	400 mg	20
Tetracaine	10-15	30 mg	1.5

*For healthy adults.

7. *Rate of metabolism and elimination.* Infants, children, patients with liver and kidney disease, the highly debilitated, and the elderly will not metabolize and/or eliminate a drug as rapidly as other patients. This obviously leads to increased systemic blood levels.

Systemic toxicity to local anesthetics is described as a descending stimulation of the central nervous system followed by depression of certain areas of the brain. It has been suggested that the entire effect of local anesthetics on the central nervous system is one of depression and that the phase of stimulation is the result of the depression of inhibitory neurons.[27,52] If the classic progression is observed, one might see the following:

1. Restlessness, apprehension, and tremors progressing to excitement and chronic convulsions
2. Increasing blood pressure and pulse rate
3. Increasing rate of respiration
4. Respiratory and cardiovascular depression with loss of reflexes and consciousness

Depression, generally the cause of death, may appear initially without signs of stimulation. Depression without the preliminary stages of stimulation has been characteristic of lidocaine toxicity.

On rare occasions, cardiovascular collapse and death have occurred after a low dose of infiltration anesthesia. Although the mechanism here is unknown, it is probably caused by cardiac arrest resulting from a direct effect on the pacemaker or sudden ventricular fibrillation.[31]

Allergic reactions. Allergic reactions to local anesthetics are not common. However, mild dermatologic reaction (urticaria or rashes), delayed reactions (serum sickness), or immediate reactions (anaphylaxis) may occur after the use of any local anesthetic. A carefully obtained medical history should disclose known sensitizations, but it is no assurance that an allergy does not exist. An allergy to any one drug will indicate that the patient is likely to be allergic to drugs with a similar chemical structure. As a rule, use of the amides is safe in patients who are allergic to the ester type of drugs and vice versa. Cross-allergenicity does not appear to exist between lidocaine and mepivacaine. Consequently, they may usually be substi-

tuted for each other. However, some individuals are allergic to several anesthetics, and no substitute is an absolute guarantee that an allergic reaction will not occur.

Reactions to the vasoconstrictor. Some individuals may show signs and symptoms after the use of a local anesthetic that are believed to be caused by the vasoconstrictor. These reactions are most likely to follow inadvertent intravenous injection and include palpitation, apprehension, and tachycardia. They are usually mild and self-limiting.

Precautions in topical anesthesia. It was mentioned earlier that some local anesthetics are absorbed very rapidly when applied topically to mucous membranes. To avoid toxic reactions from surface anesthesia, the practitioner should consider the following[22]:

1. Know the relative *toxicity* of the drug being used.
2. Know the *concentration* of the drug being used.
3. Use the *smallest volume* and the *lowest concentration* of the *least toxic* drug that will satisfy the clinical requirements.
4. Limit the *area of application* as much as possible.

The topical application of drugs is more likely to induce an allergy than would oral or parenteral administration. Consequently (1) highly allergenic drugs should never be used topically, and (2) the topical administration of parenterally useful drugs should be restricted as much as possible.

AGENTS FOR INJECTION

Procaine hydrochloride. Procaine hydrochloride (Novocain) is a para-aminobenzoic acid (PABA) ester. After its synthesis in 1905, it quickly replaced cocaine as the most used local anesthetic in both medicine and dentistry. Procaine remained the principal local anesthetic in use until the late 1950s, when the amide type of drug gained popularity.

Procaine has a quick onset and a toxicity and potency of about half that of lidocaine. It causes local vasodilation and thus has a relatively short duration of action unless used with a vasoconstrictor. Rapid hydrolysis in plasma to PABA and diethylaminoethanol makes procaine one of the safest, if not the safest, local anesthetic known. Its metabolite, PABA, interferes with the antibacterial activity of the sulfonamides; consequently, it should not be used with these drugs.

Procaine is not effective topically but is used for infiltration, block, spinal, epidural, and caudal anesthesia. It is also used intravenously in the treatment of cardiac arrhythmias and seizures of status epilepticus.[24] It is also used as an antifibrillatory agent (procaine amide) and is combined with penicillin to form procaine penicillin G. The principal use of procaine hydrochloride in dentistry today is in 2% solutions with more potent local anesthetics such as tetracaine and propoxycaine.

Lidocaine hydrochloride. Lidocaine hydrochloride (Xylocaine, Lidothesin, Octocaine) is an amide derivative of xylidine. It was introduced in 1949 and quickly became an anesthetic of considerable importance. It has to a great extent replaced procaine as the standard to which other local anesthetics are compared. It has a rapid onset, which is undoubtedly related to its tendency to spread well through the tissues. Lidocaine in 2% concentration provides profound anesthesia of long duration, especially if the solution contains a vasoconstrictor. Since lidocaine causes little or no local vasodilation, less vasoconstrictor is required than is necessary with procaine. It is twice as toxic as procaine, but with proper care the doses required in dentistry have caused little problem. There is no cross-allergenicity between lidocaine and the ester type of anesthetics, and apparently none between lidocaine and other available amides such as mepivacaine and prilocaine. Some patients appear to experience some sedation with lidocaine, and in toxic reactions one is likely to observe central nervous system (CNS) depression initially rather than the CNS stimulation characteristic of other local anesthetics.

Lidocaine is used for topical, infiltration, block, spinal, epidural, and caudal anesthesia. It is also used intravenously in the treatment of cardiac arrhythmias during surgery, to depress laryngeal and pharyngeal reflexes, to reduce the pruritus of jaundice and the pain caused by malignancy or burns, and to control the seizures of status epilepticus.[24]

In dentistry, 2% lidocaine hydrochloride is used for infiltration and block anesthesia with 1:50,000 epinephrine and 1:100,000 epinephrine and also without a vasoconstric-

tor. It is used for topical anesthesia as a 5% ointment, a 10% spray, and a 2% viscous solution.

Mepivacaine hydrochloride. Mepivacaine hydrochloride (Carbocaine) is an amide derivative of xylidine. It was introduced in the late 1950s and has become an important local anesthetic. Its rate of onset, duration, potency, and toxicity are essentially the same as those of lidocaine. There is no cross-allergenicity between mepivacaine and the ester type of local anesthetic and apparently none with the other currently available amides.

Mepivacaine hydrochloride is not effective topically but is used for infiltration, block, spinal, epidural, and caudal anesthesia. The usual dosage form in dentistry is a 2% solution with 1:20,000 levonordefrin (Neo-Cobefrin) as the vasoconstrictor. Since mepivacaine produces even less vasodilation than does lidocaine, it has been made available in a 3% solution without a vasoconstrictor. One must exercise considerable caution in using increased concentrations of a local anesthetic to eliminate the vasoconstrictor. I do not believe that the "benefit" of shorter duration warrants eliminating the vasoconstrictor, especially if the concentration of the drug is increased. In regard to the elimination of the vasoconstrictor in patients with preexisting medical problems, Reeve has said, "The excess concentration of a toxic anesthetic agent will do far more harm to the patient than the small concentration of 1:100,000 or less epinephrine used to prevent the rapid absorption of this drug into the circulating blood."[32] I agree completely with this statement.

Prilocaine hydrochloride. Prilocaine hydrochloride (Citanest) is a relatively new drug related chemically and pharmacologically to lidocaine and mepivacaine. A basic chemical difference, however, is that whereas lidocaine and mepivacaine are derivatives of xylidine, prilocaine is a derivative of toluidine. Prilocaine appears to be less potent and less toxic than lidocaine with a slightly longer duration of action. It has been shown to produce satisfactory local anesthesia with low concentrations of epinephrine and without epinephrine. Although prilocaine toxicity has been said to be 60% of that of lidocaine,[53] several cases of methemoglobinemia have been reported after its use. Although the small doses required in dental practice are not likely to present a problem in healthy, nonpregnant adults, prilocaine should not be administered to infants or to patients with methemoglobinemia, heart failure,[24] or any other condition where problems of oxygenation may be especially critical, such as in pregnancy. Methemoglobinemia can be reversed by the intravenous injection of 1% methylene blue (1 to 2 mg/kg).

Prilocaine hydrochloride is used for infiltration, block, epidural, and caudal anesthesia. It is available in dental carpules as a 4% concentration with 1:200,000 epinephrine and also as a 4% solution without a vasoconstrictor. As has been noted previously, I believe that the use of increased concentrations of a drug without the use of a vasoconstrictor is open to considerable question.

Pyrrocaine hydrochloride. Pyrrocaine (Dynacaine) is another relatively new drug, which like lidocaine and mepivacaine is an amide derivative of xylidine. The early reports on this drug are encouraging, and it appears to have qualities of onset, potency, toxicity, and duration similar to those of lidocaine and mepivacaine. It is available in carpules in 2% solutions with 1:150,000 and 1:250,000 epinephrine.

Tetracaine hydrochloride. Tetracaine hydrochloride (Pontocaine) is an ester of PABA. During the 1950s tetracaine obtained considerable use in combination with procaine for dental local anesthesia. This use decreased after the introduction of lidocaine and mepivacaine. Tetracaine has a slow onset and long duration and is generally estimated to have at least ten times the potency and toxicity of procaine. Topically, it is rapidly absorbed. In view of this drug's high toxicity and the rapidity with which it is absorbed from mucosal surfaces, great care must be exercised when it is used for topical anesthesia. As in the case of procaine and other PABA derivatives, tetracaine may reduce the effectiveness of concomitantly administered sulfonamides. It is used for topical, infiltration, block, caudal, and spinal anesthesia.

Carpules are available that contain 0.15% tetracaine HCl and 2% procaine HCl with 1:20,000 levonordefrin, 1:30,000 levarterenol, or 1:2500 phenylephrine HCl the vaso-constrictor. Tetracaine is available in various sprays, solutions, and ointments for topical application. The concentration of tetracaine in most topical preparations is 2%.

Propoxycaine. Propoxycaine (Blockain, Ravocaine) is another ester of PABA. In the late 1950s propoxycaine, like tetracaine, came to be used in combination with procaine. It is slightly less potent and less toxic than tetracaine and similarly has a long duration of action. Propoxycaine's rapid onset of action when injected and its lack of topical activity are its principal clinical differences from tetracaine.

Propoxycaine HCl is used for infiltration and block anesthesia. Dental carpules contain 0.4% propoxycaine HCl and 2% procaine HCl with 1:20,000 levonordefrin or 1:30,000 levarterenol.

Butethamine. Butethamine (Monocaine) is one of the older PABA esters and is no longer of particular importance in dentistry. It is about twice as potent as procaine and slightly more toxic. It has a more rapid onset and a slightly longer duration of action than procaine. Butethamine hydrochloride has been used for infiltration and block anesthesia at a 2% concentration with 1:50,000 epinephrine.

Metabutethamine hydrochloride. Metabutethamine hydrochloride (Unacaine) is an ester of meta-aminobenzoic acid (MABA). It has a rapid onset and a relatively short duration of action and is less potent and less toxic than procaine. Metabutethamine hydrochloride is used for infiltration and block anesthesia. It is available in carpules at a 3.8% concentration with 1:60,000 epinephrine. It may be useful for short duration anesthesia.

Meprylcaine hydrochloride. Meprylcaine hydrochloride (Oracaine) is an ester of benzoic acid. It is slightly more potent and has a toxicity approximately the same as procaine. It has a more rapid onset and a shorter duration of action than procaine. Meprylcaine hydrochloride is used for infiltration and block anesthesia. It is available in carpules at a 2% concentration with 1:50,000 epinephrine and may be useful for short duration anesthesia.

TOPICAL ANESTHETICS

Lidocaine and tetracaine are effective topical anesthetics and have been discussed previously. The following drugs, except for cocaine, have a usefulness as surface anesthetics in dentistry. Cocaine is discussed for historic reasons and because it is still used to some extent in medical practice.

Cocaine. Cocaine is an ester of benzoic acid, occurs naturally, and was the first local anesthetic. It is potent, extremely toxic, addicting, and the only local anesthetic that causes a definite vasoconstriction. Because of its toxicity and addicting properties, it is no longer used parenterally. It is used topically in medical practice but has no present application to dentistry.

Benzocaine. Benzocaine (ethyl aminobenzoate) is an ester of PABA that is chemically similar to procaine. Benzocaine lacks a basic nitrogen group and cannot be converted to a water-soluble salt for parenteral use. It is an effective and relatively safe topical anesthetic. Its safety results primarily from the fact that it is slowly absorbed from mucous membrane.

Dyclonine hydrochloride. Dyclonine hydrochloride (Dyclone) is not related chemically to the aminobenzoic acid esters but has some structural similarities to lidocaine and mepivacaine. It is an effective and relatively safe topical anesthetic but is too irritating to be injected. Dyclone is available in 0.5% and 1% solutions.

REFERENCES

1. Editorial: The other half of the picture, J.A.D.A. **32:**1031, 1945.
2. Mayer, E.: The toxic effects following the use of local anesthetics, J.A.M.A. **82:**876, 1924.
3. Mayer, E.: Fatalities from local anesthetics, J.A.M.A. **90:**1928.
4. Ruth, H. D., Haugen, F. P., and Grove, D. D.: Anesthesia Study Commission, J.A.M.A. **135:**881, 1947.
5. Dealy, F. N.: Anesthetic deaths, 5-year report, Am. J. Surg. **60:**63, 1943.
6. Adriani, J., and Campbell, D.: Fatalities following topical application of local anesthetics to mucous membranes, J.A.M.A. **162:**1527, 1956.
7. Furstenberg, A. C., Wood, L. A., Magielski, J. E., and McMahon, G. F.: An evaluation of cocaine anesthesia: the perpetuation of equivocal concepts, Trans. Am. Acad. Ophthalmol. Otolaryngol. **56:** 643, 1951.
8. Ireland, P. E., Ferguson, J. K. W., and Stark, E. J.: The clinical and experimental comparison of cocaine and pontocaine as topical anesthetics, Laryngoscope **61:**767, 1951.
9. Beecher, H. K., and Todd, D. P.: A study of the deaths associated with anesthesia and surgery: based on a study of 599, 548 anesthesias in 10 institutions, 1948-1952, Am. Surg. **140:**2, 1954.
10. Criep, L. H., and Ribeiro, C. C.: Allergy to procaine hydrochloride with 3 fatalities, J.A.M.A. **151:**1185, 1953.
11. Seldin, H. M., and Recant, B. S.: Safety of anesthesia in the dental office, J. Oral Surg. **13:**199, 1955.
12. Seldin, H. M.: Survey of anesthetic fatalities in oral surgery and a review of the etiological factors in anesthetic deaths, J. Am. Dent. Soc. Anesth. **5:**6, 1958.
13. American Dental Association: The 1962 survey of dental practice. V. Some aspects of dental practice, J.A.D.A. **67:**158, 1963.
14. Driscoll, E. J.: Anesthesia morbidity and mortality in oral surgery. Proceedings of the Conference on Anesthesia for the Ambulatory Patient, Chicago, 1966.
15. American Society of Oral Surgeons: ASOS anesthesia morbidity and mortality survey, J. Oral Surg. **32:**733, 1974.
16. Wigand, F. T.: Untoward reaction to lidocaine: report of a case, J. Oral Surg. **16:**334, 1958.
17. Morrissett, L. M.: Fatal anaphylactic reaction to lidocaine, U.S. Armed Forces Med. J. **8:**740, 1957.
18. Ningham, L. R., and Molherbe, P. H.: Xylocaine intoxication: a report of 3 recent cases, Dent. Abstr. **3:**143, 1958.
19. Medico-legal comment. Death after Xylocaine injection, Br. Med. J. **1:**280, 1952.
20. Hunter, A. R.: The toxicity of Xylocaine, Br. J. Anaesth. **23:**153, 1951.
21. Hanson, I. R., and Hingson, R. A.: Use of Xylocaine, new local anesthetic, in surgery, obstetrics and therapeutics, Anesth. Analg. **29:**136, 1950.
22. American Dental Association Council on Dental Therapeutics: Accepted dental therapeutics, ed. 37, Chicago, 1977, American Dental Association.
23. Pharmacotherapeutics in dental practice (NAVPERS 10486), Washington, D.C., 1969, U.S. Bureau of Naval Personnel.
24. American Medical Association Council on Drugs: AMA drug evaluations—1973, Chicago, 1973, American Medical Association.
25. Krantz, J. C., Jr., and Carr, C. J.: The pharmacologic principles of medical practice, ed. 7, Baltimore, 1969, The Williams & Wilkins Co.
26. Adriani, J.: The clinical pharmacology of local anesthetics, J. Clin. Pharm. Exper. Ther. **1:**645, 1960.
27. Goodman, L. S., and Gilman, A.: The pharmacological basis of therapeutics, ed. 5, New York, 1975, The Macmillan Co.
28. Campbell, D., and Adriani, J.: Absorption of local anesthetics, J.A.M.A. **168:**873, 1958.
29. Meyer, R. A., and Jokubowski, W.: Use of tripelennamine and diphenhydramine as local anesthetics, J.A.D.A. **69:**112, 1964.
30. Welborn, J. F., and Kane, J. P.: Conduction anesthesia using diphenhydramine hydrochloride, J.A.D.A. **69:**706, 1964.
31. Keesling, G. R., and Hinds, E. C.: Optimal concentration of epinephrine in lidocaine solutions, J.A.D.A. **66:**337, 1963.
32. Reeve, L. W.: Modern pharmacodynamic concepts of local anesthesia, Dent. Clin. North Am. **14:**783, Oct., 1970.
33. McCarthy, F. M.: Clinical study of blood pressure

responses to epinephrine-containing local anesthetic solutions. J. Dent. Res. **36:**132, 1957.

34. Wallace, D. A., Sadove, M. S., Spence, J. M., and Gish, G.: Systemic effects of dental local anesthetic solutions, Oral Surg. **9:**1297, 1956.

35. Tainter, M. L., and Winter, L.: Some general considerations in evaluating local anesthetic solutions in patients, Anesthesiology **5:**470, 1944.

36. Follmar, K. E., Skau, R. M., Billett, A. E., and Jorgensen, A. K.: The effects upon human blood pressure of representative local anesthetics and vasoconstrictors, Northwestern Univ. Bull. **54:**13, 1954.

37. Salman, I., and Schwartz, S. P.: Effects of vasoconstrictors used in local anesthetics in patients with diseases of the heart, J. Oral Surg. **13:**209, 1955.

38. Cheraskin, E., and Prasertsuntarasai, T.: Use of epinephrine with local anesthesia in hypertensive patients. I. Blood pressure and pulse rate observations in the waiting room, J.A.D.A. **55:**761, 1957.

39. Cheraskin, E., and Prasertsuntarasai, T.: Use of epinephrine with local anesthesia in hypertensive patients. II. Effect of sedation on blood pressure and pulse pressure and pulse rate in the waiting room, J.A.D.A. **56:**210, 1958.

40. Cheraskin, E., and Prasertsuntarasai, T.: Use of epinephrine with local anesthesia in hypertensive patients. III. Effect of epinephrine on blood pressure and pulse rate, J.A.D.A. **57:**507, 1958.

41. Cheraskin, E., and Prasertsuntarasai, T.: Use of epinephrine with local anesthesia in hypertensive patients. IV. Effect of tooth extraction on blood pressure and pulse rate, J.A.D.A. **58:**61, 1959.

42. Costich, E. P.: Study of inferior alveolar nerve block anesthesia in humans, comparing 2 per cent procaine plus 1:50,000 epinephrine, J. Dent. Res. **35:**695, 1956.

43. Dick, S. P.: Clinical toxicity of epinephrine anesthesia, Oral Surg. **6:**724, 1953.

44. Mead, S. V.: Use of epinephrine-containing anesthetic solutions in oral surgery, J. Oral Surg. **14:**79, 1956.

45. Guyton, A. C.: Textbook of medical physiology, ed. 4, Philadelphia, 1971, W. B. Saunders Co.

46. Working Conference of American Dental Association & American Heart Association on Management of Dental Problems in Patients with Cardiovascular Disease, J.A.D.A. **68:**333, 1964.

47. Special Committee of the N.Y. Heart Association, Inc.: Use of epinephrine in connection with procaine in dental procedures, J.A.D.A. **50:**108, 1955.

48. Adriani, J.: Local anesthetics. In Seminar Report, **I:**18, Fall, 1956, Philadelphia, Merck, Sharp & Dohme.

49. Costich, E. R.: The reaction of rat muscle to the constituents of procaine-epinephrine solutions in concentrations used for dental preparations, Oral Surg. **9:**205, 1956.

50. Brun, A.: Effect of procaine, Carbocaine and Xylocaine on cutaneous muscle in rabbits and mice, Acta Anaesth. Scand. **3**(2):59, 1959.

51. Monheim, L. M.: Local anesthesia and pain control in dental practice, ed. 4, St. Louis, 1969, The C. V. Mosby Co.

52. Sutherland, V. C.: A synopsis of pharmacology, ed. 2, Philadelphia, 1970, W. B. Saunders Co.

53. Aström, A., and Persson, N. H.: Some pharmacological properties of o-methyl-α propylaminopropionanilide, a new local anesthetic, Br. J. Pharmacol. **16:**32, 1961.

15

Histamine and antihistamines

BARBARA F. ROTH-SCHECHTER

HISTAMINE

Histamine is a rather ubiquitous biogenic amine. Although many of its actions are well known, its precise physiologic function and significance are not understood. It is for this reason that histamine is commonly classified as an autacoid with others such as serotonin, angiotensin, and bradykinin, that is, endogenous substances of intense pharmacologic activity whose role in the human body is not established.

Distribution, synthesis, and metabolism

Almost all mammalian tissues contain histamine and/or have the capacity to synthesize it. High concentrations are found in the intestinal mucosa, skin, and lungs, where histamine is primarily contained in mast cells.[1] Histamine is stored in the mast cell granule in physiologically inactive form. Current evidence indicates that histamine release correlates with degranulation of mast cells, is energy dependent, and requires the presence of calcium.[2] In blood, histamine is contained in basophils. In both of these "storage sites" histamine is bound to heparin. In the central nervous system, which is devoid of mast cells, histamine is most probably contained in synaptic vesicles, a finding that is consistent with the hypothesis of histamine possibly being a central transmitter.[3]

Synthesis of endogenous histamine is by way of decarboxylation of histidine by nonspecific L-amino acid decarboxylase (histidine decarboxylase), an inducible enzyme. Ingested histamine or that formed by bacteria in the gastrointestinal tract appears to be insignificant in maintaining body stores.

The two primary pathways of histamine metabolism are (1) to 1-methylhistamine by imidazole-methyltransferase (IMT) or (2) by diamine oxidase (DAO) to imidazole–acetic acid. These and additional metabolic products are excreted through the kidney.

The levels of both catabolic and anabolic enzyme systems of histamine vary considerably during different physiologic conditions, such as an increase in DAO activity during pregnancy, suggesting again a significant physiologic regulatory function of the autacoid in humans.

Pharmacologic actions

There are pronounced species differences in the actions of histamines. The following discussion deals with its actions in humans.

Histamine affects many organ systems but with different intensities and different sensitivities to drug action. Although the existence of more than one receptor for histamine had been postulated before,[4] only the synthesis of antagonists of specific histamine sites[5] made it possible to arrive at the presently accepted concept of histamine receptors. Accordingly, the actions of histamine are divided into those which are mediated by way of activation of the H_1 receptors, the H_2 receptors, or a combination of both.

1. Histamine is a powerful vasodilator and can cause extensive dilation of arterioles,

Histidine   Histidine decarboxylase   Histamine

venules, and capillaries. This effect is independent of innervation and apparently results from a direct effect on these tissues. This action of histamine can be blocked only by a combination of H_1 and H_2 histamine antagonists, and thus it is mediated by receptors of both H_1 and H_2 types.

2. Histamine will effect an increased permeability of capillaries and small veins[4] to the extent of releasing plasma proteins and fluid into extracellular space. These two main effects of histamine (vasodilation and increased capillary permeability) are primarily responsible for initiating the most deleterious sequela of histamine—cardiovascular shock. (See later.)

3. Histamine has a direct stimulatory effect on nonvascular smooth muscle. In humans the most common effect observed is bronchoconstriction, which is particularly prominent in patients suffering from various pulmonary diseases. This action of histamine is easily antagonized by the long available "classic" antihistamines known to block H_1 receptors, and therefore it is considered to involve activation of the H_1 type of receptors exclusively.

4. Almost all exocrine glands are stimulated by histamine, but to various degrees. Histamine is a powerful stimulant of gastric secretion by a direct action on parietal and chief cells. This response to histamine can be effectively antagonized by antihistaminic drugs involving H_2 receptors, and thus stimulation of gastric secretion is considered to be the typical example of activation by way of a pure H_2 receptor.

5. Histamine stimulates cutaneous nerve endings, eliciting axon reflexes. Therefore histamine causes itching, when introduced into superficial layers of skin, and pain accompanied by itching, when introduced into deeper layers of skin. At the cellular level this is apparently also mediated by membrane permeability changes, which in this case result in depolarization and initiation of nerve impulses.

Histamine release

Many physiologic and pathophysiologic reactions as well as the administration of certain drugs will result in the release of endogenous histamine. The extent of release of histamine will determine the resulting pharmacologic actions, both in severity and spectrum. Although not always clinically significant, the fact should also be kept in mind that any mechanism resulting in the endogenous release of histamine from mast cells will simultaneously result in the release of heparin, which in turn may or may not affect blood-clotting time. At present, histamine release is believed to involve activation of an enzyme, located on the mast cell membrane, that alters the permeability characteristics of the membrane to calcium ions and results in the extrusion of granules into the extracellular fluid.

Undoubtedly histamine release occurs during antigen-antibody interactions and thus is associated with some allergic reactions. Whether histamine is the *sole* mediator in any of these reactions in humans is questionable and remains to be established. Histamine has been found to be released during the initial phase of inflammatory processes, but its role appears to be transient and incomplete and not essential for the development of the most characteristic changes that produce lasting tissue damage. Almost any agent or cause that results in tissue damage also liberates histamine[6,7] including chemical, physical, thermal, or bacterial trauma.

Several drugs are known to release histamine from tissue stores. On the one hand there are "nonspecific" releasers that act by causing general tissue damage. These include, for example, surface-active agents like detergents. Interestingly, various plasma expanders (such as dextran) have also been found to release histamine in sufficient quantities to result in cardiovascular complications. The second group of drugs is of more common significance in their ability to release histamine. Their mechanism is not understood, and a wide variety of different drugs share the property. These include morphine, succinylcholine, dextrotubocurarine, epinephrine, trimethaphan, and surprisingly enough, almost all antihistamine drugs involving the H_1 receptor. Thus some of the side effects encountered with any of these drugs are directly attributable to their histamine-releasing action, and the effects observed can reach anaphylactoid proportions.

A discussion of the pharmacologic actions of histamine—directly administered or endogenously released—would be incomplete without a brief description of the anaphylac-tic-shock reaction and the symptomatology of histamine toxicity. An acute anaphylactic-shock reaction is likely to occur within min-utes after contact with an antigenic protein or precipitating agent. As mentioned earlier, histamine's direct vasodilatory effect will re-sult in a sharp fall in blood pressure, which is further intensified by the loss of fluid and plasma protein into extracellular space. This in turn will manifest itself in extensive edema formation. Thus circulation is greatly com-promised by peripheral pooling of blood, together with an increased hematocrit. Sub-sequent decreased venous return and a compensatory tachycardia can easily lead to shock and cardiovascular collapse. The spe-cific symptoms of an anaphylactic shock re-action may appear in the following order: apprehension, paresthesia, urticaria and edema, choking, cyanosis, cough, wheezing, fever, shock, loss of consciousness, coma, convulsions, and death. One should recall at this point that if histamine's action is limited locally, the well-known triple response is observed,[8] consisting of a localized red spot due to local dilation of capillaries, venules, and arterioles; a "flare" or red flush of ir-regular outline due to dilation of surrounding arterioles by way of a local axon reflex mecha-nism); and a "wheal" formed by localized ac-cumulation of edema fluid due to increased permeability of surrounding fine blood ves-sels.

Manifestations of an exogenously admin-istered overdose of histamine are more exclu-sively caused by cardiovascular and pulmo-nary symptoms. There is profound immediate hypotension and possibly life-threatening bronchoconstriction. These symptoms are ac-companied by the presence of intense head-ache, vomiting, and diarrhea.

The treatment of an acute allergic reac-tion like anaphylaxis is by physiologic an-tagonism rather than specific antihistaminic medication. Epinephrine is the drug of choice. Aminophylline also has bronchodi-lator activity and, for that reason, is used in the treatment of acute pulmonary edema as well as bronchial asthma. Steroids are used extensively as adjuncts in the management of allergic conditions to suppress any allergic inflammatory reactions. Further discussion of the treatment of an acute allergic reaction can be found in Chapter 24.

Inhibition of histamine release

Based on the knowledge of the importance of histamine release during various hyper-sensibility and allergic reactions, a sound pharmacologic approach would be a selective suppression of histamine release. There are indications that specifically in the treatment of asthma such a drug is now available: cromolyn (Aarane, Intal) itself is neither a bronchodilator nor does it relax other smooth muscles.[9] It inhibits the release of histamine and slow-reacting substance in anaphylaxis. Therefore cromolyn is prophylactically effec-tive in the management of asthma, but once the asthmatic attack has begun it is without value.

Clinical use

The only well-established clinical use of histamine and histamine-like preparations is as a diagnostic agent in the verification of achlorhydria and of pheochromocytoma, al-though for diagnosis of the latter condition better methods have been introduced during the past years.

It has been claimed that repeated admin-istration of low doses of histamine will induce tolerance to the amine. Based on this prem-ise, desensitization of allergic individuals has been attempted with histamine. Suffice it to say that, at present, the use of histamine for this purpose is highly controversial.

ANTIHISTAMINES

Although histamine was well described by Dale as early as 1911, it was 1937 by the time Bovet and his co-workers described the first compound with antihistaminic properties. These were identified by antagonism of hista-mine-induced contraction of smooth muscle and by a reduction of anaphylactic responses. The first clinically employed antihistamine was phenbenzamine (Antergan), soon to be followed by pyrilamine (Neo-Antergan), both of which are ethylenediamines. After minor modifications, diphenhydramine and tripel-ennamine were developed and introduced in the United States. Despite numerous at-tempts to improve on these initial com-pounds, they were incapable of blocking all actions of histamine, notably gastric acid se-cretion. Only with the discovery of the H_2 histamine blocking agents by Black and his colleagues[5] in 1972, a major breakthrough in antihistamine drugs was achieved. Presently, the major part of antihistaminic drugs are still those presumably acting at the H_1 receptor sites, mainly because the H_2 blocking drugs have become available only recently. The two classes of antihistaminic drugs will be discussed separately.

H_1 receptor antagonists

Chemistry. In simplified chemical terms all antihistamines involving H_1 histamine receptor sites can be looked on as structural analogs to histamine by showing the following same basic skeletal formula:

$$\text{HN} \diagdown \diagup \text{N} - CH_2 - CH_2 - N \diagup^{H} _{\diagdown H}$$

Histamine

$$R^1 \diagdown _{R^2} \diagup X - CH_2 - CH_2 - N \diagup^{R^3} _{\diagdown R^4}$$

Antihistamine

Depending on the substitution at X and type of $-CH_2-CH_2-$ bridge, H_1 blockers are classified into five large groups. These are presented in Table 15-1 for a quick grasp of their chemical, pharmacokinetic, and gross pharmacologic differences.

Absorption, metabolism, and excretion. Generally, absorption, distribution, metabolism, and excretion of H_1 blocking drugs are relatively uncomplicated and of no significant specificity. After oral and parenteral administration, they are readily absorbed. Their onset varies between 15 and 60 minutes; the duration of action of a single dose is between 3 and 12 hours, but some act much longer. Major metabolic pathways consist of hydroxylation followed by conjugation. Most of the metabolism takes place in the liver, but lung and kidney have been shown to metabolize at least some antihistamines. Most of the investigated antihistamines have been found to be excreted in the urine within 24 hours after one dose.

On long-term administration of H_1 antihistamines a certain extent of tolerance develops to their sedative effect. This tolerance is apparently caused by a combination of developing central tolerance and an induction of drug-metabolizing enzymes in the liver.

Pharmacologic actions. The pharmacologic effects and therapeutic uses of H_1 antihistaminic drugs can most easily be classified into two groups: those resulting from blocking the action of histamine at the H_1 receptor sites and those actions resulting from direct effects independent of their antihistaminic properties.

In the former type of actions these drugs will block the effects of histamine on capillary permeability and on vascular, bronchial, and other types of smooth muscle. Their mechanism is by competitive blockade at the H_1 receptor site. H_1 antihistamines are most effective in preventing histamine-induced increased capillary permeability and edema formation. It is well established that in many species H_1 antihistamines can effectively antagonize the constricting action of histamine on respiratory smooth muscle. Yet they are not very effective in protecting against anaphylactic bronchospasm in humans, a condition in which apparently other autacoids are important. Histamine-induced hypotension is only partially inhibited by H_1 antihistaminic drugs, a combination of H_1 and H_2 antihistamines being much more effective. Apparently, for the action of histamine on the vascular tree both H_1 and H_2 receptors are activated. H_1 blocking agents also block the stimulatory action of histamine on nerve endings and therefore are effective in suppressing the flare component of the triple responses and the itching associated with any histamine-mediated reaction.

The actions of H_1 antihistamines, other than those dependent on histamine blockade, are mostly of central nervous system (CNS) origin. In many instances, particularly in dentistry, antihistamines are used for these actions, their "side effects." Antihistamines have depressant as well as stimulant action on the CNS. They are sedatives of varying effectiveness and are additive with the sedation produced by other CNS depressants. Development of tolerance to this effect has been pointed out before. Many H_1 antihistamines are used freely by the public as sleep medication. In addition, with prolonged use the drugs induce various forms of oral symptoms, the most pronounced of which is xerostomia. The mechanism of this action is weak cholinergic blockade of muscarinic type.

Many but not all H_1 antihistamines have

Table 15-1. Chemical and pharmacotherapeutic properties of the various H_1 antihistamine groups

Group	Representative example	Usual adult dose (preparations available)	Duration of action (in hours)	Special properties	Other members of same group
Alkylamines	Chlorpheniramine (Chlor-Trimeton)	2-4 mg Tablets: 4 mg 8 mg 12 mg	4-6	Low incidence of moderate sedation	Dexbrompheniramine (Dimetane) Triprolidine HCl (Actidil)
Ethanolamines	Diphenhydramine (Benadryl)	50 mg Capsules: 25 mg 50 mg	4-6	High antimotion sickness activity; high incidence of pronounced sedation	Dimenhydrinate (Dramamine) Carbinoxamine maleate (Clistin)
Ethylenediamine	Tripelennamine (Pyribenzamine)	50 mg Tablets: 25 mg 50 mg Sustained-release tablets: 100 mg	4-6	Moderate incidence of pronounced sedation; gastrointestinal irritation	Pyrilamine (Neo-Antergan) Antazoline (Antistine) Methapyrilene (Histadyl, and as mixture: Co-Pyronil)
Piperazines	Chlorcyclizine HCl (Di-Paralene)	50 mg Tablets: 25 mg 50 mg	8-12	Low incidence of moderate sedation	Meclizine (Bonine) Cyclizine (Marezine)
Phenothiazines	Promethazine (Phenergan)	25-50 mg Tablets: 12.5 mg 25 mg 50 mg	4-6	Pronounced sedation; potential for all other phenothiazine side effects	Pyrathiazine HCl (Pyrrolazote) Trimeprazine tartrate (Temaril)

a pronounced antimotion sickness action. Generally, these agents also effectively control nausea and vomiting from other labyrinthine disturbances. This central antiemetic action of H_1 antihistamines is the basis for their use in the control of postsurgical nausea in dentistry.

CNS stimulation does occur on rare occasions in adults with conventional doses. Children, however, show a high incidence (50%) of this response, which manifests itself in restlessness and excitement, possibly escalating into convulsions.

H_1 antihistamines have local anesthetic activity to varying degrees. It has been stated that they are more effective local anesthetics when applied topically on denuded skin rather than as an injection for nerve block.

Adverse effects and drug interactions. The most common side effect of the H_1 antihistamine drugs is excessive sedation, which may or may not be accompanied by dizziness, tinnitus, uncoordination, blurred vision, and fatigue. Not only may these effects be hazardous to the patient's effective daytime activities but he will also be more sensitive to all other types of CNS depressant drugs. Undoubtedly a patient receiving H_1 antihistamine therapy will require less preoperative sedation than will an untreated individual.

The next most common side effects of antihistamines are gastrointestinal disturbances, such as anorexia, nausea, vomiting, constipation, and xerostomia, which can best be reduced by administering the drugs with meals.

H_1 antihistamines, as mentioned before, paradoxically are histamine releasers themselves. Allergic dermatitis is not an uncommon side effect. Other less frequent effects, apparently also from histamine release, are hypotension, palpitation, headaches, and tightness of the chest. Rare incidences of blood dyscrasias have been reported. Some antihistamines, particularly meclizine, cyclizine, and chlorcyclizine have been shown to have teratogenic effects in laboratory animals.[10] Whether this response does occur in humans and at what time course are not established. However, the potential hazard implicit in the use of these drugs in pregnant women should be appreciated.

Acute poisoning with H_1 antihistamine drugs has become relatively common because of their easy accessibility as over-the-counter drugs. Signs and symptoms are different in children than they are in adults, although in both cases they are due to central actions of the drug. In smaller children the predominant effect is excitation manifested in hallucinations, excitement, uncoordination, and convulsions. Symptoms include fever, a flushed face, and fixed, dilated pupils. Death is due to coma with cardiorespiratory collapse. In adults most commonly the convulsive phase is preceded by drowsiness. The ultimate phase is a postictal depression. In adults, fever and flushed face are rarely seen. Therapy is only symptomatic and supportive and depends exclusively on the correct diagnosis. In the case of convulsions only short-acting barbiturates are indicated.

Therapeutic uses. Once again, therapeutic uses of these drugs can best be subdivided into those caused by H_1 antihistamine action and those by actions independent on blockade of histamine receptors.

Certain acute allergic reactions such as allergic rhinitis and seasonal hay fever can effectively be controlled by H_1 antihistamines. Contrary to many initial reports and rather widespread popular belief, these antihistamines are of rather limited value in the management of the common cold. The limited relief that they afford is primarily caused by their weak atropine-like action. Obviously, under those circumstances, sedation represents the most limiting side effect. Once again, H_1 antihistamines are not the drug of choice in an anaphylactic shock reaction; physiologic antagonists like epinephrine and certain xanthines are far superior. But they are effective in relieving itching, edema, and erythema of an acute urticarial attack.

H_1 antihistamines, often in combination with corticosteroids, are sometimes useful in relieving the pain and swelling associated with certain allergic ulcers of the mouth. In this situation they are applied topically. The potential hazard of a sensitivity reaction to the antihistamine has to be weighed against the benefit of such treatment. Generally, however, these drugs are not highly allergenic.

The use of H_1 antihistamines in dentistry is primarily based on their actions independently of histamine blockade. They have been employed in preoperative sedation be-

$$\text{HN} \diagup\diagdown \text{N} -CH_2-CH_2-CH_2-CH_2-NH-\underset{\overset{\|}{S}}{C}NH-CH_3$$

Burimamide

$$CH_3$$
$$\text{HN} \diagup\diagdown \text{N} -CH_2-SCH_2-CH_2-NH-\underset{\overset{\|}{S}}{C}NH-CH_3$$

Metiamide

cause of their sedative central action and antiemetic effects. Ethanolamines and promethazine are particularly useful for this purpose (Table 15-1). They are, however, less effective than the tranquilizers and barbiturates. Promethazine has also been used clinically with meperidine, as described in Chapter 10. H_1 antihistamines have also been substituted for local anesthetics, as described in Chapter 14.

The H_1 antihistamines were once reported to control postoperative sequelae of dental surgery such as swelling, trismus, and pain.[11-14] Subsequently, well-controlled and double-blind studies did not find the antihistamines to be effective for this purpose.[15-18]

Many H_1 antihistamines, particularly diphenhydramine, dimenhydrinate, and cyclizine, are effectively used in the prevention and treatment of motion sickness. They also have been used in the control of postoperative vomiting or that induced by radiation. The use of some antihistamines in the control of nausea and vomiting of pregnancy is not considered completely safe because of their potential teratogenic action.

H_2 receptor antagonists

Chemistry. Presently, only two H_2 receptor antagonists are available, both of which have an obvious structural similarity to histamine, as indicated above. As can be seen, both drugs have an imidazole ring like histamine but differ in the side chain, which is uncharged. This is in contrast to histamine itself and the H_1 antagonists, which share a positively charged ammonium side chain. The H_2 receptor antagonists are hydrophilic molecules, which probably accounts for the lack of central nervous system effects of these drugs.

Pharmacologic actions. The mechanism of action of presently known H_2 blocking agents is by competitive blockade of those actions of histamine that are mediated by the histamine H_2 receptors, notably gastric acid secretion. Metiamide and burimamide not only block gastric acid secretion elicited by histamine infusion but also that evoked by pentagastrin. In addition, in certain model systems, burimamide has been shown to possess alpha-adrenergic blocking as well as anti-inflammatory activity. Metiamide has been found to produce agranulocytosis; however, it seems to be the only H_2 blocker with this action. The full pharmacologic spectrum of H_2 receptor blockers in humans remains to be established.

Therapeutic uses. H_2 antihistamine drugs afford significant symptomatic relief in patients suffering from peptic ulceration. Some evidence indicates that ulcer healing occurred during treatment with these drugs. This effect is thought to be due to profound reduction of gastric secretion. For the same reason H_2 blocking agents are useful in the treatment of patients with Zollinger-Ellison syndrome and other gastric hypersecretory states.

It is obvious that this class of drugs will expand greatly with progress in the understanding of histamine receptors per se. The interested reader is referred to the recent symposium on histamine H_2 receptor antagonists.[19]

REFERENCES

1. Riley, J. F., and West, G. G.: The occurrence of histamine in mast cells. In Eichler, O., and Farah, A., editors: Handbuch der experimentellen Pharmakologie. Histamine and antihistaminics, Berlin, 1966, Springer-Verlag, vol. 18/1.
2. McIntire, F. C.: Histamine and antihistamines. In Shacter, M., editor: International encyclopedia

of pharmacology and therapeutics, Oxford, 1973, Pergamon Press, Ltd., vol. 1.

3. Kahlson, G., and Rosengren, E.: Biogenesis and physiology of histamine, London, 1973, Ed. Arnold & Co., Ltd.

4. Ash, A. S. F., and Schild, H. O.: Receptors mediating some actions of histamine, Br. J. Pharmacol. Chemother. **27**:427, 1966.

5. Black, J. W., Duncan, W. A., Durant, C. J., Gannelin, C. R., and Parsons, E. M.: Definition and antagonism of histamine H_2 receptors, Nature **236**:385, 1972.

6. Spector, W. G., and Willoughby, D. A.: The inflammatory response, Bacteriol. Rev. **27**:117, 1964.

7. Spector, W. G., and Willoughby, D. A.: Vasoactive amines in acute inflammation, Ann. N.Y. Acad. Sci. **116**:839, 1964.

8. Lewis, T.: The blood vessels of the human skin and their responses, London, 1927, Shaw & Sons, Ltd.

9. Cox, J. S. C., Beach, J. E., Blair, A. M. J. N., Clarke, A. J., King, J., Lee, T. B., Loveday, D. E., Moss, G. F., Orr, T. S. C., Ritchie, J. T., and Sheard, P.: Disodium cromoglycate (Intal), Adv. Drug Res. **5**:115, 1970.

10. Sadusk, J. F., and Palmisano, P. A.: Teratogenic effect of medicine, cyclizine and chlorcyclizine, J.A.M.A. **194**:987, 1965.

11. Silverman, R. E.: The use of antihistamines in oral surgery: a preliminary report, J. Oral Surg. **11**:231, 1953.

12. Silverman, R. E.: Further clinical observations on the use of antihistamines in oral surgery, J. Oral Surg. **12**:310, 1954.

13. Blinderman, J. J.: Control of edema, pain and trismus in oral surgery with an oral antihistamine, N.Y. J. Dent. **26**:231, 1956.

14. Macchia, A. F.: Antihistamines and their value in allaying postoperative distress in the removal of impacted teeth, Oral Surg. **10**:122, 1957.

15. Szmyd, L.: A clinical evaluation of an antihistaminic preparation in oral surgery, Oral Surg. **9**:928, 1956.

16. Keesling, G. R., and Hinds, E. E.: Clinical evaluation of antihistamines in oral surgery using the double unknown technic, J. Oral Surg. **15**:279, 1957.

17. Holland, M. R., and Jurgens, P. E.: The effectiveness of an antihistamine to reduce pain following oral surgical procedures, Oral Surg. **11**:138, 1958.

18. Snyder, B. S.: Effect of antihistaminic agents on inflammatory response after surgical trauma, J. Oral Surg. **18**:319, 1960.

19. Goth, A.: Histamine H_2 receptor antagonists, Fed. Proc. **35**:1923, 1976.

16

Hormones and related substances

SEBASTIAN G. CIANCIO

Hormones are substances secreted by specific tissues and transported by way of the bloodstream to tissue target areas, where they exert an effect. They are natural secretions of the endocrine glands whose actions are essential to the maintenance of many body functions. A number of other substances are produced by various cells and tissues in the body that cannot be strictly classified as hormones, since a true physiologic role for them has not been established. However, they are naturally occurring substances with strong pharmacologic properties, and they include histamines, antihistamines, endogenous amines, angiotensin, kinins, and prostaglandins. As a group they are referred to as autacoids, a word of Greek derivation meaning self-remedy or self-medicinal agents. They have also been referred to as autopharmacologic agents and as local hormones. Autacoids are used by the body in various aspects of health and disease and are thought to be important to homeostasis. In this chapter the hormones and the most important autacoids will be discussed from the pharmacologic viewpoint, with emphasis on dental problems associated with hormonal therapy and correction of dental problems with hormone therapy.

PITUITARY HORMONES

The pituitary gland is divided into an anterior lobe (adenohypophysis) and a posterior lobe (neurohypophysis).

Anterior pituitary

The anterior pituitary produces a number of hormones that stimulate various tissues and other endocrine glands. The hormones produced by the anterior pituitary and their functions are as follows:

Adrenocorticotropin (ACTH)—stimulates secretion of adrenal corticosteroids.

Thyroid-stimulating hormone (TSH, thyrotropin)—stimulates secretion of thyroid hormones.
Follicle-stimulating hormone (FSH)—promotes development of ovarian follicles and maintains spermatogenesis.
Luteinizing hormone (LH)—induces ovulation and regulates progesterone secretion in women and testosterone secretion in men.
Growth hormone (GH, somatotropin)—promotes growth of all body cells.
Prolactin—initiates lactation and breast growth.
Melanocyte-stimulating hormone (MSH)—disperses melanin granules and increases pigmentation.

The secretion of the anterior pituitary hormones is influenced by numerous hormones of the other endocrine glands by way of a feedback system. It has also been established that anterior pituitary activity is mediated by neurohumoral substances transported to it by a vascular network from the hypothalamus directly to the pituitary.

Adrenocorticotropin (ACTH) is the principal pituitary hormone of pharmacologic importance. It will be discussed in more detail in the section relating to the adrenal gland, since its principal use is to stimulate the adrenal cortex. Thyroid-stimulating hormone (TSH) is not used therapeutically. The gonadotropins FSH and LH have been used to treat hypogonadism in males and to induce ovulation in females. Growth hormone has been used experimentally in pituitary dwarfism. Prolactin and MSH are not used therapeutically.

Posterior pituitary

The posterior pituitary secretes vasopressin and oxytocin.

Vasopressin (Pitressin) has vasoconstrictor and antidiuretic activity and has been used in the treatment of diabetes insipidus. Oxytocin (Pitocin, Syntocinon) is used to induce labor and to control postpartum hemorrhage. Oxytocin also has an effect on the metabolism of the ground substance of skin and gingiva.[1] Whether this effect is important in periodontal disease has not been investigated.

Pituitary disorders

A decrease in pituitary secretion (hypopituitarism) in the adult will result in a variety of symptoms related to a lack of pituitary hormones and includes a lack of secondary sex characteristics, lowered metabolism, and death. Failure of this gland to develop during embryogenesis results in dwarfism. Hypersecretion of the anterior pituitary results in acromegaly and gigantism.

THYROID HORMONES

The thyroid gland is the source of three hormones: thyroxin, triiodothyronine, and calcitonin. These hormones regulate growth, differentiation, and mineral and oxidative metabolism.

Thyroxin and triiodothyronine are iodine-containing derivatives of the amino acid thyronine. Iodine uptake and conversion are essential to their biosynthesis.

Certain drugs and some pathologic as well as physiologic conditions can alter the binding of thyroid hormones to proteins or can alter the amount of circulating protein. Thus the total amount of thyroid hormone bound to plasma varies from normal, depending on the degree of protein binding. The more that is bound to protein the less it is available in the free, active form and vice versa. Since there is a feedback mechanism whereby the amount of free hormone signals the gland as to the amount needed for homeostasis, compensation by the body can be made for certain fluctuations.

Regulation of thyroid function

Secretion of thyroid hormone exerts a negative feedback action on the control of secretion of thyrotropin by the adenohypophysis. This feedback system is highly efficient, and a delicate balance is maintained between the secretions of these two glands.

Normal thyroid function requires an adequate intake of iodine. If intake is inadequate, the thyroid gland becomes more active and the glandular tissue hypertrophies, resulting in enlargement of the gland. This is the common goiter seen in many iodine-deficient individuals. Obviously the treatment of this condition is simply iodine sup-

plementation. Some question has been raised concerning the possible toxic effects of iodine applied topically either as a medicament for oral disease or as a disclosing solution. If this iodine is absorbed through oral mucosa, it may alter thyroid function because of the role this element plays in thyroid gland function. However, for this to be a problem the iodine would probably have to be used on a regular basis for a long period of time.

Thyroid disorders

Undersecretion of thyroid hormone in adults is referred to as myxedema, hypothyroidism, or Gull's disease. Patients with hypothyroidism are expressionless, mentally impaired, and poor of hearing, have inadequate smooth muscle function, and may also show signs of anemia, hydropericardium, hydrothorax, and ascites. These patients will be drowsy and tired. In addition to a general state of fatigue, they may be difficult to motivate in plaque control. Furthermore, in view of their general medical problems, their dental problems may be obscure to them.

Undersecretion of thyroid hormone in children can result in cretinism. These children are dwarfed, mentally retarded, inactive, and expressionless. Undersecretion in the adult results in muscular weakness, drowsiness, expressionless face, deep voice, and mental retardation.

Oversecretion of thyroid hormone may result in diffuse, toxic goiter (Graves' disease or Badedow's disease) or toxic nodular goiter (Plummer's disease). In this condition there is nervous excitability, increased metabolism, rapid heart rate, anxiety, and apprehension. Ophthalmopathy and protruding eyes may also be associated with hyperthyroidism.

Therapeutic agents for thyroid disorders

A number of thyroid preparations are available for hypothyroidism, including thyroid tablets, thyroglobulin, levothyroxine, and liothyronine sodium. Adverse effects associated with these agents are rare. However, overdosage will produce signs and symptoms of hyperthyroidism and may precipitate angina or cardiac failure. Consequently, they must be used with caution in cardiac patients. However, large doses are indicated in coma associated with myxedema, and levothyroxine or liothyronine have been used intravenously. As the patient responds to therapy, the dose is altered.

A number of antithyroid medications are available for the treatment of hyperthyroidism. These include propylthiouracil, methylthiouracil, methimazole, and carbimazole. The most serious side effect of these drugs is agranulocytosis. Therefore, prior to dental surgical procedures, a determination should be made of the possible existence of this condition, since inhibition of wound healing may occur. It is also possible that the wound will be more susceptible to infection. Other side effects reported with these drugs include arthralgia, paresthesia (which could manifest itself in facial areas), headache, nausea, and loss or depigmentation of hair. Drug fever, hepatitis, and nephritis are rare.

In patients taking medications for thyroid dysfunction, the nature of the dysfunction should be determined, since such a determination may be essential to developing a plaque control program for the dental patient.

Calcitonin. Calcitonin is produced by parafollicular cells of the thyroid gland. Its biosynthesis and secretion are regulated by the concentration of calcium in plasma. This substance is a hypocalcemic and hypophosphatemic agent. When the calcium concentration is high, the amount of calcitonin in plasma increases and vice versa. Although it is clear that calcitonin secretion can be affected by several agents in laboratory studies, it is not known to what extent normal physiologic variations in secretion occur or if calcitonin plays a significant role in calcium homeostasis.

The action of calcitonin is primarily due to a direct inhibition of bone resorption by an alteration of the activity of osteoclasts and osteocytes.[2] It also enhances bone formation by stimulating osteoblastic activity.[3] This effect is transient, and long-term use of the hormone decreases osteoblastic and osteoclastic activity. Calcitonin also interferes with the activity of parathyroid hormone on osteolysis because of an effect it exerts on osteocytic and osteoclastic activity.

Therapeutic use. Calcitonin has been used to treat a number of skeletal diseases, including Paget's disease, in which it produces symptomatic relief. It has also been shown to reduce urinary hydroxyproline and alkaline phosphatase activity. It is effective as initial therapy in treating hypercalcemia, hyperparathyroidism, vitamin D overdose, and bone metastases of an osteolytic nature. Therapy results in a decrease in plasma calcium and phosphate, which is related to an inhibition of resorption of these substances from bone. It has also been shown to decrease glucose utilization and lactate production in bone, which is opposite to the effect of parathyroid hormone.

Side effects associated with therapy with this drug include nausea, swelling and tenderness of extremities, and urticaria.

PARATHYROID HORMONE

The parathyroid glands manufacture proparathyroid hormone, which is then converted to parathyroid hormone and is secreted as such. Parathyroid hormone functions to increase plasma calcium and lower blood phosphorus levels. This is achieved by mobilizing calcium and phosphorus from bone (increased bone resorption), increasing the absorption of calcium from the intestine, and increasing the renal tubular reabsorption of calcium while decreasing the reabsorption of phosphorus. This interrelationship for calcium is summarized in Fig. 12. The secretion of parathyroid hormone is related to levels of ionized plasma calcium; when plasma calcium levels are high or normal, less parathyroid hormone is secreted; when plasma calcium levels are low, more parathyroid hormone is secreted.

The effect on absorption of calcium from the small intestine may be a direct effect of the hormone that requires the presence of vitamin D. It may also be an indirect effect because of the accumulation of the active form of vitamin D as a result of the action of parathyroid hormone on the conversion of vitamin D to its active form.

The resorption effect of parathyroid hormone on bone is on stable, older bone and not on the labile fraction.[4] By mobilizing calcium from bone, it regulates plasma levels of calcium above 7 mg/dl. The plasma calcium below this concentration is less dependent on hormonal control and is maintained by an equilibrium that exists between extracellular fluid and the labile fraction of bone.

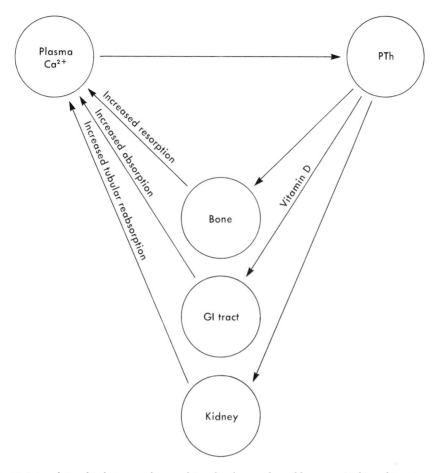

Fig. 12. Interrelationship between plasma calcium levels, parathyroid hormone (PTh), and target organs.

At the cellular level parathyroid hormone stimulates the rate of bone resorption by osteoclasts and lengthens their half-life.[5] It also increases the rate of conversion of mesenchymal cells to osteoclasts. Prolonged activity by parathyroid hormone has a paradoxical effect on bone whereby the number of bone-forming osteoblasts increases. Although the number increases, these cells are less metabolically active than normal under its influence. A number of dental studies have been concerned with the resorptive effects of this hormone on bone and the possible role it might play in periodontal disease.[6,7]

It is of interest to note that parathyroid hormone decreases the calcium content of both milk and saliva. This mechanism may be operative as a means of conserving calcium in extracellular fluid by reducing its rate of transport from extracellular fluid to milk and saliva.

Parathyroid disorders

Hypoparathyroidism is only one of the many causes of hypocalcemia and occurs relatively rarely. Another condition called pseudohypoparathyroidism is due to a lack of response of the target organs of parathyroid hormone to its action. The symptoms of these disorders include paresthesia of the extremities, muscle spasms leading to tetany, bone loss, hair loss, brittleness of fingernails and defects in dental enamel, emotional disturbances, and even death.

Hyperparathyroidism is characterized by elevated plasma levels of ionized calcium. In this condition calcium mobilized from bone is precipitated in soft tissues, and metastatic calcification is seen in the kidneys, stomach wall, bronchi, and heart muscles. This hypersecretion may lead to a bone disorder known as osteitis fibrosa, or Recklinghausen's disease of bone. Skeletal changes may be seen that vary from mild to severe. Sometimes they can be seen in dental radiographs. This decalcification, in its early stages, is associated with aching and pain in bones and joints. Since excessive amounts of calcium and phosphate are found in urine, there is a high incidence of renal calculi. There is also general muscle weakness, constipation, nausea, vomiting, and anorexia. Patients with hyperparathyroidism also have a higher than normal incidence of peptic ulcers. For this reason, when analgesics are prescribed for these patients, salicylic acid–containing drugs should be avoided.

Therapeutic uses

There are currently no valid therapeutic uses of parathyroid hormone. At one time it was used parenterally to elevate plasma calcium concentration. However, this can be accomplished with greater safety by the administration of calcium and/or vitamin D.

A diagnostic use of parathyroid hormone is in pseudoparathyroidism. As stated earlier, the target organs do not respond to parathyroid hormone. Therefore, in this test, the hormone is injected; if there is an elevation in plasma calcium, the diagnosis is then clear.

PANCREATIC HORMONES

The hormones produced by the pancreas are insulin and glucagon. They are distinctly separate hormones produced by different pancreatic cell groups and will be discussed separately.

Insulin

Beta or islet cells in the pancreas produce proinsulin, which in turn is converted to insulin through a series of metabolic changes. The major role of insulin is the maintenance of carbohydrate metabolism. In humans it affects mainly glucose, but in other animals amino and fatty acids are also affected. Its effects on glucose metabolism are as follows:

1. It aids in the transport of glucose across cell membranes into the cell.
2. It is essential in the conversion of glucose to glycogen.
3. It decreases the conversion of protein to glucose.

Other effects of insulin include enhancement of fat and protein synthesis and the promotion of amino acid uptake.

The secretion of insulin is stimulated mainly by glucose levels in plasma. This secretion is altered by other hormonal and neural stimuli, including certain gastrointestinal hormones (secretin, gastrin, pancreozymin, and gastrointestinal glucagon).

Epinephrine and norepinephrine suppress the secretion of insulin. Consequently, exercise, fear, or any other activation of the autonomic nervous system may decrease insulin secretion. Although epinephrine and norepinephrine inhibit insulin secretion, the amount in local anesthetic solutions is so small that a significant effect on the blood glucose level would not be expected. However, pain, fear, or anxiety may cause sufficient endogenous release of epinephrine to cause an increase in the blood glucose level.

The list of hormones that can affect insulin release is constantly growing. Table 16-1 lists the various hormones affecting insulin secretion. It is obvious that insulin secretion is a complex matter involving many interrelationships.

Therapeutic uses and adverse effects

Insulin is used therapeutically as replacement therapy in diabetes mellitus. It is derived from animal tissues, and the dosage is expressed in units. Most commercial preparations contain some impurities that are antigenic and have produced allergic reactions in patients. A number of forms of insulin are available and can be classified as fast-, intermediate-, and long-acting preparations. They must be given parenterally.

In patients treated with insulin, hypoglycemic reactions may occur and are usually related to a failure to eat, unaccustomed exercise or stress, and inadvertent administration of too large a dose. In view of this, dental appointments for patients taking insulin should be scheduled so they will not interfere with meals, and stressful situations should be minimized. Oral surgical procedures should be performed 1½ to 3 hours after the patient has eaten a normal breakfast and taken his regular antidiabetic medication. Dental therapy, especially surgery, should not be initiated until the diabetes is controlled.

The symptoms of hypoglycemia should

Table 16-1. Hormones and autacoids affecting insulin release

Hormone	Source	Effect on insulin release
Secretin, pancreozymin, gastrin, gastrointestinal glucagon	Gastrointestinal tract	Increase
Glucagon	Pancreas	Increase
Prostaglandins	Body cells	Increase or inhibit
Somatostatin	Hypothalamus	Inhibit

be known by the dentist. They include sweating, weakness, hunger, tachycardia, "feeling of trembling," headache, blurred vision, mental confusion, incoherent speech, and eventually coma, convulsions, and death. Treatment of hypoglycemia is by intravenous injection of glucose or glucagon or the ingestion of soluble carbohydrate or fruit juice.

A number of studies have shown that diabetic patients are susceptible to more severe periodontal disease.[8,9] It has also been suggested that these patients may be more susceptible to infection after periodontal osseous surgery. For this reason many periodontists and oral surgeons administer antibiotics postoperatively for diabetics as a prophylactic measure in cases of extensive or osseous surgery.

Research studies have shown that in diabetics elevated levels of glucose can be found in the gingival crevicular fluid.[10] It has been suggested that gingival crevicular fluid content measurements may serve as a diagnostic aid. It has also been shown that diabetic children have elevated levels of urea in gingival crevicular fluid. These data suggest that periodontal disease may be related to elevated gingival fluid levels. If this is true, these elevated levels in supposedly nondiabetic individuals may serve as predictors of periodontal disease at a later date.

Oral hypoglycemic agents

Oral hypoglycemic agents can be divided into two groups: sulfonylureas and biguanides. Drugs in the former group are tolbutamide (Orinase), acetohexamide (Dymelor), tolazimide (Tolinase), and chlorpropamide (Diabinese). In the biguanide group only one agent is available commercially, namely, phenformin (DBI, Meltrol).

The mechanism of action of the sulfonylureas is stimulation of the islet tissue to secrete insulin. In the case of biguanides it is a threefold effect: (1) increase in glucose utilization by increasing anaerobic glycolysis, (2) decrease in gluconeogenesis, and (3) inhibition of intestinal absorption of glucose.

Adverse effects. The adverse effects of sulfonylureas include blood dyscrasias, cutaneous problems, gastrointestinal disturbances, and hepatic disorders. Therefore a thorough blood picture is important prior to surgical therapy in these patients. Since hepatic dysfunction may occur, prothrombin times should be determined so that a bleeding problem can be prevented during dental surgical procedures.

The biguanides can cause nausea, vomiting, diarrhea, abdominal cramps, and a metallic sense of taste. This latter complaint is one that the dentist may encounter, and proper understanding of its etiology is important. Rather than suspecting galvanic problems, faulty restorations, or other difficulties, the dentist must consider this drug's adverse effects.

In 1970 the results of a 9-year study of the relationship between the use of oral hypoglycemics and cardiovascular disease were published.[11] Although the study has been the subject of much controversy, it appears that patients taking oral hypoglycemics have more cardiovascular problems than diabetics controlled by diet alone. Patients taking these drugs may be more susceptible to ventricular tachycardia, ventricular fibrillation, and myocardial infarction.

Glucagon

Glucagon is a hormone produced by the pancreatic alpha cells, sometimes called the "organ of Langerhans." Glucagon raises blood glucose levels by increasing the hepatic breakdown of glycogen to glucose. It may also act as a physiologic antagonist to insulin. It is important in the metabolism of glucose and is actively secreted when plasma glucose concentrations decrease. Its secretion is also stimulated by a gastrointestinal hormone pancreozymin and by epinephrine and norepinephrine.

Glucagon can be considered a hormone of fuel mobilization. When food intake is below normal, glucagon secretion is stimulated, insulin secretion is depressed, and fuels stored intracellularly are metabolized to meet the body's energy needs. Another function of this hormone is the stimulation of gluconeogenesis, thus providing the glucose needed in times of infection or stress. In high concentrations glucagon has a positive inotropic effect. This finding has been used clinically on an experimental basis to determine if this drug has any value in cardiac disorders. Therapeutically, glucagon has only limited use in the correction of hypoglycemic states resulting from hyperinsulinism.

GONADAL HORMONES

Hormones affecting sex characteristics and function are secreted by a number of organs (Table 16-2). The hormones of the ovaries, testes, and placenta are sometimes referred to as the gonadal hormones. They are interesting from a dental viewpoint, since gingival and other oral soft tissue changes have been associated with them.[12,13]

The secretions of sex hormones are affected by a feedback mechanism related to gonadotropins produced by the pituitary gland. As the gonads produce more hormone, the pituitary produces less gonadotropin. The balance between these glands, among other functions, maintains menstruation and pregnancy in the female and spermatogenesis in the male.

Estrogens

The main estrogen in humans produced by the ovary is 17β-estradiol, which is converted in the liver to estrone and estriol. During pregnancy the placenta produces the same hormone and its products in large amounts. The estrogens are responsible for the changes that take place at puberty in girls and account for many of the characteristics of the female sex. They cause growth and development of the vagina, uterus, and Fallopian tubes, breast enlargement, and pigmentation of the nipples and alveolae, fat secretions, epiphyseal changes, and growth of axillary and pubic hair. They also affect the menstrual cycle in a regulated fashion and in a manner varying with pregnancy, early stages of menstruation, and approach of menopause.

They are used pharmacologically when deficiency conditions are present and serve as replacement or supplemental therapy. In conjunction with progestins, they are widely used as birth control pills. This therapy will be discussed later in this chapter.

Adverse effects. Adverse effects associated with the estrogens include retention of salt and water and possible carcinogenesis. In 1971 and 1972 an increased incidence of vaginal and cervical carcinoma was observed in female children of mothers who had received synthetic estrogens, such as diethylstilbestrol, during the first trimester of pregnancy. Some reports have also been published associating carcinoma of the breast with estrogen therapy.

These hormones can be given orally and are readily absorbed by the gastrointestinal tract. They are also absorbed through skin and mucous membrane; therefore topical applications can be expected to exert a systemic effect by absorption through these surfaces and into the bloodstream.

Progestins

Progestins are important in the regulation of ovulation, as are the estrogens, and are also important in the development of a secretory lining of the uterus. At the end of the menstrual cycle, progestin secretion declines and the onset of menstruation occurs. Progestins also cause a proliferation of the mammary gland acini. This change is most pronounced during pregnancy and, to a lesser extent, during one phase of the menstrual cycle.

The natural progestin produced by the body is progesterone. Synthetic oral hormones available with similar effects include megestrol acetate (Megace), dydrogesterone

Table 16-2. Sex hormones

Hormone	Major gland	Minor gland(s)
Estrogens	Ovary	Testes, placenta
Progestins	Ovary	Testes, adrenal cortex, placenta
Androgens	Testes	Ovary, adrenal cortex

(Duphaston, Gynorest), norethindrone (Micronor, Nor-Q.D., Norlutin), norethindrone acetate (Norlutate), and ethisterone (Duosterone).

Synthetic progestins are used therapeutically as oral contraceptives, to control uterine bleeding, in dysmenorrhea, in endometriosis, for the relief of premenstrual tension, in the prevention of natural abortion, as suppressors of postpartum lactation, and as palliative agents in uterine carcinoma.

Oral contraception

The use of various oral contraceptives is common practice for many women throughout the world. Research is currently being carried out on oral male contraceptives that may result in an effective drug for men in the near future.

Oral contraceptives in use today are estrogen- or progesterone-like substances, either singly or in combination, and they are about 99% effective. Some medications are given daily between days 5 and 25 of the menstrual cycle, some are given on a sequential basis (estrogen for 14 to 16 days and combination for 5 to 6 days), and others have been formulated as single dose preparations taken daily on a continual basis. This latter group has been referred to as "minipills" (progesterone alone). Investigations are currently under way to develop a "morning-after" pill. At the present time diethylstilbestrol has been approved, but because of its possible carcinogenicity it is limited to emergencies such as rape.

When estrogen and progestin are administered together, inhibition of ovulation occurs. This appears to be caused by a suppression of the production of gonadotropins (follicle-stimulating hormone and luteinizing hormone) by the anterior pituitary gland. It is thought that this effect is mainly due to the estrogen component and that progesterone aids during the withdrawal bleeding stage of the cycle to regulate and control this bleeding.

The use of progestins alone does not inhibit ovulation but appears to be helpful in altering the structure of the endometrium and the consistency of cervical mucus without altering ovulation. The effect on the uterine wall probably minimizes implantation of the egg; the effect on cervical mucus may inhibit activity of sperm. In this way pregnancy is prevented.

Adverse effects associated with the use of these drugs include nausea, dizziness, headache, weight gain, breast discomfort, brownish spots on the face (chloasma), gallbladder disorders, blood pressure elevation, ocular disturbances, liver damage, and gingival bleeding.

Women taking oral contraceptives have an increased tendency toward thrombophlebitis and other thromboembolic disorders. There is also some indication that certain oral contraceptives may increase the risk of myocardial infarction. It has been noted that these patients have accelerated blood clotting and increased blood concentrations of some clotting factors. It has also been reported that the incidence of thromboembolic disorders increases between fourfold and tenfold with the use of combined or sequential oral contraceptives. A few studies have suggested that these drugs may produce both benign and malignant tumors, but other studies have suggested a decreased incidence of tumors when these drugs are used regularly. Therefore this should be considered an open question at this time.

Dental considerations. A number of studies have suggested that oral contraceptives may result in an increase in the incidence of gingival inflammation and bleeding due to (1) proliferation of blood vessels in marginal gingivae, (2) decrease in clotting ability of the patient's blood, and (3) alteration in permeability of blood vessels. Other studies have disagreed with the foregoing. Until this question is resolved, the possible relationship between oral contraceptives and gingival bleeding should be kept in mind when evaluating gingival problems in patients taking oral contraceptives.

It has also been suggested that oral contraceptives may alter immunologic mechanisms. If this is true, the decrease in an individual's immunologic defenses to plaque bacteria and their products may result in the initiation and/or progression of periodontal disease.

Androgens

Androgens, notably testosterone, are responsible for most male sexual characteristics. They also have a strong anabolic effect. Testosterone is produced mainly by the testes and is converted at the receptor site to dihydrotestosterone, which is more active than the parent compound. A feedback system is present between this gland and the anterior pituitary similar to that described for the estrogens. A number of synthetic androgens are available. These drugs are used when replacement therapy is necessary because of lack of production by the testes. They have also been used in the palliative treatment of breast cancer, menstrual disorders, anemia, and suppression of lactation.

Adverse effects associated with the use of synthetic androgens include masculinization in the female, generalized edema, liver damage, fever, and stomatitis from buccal and sublingual preparations. This latter problem may be first detected by the dentist during a routine dental visit.

Investigations are currently under way relative to the use of these agents in conjunction with a progestin as a male oral contraceptive. The rationale for such usage is to decrease gonadotropin secretion and spermatogenesis and still maintain the secondary male traits.

ADRENAL HORMONES

The adrenal gland produces hormones from both the medulla and the cortex. The medullary secretions of the adrenal are discussed in Chapter 13. Because of the important clinical implications of adrenocorticosteroids in dental practice, they will be discussed separately in Chapter 17.

AUTACOIDS
Prostaglandins

Prostaglandins are not hormones but are among the most important autacoids and have been detected in most body tissues and fluids. There are six main classes of these agents: E, F, A, B, C, and D, of which the E and F groups are predominant. Clinically, they are cyclic, oxygenated fatty acids and have a diversity of effects. Prostaglandins are derived from essential fatty acids, which are, in turn, converted to one of three complex fatty acids: 8, 11, 14-eicosatrienoc acid; 5, 8, 11, 14-eicosatetraenoic (arachidonic) acid; or 5, 8, 11, 14, 17-eicosapentaenoic acid. Their activities include vasodilation, increased heart rate and cardiac output, increased capillary permeability, alteration of smooth muscle contraction, inhibition of gastric secretion and increased mucous secretion in the intestine, increased renal blood flow, sedation, stimulation of pain fibers, and effects on a number of endocrine gland secretions. The E group are interesting to dental practitioners, since these prostaglandins exert parathyroid hormone–like effects that result in a mobilization of calcium from bone in tissue culture.[14] Therefore it is possible that they also do the same in vivo. A number of investigations are under way to investigate the role these compounds may play as an etiologic factor in periodontal disease.[15]

There appears to be no single receptor for prostaglandins; however, it is believed that specific receptors exist for the various agents. Interestingly enough, these receptors may produce one effect with one class of prostaglandin and an opposite effect with a member of another class. By the use of this antagonism, special receptors have been identified for prostaglandins.

The prostaglandins are released by a host of mechanical, thermal, chemical, bacterial, and other traumatic effects and appear to be important in inflammation. It is thought that the more chronic the inflammation the more prominent is their role. In this respect they may be involved in the initiation and/or progression of periodontal disease.

The prostaglandins are currently used mainly as agents to induce abortions. They have their greatest use for inducing abortion in midtrimester. It is also possible that they may play a role in future contraceptives as a "morning-after" pill.

On a limited basis prostaglandins are being used to treat bronchial asthma and as an antiulcer agent. In the future they may also be used as antihypertensive agents.

In view of the multiplicity of effects of prostaglandins, it has been postulated that certain pathologic conditions can be improved by the administration of antagonists. It has been demonstrated that aspirin and similar anti-inflammatory drugs of the nonsteroid class interfere with the synthesis and release of these compounds. At the present time drugs belonging to the following groups have been shown to be inhibitors of prostaglandins: fenamates, phenylbutazone, aspirin, and prostynoic acid.

Kinins

Kinins are polypeptides and are distributed in a variety of body tissues. Kallidin and bradykinin are members of this group, are found in plasma, and may play a role in dental diseases. They are both derived from a common precursor, kinogen by the action of proteolytic enzymes (kininogenases), such as those labeled kallikrein. Other kininogenases include trypsin, plasmin, and components of certain snake venom.

The plasma kinins appear to be important in blood clotting, fibrinolysis, and complement activity. Once formed, their inactivation is rapid. They also cause vasodilation, increase capillary permeability, produce edema, evoke pain by an effect on nerve endings, and contract or relax a variety of extravascular smooth muscles. It is possible that these agents mediate pulpal pain and that inhibitors of them may be useful dental therapeutic aids in the future.

No specific antagonists are yet available. However, some drugs are known to inhibit kinin-evoked responses. It has been reported that salicylates and glucocorticoids inhibit kallikinin activation and may play a role in future therapy. Also, investigations are now in progress relative to antagonists to the kinins and their possible clinical usage.

REFERENCES

1. Schultz-Haudt, S. D.: Anatomy and physiology of the periodontal structures—review of the literature, World Workshop in Periodontics, Ann Arbor, 1966, The University of Michigan Press.
2. Raisz, L. G.: Physiologic and pharmacologic regulation of bone resorption, N. Engl. J. Med. **282:**909, 1970.
3. Hirsch, P. F.: Thyrocalcitonin, Physiol. Rev. **49:**548, 1969.
4. Goodman, L. S., and Gilman, A., editors: The pharmacological basis of therapeutics, ed. 5, New York, 1975, The Macmillan Co.
5. Rasmussen, H., and Bordier, P.: The physiological and cellular basis of metabolic bone disease, Baltimore, 1974, The Williams & Wilkins Co.
6. Rosenberg, E. H., and Guralnick, W. C.: Hyperparathyroidism, Oral Surg. **15**(supp. 2):84, 1962.
7. Silverman, S., Gordon, G., Grant, T., Steinbach, H., Eisenberg, E., and Manson, R.: The dental structures in primary hyperparathyroidism, Oral Surg. **15:**426, 1962.
8. Cohen, D. W., Friedman, L. A., Shapiro, J., and Kyle, G. C.: Studies on periodontal patterns in diabetes mellitus, J. Periodont. Res. **4**(supp.):35, 1969.
9. Belting, C. M., Hinicher, J. J., and Dummett, C. O.: Influence of diabetes mellitus on the severity of periodontal disease, J. Periodontol. **35:**476, 1964.
10. Kjellman, O.: The presence of glucose on gingival exudate and resting saliva of subjects with insulin-treated diabetes mellitus, Swed. Dent. J. **63:**11, 1970.
11. Collaborative Group for the Study of Stroke in Young Women: Oral contraceptives and stroke in young women: associated risk factors, J.A.M.A. **231:**718, 1975.
12. Lindhe, J., and Hugoson, A.: The influence of estrogen and progesterone on gingival exudation of regenerating dentogingival tissues, Paradontology **23:**16, 1969.
13. Lindhe, J., Attstroem, R., and Bjoern, A.: The influence of progestogen on gingival exudation during menstrual cycles: longitudinal study, J. Periodont. Res. **4:**97, 1969.
14. Raisz, L. G.: Physiologic and pharmacologic regulation of bone resorption, N. Engl. J. Med. **282:**909, 1970.
15. Goodson, J. M., and Brunetti, A.: Biosynthesis of prostaglandin E_2 by gingival homogenates, IADR Abstracts **53:**181, 1974.

17

Adrenocorticosteroids

SAM V. HOLROYD

The adrenal cortex secretes a number of steroids that are essential to life. For convenience these may be classified as *glucocorticoids*, which primarily affect carbohydrate metabolism and the inflammatory response, and *mineralocorticoids*, which principally affect water and electrolyte balance. The glucocorticoids are secreted in response to stimulation of the cortex by the pituitary trophic hormone (ACTH). The mineralocorticoids are under the influence of body electrolyte balance.

In deficiency states of the adrenal cortex (Addison's disease) the corticosteroids (corticoids) may be administered as replacement therapy. However, the principal pharmacologic use of these steroids and their synthetic derivatives is as anti-inflammatory agents.

The major natural adrenocorticosteroids are as follows:

Glucocorticoids (anti-inflammatory and catabolic effects)
Cortisol, or hydrocortisone (Cortef, Cortenema, Cortifan, Cortril, Hydrocortone, Solu-Cortef)
Corticosterone (of no pharmacologic importance)
Cortisone (Cortogen, Cortone)
Mineralocorticoids (sodium retaining, potassium depleting)
Aldosterone (of no pharmacologic importance)
Desoxycorticosterone (Cortate, Decortin, Doca, Percorten)

Since the principal therapeutic application of the adrenocorticosteroids is as anti-inflammatory agents, a considerable effort has been made to develop drugs that are anti-inflammatory but produce a minimum of the other effects typical of the naturally occurring adrenal steroids. These recently synthesized corticosteroids include prednisone (Deltasone, Deltra, Meticorten, Paracort, Servisone), prednisolone (Delta-Cortef, Hydeltrasol, Meticortelone, Nisolone, Sterane, Sterolone), methylprednisolone (Medrol), triamcinolone (Aristocort, Kenacort), betamethasone (Celestone, Valisone), dexamethasone (Decadron, Deronil, Dexameth, Hexadrol), fluocinolone (Synalar), fluorometholone (Oxylone), paramethasone (Haldrone, Stemex), fluprednisolone (Alphadrol), flurandrenolide (Cordran), and fludrocortisone (Florinef).

The naturally occurring and synthetic adrenocorticoids contain the following basic steroid nucleus:

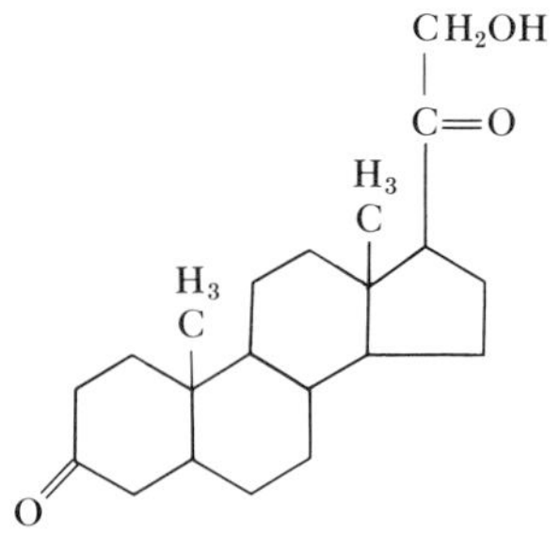

A minor modification of this nucleus produced the synthetic corticoid, triamcinolone, diagrammed below, which has had some popularity as a topical agent in dental practice.

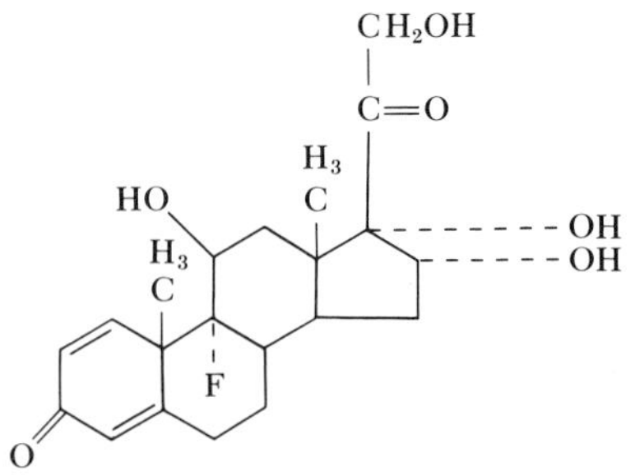

☐ The opinions or assertions contained herein are the private ones of the writer and are not to be construed as official or as reflecting the views of the Navy Department or the naval service at large.

ADMINISTRATION AND BODY HANDLING

Glucocorticoids are available in a large number of preparations for oral, intramuscular, intravenous, and topical use. After absorption some, and probably all, of the corticosteroids become bound to plasma proteins and are distributed throughout the body. Metabolism occurs primarily in the liver, and very little corticosteroid is excreted unchanged from the kidney. Prolonged blood levels may be anticipated in patients with liver or kidney disease.

PHARMACOLOGIC EFFECTS

The adrenocorticosteroids have broad pharmacologic effects and function to maintain numerous homeostatic balances. They affect many fundamental body processes such as the synthesis and activity of a number of enzymes, membrane function and permeability, and ribonucleic acid (RNA) synthesis.[2] Through these and other mechanisms they have pronounced effects on body function. Abnormally high or low corticosteroid blood levels affect the equilibrium of many physiologic systems. Although both the glucocorticoids and the mineralocorticoids have essentially the same pharmacologic actions, there is a significant variation in the degree to which they produce a particular effect. The glucocorticoids have a pronounced effect on carbohydrate metabolism, protein metabolism, and the inflammatory response. The

Table 17-1. Relative potencies of the systemic corticosteroids*

Steroid	Glucocorticoid potency	Mineralo- corticoid potency
Hydrocortisone	1.0	++
Cortisone	0.8	++
Prednisolone	4.0	+
Prednisone	4.0	+
Methylprednisolone	5.0	0
Triamcinolone	5.0	0
Paramethasone	10.0	0
Fluprednisolone	10.0	0
Dexamethasone	30.0	0
Betamethasone	30.0	0
Fludrocortisone†	15.0	++++

*Modified from American Medical Association Council on Drugs: AMA drug evaluations, ed. 2, Acton, Mass., 1973, Publishing Sciences Group, Inc.
†Used only for mineralocorticoid effect.

mineralocorticoids' most potent effect is on electrolyte and water balance.

The relative potencies of the systemic corticosteroids are shown in Table 17-1.

The adrenal steroids, and particularly the glucocorticoids, affect carbohydrate metabolism catabolically by increasing gluconeogenesis and decreasing the utilization of glucose. Consequently, an obvious result of excessive blood levels of the corticosteroids is hyperglycemia. Adrenal inadequacy with the resulting deficiency of corticosteroids, as is seen in Addison's disease, would conversely lead to hypoglycemia. The glucocorticoids inhibit protein synthesis or increase protein catabolism or both. Abnormally high levels of corticoids may thus lead to a negative nitrogen balance, a cessation of growth, and impaired wound healing. The adrenal steroids also appear to increase fat deposition.

The adrenal steroids, particularly the mineralocorticoids, act on the renal tubules to increase sodium retention and potassium excretion. Alterations in sodium and potassium excretion result in electrolyte imbalance. Since water retention is associated with sodium retention, excessive concentration of the mineralocorticoids may lead to edema and hypertension. Conversely, inadequate blood levels of the mineralocorticoids may lead to dehydration and hypotension, as is characteristic of Addison's disease.

The glucocorticoids, and to a limited extent the mineralocorticoids, depress the inflammatory response. Capillary dilation, exudation, and cellular proliferation are reduced. The adrenal steroids, and again particularly the glucocorticoids, tend to suppress allergic reactions.

Changes in blood levels of adrenocorticosteroids, whether attributable to adrenocortical hyperfunction (Cushing's syndrome), hypofunction (Addison's disease), or the administration of corticosteroid, have other widespread effects on the body. Imbalances in corticosteroid levels may modify enzyme activity, alter mental and myocardial functions, modify gastric secretion, induce muscle weakness, and inhibit the phagocytic properties and activities of blood cells. High corticoid levels may inhibit new bone formation because of the impaired absorption of calcium from the gastrointestinal tract.

Relationship to corticotropin. Corticotropin (adrenocorticotropic hormone, ACTH), which is produced by the anterior pituitary, is essential for maintenance of the structure and function of the adrenal cortex. ACTH stimulates the formation and release of adrenal steroids, particularly the glucocorticoids, and is used clinically to increase the blood level of the corticoids. Some authorities consider the use of corticotropin to represent a more natural means of obtaining an increased body concentration of adrenal steroids than direct administration of those steroids. However, direct administration generally provides a more predictable response, and with the advent of the newer, synthetic corticoids, more specific effects can be obtained. Consequently, the use of ACTH has declined somewhat in recent years.

The glucocorticoids suppress the secretion of ACTH by the pituitary. Thus a negative feedback mechanism exists, and a balance between ACTH and the corticosteroids is maintained. It is of considerable importance to note at this point that administration of the glucocorticoids, by depressing the secretion of ACTH, can result in atrophy of the adrenal cortex.

ADVERSE REACTIONS

Short courses of low dosages of the corticosteroids are essentially safe, but higher doses given over relatively long periods may cause extensive and dangerous adverse reactions.

Commonly during long-term corticosteroid therapy the milder signs of Cushing's syndrome appear, including rounding and puffiness of the face, hirsutism, development of purplish striae on the abdomen, menstrual abnormalities, and some redistribution of body fat from the extremities to the trunk. Since some glucocorticoids tend to stimulate the appetite, patients often gain weight. Behavioral and personality changes, euphoria, and other mental changes, which vary from agitation to depression, are also seen relatively often in patients receiving long-term or high-dosage corticosteroid therapy.

The effects of hyperglycemia and a negative nitrogen balance may become widespread and serious. Muscular weakness, osteoporosis, peptic ulcer, delayed wound healing, and a lowered resistance to infection may be experienced. The lowered resistance to infection is particularly significant in viral and fungal infections where antimicrobial control may be limited.

The effects of the corticosteroids on electrolyte balance, although predominately a problem with the mineralocorticoids, may also be seen with the glucocorticoids, particularly cortisol and cortisone. Water retention resulting from sodium retention produces edema and may cause an increase in blood pressure. Symptoms of the excessive loss of potassium may also occur. The significance of corticoid-induced adrenocortical atrophy has previously been mentioned. In these cases symptoms of adrenal insufficiency may follow a rapid withdrawal of corticosteroid therapy or may emerge in times of stress. This problem can be acute and may present serious difficulties. One must also remember that the adrenal steroids may, through their anti-inflammatory action, mask the appearance of disease and delay diagnosis.

Without careful medical evaluation and observation the adrenal steroids should not be used in the presence of systemic infections (especially viral and fungal infections), active or arrested tuberculosis, peptic ulcers, diabetes mellitus, congestive heart failure, glaucoma, osteoporosis, and psychotic tendencies.

Adrenal crisis. The widespread body effects of the adrenal steroids are necessary as compensatory mechanisms against stressful situations. During stress, ACTH is released to stimulate the increased secretion of the adrenal steroids. If an adequate flow of corticoids is not forthcoming, a physiologic adjustment to stress is impossible and an adrenal crisis is said to occur. An adrenal crisis can be precipitated by dental procedures and may be manifested by weakness, syncope, and cardiovascular collapse with acute shock. Consequently, a patient with Addison's disease or one who has been taking adrenal steroids for some time should be treated only after consultation with the patient's physician as to the need for adjusting the intake of adrenocorticoids. Stress must be minimized for these patients.

THERAPEUTIC USES

The adrenal steroids are administered as replacement therapy in cases of hypofunction of the adrenal cortex. Cortisol or cortisone is used to restore the glucocorticoid effects, and in most cases desoxycorticosterone is used to alleviate the mineralocorticoid deficiency.

The more extensive use of the corticosteroids is in the treatment of a wide variety of inflammatory and severe allergic conditions. Because of the large number of undesirable potentialities involved in therapy with the adrenal steroids, it has been stated that they should be administered only to patients experiencing severe symptoms that have not responded to more benign measures or to patients suffering from life-threatening conditions.[4] This does not preclude the relatively safe, short-term, low-dosage use of steroids, but therapy with these drugs should be carried out cautiously and with full respect for their diverse pharmacologic actions.

Although cortisone and cortisol have been used extensively for their anti-inflammatory effects, the newer synthetic steroids (that is, prednisone, prednisolone, triamcinolone, and others) are more specific anti-inflammatory agents and have less effect on electrolyte and water balance. Conditions that have been treated with corticosteroids include adrenal hypofunction (Addison's disease), rheumatoid arthritis, rheumatic fever, lupus erythematosus, scleroderma, inflammation of joints and soft tissues, acute bronchial asthma, severe and acute allergic reactions, and severe allergic dermatoses.

The dentist's responsibility in regard to corticosteroid therapy lies in two areas: (1) care of the patient whose physician has prescribed the drugs and (2) use of the drugs in dental practice.

Since these potent drugs are widely prescribed medically, the dental practitioner must be on the alert for the patient who is taking adrenal steroids; and he must know how these drugs have, or may have, modified the patient's physiologic functions. Consultation with the patient's physician in these cases is highly desirable and is imperative if the patient is to undergo surgery or any stressful procedure.

Individuals taking corticosteroids are likely to have a lowered resistance to infection so that special consideration must be given to aseptic dental technique. Prophylactic antibiotic therapy may be indicated in many surgical situations involving these patients. Appropriate consideration should also be given to the fact that wound healing may be delayed.

Krohn[5] has reported that patients taking ACTH or corticosteroids do not have a greater incidence or severity of periodontal disease than do comparable patients not taking these drugs. However, one must not rule out the fact that the effects of corticosteroid therapy may be reflected in the oral tissues. Osteoporosis of alveolar bone, degeneration of the fibers of the periodontal ligament, and increased destruction of the periodontal tissues associated with inflammation have been demonstrated in experimental animals.[6]

The second aspect of the dentist's responsibility in regard to corticosteroid therapy involves the use of these drugs in the dental office. Adrenal steroids are of great value in severe allergic reactions. Consequently, they should be a part of the dentist's emergency kit. The actual administration of these drugs in allergic reactions is discussed in Chapter 24. To relieve the acute symptoms of rheumatoid arthritis or osteoarthritis of the temporomandibular joint, the adrenal steroids have been injected into the intra-articular space. Pain may be relieved and mandibular movement improved by the injection of hydrocortisone acetate. Prednisolone acetate has also been used for intra-articular injection.[7]

The adrenocorticosteroids have been applied locally in a number of dental conditions. Reports of their use in pulp capping and pulpotomy procedures have been encouraging but are as yet inconclusive. Paramethasone[8] and prednisolone[9] have been used topically with success in treating hypersensitive cervical dentin. The prednisolone solution used consisted of 25% parachlorophenol, 25% metacresyl acetate, 49% gum camphor, and 1% prednisolone. The sensitive teeth were dried, and the solution was applied constantly for 2 minutes, after which the patient rinsed with water.

Adrenal steroids have been used to reduce edema, trismus, and pain after oral surgical procedures. Linenberg[10] and Messer and Keller[11] have reported that dexamethasone is effective in this regard. Present evidence of the effectiveness and safety of adrenal steroids in the control of postoperative edema in oral surgery is essentially that of clinical observations rather than that of controlled double-blind studies.

Perhaps the most widespread use of the corticosteroids in dental practice has been as a topical application in the treatment of various ulcerative and inflammatory soft tissue lesions. Some success has been reported with the use of estradiol benzoate and ACTH[12] and of 0.5% prednisolone ointment[13] in the treatment of desquamative gingivostomatitis.

Although the corticosteroids are specifically contraindicated for herpetic lesions,[14] they have been used with some success in severe cases of recurrent aphthous stomatitis. Relief from a severe, constant aphthous condition has been reported with 2.5 mg hydrocortisone hemisuccinate lozenges dissolved in the mouth four times per 24 hours during exacerbations and twice per 24 hours during remissions.[15] The application of a hydrocortisone acetate–antibiotic lozenge (Hydrozets) to aphthous lesions four times per 24 hours for 5 to 7 days was reported to have reduced pain and healing time in about 60% of the patients. However, the antibiotics in the steroid–antibiotic lozenge had no effect when used alone.[16]

REFERENCES

1. Pharmacotherapeutics in dental practice, NAVPERS 10486, Washington, D.C., 1969, U.S. Bureau of Naval Personnel.
2. Sutherland, V. C.: A synopsis of pharmacology, Philadelphia, 1970, W. B. Saunders Co.
3. American Medical Association Council on Drugs: AMA drug evaluations, ed. 2, Acton, Mass., 1973, Publishing Sciences Group, Inc.
4. American Medical Association Council on Drugs: New drugs 1967, Chicago, 1967, American Medical Association.
5. Krohn, S.: Effect of the administration of steroid hormones on the gingival tissues, J. Periodontol. **29:**300-306, 1958.
6. Glickman, I., Stone, I. C., and Chawla, T. N.: The effect of the systemic administration of cortisone upon the periodontium of white mice, J. Periodontol. **24:**161-166, 1953.
7. American Dental Association Council on Dental Therapeutics: Accepted dental therapeutics 1969/1970, ed. 33, Chicago, 1969, American Dental Association.
8. Lawson, B. F., and Huff, T. W.: Desensitization of teeth with a topically applied glucocorticoid drug: a preliminary study, J. Oral Ther. **2:**295-299, 1966.
9. Bowers, G. M., and Elliott, J. R.: Topical use of prednisolone in periodontics, J. Periodontol. **35:**486-488, 1964.
10. Linenberg, W. B.: The clinical evaluation of dexamethasone in oral surgery, Oral Surg. **20:**6-28, 1965.
11. Messer, E. J., and Keller, J. J.: The use of intraoral dexamethasone after extractions of mandibular third molars, Oral Surg. **40:**594-598, 1975.
12. Dreizen, S., Stone, R. E., and Spies, T.D.: A note on the use of pituitary adrenocorticotrophic hormone (ACTH) and estradiol benzoate (Progynon B) in the treatment of gingivitis associated with endocrine imbalance, Surg. Gynecol. Obstet. **90:**580-582, 1950.
13. Zegarelli, E. V., Kutscher, A. H., and Silvers, H. F.: Prednisolone in the treatment of incapacitating desquamative stomatitis: case report, J. Periodontol. **28:**310-313, 1957.
14. Burket, L. W.: Oral medicine, ed. 5, Philadelphia, 1965, J. B. Lippincott Co., p. 109.
15. Burket, L. W.: Oral medicine, ed. 5, Philadelphia, 1965, J. B. Lippincott Co., p. 117.
16. Graykowski, E. A., Barile, M. F., Lee, W. B., and Stanley, H. R., Jr.: Recurrent aphthous stomatitis: clinical, therapeutic, histopathologic, and hypersensitivity aspects, J.A.M.A. **196:**637-644, 1966.

18
Antineoplastic drugs

WILLIAM K. BOTTOMLEY

Antineoplastic agents are medications that currently are used almost exclusively by physicians. However, even though dentists do not prescribe these drugs, they are frequently asked to evaluate and treat the oral sequelae that may be induced by their use. Therefore it is essential that the dentist be familiar with these agents, their mechanisms of action, and the management of their oral toxic manifestations.

USE OF ANTINEOPLASTIC AGENTS

Antineoplastic agents, sometimes referred to as "chemotherapeutics," are used clinically to destroy and to suppress the growth and spread of malignant cells. In the past these agents were used when a neoplasm had not been controlled by either surgery or radiation or a combination of both approaches. Today, however, as a result of collective experiences and concerted clinical investigation, antineoplastic agents are employed at all levels of cancer treatment. In addition, they are considered to be the primary treatment for a number of malignancies, such as acute and chronic leukemia, choriocarcinoma, multiple myeloma, and Burkitt's lymphoma. When surgery and radiation are not curative, antineoplastic agents may provide a therapeutic means for cure, a longer remission or disease-free interval, decreased morbidity, and a resultant improved quality of life. The value of antineoplastics in reducing the size of neoplastic tumors prior to surgery or radiation therapy, or in ensuring a cure subsequent to these procedures, is gaining oncologic appreciation. Consequently, antineoplastics are being employed with increasing frequency.

MECHANISMS OF ACTION

The efficacy of antineoplastic agents is based primarily on their ability to interfere with the metabolism or the reproductive cycle of the tumor cells, thereby destroying them. The reproductive cycle of a cell is considered to consist of four stages (Fig. 13) as follows:

1. G_1 ("gap" 1), which is the postmitotic or pre–deoxyribonucleic acid (DNA) synthesis phase
2. S, which is the period of DNA synthesis
3. G_2 ("gap" 2), which is the premitotic or post–DNA synthesis phase
4. M, which is the period of mitosis

Cells in a resting stage, or not in a process of cell division, are described as being in the G_0 stage. Cells enter the cycle from the G_0 stage. In some tumors a large proportion of the cells may be at the G_0 level.

Most antineoplastic agents are labeled either "cycle dependent," indicating that they are effective only at specific stages in

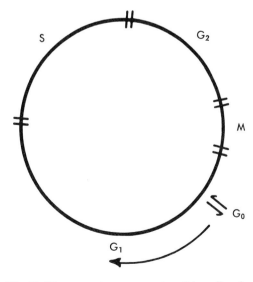

Fig. 13. Diagrammatic representation of the cell cycle.

173

the mitotic cycle, or "cycle independent," indicating that they are effective at all levels of the cycle. For example, the alkylating agents interfere with the malignant cells during all phases of the reproductive cycle as well as the resting stage (G_0) and are therefore classified as cycle independent.

Agents of widely different mechanisms of action are often employed together to inhibit the reproduction of neoplastic cells in all phases and to gain therapeutic advantage for the host. Mixtures of these agents may act synergistically, leading to enhanced cytotoxicity with fewer side effects. This is the rationale for combination drug therapy.

CLASSIFICATION

Six major groups of antineoplastic drugs are in use today.

Alkylating agents

The group of alkylating agents includes, among others, busulfan (Myleran), chlorambucil (Leukeran), cyclophosphamide (Cytoxan, Endoxan), mechlorethamine (nitrogen mustard), and melphalan (Alkeran). The alkyl radical of these drugs reacts with DNA in all phases of the cell cycle, thereby preventing cell reproduction. They are most effective in chronic leukemias, lymphomas, myelomas, and carcinomas of the breast and ovary.

Antimetabolites

Agents representative of this group are mercaptopurine (Purinethol), methotrexate, fluorouracil (5-FU), and cytosine arabinoside (Cytosar). They attack the cells in the S period of the reproduction cycle by interfering with the biosynthesis of the purine or pyrimidine bases. The antimetabolites have been used to treat the entire spectrum of cancers.

Synthetic organic agents

The synthetic organic agents are a miscellaneous group that include procarbazine (Matulane); hydroxyurea (Hydrea); mitotane (Lysodren); and the nitrosoureas 1,3-bis(2-chloroethyl)-1-nitrosourea (BCNU), (1)-(2) chloroethyl(-3-cyclohexyl-1-nitrosourea) (CCNU), and methyl-CCNU. Procarbazine is used in combination chemotherapy for Hodgkin's disease. It acts by inducing the formation of free radicals in tissue similar to the effect of radiation therapy. Hydroxyurea is useful in chronic myelocytic leukemia. Mitotane is employed in the treatment of inoperable adrenal cortex carcinoma.

Plant alkaloids

Vinblastine (Velban) and vincristine (Oncovin) comprise those agents which act by arresting cells in metaphase. Since they have little bone marrow toxicity, they are frequently used in combination regimens for the treatment of a wide variety of malignancies.

Antibiotics

Several of the antibiotics administered for antineoplastic therapy are actinomycin D (dactinomycin), doxorubicin hydrochloride (Adriamycin), mithramycin (Mithracin), mitomycin-C (Mitomycin), and bleomycin sulfate (Blenoxane). These are effective in the treatment of a variety of solid tumors.

Hormones

Androgens. Dromostanolone (Drolban), fluoxymesterone (Halotestin), and testosterone (Oreton) are representative androgens whose primary use is for palliation in patients with inoperable carcinoma of the breast.

Adrenal corticosteroids. The steroids prednisone (Deltasone, Meticorten), prednisolone (Delta-Cortef, Meticortelone), cortisone acetate (Cortone), and hydrocortisone (Cortef, Hydrocortone) are used alone or in combination therapy for acute leukemias. They interrupt the cell cycle at the G_1 stage.

Estrogens. The estrogens diethylstilbestrol (DES) and ethinyl estradiol (Estinyl) are considered as reliable palliative therapy in patients with carcinoma of the breast, especially in the postmenopausal patient.

ADVERSE DRUG EFFECTS

Rapidly growing cells, such as neoplastic cells, are more susceptible to inhibition or destruction by antineoplastic agents. The most serious difficulty in antineoplastic therapy stems from the lack of selectivity between tumor tissue and normal tissue. Some normal cells exhibit a faster reproduction cycle than do slowly growing tumor cells. In an effort to eradicate a malignancy, certain normal cells are also destroyed, resulting in clinically expressed adverse effects. Since the cells of the gastrointestinal tract, bone marrow, and hair follicles are among the faster growing normal cells, the early clinical manifestations of side effects are associated with the loss of these cells.

The principal adverse effects are as follows:

1. There is a suppression of bone marrow activity resulting in leukopenia, thrombocytopenia, and anemia. The degree of cytopenia that results depends on the drugs being employed, the condition of the bone marrow at the time of administration, and other contributing factors.

2. Gastrointestinal disturbances may occur, resulting from sloughing of the gastrointestinal mucosa. Clinically, these disturbances are expressed as nausea, stomatitis, vomiting, and hemorrhagic diarrhea.

3. Cutaneous reactions may occur infrequently, varying from mild erythema and maculopapular eruptions to exfoliative dermatitis and Stevens-Johnson syndrome. Alopecia is frequent, but the hair usually regrows when therapy is discontinued.

4. Hepatotoxicity occurs principally with the antimetabolites, for example, methotrexate, but it may occur with other agents as well.

5. Neurotoxic effects may develop, such as peripheral neuropathy, ileus, inappropriate antidiuretic hormone secretion, and convulsions, which are chiefly associated with vincristine or vinblastine administration.

6. Renal tubular impairment, occurring secondary to hyperuricemia, is due to rapid cell destruction and the release of nucleotides. For example, the treatment of leukemias and lymphomas often results in rapid tumor destruction with a consequent high uric acid level. Allopurinol (Zyloprim) is administered routinely prior to the initiation of a regimen of antineoplastic agents to prevent hyperuricemia.

7. Immune deficiency may occur, resulting in an enhanced susceptibility to infection and/or a second malignancy, since many antineoplastic agents have an immunosuppressant effect.

8. Inhibition of spermatogenesis and oogenesis is frequent, at least temporarily. Mutations within the germ cells may occur, and the menstrual cycle may also be inhibited. The patient can recover after discontinuation of the drug.

9. Adverse effects on oral tissue may develop. These are discussed below.

Oral considerations

Oral complaints precipitated by side effects of the antineoplastic agents are primarily those of discomfort, sensitivity of teeth and gums, pain, ulceration, gingival hemorrhage, dryness, and impaired taste sensation. Because of the complicated interaction of the antineoplastic agents with the body system, oral symptoms are best treated topically.

The most important therapeutic consideration is to attempt to prevent toxicity. When the decision has been made to institute antineoplastic therapy, appropriate maintenance of the oral cavity should receive priority attention. Plaque control instructions and their periodic reinforcement are essential to prevent or attenuate the anticipated oral complications. Commercial mouthwashes tend to dry the oral tissues and interfere with the delicate balance of the oral flora, and therefore they should be avoided. An alkaline saline rinse of warm water flavored with salt and sodium bicarbonate is a simple, effective remedy that can be used for oral flushing. A soft toothbrush will reduce the possibility of gingival or mucosal irritation or abrasion. Oral irrigating devices, if used, should be regulated to low pressure only to prevent initiating or exacerbating gingival hemorrhage. Gingival hemorrhage is an indication of some degree of ulceration of the crevicular lining. This should *not* be interpreted as a signal to discontinue brushing. Judicious brushing should be continued, or the local irritants produced by the unmolested plaque will promote the diseased state of the gingival crevice, resulting in increased hemorrhage and pain.

Candidiasis. Frequently, the altered oral environment allows the opportunistic overgrowth of *Candida albicans*. Since this is a predictable occurrence, nystatin (Mycostatin) therapy is often instituted simultaneously with the administration of antineoplastic agents. Rinses with 2 ml of an oral suspension of 100,000 μ/ml four times per 24 hours may be adequate to control the infection. If the oral candidiasis is persistent, an often efficacious therapeutic modality is to allow vaginal suppositories to slowly dissolve in the buccal vestibule, thereby allowing a constant supply of the antifungal agent to come in contact with the infectious agent.

Xerostomia. Another side effect of antineoplastic agents is reduced salivary gland activity. Sequelae of this condition are sensitivity of the teeth and the mucous membranes. Frequent (for example, every 2 hours) oral rinses with a 0.5% aqueous solution of sodium carboxymethyl cellulose will often relieve these symptoms.

Ulcerations. Ulcerations of the oral mucous membranes occur most commonly with methotrexate, fluorouracil, actinomycin D (dactinomycin), doxorubicin hydrochloride (Adriamycin), and bleomycin. However, any antineoplastic agent that significantly depresses the marrow can induce oral ulceration as a sequelae to leukopenia. The characteristic oral lesion is a cratered ulceration with a wide, diffuse, erythematous border reflecting severely compromised host resistance to any tissue insult.

An effective regimen to bathe the tissues, guard against secondary infection, and control the *Candida* in the ulcerations comprises alternating rinses of 2 ml nystatin oral suspension, alkaline saline solution, and 0.5% providone-iodine solution, with 1-hour intervals between rinses.

Gingival hemorrhage. Constant, low-grade gingival hemorrhage frequently occurs when a thrombocytopenia develops either as a result of the disease process or the therapy. Periodontal packs may reduce the blood loss and mechanically contribute to local clotting. When the marrow is depressed to the degree that oral hemorrhage and ulcerations are not controllable on a local basis, systemic therapy may be necessary. The temporary discontinuation of the antineoplastic agents and transfusions of platelet packs will often quickly improve the oral health.

ELECTIVE DENTAL TREATMENT

Generally, elective dental procedures should not be performed when patients are receiving antineoplastic therapy, especially if the patient is experiencing acute adverse side effects. If possible, multiple extractions should be avoided. Before any extractions the coagulation status of the patient should be carefully evaluated so that appropriate measures can be used at the time of surgery for anticipated complications. In a situation where a coagulopathy exists and an extraction is necessary, packing the socket with oxidized regenerated cellulose and suturing as indicated will tend to minimize postoperative difficulties.

Dental treatment of leukemic patients preferably should be performed during the remission phase.

There is a lack of consensus about antibiotic prophylactic coverage for required dental treatment on these patients. In support of antibiotic coverage is the observation that susceptibility to infection is increased in individuals who are receiving chemotherapy. On the other hand, the use of antibiotics may result in superinfection that may be difficult to manage. The decision about their use should be reached by mutual agreement with the referring physician.

REFERENCES

1. Holland, J. F., and Frei, E., III: Cancer medicine, Philadelphia, 1973, Lea & Febiger.
2. American Medical Association Council on Drugs: AMA drug evaluations, ed. 2, Acton, Mass., 1973, Publishing Sciences Group, Inc.
3. Cole, W. H.: Chemotherapy of cancer, Philadelphia, 1970, Lea & Febiger.
4. Ansfield, J.: Chemotherapy of malignant neoplasms, ed. 2, Springfield, Ill., 1973, Charles C Thomas, Publisher.
5. Greenwald, E. S.: Cancer chemotherapy, ed. 2, Flushing, N.Y., 1973, Medical Examination Publishing Co., Inc.
6. Carl, W., and Schaaf, N. G.: Proceedings: dental care for the cancer patient, J. Surg. Oncol. 6(4): 293-310, 1974.
7. Clinical oncology for medical students and physicians, ed. 4, Rochester, N.Y., 1974, University of Rochester School of Medicine and Dentistry.

19

Cardiovascular drugs

TOMMY W. GAGE

Cardiovascular disease is an inclusive term referring to a variety of diseases of the heart and blood vessels. These diseases include, among others, hypertension (high blood pressure), angina pectoris, heart muscle disease, stroke, and heart failure. Cardiovascular disease is the leading cause of death in the United States. It is estimated that as many as 28 million Americans have cardiovascular disease, and some 4 million experience angina or heart attack each year. With the development of cardiac care units, comprehensive drug therapy, and intensive screening for cardiovascular diseases, many patients are now living longer, more productive lives. These factors help to explain why cardiovascular disease affects such a large segment of the dental patient population.

Because patients take cardiovascular drugs for long periods of time, a knowledge of the drugs employed to treat cardiovascular patients should provide the dentist with more confidence in the management of these patients and in the avoidance of potential drug interactions. The following cardiovascular drugs will be discussed in this chapter[1]: cardiac glycosides, antiarrhythmics, antianginal agents, antihypertensives, diuretics, and anticoagulants.

CARDIAC GLYCOSIDES
Review of congestive heart failure

The function of the heart is to act as a pump to ensure an adequate circulation of blood to meet the oxygen needs of all body tissues. Circulation needs are variable, such as that dictated by exercise, and the heart must have enough myocardial reserve to meet this demand. Part of the myocardial reserve can be explained by the automatic neurohumoral and intrinsic mechanisms that result in an increased rate and contractility. The heart adjusts its cardiac output in re-

lationship to the end diastolic volume. Increased ventricular filling lengthens and increases the tension of the cardiac muscle, thereby increasing the force of contraction (Starling's law) within physiologic limits. In a normal heart all of these compensatory mechanisms work together to ensure an adequate cardiac output and circulation.

The failing heart is characterized by an inefficient pumping mechanism with an inadequate cardiac output, resulting in a less than satisfactory circulation. A number of different forms of injury to the heart, that is, rheumatic heart disease, myocardial lesions, or arrhythmias may contribute to heart failure. If heart failure is accompanied by an increased left ventricular filling pressure, increased hydrostatic pressure in the pulmonary capillaries can lead to pulmonary edema and congestion. If the failure occurs on the right side of the heart, systemic congestion occurs with edema in the extremities. Other organ systems such as the liver and kidney will respond to the reduced circulation in an adverse manner, further complicating the disorder. Both right and left ventricular failure may occur in the same patient. Patients with chronic congestive heart failure manifest symptoms of shortness of breath, an enlarged heart, and edema. Pulmonary congestion may require that the patient sleep on stacked pillows to ensure comfortable breathing. Congestive heart failure is the result of the failure of the myocardium to function as a pump and maintain an adequate circulation.[2]

Digitalis

The most important group of drugs in the treatment of congestive heart failure were first described by William Withering in 1785 and are called the cardiac or digitalis glycosides. The term *glycoside* is given to this

Table 19-1. Differences among more commonly used cardiac glycosides*†

Preparation	Source	Routes	Oral onset	Duration	Oral maintenance dose per 24 hours
Digitalis leaf	*D. purpurea*	Oral	Slow	Long	100-200 mg
Digitoxin	*D. purpurea*	Oral, IV	Slow	Long	0.05-0.2 mg
Digoxin	*D. lanata*	Oral, IV	Fast	Medium	0.125-0.5 mg
Acetyldigitoxin	*D. lanata*	Oral	Medium	Medium	0.1-0.2 mg
Deslanoside	*D. lanata*	Oral, IV	Fast	Medium	0.4-0.5 mg
Ouabain	*Strophanthus gratus*	IV	IV only	Short	

*Data from Dr. D. T. Watts, Richmond, Va.
†The previously mentioned glycosides gitalin and lanatoside C are not listed because they are infrequently used.

group of drugs because the active molecule portion (the aglycone) is connected by a glycosidic linkage to a variety of sugar molecules. All of the glycosides have the same fundamental action on the heart. The sugar moiety is important in determining water solubility, which in turn accounts for the differences in potency, route of administration, onset and duration of action, and rate of excretion of the various glycosides. All of the glycosides are of botanical origin, coming from *Digitalis purpurea*, *D. lanata*, and *Strophanthus gratus*, the source of ouabain.

A large number of cardiac glycosides are available for clinical use. The two most widely prescribed are digitoxin (Crystodigin, Digitaline, Nativelle, Purodigin) and digoxin (Davoxin, Lanoxin). Powdered or whole digitalis leaf (Digifortis, Digitoria, Pil-Digis) preparations are not used as extensively as they once were. Other glycosides available but encountered less frequently include gitalin (Gitaligin), ouabain, lanatoside C (Cedilanid), acetyldigitoxin (Acylanid) and deslanoside (Cedilanid-D). Differences among the more important cardiac glycosides are shown in Table 19-1. The antiarrhythmic use of the glycosides is discussed later in this chapter.[3]

Pharmacologic effects. The principal effect of the cardiac glycosides on the failing heart is to increase the force of contraction of the myocardium, which is termed the *positive inotropic effect.* The improvement in contractile force makes the heart more efficient as a pump, increasing the stroke volume and cardiac output. As a result of this improved pumping action, other compensatory changes occur such as a reduction in heart size with a decrease in heart rate and venous

pressure. All of these events occur provided there is still sufficient cardiac reserve present and cardiac function is not severely impaired. The action of digitalis is directly on the heart cell except for the decrease in rate, which is accounted for, at least in part, by an indirect vagal slowing. It should be pointed out that the positive inotropic effects of digitalis are seldom observed in a normal heart or in a heart in which myocardial cell damage is the cause of failure.

In addition to the direct effect of digitalis on the myocardium, there are effects on the electrophysiologic properties of the heart that are dose dependent. These dose-dependent events are most significant when toxicity to digitalis occurs. Low doses of digitalis increase cardiac excitability, and high doses decrease excitability. Changes in conduction velocity are variable depending on the specific heart tissue, but some increase in conduction velocity is observed in the atria with a decrease in the A-V nodal tissues. There is an increase in automaticity of the ventricles (chronotropic effect) and in ectopic pacemaker activity. This latter event becomes more evident with toxic doses.

Another effect of digitalis is the reduction in edema that occurs with its use. The diuresis that occurs is largely the result of an improved circulation and a decrease in venous pressure, causing an improved glomerular filtration rate. The net result is a more efficient kidney function that reduces the edematous fluid accumulation.

The mechanism of action of digitalis on the myocardium as well as changes in the electrical activity of the heart are probably the same, although the exact mechanism is still unclear. One concept relates a facilitation of the excitation-coupling mechanism with an increased availability of Ca^{++} ion for the contractile elements as influenced by digitalis. A second and perhaps more widely accepted view is that digitalis inhibits a Na^+, K^+-ATPase enzyme responsible for the energy dependent transport of Na^+ and K^+ across the myocardial cell membrane.[4]

Absorption, metabolism, and doses. The route of administration of the cardiac glycosides is usually determined by the urgency of the clinical situation. Since patients normally take digitalis on a lifetime basis, the oral route is preferred for the convenience of self-administration. With the exception of ouabain, most of the cardiac glycosides are well absorbed when given orally. Digitoxin is the most efficiently absorbed, followed by digoxin. The whole leaf glycoside preparations are not as well absorbed but sufficiently to be useful. With earlier commercial preparations, the bioavailability of marketed digoxin products presented some problems in therapy. A more recently implemented digoxin certification program has largely remedied this problem while at the same time modifying older dosage schedules.[5]

A number of cardiac glycoside preparations are available for parenteral use. Pain and irritation on injection limit the intramuscular and subcutaneous routes of administration. The preferred but also the most dangerous route is intravenous. Both ouabain and digoxin are suitable for rapid plasma levels required for demanding clinical situations. After stabilization with parenteral doses, the patient can be switched to the oral route for more convenience in maintenance.

Digitoxin has the longest duration of action with the slowest onset. This may be accounted for by its high plasma protein binding affinity and its slower metabolism by the liver. Digoxin is not bound to plasma protein in as high a quantity and is excreted by the kidney largely unmetabolized. The presence of liver or kidney disease can influence the duration of action of these glycosides. A drug, such as phenobarbital, that is a potent liver enzyme inducer could also alter the effects of digitoxin by speeding its metabolism.

The establishment of a dose of digitalis sufficient to provide symptomatic relief of congestive heart failure must be based on the individual patient's needs. Two basic means of providing adequate plasma levels of the cardiac glycosides are employed. The classic dosage technique requires that an initial loading or digitalization dose be started first. This initial dose is several times the maintenance dose and is necessary because of the slow tissue accumulation of the glycoside. Once the effective plasma level is established, daily maintenance doses can then be started based on the rate of elimination of the glycoside. Doses are just sufficient to replace the daily loss, since the effects of repeated doses are cumulative.

Another dosage technique can be used provided the clinical situation is favorable. The patient is hospitalized, and the maintenance dose only is administered over several days until the cumulative drug effects are evident. This method is slower in establishing therapeutic levels but may avoid some of the toxic reactions associated with digitalization. These dosage techniques are suitable for patients who have not been taking digitalis. If the patient is taking digitalis and requires an additional amount of glycoside, careful use of smaller doses is required.[6]

Adverse effects. The digitalis glycosides are important therapeutic agents in congestive heart failure, but dosage adjustment can be a problem because the margin of safety is low. Even slight changes in dosage, alterations in metabolism, or absorption can be sufficient to trigger toxic symptoms. These symptoms are similar for all the glycosides and are more evident in the long-term user. The signs of early toxicity to digitalis could be easily detected by the alert dental practitioner, and they would include anorexia (loss of appetite) and nausea and vomiting; copious salivation may also be evident. The importance of recognizing early toxicity is more fully appreciated when one realizes that a reduction in dosage is sufficient to reduce the toxicity. More serious cardiac irregularities develop with continued doses or with a too rapid initial loading. These reactions include arrhythmias that can progress to ventricular fibrillation. Neurologic signs of toxicity include headache, drowsiness, and visual disturbances. At least one neurologic sign of some significance to the dentist is pain in the lower face that resembles somewhat the pain associated with trigeminal neuralgia.

In the chronic heart failure patient, digitalis therapy is often combined with a diuretic, low-sodium diet, and limited exercise. Diuretics can produce a hypokalemia, making the myocardium more sensitive to the toxic effects of digitalis. Weakness, faintness, and xerostomia may be observed in the patient. If liver damage results from a chronic congestive failure, drug metabolism may be reduced along with interference in normal coagulation processes.[7]

Drug interactions

The cardiac glycosides are commonly encountered drugs, and therefore drug interactions are likely. The effects of hypokalemia caused by diuretics have already been discussed. Amphotericin B may also lower potassium levels and could be a potential hazard. Other drugs employed by the dentist that are possible interactants include the barbiturates, which increase the metabolic activity of liver enzymes and increase the rate of digitoxin conversion to digoxin. The importance of this interaction seems to be minimal. Propantheline (Pro-Banthine), an anticholinergic agent occasionally employed to reduce salivary flow, may increase digoxin absorption in those patients taking slow-release digoxin preparations. Sympathomimetic drugs with beta-adrenergic activity may produce additive effects with digitalis in causing ectopic pacemaker activity.[8]

ANTIARRHYTHMIC AGENTS
Review of cardiac physiology

The function of the heart is dependent on rhythmic contractions of the cardiac muscle. The sequence of events in the contraction process requires the atrial muscle to contract at a sufficient interval before the ventricular muscle to assure complete ventricular filling. This is necessary to have an adequate cardiac output. The contraction rhythm is dependent on specialized conductive fibers that constitute part of the cardiac muscle.

The rate of cardiac contraction (beats per minute) is subject to regulation by the autonomic nervous system in response to demands by the organism. Vagal nerve (parasympathetic) stimulation causes a decrease in the S-A nodal rate and a decrease in A-V node excitability. This results in a slowing of the cardiac rate, and vigorous vagal stimulation can cause complete stoppage of the heart. The cardiac accelerator nerves (sym-

pathetic) have the opposite effect; they increase S-A nodal rhythm and thereby increase the number of beats per minute.

Normal cardiac rhythm may be altered by disease or cardiac injury. The altered patterns of rhythm are referred to as cardiac arrhythmias. The causes of arrhythmias are related to many factors, such as the development of an ectopic pacemaker, blockage or alterations in the impulse-conducting systems, and abnormal pacemaker rhythms.[9] The types of cardiac arrhythmias are shown in Table 19-2.

Drugs in current use

Quinidine. Quinidine, the dextroisomer of quinine, is one of the oldest and most commonly employed drugs in the treatment of cardiac arrhythmias. Quinidine is an alkaloid obtained from cinchona bark with pharmacologic actions similar to those of quinine. Its various salts are marketed as Quinaglute, Cardioquin, Quinidex, Quinora, and generically. Its myocardial depressant action accounts for its principal medical usefulness. Quinidine has both a direct and indirect action on the heart. Its direct actions are characterized by a decrease in excitability, conduction velocity, and automaticity. The refractory period is increased, hence its ability to slow increased rates of cardiac rhythm. The indirect effects of quinidine are best described as atropine-like, in that vagal influence on the myocardium is reduced. For quinidine to function as an effective antiarrhythmic agent, the clinician must adjust the dose so that the indirect effects do not complicate the cardiac condition.

Usual oral doses may cause nausea and vomiting. Hypersensitivity reactions occur rarely, with the most serious being thrombocytopenia purpura. Large doses of quinidine cause tinnitus, impaired hearing, and headache characterized as cinchonism. Intravenous or intramuscular doses can produce arterial hypotension. A paradoxical ventricular tachycardia can occur during the treatment of atrial flutter and fibrillation presumably as a result of its indirect action on A-V conduction. Specific contraindications to its use include complete A-V block and in cases of known hypersensitivity.

Quinidine is used for the treatment and prevention of atrial flutter and fibrillation, ventricular tachycardia, and premature sys-

Table 19-2. Types of cardiac arrhythmias[10]

Sinus bradycardia (less than 60 beats/min)	If uncomplicated by other disease, it may not be a problem; syncope may be common
Sinus tachycardia (more than 100 beats/min)	Gradual onset, if prolonged may be from cardiac disease and lead to cardiac failure
Sinus arrhythmia	Alternate changes in rate related to vagal tone
Wandering pacemaker	From shifting of pacemaker from S-A node to atria to A-V node; may be related to vagal tone
Premature contractions (impulses from any part of the heart evoking a beat)	May be from cardiac disease or drugs; importance and treatment depends on cause
Paroxysmal tachycardia (sudden rate increase because of ectopic pacemaker)	May be atrial, nodal, or ventricular; palpitations and heart failure may be observed; angina-like pain
Atrial flutter (rapid—200 to 300 beats/min)	Incomplete ventricular filling, ectopic atrial focus; syncope and weakness
Atrial fibrillation (rapid, irregular depolarization, 300 to 500 beats/min)	Decreased cardiac reserve; palpitations and thromboembolism
Ventricular fibrillation (rapid, uncoordinated beats, no pumping action)	Requires heroic defibrillatory treatment; sudden death
Pulse alternans (alterations in arterial pulse, small then large)	Requires diagnosis of various types of cardiac diseases

toles. Quinidine sulfate is the preferred oral dosage form, and quinidine gluconate is used for intravenous injections.[11]

Procainamide. Procainamide is a derivative of the local anesthetic procaine, having an amide group instead of the ester linkage. It is marketed as procainamide hydrochloride (Pronestyl Hydrochloride). The response of cardiac muscle to procainamide is similar to that of quinidine. It can be used for the same types of arrhythmias as quinidine and serves as a valuable agent that can be given during emergencies associated with ventricular arrhythmias. Like quinidine it is effective when given orally or intravenously. Intravenous doses must be given slowly to avoid toxic reactions such as alarming increases in ventricular rate and central nervous system reactions of convulsions and hyperexcitability. Deaths have been reported with improper use. Oral doses may provoke nausea and vomiting, and hypersensitivity reactions may be observed. Procainamide is contraindicated in patients with complete or incomplete A-V block.[12]

Other antiarrhythmic agents. There are a number of other drugs that are used in treating cardiac arrhythmias. Their action is discussed briefly here, since their basic pharmacology and uses have been described in more detail in other chapters of this book.

Lidocaine. Lidocaine hydrochloride is a local anesthetic that is useful in the treatment of ventricular premature beats and tachycardia. It finds its greatest use in those patients recovering from cardiac surgery or myocardial infarctions. Its principal advantage is its short duration of action and, reportedly, a reduction in the amount of hypotension occurring with other antiarrhythmic drugs. It is given intravenously in a single dose of 1 mg/kg up to 100 mg. The patient is then maintained with infusions of 1 to 3 mg/min as required. Toxic reactions ranging from drowsiness and dizziness to convulsions can occur. Lidocaine hydrochloride solutions used to treat arrhythmias should not be confused with the dental anesthetic solution, since these preparations contain no epinephrine and are buffered differently.[12]

Phenytoin. * Phenytoin (diphenylhydantoin, Dilantin) is a commonly used antiepileptic agent that has been studied in recent years as a possible antiarrhythmic agent. It works best in arrhythmias associated with the ventricles and particularly if the arrhythmia is induced by digitalis. Research claims indicate that this drug has an action unlike that of quinidine, procainamide, and lidocaine because it does not depress excitability or improve A-V conduction but depresses automaticity. Apparently, phenytoin exerts little effect on atrial arrhythmias, with the

---

*New name for diphenylhydantoin.

Table 19-3. Summary of the effects of antiarrhythmic drugs on the myocardium

Antiarrhythmic drug	Automaticity		Conduction velocity	Refractory period
	Atrium	Ventricle		
Quinidine	Decrease	Decrease	Decrease	Increase
Procainamide	Decrease	Decrease	Decrease	Increase
Lidocaine	No effect	Decrease	No effect	Decrease
Phenytoin	Decrease	Decrease	Increase	Decrease
Propranolol	Decrease	Decrease	Decrease	Decrease
Digitalis	Decrease	Slight increase	Decrease	Atrium—increase; ventricle— decrease

exception of paroxysmal atrial tachycardia associated with digitalis intoxication. Many clinicians believe that more studies are required before an adequate conclusion can be reached regarding its overall effectiveness. Toxic reactions associated with rapid intravenous injection of large doses of phenytoin include bradycardia, A-V nodal block, and ventricular standstill.[13]

Digitalis. The digitalis drugs, or cardiac glycosides as they are also known, are probably among the oldest of all drugs used in the treatment of cardiac disease. Although their principal use is related to the restoration of the failing heart in congestive heart disease, they are also employed in the treatment of atrial arrhythmias. Digitalis drugs reduce the automaticity of the atria and slow conduction through the A-V bundle, thereby reducing ventricular rate. Digitalis slows atrial flutter and fibrillation and terminates paroxysmal atrial tachycardia; however, the other antiarrhythmic agents quinidine, procainamide, and lidocaine must be used in combination with digitalis to produce the desired sinus rhythm. Dosages of digitalis for patients are based on individual requirements. There are numerous commercial forms of digitalis available, all of which have the same basic action on the myocardium.

Autonomic agents. Autonomic drugs do not occupy the same importance in the treatment of arrhythmias as do other drugs. The most commonly employed agent is a beta-blocking drug known as propranolol hydrochloride (Inderal). Its use is relatively new, and more clinical experience is required before definitive judgment can be made on its efficacy. Its primary usefulness is in the treatment of arrhythmias induced by digitalis or anesthetic agents. Although it has been used in almost every type of arrhythmic disorder, it is not suitable to use in arrhythmias induced by myocardial failure, bradycardia, or complete A-V block. Its basic action is more of reducing automaticity of an ectopic focus, and it slows A-V conduction.

Epinephrine and isoproterenol hydrochloride (Isuprel) are direct cardiac stimulants that increase automaticity and the force of contraction. Epinephrine can induce ventricular arrhythmias and angina pectoris when employed in the wrong cardiac disease. Isoproterenol is the drug of choice in complete heart block because it functions as a direct beta stimulant to the myocardium.

Anticholinergic drugs such as atropine are used to treat slow cardiac rates when ventricular pumping is so diminished as to cause serious hemodynamic changes. The action of atropine is that of reducing or blocking vagal slowing of the heart.[14]

A summary of the basic effects of the antiarrhythmic agents is given in Table 19-3.

ANTIANGINAL DRUGS

Angina pectoris is a common cardiovascular disease affecting a large segment of the population. It is characterized by pain or discomfort in the chest that frequently radiates to the left arm and shoulder. Pain may also be reported in the neck, back, and lower jaw. Lower jaw pain can be of such an intensity that it may be confused with a toothache. The cause of angina is related to a failure of the coronary arteries to supply a sufficient amount of oxygen to the myocardium on demand. It is easy to see why anginal pain can be precipitated by the stress induced by physical exercise. Emotional states that trigger catecholamine release, such as the anxiety and apprehension of a dental appointment, could also provoke episodes of angina in certain patients. Coronary atherosclerosis is associated with angina and, if sufficiently severe, may dictate coronary artery surgical bypass rather than drug therapy. The basic effects of drugs in relieving the pain of angina are based on the use of vasodilators to improve coronary blood flow and agents that reduce the work load on the myocardium, thereby lowering the oxygen requirements of the myocardium. The drugs normally employed for angina therapy are classified as follows[15]:

Nitrites
  Amyl nitrite
  Sodium nitrite
Nitrates
  Glyceryl trinitrate (nitroglycerin)
  Pentaerythritol tetranitrate (Duotrate, Peritrate)
  Isosorbide dinitrate (Isordil)
  Erythrityl tetranitrate (Cardilate)
Others
  Ethyl alcohol
  Xanthines
  Nicotinic acid
  Propranolol (Inderal)
  Dipyridamole (Persantine)
  Papaverine

Nitrites and nitrates

The nitrites and nitrates are really different chemical classes of drugs, but because of basic pharmacologic effects, they can be discussed collectively. Often there is no distinction made between these terms. These drugs relax vascular smooth muscle with variations in time of onset, potency, and duration of action. At one time these drugs were termed *coronary artery vasodilators*, and this was their presumed mechanism in the relief of angina. It is now recognized that they relax vascular smooth muscle throughout the body, reducing the work load (resistance) against which the heart has to pump. This would reduce the metabolic oxygen demand of the myocardium and hence bring about relief of pain.[16]

Because these drugs produce vascular relaxation, hypotension and fainting are common side effects. Headache is also reported, and tolerance develops with long-term use of these drugs. Methemoglobinemia occurs with the use of sodium nitrite, which is no longer employed in angina therapy.

Amyl nitrite. Amyl nitrite is a highly volatile substance administered by inhalation only. It is the most rapidly acting of the antianginal drugs, producing effects in a few seconds. It has no real advantages over nitroglycerin, and the odor is objectionable, especially in the closed atmosphere of a dental operatory. Because amyl nitrite is administered by inhalation, dosage regulation is variable and will affect the attending personnel as well as the patient. As a result, hypotension with fainting and headache is not uncommon. Amyl nitrite is packaged in thin glass ampules wrapped in gauze so that they may be easily and safely crushed with finger pressure.

Glyceryl trinitrate (nitroglycerin). Nitroglycerin is the most commonly employed drug and perhaps the drug of choice in angina therapy. It is administered sublingually and has a rapid onset of action. Its effects can last up to 30 minutes. An ointment form of nitroglycerin is also available for use, and when applied to the skin it is absorbed for a therapeutic effect. Nitroglycerin is usually given in doses that range from 0.2 to 0.6 mg. Although this is a useful drug to have in the dental emergency drug locker, most dentists will probably find that angina patients keep nitroglycerin readily available for use. The prophylactic use of nitroglycerin in preventing an anginal attack remains questionable.

Other nitrates. The other nitrates, isosorbide dinitrate and erythrityl tetranitrate, can also be given both orally and sublingually but are usually slower in their onset of action when compared with nitroglycerin. Pentaerythritol tetranitrate is a longer acting nitrate that has been promoted for the prophylactic prevention of anginal attacks. There is little evidence that this drug, or other similar long-acting nitrites, are really effective in the prevention of angina attacks. All of the nitrates are available under numerous trade names; only those more commonly known have been listed.[16]

Other antianginal agents

A large variety of other drugs from time to time have been used to treat the symptoms of angina. Most act to cause peripheral vasodilation or relax vascular smooth muscle (papaverine). Dipyridamole, although slow in onset, is reported to dilate coronary arteries without affecting peripheral vessels. The FDA has approved the use of propranolol, a beta-blocking agent, for use in angina.

Propranolol is said to decrease anginal pain through the mechanism of decreasing cardiac work and metabolic oxygen consumption. Only selected patients who do not respond to conventional therapy are candidates for this use of propranolol.[17]

ANTIHYPERTENSIVE AGENTS
Hypertension

Hypertension is apparently the most common of all cardiovascular diseases, affecting some 24 million Americans. It is a clinical finding related to a variety of complex causes and, if progressive, becomes a dangerous disease. Hypertension does not usually produce any outward symptoms until some damage has occurred to the heart, kidney, brain, or retina. Untreated hypertensive patients are more likely to have kidney disease, heart disease, and cerebrovascular accidents. Fortunately, early detection and treatment of hypertension with drug therapy reduce the possibilities of damage to vital organs and extend the lifetime of many patients.

Hypertensive disease is generally divided into at least three categories based on cause or progression of the disease. The first group includes approximately 90% of the diagnosed hypertensive patients who have essential or primary hypertension. The exact etiology is unknown in most of these cases. In the second group of approximately 10% of hypertensive patients, the cause can be associated with a specific disease process, such as medullary tumor. In this category the term *secondary hypertension* is used. The third group of hypertensive patients are those with malignant hypertension. Blood pressures are very high, and there is usually evidence of retinal and renal damage. Only a small number of patients are actually in this group, and some believe it to be a more severe progression of essential hypertension.[18]

Drug therapy is directed at the two most important factors that influence blood pressure, namely peripheral resistance and the vascular fluid volume. Active drug therapy usually begins as diastolic pressures range above 90 mm Hg. Initial therapy is normally begun with one of the thiazide diuretics and a weight reduction diet when obesity is present. Other drugs are added as the situation dictates. The exact combination of drugs eventually selected for a specific patient is determined by the response to the drugs in terms of reducing the hypertensive state as well as the complications of other disease processes. Anxiety states concurrent with hypertensive disease require the use of sedative types of drugs not directly related to vascular disease. It is not unusual in questioning dental patients about drug usage to discover that many of them may be taking five or six different drugs for their hypertension. Therefore it should be apparent that some basic knowledge of antihypertensive drugs is essential in evaluation of the hypertensive dental patient.

A large number of drugs are currently available for the treatment of hypertension. They will be presented in the following sequence: diuretics, neuronal blockers, centrally acting drugs, direct-acting vasodilators, ganglionic blockers, and finally, a miscellaneous category. Certain diuretics are included as antihypertensive drugs as well as agents to reduce edema associated with other cardiovascular diseases. It is also recognized that diuretics are useful in other disease entities where edema is a prominent feature.

Diuretics
Review of renal physiology

The basic role of the kidney is to filter metabolic products from the plasma and to control sodium, potassium, and hydrogen ions and body water within rather narrow limits. The nephron is the functional unit of the kidney consisting of a glomerular filtering membrane and the proximal tubule, loop of Henle, and the distal tubule across which ions are exchanged. The amount of sodium filtered is a function of the plasma concentration as well as the filtration pressure. The proximal tubule actively reabsorbs approximately 70% of the filtered sodium with chloride, water and bicarbonate accompanying the reabsorption. The ascending loop of Henle also reabsorbs a portion of the sodium ion remaining in the tubule but without the accompanying water. The distal tubule and the collecting ducts serve to make the final and critical adjustment of sodium ion reabsorption. Potassium and hydrogen ions are exchanged for sodium so that more sodium is reabsorbed for the body. Aldosterone, a hormone that increases sodium retention, has its effect on the distal tubule where final volume adjustments are made. A disease process that would tend to reduce the efficiency of the kidney to regulate ion exchange could lead to sodium retention and edema.[19]

Diuretics are an important group of drugs employed in the management of a variety of disorders in which edema is a prominent finding. Such disorders would include congestive heart failure, hypertension, cirrhosis of the liver, pregnancy, and some renal diseases. The basic effect of diuretic therapy is to increase the excretion of excess sodium ion, thereby reducing extracellular fluid accumulation. The reduction of blood volume is one means of reducing blood pressure. The most important class of diuretics in contemporary use are the thiazides. However, it must be emphasized that although the thiazides do reduce fluid volume by diuresis, their most important antihypertensive effect is the direct relaxation of vascular smooth muscle.

Thiazides

The thiazide diuretics (benzothiadiazides) are the most important category of drugs for use in hypertension. It is estimated that of the mild hypertensive patients, the condition of approximately 40% to 70% may be adequately managed with thiazides. This group of drugs evolved out of research designed to develop more potent diuretics of the carbonic anhydrase inhibitor type. They have a basic chemical resemblance to the sulfonamide type of drugs. The first thiazide diuretic marketed was chlorothiazide, and its success as a therapeutic agent stimulated the search and development of a large number of thiazide diuretics. Their principal pharmacologic effects are the same, differing from one another in potency and duration and onset of action. A number of thiazide diuretics and their single oral adult doses are listed in Table 19-4.

The mechanism of action of the thiazide diuretics at the cellular level is not established. However, the pharmacologic effects of diuresis and reduction of arterial blood pressure can be discussed. The diuretic effect occurs as a result of the inhibition of Na^+ reabsorption in the distal tubule. Chloride anion and water accompany the sodium ion resulting in an increased urine volume. The inhibition of sodium reabsorption in the distal tubule occurs at a site different from that of the K^+ and Na^+ exchange. Because of an increased amount of sodium available for exchange with potassium, more potassium is excreted than normal. For this reason aldosterone antagonists are sometimes combined with a thiazide to conserve potassium. The carbonic anhydrase–inhibiting properties of the thiazides are not important for diuresis.

The antihypertensive effect of the thiazides was not recognized until after their use as diuretics. This effect became evident in some hypertensive patients because a certain amount of edema recurred without an accompanying increase in blood pressure. Also, diazoxide, a thiazide without diuretic effects, was shown to lower blood pressure by a direct effect on arterial smooth muscle. Other studies have shown that thiazide diuretics can inhibit the vasopressor response of certain vasoconstrictors. Therefore the antihypertensive effect of the thiazides is related to a reduction of arterial blood pressure by a direct effect on the arteriole.

All of the thiazide diuretics are well absorbed when given orally. Chlorothiazide is the most slowly absorbed and rapidly excreted. Hydrochlorothiazide is more rapidly absorbed, as is polythiazide, and they are also longer acting than chlorothiazide. The onset of action of the orally administered drugs is approximately 1 hour, with a duration lasting up to 24 hours or longer. The intravenously administered thiazides have a short duration of action. They are concentrated in the kidney, which is also the major organ concerned with the excretion of these drugs. Intervals of doses and duration of action are determined, for the most part, by the excretion rates of the various thiazides.

Table 19-4. Thiazide diuretics and single oral doses for an antihypertensive effect

Thiazide diuretic	Usual oral adult dose
Chlorothiazide (Diuril)	500 mg
Hydrochlorothiazide (HydroDiuril, Esidrix, Oretic)	50 mg
Benzthiazide (Exna)	50 mg
Hydroflumethiazide (Saluron, Diucardin)	50 mg
Bendroflumethazide (Naturetin)	5 mg
Methyclothiazide (Enduron, Aquatensen)	5 mg
Trichlormethiazide (Naqua, Metahydrin)	4 mg
Cyclothiazide (Anhydron)	2 mg
Polythiazide (Renese)	2 mg

Adverse reactions associated with the thiazides are based on changes in plasma electrolytes. Their long-term use can lead to hypokalemia, and potassium chloride supplementation is often required to replace potassium ions. Hypokalemia can be of critical importance if thiazides and digitalis are combined, since lowered serum potassium increases the toxicity of digitalis. High doses of thiazides can produce anorexia with heartburn, which could be a source of confusion when they are combined with digitalis therapy because these toxic symptoms are similar for both drugs. Thiazides also increase uric acid retention, producing a hyperuricemia that can adversely affect the gout patient. Thiazide therapy can produce hyperglycemia in certain individuals, but the cause is largely unknown. Other adverse reactions such as hypersensitivity-induced skin rashes may be observed. The increased toxicity of digitalis, gastric irritation occurring with potassium chloride supplements, potentiation of other antihypertensive agents, and hyperglycemia in patients taking oral antidiabetic agents are the most important drug interactions associated with thiazide use.[20]

Diuretics with thiazide-like activity

Furosemide. Furosemide (Lasix) is a sulfonamide moiety–containing diuretic of high potency. Whereas some of its diuretic effects can be related to the inhibition of Na^+ reabsorption in the distal tubule, its principal site of action is on the ascending loop of Henle. The ascending loop of Henle functions in the countercurrent flow mechanism to conserve sodium and adjust the final urine concentration in the collecting tubules. Furosemide blocks this function, producing a rapid diuresis and dilute urine. It is such a potent diuretic that oral doses of 40 to 80 mg/24 hr are highly effective. In an emergency, doses of 20 mg are given by intravenous or intramuscular injection.

The thiazides are better day-to-day antihypertensive drugs, but furosemide also has antihypertensive properties similar to those of the thiazides. It, too, is employed as a single drug in hypertension, and like the thiazides it potentiates other antihypertensive drugs. Furosemide finds its greatest application in those edematous and hypertensive states that constitute an emergency situation. Adverse effects associated with

furosemide are associated with serum electrolyte imbalance.

Ethacrynic acid. Ethacrynic acid (Edecrin) is a diuretic with a potency like that of furosemide. It differs from the thiazides and furosemide chemically in that no sulfonamide moiety is in the structure. The major site and type of pharmacologic action are the same as those of furosemide with some effects on the proximal and distal tubular reabsorption mechanism. The principal indication for ethacrynic acid is severe edematous disease states, although there is some caution to be observed in patients with renal failure. Adverse effects resemble those for furosemide.

Chlorthalidone. Chlorthalidone (Hygroton) is a sulfonamide type diuretic chemically unrelated to the thiazides but possessing the same basic pharmacological effects. Quinethazone (Hydromox) and metolazone (Zaroxolyn) are other members of this type of diuretic. Uses and effects are similar to those of the thiazides.

Carbonic anhydrase inhibitors. The carbonic anhydrase inhibitors were used in combination with mercurial diuretics before the development of the thiazides. Their use has diminished, but they still have significant therapeutic value. The currently available drugs include acetazolamide (Diamox), ethoxzolamide (Cardrase), dichlorphenamide (Daranide), and methazolamide (Neptazane). Acetazolamide is the most frequently prescribed of this category. Like the thiazides, these drugs are structurally related to the sulfonamides.

The mechanism of action of these drugs is inhibition of the enzyme carbonic anhydrase. Carbonic anhydrase is the enzyme catalyzing the reaction of water and carbon dioxide to carbonic acid, illustrated as follows:

$$CO_2 + H_2O \xrightarrow[\text{anhydrase}]{\text{Carbonic}} H^+ + HCO_3^-$$

This reaction occurs in the distal tubule of the kidney and provides hydrogen ions that can be exchanged for sodium. This is another mechanism whereby the distal tubular segment of the nephron conserves sodium. As the carbonic anhydrase enzyme is inhibited, fewer hydrogen ions are available for exchange with sodium, and diuresis results. There is also an accompanying increase in potassium and bicarbonate loss. To minimize the loss of bicarbonate and the development of acidosis, the drugs are given on alternate days.

Adverse reactions to these diuretics are infrequent, but paresthesia of the face and extremities, drowsiness, and gastrointestinal effects have been known to occur. Because the drugs resemble the sulfonamides, a similar renal toxicity has been reported. Other adverse effects include hypersensitivity reactions and bone marrow depression.

The carbonic anhydrase inhibitors have been used to manage a variety of edematous states associated with cardiovascular diseases. However, they are not used specifically as antihypertensive agents. Acetazolamide is currently used to reduce fluid accumulation in glaucoma and has been tried in epilepsy.[21]

Potassium-conserving diuretics

There are a number of homeostatic mechanisms concerned with sodium ion regulation and volume of the circulatory system. One of the most important systems is that of the renin-angiotensin mechanisms. Renin is released from the kidney in response to a decrease in blood flow through the kidney. Renin catalyzes the conversion of angiotensinogen to angiotensin I. Another enzyme acts to convert angiotensin I to angiotensin II, which can then act directly on the kidney, increasing sodium retention or through an increase in peripheral resistance and elevation of blood pressure. Angiotensin II can also stimulate the adrenal cortex to produce aldosterone. Aldosterone increases sodium retention by the kidney, which in turn increases water retention and increases vascular fluid volume. This process results in a conservation of sodium at the expense of potassium. At least one theory on the etiology of hypertension is related to higher than normal levels of aldosterone.

Spironolactone. Spironolactone (Aldactone-A) is structurally similar to the hormone aldosterone and exerts its diuretic effect by a direct antagonism of aldosterone on the distal tubule. The net effect is an increase in sodium ion excretion and conservation of potassium. Since this action takes place at a location different from that associated with the thiazides, spironolactone can be combined with the thiazides to conserve potassium and prevent hypokalemia in hypertensive diseases associated with elevated aldo-

sterone plasma levels. A recent warning has appeared with the official package insert of a thiazide and spironolactone diuretic combination implicating spironolactone as a tumorigen in rats. Consequently, there are certain limitations to the indications for the use of this type therapy.[22]

Triamterene. Triamterene (Dyrenium) is also a potassium-sparing diuretic with a mechanism of action related to the blocking of aldosterone effects on the kidney. The general indications for its use are similar to those of aldosterone in supporting other diuretics in refractory cases of edema.

Other diuretics

There are many drugs with a diuretic effect that are used in the management of edema associated with cardiovascular disease. Among these agents are the mercurial diuretics, perhaps the oldest and most potent of all the diuretic agents. At one time these agents were the front line in diuretic therapy, but now only two clinically useful agents remain, chlormerodrin (Neohydrin) and mercaptomerin (Thiomerin). Mercaptomerin is administered by injection, and chlormerodrin is given orally. Side effects such as stomatitis, cardiac and renal toxicity, and gastric irritation and weakness as well as the use of the thiazides have now limited their application in clinical medicine. These drugs also reduced the reabsorption of sodium ion in the tubule.

Other diuretics include the osmotic nonelectrolytes mannitol, glucose, and urea. The diuretic effects of caffeine and theophylline are well known to tea and coffee consumers. The diuretic effects of digitalis are described in an earlier part of this chapter. The listing of other diuretics is included for completeness and to show that many agents are of value in the management of edema due to a wide variety of causes.[23]

Neuronal blockers—agents blocking norepinephrine release

Guanethidine. Guanethidine (Ismelin) is an antihypertensive agent that blocks the release of norepinephrine from adrenergic nerve terminals by a direct effect on the neuron. Consequently, norepinephrine is not released in response to adrenergic stimulation. Additionally, the amount of norepinephrine normally stored in synaptic vesicles is reduced. Both of these mechanisms reduce the amount of norepinephrine available to interact with the receptor site, resulting in a reduced sympathetic tone with a resultant decrease in blood pressure. Guanethidine has a rather long onset of action after oral doses (up to 3 days), and because guanethidine accumulates in the adrenergic nerve terminal, its effects are present for a long time (up to 2 weeks). The main indication for the use of guanethidine is in cases of resistant mild hypertension and severe hypertensive crisis. Patients taking guanethidine over a period of time tend to show sodium retention with edema. For this reason guanethidine is usually combined with a diuretic to minimize this response.

Patients taking guanethidine may show episodes of hypotension when making sudden positional changes, such as that encountered on arising from the dental chair. Other side effects include diarrhea, interference with ejaculation in men, and cardiac problems in patients with a marginal cardiac reserve. Muscle weakness may also be a complaint. A specific contraindication to the use of guanethidine is the presence of the adrenal medullary tumor pheochromocytoma. The action of guanethidine can be diminished by dextroamphetamine, chlorpromazine, and the tricyclic antidepressants. The effects of indirect-acting sympathomimetics are reduced in the presence of guanethidine. Cold remedies that contain direct-acting sympathomimetics in their formulation may produce a hypertensive episode as a result of increased sensitivity of the adrenergic receptor. Alcohol will potentiate the hypotensive effects of guanethidine.

Pargyline. The monoamine oxidase inhibitor (MAOI) pargyline has been observed to lower blood pressure in certain cases. The central effects of pargyline are related to the inhibition of norepinephrine metabolism and do not account for the paradoxical lowering of blood pressure. At least one theory on its antihypertensive effects is related to a guanethidine-like response in inhibiting nerve impulse–induced release of norepinephrine. Pargyline has a limited usefulness in hypertension because of the many adverse reactions and drug interactions associated with the MAOI type of drugs. Also, better antihypertensive drugs are available, but its use may be observed on occasion. The pharmacology of the MAOI drugs are discussed more fully in Chapter 7.[24]

Rauwolfia. The development of the rauwolfia alkaloids in therapy is something like that of digitalis, in that extracts of the *Rauwolfia serpentina* plant were used for years as a part of Hindu folk medicine. In the 1950s, rauwolfia was recognized as a tranquilizer and subsequently as a drug that would lower blood pressure in a hypertensive patient. The principal alkaloid of rauwolfia is reserpine (Serpasil). Other alkaloids of rauwolfia or rauwolfia preparations include deserpidine (Harmonyl), rescinnamine (Moderil), alseroxylon (Rauwiloid), which is a whole root extract, and a dried root preparation (Raudixin).

The mechanism of action of reserpine is one of depleting norepinephrine stores from the adrenergic nerve terminal. Its central effects include an effect on 5-hydrotryptamine in addition to depletion of norepinephrine stores. Like other drugs in this group its central effects are not related to its antihypertensive effects. Reserpine, like guanethidine, has a cumulative effect with a delayed onset of action and a prolonged duration. Reserpine is seldom useful as a single agent in controlling hypertension.

Adverse effects associated with the use of reserpine include diarrhea, bad dreams, sedation, and even psychic depression leading to suicidal tendencies. Reserpine causes an increase in gastric acid production, leading to gastrointestinal upset and aggravation of peptic ulcer if present. An additional and unexpected adverse effect in long-term users is a suspected increase in breast cancer as reported in 1974.[25] Reserpine will potentiate other depressant type of drugs, and an occasional extrapyramidal side effect may be observed.

Centrally acting agents

Methyldopa. Alpha-methyldopa (Aldomet) is a frequently encountered antihypertensive agent and, like guanethidine, is usually combined with a diuretic for more beneficial results. The manner in which methyldopa acts is still somewhat of a question. It has been related to an interference with norepinephrine formation and a neuronal blocking action like that of guanethidine. Currently, it is generally believed that methyldopa exerts an antihypertensive action by a central effect. In the synthesis pathway for norepinephrine, the enzyme dopa decarboxylase catalyzes the reaction of dopa to dopamine. Norepinephrine, the potent vasoconstrictor released from storage vesicles in the nerve ending, is then formed from dopamine. It appears that alpha-methyldopa is also a dopa decarboxylase substrate leading to the formation of alpha-methylnorepinephrine. Alpha-methylnorepinephrine is a much less effective neurotransmitter and replaces norepinephrine in the storage vesicles. In this way alpha-methylnorepinephrine behaves as a false transmitter substance. Dentists will recognize that the vasoconstrictor levonordefrin, used in local anesthetic preparations, is also known as alpha-methylnorepinephrine. Blood pressure is believed to be lowered by stimulation of alpha-adrenergic receptors that act to lower blood pressure centrally.

Methyldopa can be given by mouth or by intravenous injection with effects lasting up to 24 hours. The adverse effects are similar to those associated with other antihypertensive agents and would include postural hypotension, gastrointestinal upset, extrapyramidal tremors, vertigo, and psychic depression. Sedation is a common side effect. Excretory products of methyldopa can give a direct positive Coombs' test and interfere with the diagnosis of pheochromocytoma. Its use is contraindicated in patients with active liver disease. Methyldopa is useful in most hypertensive disease states and is of most benefit in those patients with renal damage.

Clonidine. Clonidine (Catapres) is one of the newer centrally acting antihypertensive agents. The site of action appears to be alpha-inhibitory receptors located in the medulla. The antihypertensive effect is dependent on the use of low doses, since high doses may cause an increase in blood pressure. It appears that central receptors are much more sensitive to the drug than peripheral receptors.

Adverse effects associated with the use of clonidine include dryness of the mouth, drowsiness, and sedation. Other effects resemble those of other antihypertensive agents.

Direct-acting vasodilators

Hydralazine. Hydralazine hydrochloride (Apresoline) exerts its antihypertensive effect by a direct action on arterioles, reducing peripheral resistance. A concurrent increase in cardiac rate and output is also observed. Hydralazine is usually given orally but can also be administered parenterally to hospitalized patients.

Hydralazine is a useful antihypertensive agent but appears to be more suitable when combined with other agents such as the thiazide diuretics reserpine and guanethidine. Indeed, it is not unusual to find patients taking such a combination. However, it does appear that the side effects produced by hydralazine limit its usefulness. Among these effects are cardiac arrhythmias, angina, headache, dizziness, and postural hypotension. A more serious effect is a toxic reaction with features similar to those of lupus erythematosus.

Other vasodilators. There are at least three other drugs that are thought to resemble hydralazine in terms of mechanism of action. These drugs are Guancydine and Minoxidil, both considered as investigative drugs as of this writing, and prazosin (Minipress). Prazosin is administered orally in smaller doses than hydralazine. Side effects associated with its use include syncope, dizziness, palpitation, and weakness; headache may also be a complaint. The exact role of these newer agents in hypertension will evolve with clinical experience.

Diazoxide. Diazoxide (Hyperstat) is a direct-acting dilator that has a rapid effect when given intravenously. Chemically it is a thiazide without the diuretic properties. It is intended for use only in hospitalized patients for emergency reduction of high blood pressure in malignant hypertension.

Sodium nitroprusside. Sodium nitroprusside (Nipride) is a rapidly acting antihypertensive agent that has a direct effect on vascular smooth muscle. Like diazoxide it is intended for use in hospitalized patients for the management of hypertensive emergencies. It is given by slow intravenous infusion.

Ganglionic blocking agents

The ganglionic blocking agents were among the first drugs used in the management of hypertensive disease. The currently available drugs for clinical use are mecamylamine (Inversine), pentolinium tartrate (Ansolysen), and trimethaphan (Arfonad). Three other drugs in this same class, but seldom if ever used today, include hexame-

Table 19-5. Sites of action of antihypertensive drugs

Antihypertensive drugs	Site of action
Direct-acting drugs	
Hydralazine (Apresoline)	Has direct effect on arteriole, producing dilation
Diazoxide (Hyperstat)	
Sodium nitroprusside (Nipride)	
Thiazide diuretics	
Prazosin (Minipress)	
Neuronal blockers	
Guanethidine (Ismelin)	Blocks sympathetic neuron and norepinephrine release
Reserpine (Serpasil)	
MAOI (pargyline)	
Centrally acting drugs	
Alpha-methyldopa (Aldomet)	Acts in the CNS to reduce sympathetic tone
Clonidine (Catapres)	
Ganglionic blockers	
Mecamylamine (Inversine)	Blocks sympathetic ganglia
Pentolinium tartrate (Ansolysen)	
Trimethaphan (Arfonad)	
Hexamethonium	
Adrenergic receptor blockers	
Propranolol (Inderal)	Beta receptor blocker
Phenoxybenzamine (Dibenzyline)	Alpha receptor blocker
Phentolamine (Regitine)	Alpha receptor blocker
Other antihypertensive	
Veratrum alkaloids	Sensitizes baroreceptor reflex—slowing of heart

thonium, chlorisondamine, and trimethidinium.

The mechanism of action and pharmacologic effects of these agents are similar and can be discussed as a group. The ganglionic blocking agents act at the ganglia formed by the synapse of preganglionic and postganglionic autonomic neurons. These drugs act at the receptor site for acetylcholine that is located on the postganglionic fiber and essentially block ganglionic transmission. Therefore the system response will be related to the predominant action of either the sympathetic or parasympathetic division. In the arterioles and veins, inhibition of sympathetic tone occurs with vasodilation and a reduction in blood pressure.

The blockade of parasympathetic effects accounts for most of the side effects of the ganglionic blocking drugs. They include tachycardia, xerostomia, and a decreased amount of sweating. Among the most serious adverse effects is postural hypotension that can lead to syncope, and a patient could demonstrate such an effect on standing after a long dental appointment. Other severe side effects include constipation, urinary retention, and paralytic ileus.

The use of these drugs has greatly diminished with the availability of more effective and less dangerous antihypertensive drugs. Mecamylamine and pentolinium are usually given orally to help support other drugs in hypertensive therapy. Trimethaphan is a very rapidly acting agent that is used intravenously for severe hypertensive episodes.[26]

Other antihypertensive agents

Although the aforementioned drugs are the most often employed in hypertensive diseases, two other groups should be included for completeness. The *Veratrum* alkaloids have an action of sensitizing the baroreceptor nerve endings to stretch. Thus, in response to elevated blood pressure, they would produce a reflex slowing of the heart. A summary of the antihypertensive drugs and their sites of action is found in Table 19-5.

Adrenergic receptor blocking agents

The adrenergic receptor blocking drugs can be divided into two distinct groups, depending on which receptor, alpha or beta, is blocked. The alpha receptor blocking drugs in this category include phenoxybenzamine

(Dibenzyline) and phentolamine (Regitine). Both have been used in the treatment and diagnosis of hypertension associated with pheochromocytoma. They act to block the effects of norepinephrine at the alpha receptor.

Although the beta-blocking agent propranolol (Inderal) is discussed near the end of the antihypertensive drugs, this by no means implies a lesser role in the management of hypertension. Indeed, experimental evidence on this use of propranolol has been accumulating for a number of years. It is used in combination with thiazides in a similar manner to other drug combinations used in hypertension. The mechanism whereby propranolol exerts its effect is believed to be related to a reduction in cardiac output. A second postulated mechanism is related to the inhibition of renin secretion, which may offer a means to control this form of secondary hypertension.

A number of adverse effects have been reported with propranolol, many of which are dose related. They include bradycardia, paresthesia of the hands, weakness, fatigue, gastrointestinal symptoms, and bronchospasm. Contraindications include bronchial asthma, allergic rhinitis, and cardiogenic shock and when a patient is taking MAOI–type drugs. Those patients requiring general anesthesia and at the same time receiving propranolol require the expert management of an anesthesiologist, since special problems are encountered with reflex cardiovascular function.[27]

ANTICOAGULANTS
Review of the clotting mechanism

Hemostasis is a defense mechanism designed to prevent the loss of blood from injury to a blood vessel. The leaking vessel is plugged by a complicated process of clot formation. The clotting mechanism is initiated when vascular injury releases a special tissue component known as thromboplastin. Thromboplastin in combination with factors V, VII, and X and calcium ions form the extrinsic prothrombin to thrombin and finally fibrinogen to fibrin. Fibrin, along with vascular spasm, platelets, and red blood cells, form the final clot rapidly.

As long as the blood vessel remains smooth and intact, circulating blood will not clot. However, should internal injury to the vessel occur and a roughened surface develop,

intravascular clotting will also occur. This process involves an intrinsic prothrombin activator consisting of a platelet factor, factors V and VIII through XII, and calcium ions. Once again the prothrombin activator is necessary for the conversion of prothrombin to thrombin. Thrombin enzymatically converts fibrinogen to fibrin, and thus there is clot formation. Intravascular clotting is a slower process, requiring several minutes for a clot to develop.

Many of the factors required in the clotting process are protein in nature and synthesized by normal metabolic processes. It is important to point out that factors VIII, IX, and X and prothrombin require vitamin K to be synthesized. Therefore one of the mechanisms of anticoagulant drug action involves interference with vitamin K. The preceding clotting processes have been greatly simplified.[28]

Usefulness of anticoagulants

Although the clotting processes just mentioned appear simple, the exact mechanism of intravascular clotting still remains a difficult problem area. Suffice it to say, however, that intravascular clots do occur because of vascular diseases or changes in the blood. These clots, or thrombi, tend to break loose, forming emboli that can lodge in smaller vessels to the major organs such as the heart, brain, or lungs, thereby producing severe and fatal thromboembolic diseases. Anticoagulant therapy provides a way in which the incidence of intravascular clotting may be reduced and may prevent life-threatening situations. However, one must keep in mind that anticoagulant therapy has to be adjusted to suit each patient's need. Constant supervision of the patient is required while the correct dosage and regimen for each situation is established. If the dose of anticoagulant is too large, hemorrhage may occur, or if the dose is too small, the danger of the embolism remains.

Drugs in current use

Heparin. Heparin is one of the most commonly employed anticoagulant agents. It is a mucopolysaccharide consisting of glucosamine and glucuronic acid units in alternate linkages. Heparin acts as an antithromboplastin, preventing the enzymatic conversion of prothrombin to thrombin. It is given by intramuscular, intravenous, or subcutaneous administration and has a brief but rapid duration of action. Because it can be administered intravenously, it can have an immediate effect on clot formation. Since it cannot be used orally, its use is limited to hospital situations, and it is expensive.

Adverse effects are associated with overdosage, leading to internal hemorrhage and an occasional hypersensitivity reaction. Commercial heparin is obtained from beef sources.[29]

Coumarins. The coumarins are a group of chemically related drugs having a common mechanism of action; they are also referred to as the oral anticoagulants. In contrast to heparin these agents are commonly given by the oral route, but because of absorption irregularities, dosage adjustment is complicated. These agents act as vitamin K antimetabolites, thereby interfering with the synthesis of factors VII, IX, and X and prothrombin. There is a delay in onset of action of these agents until the usual plasma stores of these clotting agents are depleted. These agents are generally employed in long-term therapy because they are less expensive and more convenient to use than heparin.

Adverse effects with these agents are mostly related to overdosage and hemorrhage. A more important consideration is the interaction of other drugs with the oral anticoagulants. Drugs that increase the effect of the coumarin anticoagulants include the antibiotics, phenylbutazone, and the salicylates. Phenobarbital may reduce their effectiveness by enzyme induction and hence destruction of the anticoagulant.[30]

The following is a list of the most commonly used, coumarin-like anticoagulants.

Ethyl biscoumacetate (Tromexan)
Bishydroxycoumarin (dicumarol)
Warfarin (Coumadin, Panwarfin)
Phenprocoumon (Liquamar, Marcumar)
Acenocoumarol (Sintrom)

Indandiones. The indandiones are a group of oral anticoagulants with an action similar to that of the coumarins. Medical use of the indandiones becomes a matter of judgment on the part of the physician as well as a consideration of side effects. Some of the indandione derivatives available for clinical use include diphenadione (Dipaxin), phenindione (Danilone, Hedulin), and anisindione (Miradon).

REFERENCES

1. Kolata, G. B., and Marx, J. L.: Epidemiology of heart disease: searches for causes, Science **194:**509-512, 1976.
2. Silber, E. N., and Katz, L. N.: Heart disease, New York, 1975, The Macmillan Co.
3. Huffman, D. H., and Azarnoff, D. L.: The use of digitalis, Ration. Drug Ther. vol. 8, no. 1, 1974.
4. Selzer, A.: Drug therapy. In Selzer, A.: Principles of clinical cardiology, Philadelphia, 1975, W. B. Saunders Co.
5. Revised digoxin dosage, FDA Drug Bull. **6:**31, Aug.-Oct., 1976.
6. Aviado, D. M.: The treatment of congestive heart failure. In Aviado, D. M., editor: Pharmacologic principles of medical practice, ed. 8, Baltimore, 1972, The Williams & Wilkins Co.
7. McCallum, C. A., and Harrison, J. B.: Pharmacological considerations in dental treatment for the patient with systemic disease, Dent. Clin. North Am. **14:**663-680, 1970.
8. Evaluations of drug interactions, ed. 2, Washington, D.C., 1976, The American Pharmaceutical Association.
9. Rushmer, R. F.: Cardiovascular dynamics, Philadelphia, 1970, W. B. Saunders Co.
10. Lyght, C. E., editor: The Merck manual, Rahway, N.J., 1968, Merck & Co., Inc.
11. Moe, G. K., and Abildskov, J. A.: Antiarrhythmic drugs. In Goodman, L. S., and Gilman, A. Z., editors: The pharmacological basis of therapeutics, ed. 5, New York, 1975, The Macmillan Co.
12. Melmon, K. L., and Morrelli, H. F., editors: Clinical pharmacology, New York, 1972, The Macmillan Co.
13. American Medical Association Council on Drugs: AMA drug evaluations—1973, Chicago, 1973, American Medical Association.
14. Hayes, A. H.: The action and clinical use of the newer antiarrhythmic drugs, Ration. Drug Ther. vol. 6, no. 7, 1972.
15. Parmley, W. W.: Therapy of angina pectoris, Ration. Drug Ther. vol. 9, no. 3, 1975.
16. Needleman, P.: Organic nitrate metabolism, Annu. Rev. Pharmacol. Toxicol. **16:**81-93, 1976.
17. FDA approves propranolol in angina pectoris, FDA Drug Bull. Jan., 1974.
18. Marx, J. L.: Hypertension: a complex disease with complex causes, Science **194:**821-825, 1976.
19. Pitts, R. F.: Physiology of the kidney and body fluids, Chicago, 1966, Year Book Medical Publishers, Inc.
20. Nies, A. S.: Cardiovascular disorders. I. Alteration of cardiac function without shock. In Melmon, K. L., and Morelli, H. F., editors: Clinical pharmacology, New York, 1972, The Macmillan Co.
21. Gantt, C. L.: Diuretic therapy, Ration. Drug Ther. vol. 6, no. 18, 1972.
22. New aldactone/aldactazide warning and revised indications, FDA Drug Bull. **6:**33, Aug.-Oct., 1976.
23. Mudge, G. H.: Diuretics and other agents employed in the mobilization of edema fluid. In Goodman, L. S., and Gilman, A., editors: The pharmacological basis of therapeutics, ed. 5, New York, 1975, The Macmillan Co.
24. Briggs, A. H., and Holland, W. C.: Antihypertensive drugs. In DiPalma, J. R., editor: Drill's phar-

macology in medicine, ed. 4, New York, 1971, McGraw-Hill Book Co.

25. Armstrong, B., Stevens, N., and Doll, R.: A retrospective study of the association between the use of Rauwolfia derivatives and breast cancer in English women, Lancet 2:672, 1974.

26. Bourne, H. R., and Melmon, K. L.: Guides to the pharmacologic management of essential hypertension, Ration. Drug Ther. vol. 5, no. 4, 1971.

27. Zacharias, F. J., Cowen, K. J., Prestt, J., et al.: Propranolol in hypertension: a study of long-term therapy, 1965-1970, Am. Heart J. **83:**755-761, 1972.

28. Guyton, A. C.: Textbook of medical physiology, Philadelphia, 1966, W. B. Saunders Co.

29. Modell, W., editor: Drugs of choice, 1976-1977, St. Louis, 1976, The C. V. Mosby Co.

30. Martin, E. W., editor: Hazards of medication, Philadelphia, 1971, J. B. Lippincott Co.

20
Antimicrobial agents

SAM V. HOLROYD

BARBARA REQUA-GEORGE

The control of infection represents one of the most important aspects of pharmacotherapeutics. Oral infections can spread rapidly and undoubtedly account for the majority of severe illnesses and fatalities that occur in the practice of dentistry. The *prevention* of postoperative dental infections requires proper attention to surgical and aseptic technique. The *treatment* of dental infections requires a complete awareness of the patient's medical history, an understanding of the fundamentals of infection, and a knowledge of the pharmacology of available drugs. Before discussing the individual antimicrobial agents, certain terms will be defined:

antibiotic agents Chemical substances produced by microorganisms that have the capacity, in dilute solutions, to produce antimicrobial action.

antimicrobial agents Substances that kill or suppress the growth or multiplication of microorganisms. Antimicrobial agents may be antibacterial, antiviral, or antifungal.

antibacterial agents Substances that destroy or suppress the growth or multiplication of bacteria. They are classed as antibiotic or synthetic agents.

Some clinically oriented information relating to infection needs to be briefly reviewed next.

INFECTION

Infection has been defined as "invasion of the body by pathogenic microorganisms and the reaction of the tissues to their presence and to the toxins generated by them."[1] One must remember that the simple presence of a pathogen does not constitute "invasion." The oral cavity and in fact the entire gastrointestinal tract, respiratory tract, and skin

are all inhabited by microorganisms, many of which are potentially pathogenic. The manifestation of infection as a disease state presupposes that the pathogen obtains an environment suitable for its growth and multiplication. The principal factors that determine the likelihood of a microorganism causing an infection are (1) virulence of the microorganism, (2) number of organisms present, and (3) resistance of the host. Host resistance should be considered as having both local and systemic components. Locally, tissue trauma, inadequate wound closure, and lack of blood clot retention are important. Systemically, one is confronted with a number of conditions that decrease resistance to infection. These predisposing conditions occur in patients with diabetes, leukemia, Addison's disease, immunoglobulin deficiencies, malnutrition, agranulocytosis, and various other blood dyscrasias. Alcoholics, patients who have been taking adrenal steroids, immunosuppressive or cytotoxic drugs, and those debilitated for any reason also have a decreased resistance to infection.

A wide variety of microorganisms may cause infections of the oral structures. An excellent and condensed description of the normal oral flora, virulence and resistance factors, and the organisms involved in dental infections is presented by Burnett.[2] He concludes that most dental infections are caused by streptococci and staphylococci and will respond to antimicrobial agents with a predominately gram-positive spectrum. It is important to note that since the advent of penicillin the percentage of dental infections caused by staphylococci, particularly the penicillinase-producing staphylococci, has been increasing. There is also evidence that an increasing percentage of oral infections are being caused by gram-negative organ-

☐ The opinions or assertions contained herein are the private ones of the writers and are not to be construed as official or as reflecting the views of the Navy Department or the naval service at large.

isms.[3] With this in mind the selection of the proper antibiotic cannot be made arbitrarily.

INDICATIONS FOR ANTIMICROBIAL AGENTS

Considerable indecision exists relative to determining a need for antimicrobial agents. Although it is not within the scope or intent of this text to discuss indications in detail, some generalizations should be stated.

Therapeutic indications

All infections do not require antimicrobial therapy. Unfortunately, there is no simple rule that can be employed to give an immediate yes or no answer in regard to the need for therapy. The basic question is "Does this particular patient need the assistance of antimicrobial agents to resolve this particular infection?" The decision to use or not to use can be made only after considering all those factors that would tend to indicate a need against those which tend to obviate a need. The following should be evaluated:

1. *The patient.* One should never lose sight of the fact that the best defenses against pathogens are host responses. Properly functioning defense mechanisms in the healthy patient are of primary importance. The lack of these defenses, which may occur in conditions previously mentioned, must receive close attention. The presence or absence of systemic manifestations such as fever, malaise, and lymphadenopathy are indicators of how well the patient is doing without antimicrobial therapy.

2. *The infection.* The virulence and invasiveness of the etiologic microorganism are important in determining the acuteness, severity and spreading tendency of the infection. Obviously, the acute, severe, rapidly spreading infection should generally be treated with antimicrobial agents. At the other end of the spectrum is the mild localized infection where drainage can be established. Most cases lie somewhere between these extremes. In these cases the decision can only be based on the clinician's capability to balance the patient's need for pharmacologic assistance against the potential toxicity of an antimicrobial agent.

Prophylactic indications

A definite indication for prophylactic antibiotic coverage exists when patients with rheumatic or congenital heart disease or those with heart prostheses are to undergo procedures that may precipitate a bacteremia. This prophylaxis is against bacterial endocarditis and is discussed in more detail in Appendix C. Other prophylactic uses of antimicrobial agents in dental practice are not so definitive. In fact, some studies question the validity of antibiotic coverage in the prevention of bacterial endocarditis.[4] Although some clinicians suggest antibiotic prophylaxis for patients with total hip replacements,[5] coronary bypass operations, and Teflon implants, the value of treatment in these situations is not clear. In one specialized situation, the compound mandibular fracture,[6] the use of prophylactic antimicrobial agents decreased the rate of infection. Some clinicians employ antibiotic coverage for surgical patients in an attempt to avert postsurgical infection, enhance the surgical results, and reduce postoperative discomfort. This philosophy has been discussed in some detail[7] and can be summarized as follows: Although parallel dental studies are not available, the failure of prophylactic antibiotic coverage to prevent postsurgical infections is well documented in the medical literature.[8-21] The following analysis relating to periodontics pertains.

Most patients who undergo periodontal surgery are not going to develop a postoperative infection. Infections that do evolve might have been prevented by prophylactic antibiotics if the invading organism was susceptible to the particular drug selected. It is apparent from medical studies that some individuals who would not have developed a postoperative infection may do so if prophylactic antibiotics *are* used. The mechanism of this may be related to alterations in the normal flora which were induced by the antibiotic. Thus, in the final analysis, one must balance the infections he *prevents* with antibiotics against the infections he *causes* with antibiotics. If the medical literature on this subject accurately reflects the situation in periodontal surgery, the gains and losses in using antibiotics to prevent postsurgical infection are approximately equal. One's capacity to gain more than he loses from using antibiotics to prevent postsurgical infections is likely to be proportional to his ability to predict the likelihood of a postoperative infection in a particular case.[7]

Although there is some indication that prophylactic antibiotics may enhance healing[22-24] and reduce postoperative discomfort,[25] this area of antibiotic use is strictly speculative at the present time. Such use is not recommended.

BACTERICIDAL AS OPPOSED TO BACTERIOSTATIC ANTIMICROBIAL AGENTS

The following discussion of antimicrobial drugs refers to the various agents as being bactericidal or bacteriostatic. It is of clinical importance that one is familiar with this distinction. *Bactericidal* drugs kill bacteria; *bacteriostatic* drugs retard the growth of bacteria, leaving final elimination to body defense mechanisms. It is apparent that bacteriostatic agents are relatively ineffective in the patient whose defense mechanisms are severely impaired. Drugs that may be only bacteriostatic at low concentrations against some microorganisms, may be bactericidal at higher concentrations against the same or other microorganisms. Thus the labeling of a drug as bactericidal or bacteriostatic is far from absolute.

ANTIBIOTIC SENSITIVITY TESTS

Ideally, all infections requiring antibiotic therapy would be cultured and antibiotic sensitivity tests conducted. This is the only way in which you can ensure that a particular drug will kill or inhibit the growth of an infecting microorganism. These in vitro tests will not illustrate relative in vivo potency of the drugs or will they differentiate between bactericidal and bacteriostatic effects. They will only show which drugs adversely affect the growth of the microorganisms on the culture plate. This can generally be accepted as evidence that they will or will not adversely affect the microorganisms in vivo.

In most dental infections, antibiotic therapy is started before the results of sensitivity tests are available. Although test results can usually be obtained in 12 to 24 hours, even this delay in starting antibiotics against a severe infection could be detrimental to the patient. The advantage of sensitivity tests in these cases is that if the drug selected is not effective against the etiologic agent, an early correction in therapy is possible. Also, the severe infection, which does not respond to the antibiotic chosen, will be more difficult to identify if cultured only after a therapeutic failure.

SUPERINFECTION

Superinfection (also called suprainfection) is caused by the proliferation of microorganisms that are different from those causing the original infection. Antibiotics are not so specific that they "hit" only the offending pathogen. Consequently, the normal flora is altered and microbial equilibriums are disrupted. This predisposes to the emergence of organisms that are not affected by the antibiotic being used. For instance, the use of penicillin to combat a sensitive type of streptococcus may alter the bacterial flora, allowing insensitive (*Pseudomonas aeruginosa*) or resistant (penicillinase-producing staphylococci) organisms to produce a concurrent infection. More frequently, superinfection is caused by broad-spectrum drugs such as the tetracyclines. The emerging pathogen in these cases is often the fungus *Candida albicans*. The pathogenic organism emerging in a superinfection is usually more difficult to eradicate than the original organism being treated. The fact that the clinician can *cause* as well as *eliminate* infections with antibiotics emphasizes the importance of determining a definite *need* prior to the use of these drugs.

DURATION OF DOSAGE

An antimicrobial agent should be continued long enough to prohibit a regrowth of the causative microbe but not so long as to induce toxic drug symptoms or alter the normal flora to the extent that superinfection results. It is generally conceded that the administration of antimicrobial drugs should continue for 48 hours after the symptoms of infection are absent. If beta-hemolytic streptococci are the causative organisms, antibiotic therapy, usually penicillin in this case, should be continued for at least 10 days. Antimicrobial therapy for osteomyelitis should be continued for at least 14 days after fever and tenderness are absent and drainage has ceased.[26] In patients with a depressed immune system or history of prolonged healing, antibiotic coverage usually needs to be continued longer than in the normal patient.[27]

BEGINNING OF SYSTEMIC ANTIMICROBIAL THERAPY

In 1932, Gerhard Domagk observed in Germany that the azo dye Prontosil protected mice against infection by streptococci. This milestone in medical history led to the development of the sulfonamides and marked the beginning of systemic antimicrobial therapy.

In 1940, Chain, Florey, and co-workers (England) made the following observation: "In recent years interest in chemotherapeutic effects has been almost exclusively focused on the sulfonamides and their derivatives. There are, however, other possibilities, notably those connected with naturally occurring substances."[28] Fleming (England) in 1928 observed that a mold produced a naturally occurring substance which inhibited the growth of certain bacteria.[29] He had named this substance "penicillin" and suggested that it might be useful for the application to infected wounds. In their classic paper Chain, Florey, and co-workers reported in vivo animal studies that indicated the low toxicity and systemic antibacterial effectiveness of penicillin.[28] The excitement that had begun with the sulfonamides was being transferred to the "antibiotics." Today, as each new "therapeutic advancement in the treatment of infection" (antibiotic) is marketed, this excitement is again transferred.

DRUGS AVAILABLE

As noted earlier, antimicrobial agents may be antibacterial, antifungal, or antiviral. Agents effective against bacteria may be either antibiotics or synthetic antibacterials, such as the sulfonamides, which are not antibiotics in the true sense of the definition. The following drugs are considered in this chapter; more detailed descriptions are given those drugs of greater importance in the practice of dentistry:

Antibiotics effective primarily against gram-positive organisms
  Penicillins
  Erythromycin
  Cephalosporins
  Lincomycin
  Clindamycin
Broad-spectrum antibiotics
  Tetracyclines
  Chloramphenicol
Aminoglycoside antibiotics
  Neomycin
  Streptomycin

Kanamycin
Gentamicin
Tobramycin
Amikacin
Other antibiotics
  Vancomycin
  Spectinomycin
  Novobiocin
  Colistin
Topical antibiotics
  Bacitracin
  Polymyxin B
  Neomycin
Antifungal agents
  Nystatin
  Amphotericin B

Candicidin
Griseofulvin
Flucytosine
Synthetic antibacterial agents
  Sulfonamides
  Trimethoprim-sulfamethoxazole
Urinary tract antiseptics
  Methenamine
  Nitrofurantoin
  Nalidixic acid

Agents used in the treatment of tuberculosis
  Isoniazid
  Ethambutol
  Streptomycin
  Aminosalicylic acid
  Rifampin
Antiviral agents
  Idoxuridine
  Amantadine

ANTIBIOTICS EFFECTIVE PRIMARILY AGAINST GRAM-POSITIVE ORGANISMS
Penicillins

All penicillins can be divided into three main groups. The first group contains the penicillin G salts and penicillin V; the second group includes the penicillinase-resistant penicillins; and the third group encompasses the wider or broader spectrum penicillins. The penicillins have many properties in common and will be discussed together.

Source and chemistry. The naturally occurring penicillins are produced by the mold *Penicillium notatum* and related species. The semisynthetic penicillins are produced by chemical alteration of naturally produced precursors. All penicillins contain the nucleus 6-aminopenicillanic acid, which by itself has little antibacterial activity.

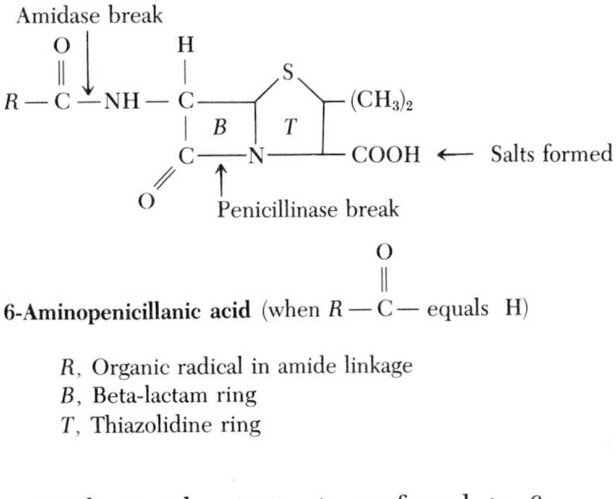

6-Aminopenicillanic acid (when $R - C -$ equals H)

R, Organic radical in amide linkage
B, Beta-lactam ring
T, Thiazolidine ring

Antibacterial activity is conferred to 6-aminopenicillanic acid by the addition of organic groups at R. This addition distinguishes the various penicillins. Penicillin is inactivated by any reaction that removes the R group or, as in the case of penicillinase, that breaks the beta-lactam ring. Salts of penicillin are formed by reactions at the thiazolidine carboxyl group.

Of the naturally occurring penicillins (G, K, O, X, F, and dehydro-F), only penicillin G (benzylpenicillin), which was the original compound, is of particular clinical importance. As the name implies, the R substitution is a benzyl group. Penicillin G is widely used as the potassium, procaine, and benzathine salts, which vary in duration of action. Other R substitutions have produced the semisynthetics: penicillin V (phenoxymethyl penicillin) and phenethicillin (phenoxyethyl penicillin), which are more stable in gastric acid than is penicillin G; methicillin, oxacillin, nafcillin, cloxacillin, and dicloxacillin, which are penicillinase resistant; ampicillin, hetacillin, and amoxicillin, which have a broader spectrum than other penicillins; and carbenicillin, which is uniquely effective against *Pseudomonas aeruginosa*. Additional differences between penicillin G and the semisynthetic drugs will be presented later.

Administration and body handling. Penicillin is administered by all the usual routes. However, because of its great allergenicity, penicillin should *not* be used topically. The Council on Dental Therapeutics of the American Dental Association has classified the following as unacceptable preparations: penicillin troches, lozenges, ointments, pastes, topical powders, and dental cones.[53]

Penicillin is most frequently administered orally. When administered orally, about 30% of penicillin G is absorbed under favorable conditions. Penicillin V is often substituted for penicillin G when oral administration is desired because with an equal oral dose the penicillin V achieves plasma concentrations two to five times greater than those achieved by penicillin G, and there is less interference from food. Both preparations achieve peak blood levels in less than 60 minutes and are excreted with a half-life of about 30 minutes. The oral route provides the advantages of convenience and a lessened likelihood of life-threatening allergic reactions. However, there are certain limitations when compared with parenteral use: (1) blood levels are more slowly obtained; (2) variations in gastric breakdown and absorption by the small intestine make blood levels less predictable; and (3) failure of the patient to follow instruc-

tions may result in inadequate blood levels. Since penicillin is broken down in gastric fluid, it is best administered 1 hour before or 2 hours after meals. The parenteral route should be used in the more serious infections in which penicillin is indicated and in those cases where patient cooperation is questionable. In prophylaxis against bacterial endocarditis for patients with rheumatic or congenital heart disease, the parenteral route is also preferred. Certain acid-labile penicillins, such as methicillin and carbenicillin, can only be administered parenterally.

After absorption, penicillin becomes distributed throughout the body, but ordinarily penetration is relatively poor into the central nervous system, bone, and the synovial, pleural, and pericardial fluids. Penicillin penetrates blood clots but does not permeate pus to any significant extent.[27,29] It crosses the placental barrier, but little appears to be excreted in saliva.

Although penicillin is metabolized by the liver, the rapid decline of a blood level results from rapid renal clearance. Penicillin is actively secreted by the renal tubules. In renal disease, high blood levels may result from failure to excrete the drug.

Antibacterial activity and spectrum. Penicillin is a highly potent bactericidal agent but may only be bacteriostatic at low blood levels. It acts by interfering with the synthesis of the bacterial cell wall. It not only inhibits the formation of cross linkages in the cell wall but also inhibits cellular enzymes with mucopeptide hydrolase activity. Consequently, rapidly multiplying bacteria are the most vulnerable. Its relatively narrow antibacterial spectrum includes most gram-positive cocci (streptococci, staphylococci, pneumococci), spirochetes, actinomycetes, and certain gram-negative cocci such as *Neisseria gonorrhoeae* and *N. meningitidis*. Ampicillin and carbenicillin have broader spectra, which include additional gram-negative bacteria. Bacterial resistance to penicillin develops quickly and frequently.

The antibacterial activity of penicillin preparations is standardized as international units. One unit has the activity of 0.6 μg penicillin G (1 mg penicillin G equals 1667 units). Thus 125, 250, and 500 mg contain approximately 200,000, 400,000 and 800,000 units, respectively.

Adverse reactions. Penicillin has an almost nonexistent toxicity, and extremely large doses of penicillin G have been tolerated without adverse effects. However, massive intravenous doses have been reported to cause a depression of consciousness and myoclonic jerking movements,[30,31] which are a manifestation of its direct central nervous system irritation. Very large doses of penicillin G have been associated with renal damage,[32,33] manifesting as fever, eosinophilia, rashes, albuminuria, and a rise in blood urea nitrogen (BUN). A penicillin-induced hemolytic anemia has also been reported.[34,35] Hematuria, proteinuria, and depression of red bone marrow have been associated with methicillin, and cholestatic hepatitis has followed the use of oxacillin.[36] It is generally acknowledged that the penicillinase-resistant penicillins are significantly more toxic than penicillin G.

Allergic reactions present the greatest danger in penicillin therapy. These reactions may be (1) mild and strictly dermatologic in nature, (2) a delayed serum sickness response, or (3) a severe and immediate anaphylactic reaction. The allergic potentiality should be vividly in the mind of the clinician each time he writes a prescription for or administers penicillin. It has been estimated that 2.5 million people in the United States are allergic to penicillin[37] and that reactions may occur in 5% to 10% of those people receiving it.[38] In 1966 a hospital survey showed allergic reactions in 7.8% of patients receiving penicillin.[39] Since the mechanism of penicillin allergy is complex, testing for the presence of an allergy is also difficult. Penicillin derivatives or breakdown products of the penicillin molecule act as haptens and combine with body proteins to form an antigen. The most important breakdown product is the penicilloyl derivative. Since it readily combines with body proteins, it is called the "major antigenic determinant"[40]; other products are called "minor antigenic determinants." For skin testing procedures the major antigenic determinant is combined with polymerized lysine, forming penicilloyl polylysine (PPL). The reliability of skin testing is increased by combining PPL with a minor determinant mixture. The testing of patients for penicillin allergy can cause an anaphylactic reaction so that it is recommended that testing only be done by trained people in a situation where emergency equipment is immediately available. In one study only 21% of those with a clinical allergic reaction had a positive PPL skin test, and all showed a negative skin test to penicillin G. This demonstrates that these skin tests are not yet completely reliable. It is important to note that patients with other allergies are more likely to be allergic to penicillin.

Not only is the incidence of allergic reactions to penicillin high but the consequences are often serious. It has been estimated that the anaphylactic reaction occurs in between 0.004% and 0.04% of penicillin-treated patients,[41,42] with mortality approaching 10%.[43]

Welch and associates[44] found that about 9% of the severe reactions that they surveyed were fatal. A projection of statistics[45] from the work of Welch[46] indicates that from 100 to 300 deaths probably occur annually in the United States from allergic reactions to penicillin. There is also evidence that some patients who survive severe reactions suffer permanent brain damage from the anoxia of the attack.[47] Although the chance of a serious allergic reaction to penicillin is greater after parenteral administration, anaphylactic shock and deaths after oral use have also been reported.[48-53]

The practitioner should always keep in mind that minor allergic reactions to penicillin after one exposure may be followed by more severe reactions on subsequent exposures. Any history of allergic symptoms to penicillin is sufficient contraindication to its use, and another drug should be employed. However, a negative history is no guarantee that penicillin allergy does not exist.

Uses. Penicillin is the most important antibiotic in medical and dental practice. Its importance results from its great bactericidal potency against many microorganisms that cause serious infections in humans. Penicillin is particularly valuable in life-threatening infections because its almost complete lack of toxicity allows massive blood levels to be used.

Penicillin is effective against most dental infections. It is the drug of choice in the prophylaxis of patients with a past history of bacterial endocarditis, rheumatic fever, or valvular heart disease without penicillin allergy (Appendix C). In view of penicillin's special value in serious infections, its great allergenicity, and the frequency with which bacterial resistance develops, it should be *selected* on the basis of a *clearly* established need and not automatically accepted as the drug of choice. *Accepted Dental Therapeutics 1975* states: "The systemic use of penicillin is indicated in severe infections that are caused by penicillin-sensitive organisms."[53] When the infecting agent is resistant to penicillin, other antibiotics *must* be considered; and where a potent bactericidal agent is not required, other antibiotics *may* be considered.[54]

Preparations and dosages

Na and K penicillin G. Sodium and potassium penicillin G are available in crystalline form for IM and IV use. When used parenterally, peak blood levels are rapidly obtained and rapidly lost. The usual adult IM dose of Na or K penicillin G is 300,000 to 600,000 units every 3 to 4 hours. Much higher doses and the IV route have been used in more severe infections. The sodium and potassium salts have identical antibacterial activity. The sodium salt, in very high doses, can be detrimental to cardiac patients taking low-sodium diets, whereas the potassium salt can cause hyperkalemia in patients with renal failure.

Oral preparations of buffered K penicillin G are commonly used for convenience in cases where high blood levels of a predictable nature are not required. Preparations and dosages are shown in Table 20-1.

Procaine penicillin G. Procaine penicillin G is released more slowly from the injection site than is the potassium salt because of its decreased solubility. Blood levels obtained with the procaine salt are lower and more slowly attained and have a longer duration than the levels that would result from an equal dose of the potassium salt. The usual adult IM dose of procaine penicillin G is 300,000 U/12 hr or 600,000 U/24 hr. It is not used orally.

Procaine penicillin G is available in suspensions for IM use as 300,000, 500,000, and 600,000 U/ml (Crysticillin, Duracillin, Pentid-P, Wycillin). It is also available in combination with benzathine penicillin for deep IM injections as 150,000 or 300,000 U/ml (Bicillin C-R).

Benzathine penicillin G. Benzathine penicillin G is released more slowly from the in-

Table 20-1. Oral preparations and dosages of penicillin G and V and phenethicillin

Drug	Preparations
K penicillin G (Kesso-Pen, Pentids, Pfizerpen G, Sugracillin)	Tablets: 125, 150, 250, and 500 mg Oral liquids: 75, 125, 150, and 250 mg/5 ml
Penicillin V (Compocillin V, Pen-Vee, V-Cillin)	Chewable tablets: 125 and 250 mg Oral liquid: 180 mg/5 ml
K Penicillin V (Betapen-VK, Compocillin-VK, Ledercillin VK, Penapar VK, Pen-Vee K, Pfizerpen VK, Robicillin VK, Uticillin VK, V-Cillin K, Veetids)	Tablets: 125, 250, 500 mg Oral liquids: 125 and 250 mg/5 ml Drops: 125 mg/2.5 ml dropperful
K phenethicillin (Syncillin)	Tablets: 125 and 250 mg Oral liquid: 125 mg/5 ml

DOSAGE: The oral dosage of penicillin G and V and phenethicillin should be determined according to the sensitivity of the etiologic microorganism and the severity of the infection and should be adjusted according to the clinical response of the patient. The usual dose for adults and children over 12 years of age for oral infection is 250 to 500 mg (400,000 to 800,000 units) every 6 to 8 hours. The dose for children under 12 years should be calculated according to weight or body surface area. The recommended dosage for infants and small children is 25,000 to 90,000 U/kg/24 hr in three to six divided doses.

jection site than is the procaine salt. The blood levels obtained are lower, more slowly attained, and maintained longer than the levels that would result from an equal dose of the procaine salt. Benzathine penicillin G would be used when low penicillin blood levels are acceptable but are required over a relatively long duration. This dosage form is often used for long-term prophylaxis of rheumatic heart disease. It is not recommended for prophylaxis during dental procedures. The usual adult dose of benzathine penicillin G is 900,000 to 1,200,000 units IM. This dose provides blood concentrations that are effective in some cases for up to 10 days, and detectable blood levels may be observed for up to 30 days.

Benzathine penicillin G is available in suspension for deep IM use as 300,000 or 600,000 U/ml (Bicillin, Permapen) and in combination with procaine penicillin G (Bicillin C-R).

Penicillin V and phenethicillin. Penicillin V and phenethicillin are available for oral use, and they produce higher blood levels than equal amounts of penicillin G given orally. Neither penicillin V nor phenethicillin has proved to be of greater therapeutic value than penicillin G given in higher dosages.[55] The potassium salt of penicillin V is more soluble than the free acid and therefore gives somewhat better absorption. Preparations and dosages are shown in Table 20-1.

Penicillinase-resistant penicillins. The following drugs are semisynthetic penicillins that are penicillinase resistant:

Methicillin (Staphcillin)
Oxacillin (Prostaphlin)
Nafcillin (Unipen)
Cloxacillin (Tegopen)
Dicloxacillin (Dynapen, Pathocil, Veracillin)
Flucloxacillin

These drugs should be reserved for use only against sensitive staphylococci known to be resistant to penicillin G. Compared to penicillin G, they are less effective against nonpenicillinase-producing microbes, are more toxic, and cause more side effects. Principal adverse effects include mild and serious allergic reactions, gastrointestinal upset, infrequent and usually transient bone marrow depression, and some signs of abnormal renal and hepatic function. Safety for their use in pregnancy has not been established. Patients allergic to penicillin G are extremely likely to be allergic to these drugs.

Since methicillin is acid labile, it cannot be used orally. If an oral preparation is needed, oxacillin, cloxacillin, or dicloxacillin can be administered. Both cloxacillin and dicloxacillin are better absorbed than oxacillin. Flucloxacillin, not yet available in the United States, may supercede the other agents for oral administration of a penicillinase-resistant penicillin.[56] Because of the infrequency with which the penicillinase-resistant penicillins are used in dentistry, their preparations and dosages are not presented.

Wider spectrum penicillins. Ampicillin, hetacillin, and amoxicillin are the three penicillins with a broader spectrum of activity. Carbenicillin also has a broader spectrum of action but includes specificity for *Pseudomonas*.

AMPICILLIN. Ampicillin (Alpen, Amcill, Omnipen, Penbritin, Polycillin, Principen, Supen, Totacillin) has a slightly broader spectrum of activity than penicillin G. It is not penicillinase resistant. Its spectrum includes some gram-negative organisms, but it should not be considered a broad-spectrum drug. Safety for the use of ampicillin in pregnancy has not been established. Adverse reactions are the same as for the penicillinase-resistant semisynthetics.

Ampicillin has one unusual property that makes it different from other penicillins. It tends to cause rashes with a greater degree of frequency (7.7% compared with 2.7% with other penicillins),[57] and their incidence may also be dose related.[58-60] It appears that these rashes are specific for ampicillin and do not indicate a true penicillin hypersensitivity,[61] and in fact they may be toxic in nature.[58,60] It has also been noted that patients with glandular fever have an extremely high percentage (95%) of rashes if given ampicillin.[62,63] The occurrence of this ampicillin-related rash is now not considered to be a contraindication to future treatment with the penicillins.[60] As with all penicillins, the major adverse reaction is its allergenicity. Patients who are allergic to other penicillins are likely to be allergic to ampicillin also. Since there is some evidence that an increasing number of dental infections are caused by gram-negative microbes, ampicillin may have occasional use in dental practice. It should not be used as a substitute for penicillin G unless sensitivity tests indicate a need.

Ampicillin is available for parenteral use and also in the following oral preparations: capsules of 250 and 500 mg, oral suspensions of 125 and 250 mg/5 ml, and pediatric drops of 100 mg/ml. The usual adult oral dose is 250 to 500 mg/6 hr. A suggested dosage for children under 50 pounds is 50 mg/kg/24 hr divided into four equally spaced doses. An oral dose produces a peak serum level in 2 hours, a half-life of 90 minutes, and is detectable for about 4 hours after administration. It is preferable to administer ampicillin on an empty stomach, since food decreases its absorption.

HETACILLIN. Hetacillin (Versapen) is another semisynthetic penicillin that is hydrolyzed in the body to ampicillin and acetone. The only antibacterial activity is that provided by the ampicillin. Stated advantages over using ampicillin directly are unfounded.[64]

AMOXICILLIN. Amoxicillin (Amoxil, Larotid, Polymox) has an antibacterial action equivalent to ampicillin. It is better absorbed and therefore gives higher blood levels. Food does not seem to interfere with absorption. Taken orally, a peak level is reached in 2 hours, with a half-life of 90 minutes. It is useful in the same situations as ampicillin.

Carbenicillin. Carbenicillin (Geopen, Pyopen), another semisynthetic penicillin, has special indications. Adverse effects are the same as for the penicillinase-resistant semisynthetics. Additionally, uremic patients have shown hemorrhagic manifestations with altered clotting and prothrombin times. Safety for use in pregnancy has not been established. It is not penicillinase resistant and is only used parenterally. Its special therapeutic importance is in infections by *Pseudomonas aeruginosa.* Microorganisms develop resistance to carbenicillin quickly and frequently. This drug should be reserved for use against serious infections by *P. aeruginosa* and by sensitive strains of *Proteus* that are resistant to ampicillin.[65]

Carbenicillin indanyl. Carbenicillin indanyl (Geocillin) is an acid-stable ester of carbenicillin that is suitable for oral use. The antimicrobial spectrum is equivalent to that of carbenicillin, and resistance develops quickly. Although low levels of the drug are obtained in the serum, the drug is excreted in the urine. Therefore its usefulness is limited to the treatment of urinary tract infections caused by susceptible organisms.

Erythromycin

Erythromycin was isolated from a strain of *Streptomyces erythreus* in 1952. It is an organic base with a high molecular weight.

Administration and body handling. Erythromycin is usually administered orally as the free base, in various salt forms, or as insoluble esters. Intravenous and intramuscular forms are available. Since erythromycin is broken down in gastric fluid, it is best administered when the stomach is empty: 1 hour before or 2 hours after meals. The peak blood level is obtained in from 1 to 4 hours, depending on stomach emptying time. The tablet is usually enteric coated or supplied as an insoluble ester so that the drug is not broken down extensively in the stomach acid. Although different salts and esters provide different blood levels, no therapeutic

differences between them have been demonstrated.[66,67] Erythromycin is distributed to most body tissues, particularly the liver where it is concentrated, excreted in bile, and partially reabsorbed. Although most is excreted in the urine in the form of metabolic products, some is excreted in the feces.

Antibacterial activity and spectrum. Erythromycin is believed to interfere with bacterial protein synthesis. Its antibacterial spectrum closely resembles that of penicillin. It is active against most gram-positive bacteria, some gram-negative bacteria, certain strains of *Rickettsia* and *Actinomyces*, protozoa, and some large viruses. Although erythromycin is essentially a bacteriostatic drug, it is bactericidal against rapidly multiplying hemolytic streptococci and staphylococci.[29] Bacterial resistance occurs but not as frequently as is seen with penicillin and streptomycin. But, in some hospitals as many as 50% of staphylococci are not inhibited by erythromycin.[68]

Adverse reactions. Adverse reactions to the usual dosages of erythromycin are infrequent and generally mild. Side effects are generally gastrointestinal in nature and include stomatitis, abdominal cramps, nausea, vomiting, and diarrhea. These effects usually disappear when the drug is discontinued.

Table 20-2. Erythromycin preparations

Drug	Preparations
Erythromycin (E-Mycin, Ilotycin)	Enteric-coated tablets: 100 and 250 mg
Erythromycin stearate (Erythrocin s.)	Tablets: 100 and 250 mg
Erythromycin estolate (Ilosone)	Capsules: 125 and 250 mg Chewable tablets: 125 mg Drops: 100 mg/ml Liquid: 125 and 250 mg/5 ml
Erythromycin ethyl succinate (E.E.S.-400, Erythrocin e.s., Pediamycin)	Liquid and drops: 200 and 400 mg/5 ml Chewable tablets: 200 mg Tablets: 400 mg Intramuscular
Erythromycin lactobionate (Erythrocin Lactobionate)	Intravenous
Erythromycin gluceptate (Ilotycin Gluceptate)	Intravenous

Allergic reactions are infrequent and generally mild. Urticaria and rashes occur, but anaphylaxis and other serious allergic reactions are rare. Teratogenic effects have not been attributed to erythromycin.

Adverse effects on the hematologic and renal tissues have not been reported. Cholestatic jaundice and changes in liver function tests have occurred with erythromycin estolate. This is believed to be caused by a hypersensitivity type of reaction. It has occurred in some patients after a few days of treatment but usually follows 1 or 2 weeks of therapy. Erythromycin estolate is probably the most toxic form of erythromycin and presents the only significant hepatic effect of the erythromycins.

Uses, preparations, and dosages. Erythromycin is active against essentially the same microorganisms as penicillin. It is a satisfactory alternate for infections that do not require the high blood levels obtainable with penicillin[55] and is also of value in patients who are allergic to penicillin. Erythromycin will be active against most organisms that cause dental infections. It may fill an important need in dental practice (1) when penicillin is ineffective or cannot be used, (2) in patients with a high predisposition to allergy, and (3) in situations where the bactericidal potency of penicillin is not required. The various preparations of erythromycin are presented in Table 20-2. The usual oral doses are shown in Table 20-3.

Cephalosporins

Seven cephalosporins are currently marketed in the United States. The two available for oral use in the treatment of systemic infections are cephalexin and cephradine. The others discussed are too poorly absorbed orally to be useful for outpatient therapy.

Cephalothin. Sodium cephalothin (Keflin) is a semisynthetic antibiotic whose precursors are derived from several species of the fungus *Cephalosporium.* Its chemical structure and mechanism of action are similar to those of penicillin. Sodium cephalothin is not absorbed orally; consequently, it is used primarily intravenously. Wide tissue distribution is obtained. Approximately 60% of cephalothin is protein bound, and it is excreted in the urine with a half-life of less than 1 hour.[69] Cephalothin is a potent bactericidal agent against many gram-positive and gram-negative microbes including penicillinase-producing staphylococci. *Pseudomonas* is notably resistant.

Cephalothin is usually well tolerated. Although neutropenia has occurred, hematologic tolerance is favorable. Thrombophlebitis has occurred after infusion of over 3 days' duration, and there is irritation after intramuscular injections. Superinfection has resulted after prolonged use. Hepatic toxicity has not presented a problem. Until recently, nephrotoxicity was not considered to be a problem. Evidence now suggests that nephrotoxicity may occur under certain condi-

Table 20-3. Usual oral dosages of erythromycin*

Drug	Adult	Children
Erythromycin base and erythromycin stearate	250 mg/6 hr	15 mg/lb/24 hr in four or five divided doses
Erythromycin estolate	250 mg/6 hr	Under 25 pounds: 5 mg/lb/6 hr 25-50 pounds: 125 mg/6 hr Over 50 pounds: Adult dose
Erythromycin ethyl succinate	400 mg/6 hr	Under 10 pounds: 20 mg/lb/24 hr in four divided doses 10-15 pounds: 50 mg/6 hr 15-25 pounds: 100 mg/6 hr 25-50 pounds: 200 mg/6 hr Over 50 pounds: 200 mg five times every 24 hours

*Higher dosages have been recommended for severe infections. Where higher dosages are necessary, the practitioner should monitor the patient's response and ensure that maximal doses as recommended by the manufacturer are not exceeded.

tions, for example, preexisting renal disease.[70] Safety for the use of cephalothin during pregnancy has not been established. Allergy occurs infrequently and may be manifested as a rash, hives, or anaphylaxis. About 5% of patients receiving cephalothin develop hypersensitivity reactions, including fever, eosinophilia, serum sickness, rashes, or anaphylaxis. When large doses (12 Gm/24 hr) are given, a direct positive Coombs' reaction is frequently noted. The incidence of hypersensitivity reactions to the cephalosporins is higher in patients who have a history of penicillin allergy. The estimate of the degree of cross-sensitivity varies widely but seems to be low.

Sodium cephalothin is of particular value in severe infections that are treated on an inpatient basis and should be reserved for this use. Cephalothin has been used effectively against bacterial endocarditis and consequently should be considered an alternative in prophylaxis against subacute bacterial endocarditis when penicillin and erythromycin cannot be used. The usual adult intramuscular or intravenous dose is 0.5 to 1 Gm every 4 to 6 hours.

Cephalexin. Cephalexin monohydrate (Keflex) is an acid-stable, orally effective cephalosporin. It is well absorbed in the upper intestine, becomes distributed throughout the tissues, and has a bacterial activity and spectrum similar to that of cephalothin. A peak serum level is reached in 1 hour and food may delay absorption. It is mainly excreted in the urine unchanged with a half-life of 40 minutes.

Early observation indicates that cephalexin has a low incidence of adverse effects. Most adverse reactions have been gastrointestinal in nature; principally, they are diarrhea, nausea, and vomiting. Abdominal pain, anorexia, dyspepsia, and stomatitis have occurred. Allergic reactions have been limited and are essentially dermatologic in nature. Cross-allergenicity with other cephalosporins probably exists. Cephalexin should be used cautiously in patients allergic to penicillin. Although eosinophilia and neutropenia have been observed, hematologic, renal, and hepatic tolerance has been favorable. Renal damage occurs only rarely. Superinfection may occur after prolonged use, and safety during pregnancy has not been established.

Cephalexin has been effective against respiratory, soft tissue, and urinary tract infections caused by susceptible microorganisms. Although its place in dental practice has not been established, it may be an orally useful agent against sensitive organisms when other better known bactericidal antibiotics are ineffective or cannot be used. It is available in a 250 mg capsule and as an oral liquid containing 125 mg/5 ml. The usual adult oral dose is 250 mg/6 hr. The recommended dose for children is 25 to 50 mg/kg/24 hr divided into four doses.

Cephaloridine. Cephaloridine (Loridine) is a semisynthetic antibiotic closely related chemically and pharmacologically to cephalothin. Its method of administration is usually intramuscular. Its antibacterial spectrum and uses are the same as those of cephalothin. Its bactericidal potency is generally equal to that of cephalothin except that the latter is somewhat more effective against penicillinase-producing staphylococci. The adverse reactions that relate to cephalothin also apply to cephaloridine. Additionally, doses of cephaloridine above 4 Gm/24 hr have caused fatal cases of renal tubular necrosis, and usual dosage levels are more often associated with superinfections with *Pseudomonas* than if cephalothin is used.[71]

The indications for cephaloridine are the same as those of cephalothin. However, in view of its greater ability to cause adverse reactions and its decreased effectiveness against some staphylococci, it would be difficult at this time to justify the selection of cephaloridine over cephalothin in situations where the latter can be used. Its only advantage seems to be the ability to be used IM with less discomfort than with cephalothin. The usual adult IM or IV dose of cephaloridine is 0.5 to 1 Gm every 6 to 8 hours.

Cephaloglycin. Cephaloglycin (Kafocin) is a cephalosporin with chemical and pharmacologic properties similar to those for the other members of the group. Although it can be used orally, effective antibacterial activity is only obtained in the urine. Consequently, its only current usefulness is in urinary tract infections.

Cefazolin. Cefazolin (Ancef, Kefzol) is another cephalosporin administered IM or IV. Its antibacterial activity and adverse reactions are similar to those of other cephalosporins. When given IM, it produces less pain than the other cephalosporins. The adult dosage in patients with normal renal function is 500 mg to 1 Gm every 6 to 8 hours.

Cephradine. Cephradine (Anspor, Velosef), another cephalosporin, may be given orally, IM, or IV. Its activity and adverse reactions are similar to those of cephalexin. The recommended adult dose is 250 mg/6 hr.

Cephapirin. Cephapirin (Cefadyl), another cephalosporin, is useful IM or IV.

Lincomycin

Lincomycin (Lincocin) is a relatively new antibiotic that was derived from *Streptomyces lincolnesis.* With the exception of its more recently marketed derivative clindamycin, the chemical structure of lincomycin is distinctly different from that of other antibiotics.

Administration and body handling. Lincomycin hydrochloride monohydrate is used orally, intramuscularly, and intravenously. Oral administration of 500 mg produces a peak blood level in 2 to 4 hours. Given orally, approximately 20% to 35% of the drug is absorbed, and it has a half-life of 4 to 5 hours.[72] Lincomycin becomes distributed throughout most body tissues including bone. It is eliminated largely in the active form in feces after biliary excretion. Some active drug is eliminated in urine.

Antibacterial activity and spectrum. The antibacterial spectrum of lincomycin includes most gram-positive pathogens and has been used successfully against staphylococci that were resistant to penicillin. It has also been reported to be effective in cases of actinomycosis.[73] Its antibacterial action appears to result from an interference with bacterial protein synthesis by binding at the 50 S subunit of the bacterial ribosome. Although it is essentially a bacteriostatic drug, it is bactericidal against some organisms at blood levels that are obtainable by oral administration. Bacterial resistance has not yet presented a significant clinical problem. There is some evidence of therapeutic antagonism between lincomycin and erythromycin[74] because of competition for the same binding site on the bacteria. Consequently, these drugs should not be administered simultaneously.

Adverse reactions. Lincomycin has a moderate toxicity and a few serious toxic effects have occurred during short-term therapy. Troublesome side effects include diarrhea, nausea, vomiting, enterocolitis, and abdominal cramps. Diarrhea, which occurs rather frequently, may be severe and persistent. Some patients develop pseudomembranous colitis, which can be fatal, and is associated with severe persistent diarrhea associated with passage of blood and mucus. These gastrointestinal effects probably result from the fact that relatively high concentrations of active drug continue through the gastrointestinal tract and disturb the normal enteric flora. Glossitis, stomatitis, headache, dizziness, and superinfection by *Candida albicans* are also sometimes associated with its use. Reversible hematologic effects (neutropenia, leukopenia, thrombocytopenic purpura) and abnormal liver function tests have been reported. Allergic reactions to lincomycin have not yet presented a significant clinical limitation, but skin rashes, urticaria, angioneurotic edema, serum sickness, and anaphylaxis have occurred. Safety for use in pregnant women and the newborn has not been established. Since this is a relatively new drug, blood studies and liver function tests should be carried out in cases of prolonged use.

Uses, preparations, and dosages. Lincomycin has been used as a substitute for penicillin and erythromycin and has shown particular efficacy in acute and chronic osteomyelitis. Favorable reports of its use in dentistry have been published, showing its effectiveness in many dental infections.[75,76] In cases where a potent bactericidal agent is required, it should not be substituted for penicillin or sodium cephalothin unless these drugs are ineffective or cannot otherwise be used. Lincomycin should receive consideration in cases of osteomyelitis. In cases where a gram-negative organism is involved, lincomycin will not be effective. It may be more effective against some staphylococci infections than erythromycin.

Lincomycin HCl monohydrate (Lincocin) is available in parenteral solutions for intravenous and intramuscular use. It is available orally as 250 and 500 mg capsules and as an oral liquid containing 250 mg/5 ml. The usual adult oral dose of lincomycin HCl is 500 mg every 6 to 8 hours. The recommended dose for children over 1 month of age is 15 mg/lb/24 hr total, divided into three or four equal doses.

Clindamycin

Clindamycin is a new semisynthetic antibiotic that was produced by chemical modification of the lincomycin molecule.

Administration and body handling. Clindamycin is used orally, intramuscularly, and intravenously. After oral administration it is rapidly and almost completely absorbed. There is some indication that a 150 mg oral dose provides a peak blood level in about 45 minutes with a half-life of about 2 hours. An effective blood level is maintained for about 6 hours. Like lincomycin, clindamycin becomes widely distributed in the tissues, including bone. Unlike lincomycin, most clindamycin is excreted as inactive metabolites, with relatively little active drug being eliminated in the urine or feces.

Antibacterial activity and spectrum. The antibacterial spectrum of clindamycin is slightly broader than that of lincomycin. It includes most gram-positive pathogens plus a few gram-negative bacteria. It can be considered a bactericidal drug, although as with any antibiotic, it is bacteriostatic at low dosages. There is evidence that clindamycin is more active than lincomycin and at least as active as erythromycin against beta-hemolytic streptococci, *Streptomyces viridans, Diplococcus pneumoniae,* and *Staphylococcus aureus.*[77] Its mechanism of action is by inhibition of bacterial protein synthesis by binding to the 50 S subunit of the bacterial ribosome. At this time bacterial resistance to clindamycin has not been found to develop rapidly. Cross-resistance with lincomycin has been reported. As with lincomycin, an antagonistic relationship has been observed between clindamycin and erythromycin.

Adverse reactions. Present knowledge indicates that clindamycin is usually well tolerated. Studies have not demonstrated irreversible hematologic, hepatic, renal, dermatologic, or neurologic abnormalities. Transient leukopenia, eosinophilia, and abnormal liver function tests as well as agranulocytosis and thrombocytopenia have been reported. The most commonly observed side effects are gastrointestinal in nature. The manufacturer reported that diarrhea and loose stools were observed in 3% of patients in initial clinical trials. More recently, the incidence of diarrhea has been found to be between 5% and 20%, with some studies showing a low incidence[78] and others showing that diarrhea with clindamycin is as common as that with lincomycin.[79] One recent study reported a 7% incidence of diarrhea.[80]

A more serious consequence associated with the diarrhea has been the development of pseudomembranous colitis, characterized by severe, persistent diarrhea and the passage of blood and mucus.[81,82] It has been fatal in some patients. The colitis may not be specific for clindamycin and lincomycin but may also occur with other antibiotics such as tetracycline and ampicillin.[83] Pseudomembranous colitis should be treated with fluid and electrolytic replacement and the discontinuation of the drug. Systemic corticosteroids have sometimes proved helpful. Narcotic derivatives such as diphenoxylate with atropine (Lomotil) may exacerbate the condition and should not be used. This condition may begin during or as long as several weeks after cessation of clindamycin therapy.

Clindamycin is likely to accumulate in patients with renal insufficiency. Consequently, serum levels should be determined periodically in these patients. To date allergic reactions have been minimal, but skin rashes, urticaria, and other allergic manifestations have occurred. Cross-sensitization with lincomycin has not been demonstrated but would be predicted to occur. Safety for use in pregnant women has not been established. Since this is a new drug, blood studies and liver function tests should be carried out in cases of prolonged use.

Uses, preparations, and dosages. Clindamycin has been recommended for most gram-positive infections, particularly streptococci, *D. pneumoniae,* and staphylococci. If early observations are accurate, this drug should provide bactericidal potency against many gram-positive pathogens and should be effective against many dental infections, including osteomyelitis.

Oral clindamycin will probably replace lincomycin in the treatment of serious infections where less toxic antimicrobial agents are not indicated. The advantages of clindamycin over lincomycin include the following: better oral absorption, the possibility of a decreased incidence of diarrhea with oral administration, a greater in vitro activity against susceptible pathogens, and probably greater safety when used in patients with renal insufficiency.

Clindamycin HCl hydrate (Cleocin) is

available in capsules containing 75 and 150 mg. Clindamycin palmitate HCl (Cleocin palmitate) is available for oral suspension (75 mg/5 ml) in 30, 80, and 200 ml bottles. The recommended adult, oral dosage of clindamycin HCl hydrate in mild to moderate infections is 150 to 300 mg/6 hr, and in severe infections 300 to 450 mg/6 hr. The recommended dosage for children in mild to moderate infections is 4 to 8 mg/lb/24 hr divided into three or four equal doses, and in severe infections 8 to 10 mg/lb/24 hr divided into three or four equal doses.

BROAD-SPECTRUM ANTIBIOTICS
Tetracyclines

Chlortetracycline was isolated from *Streptomyces aureofaciens* in 1948. Other tetraclines have been derived from several species of *Streptomyces*, and some members are produced synthetically. All tetracyclines are closely related chemically and have a structure similar to that of tetracycline itself, as shown below:

Administration and body handling. Although parenteral preparations are available, the tetracyclines are usually administered orally. Gastrointestinal absorption is incomplete but fairly rapid. Wide tissue distribution is obtained. The tetracyclines are secreted in saliva and to a very minor extent in the milk of lactating mothers. In the latter case mothers taking up to 2 Gm/24 hr are not likely to eliminate enough tetracycline in milk to affect the teeth or bones of a breast-fed child.[84]

The tetracyclines are concentrated by the liver and are excreted in bile, feces, and urine. Elimination of a 250 mg dose is not complete after 6 hours. Consequently, some cumulation occurs but is ordinarily not a problem in therapy of under 10 days' duration. Oral absorption is decreased by the concomitant administration of antacids containing divalent cations such as aluminum, calcium, and magnesium and should not be administered with these preparations. Foods

having a high calcium content, such as dairy products, also decrease the oral absorption of tetracyclines. The mechanism involved is apparently the chelation of tetracycline with aluminum, calcium, and magnesium. However, a significant increase in gastric pH resulting from the use of antacids might also be a factor in the reduced absorption of tetracycline.[85]

Antibacterial activity and spectrum. The tetracyclines are bacteriostatic antibiotics and are believed to interfere with the synthesis of bacterial protein. As broad-spectrum antibiotics, they are effective against a wide variety of gram-positive and gram-negative microorganisms, rickettsias, spirochetes, some protozoa, and some large viruses. All tetracyclines appear to have essentially the same antibacterial potency against the same microorganisms. It is reasonable to assume that an infection that will respond to one tetracycline will respond to the others. Bacterial resistance to the tetracyclines develops slowly and is not a significant clinical problem. However, cross-resistance between tetracyclines is probably complete.

Adverse reactions. The usual dosage levels of tetracyclines seldom produce serious toxic reactions. Renal impairment leads to accumulation and increases the likelihood of hepatic damage. Doxycycline is the one tetracycline that does not accumulate in renal failure. The incidence of liver damage increases with the intravenous use of tetracyclines and deaths have occurred,[86,87] especially in pregnant women.[88,89] It has been recommended that the practitioner not use over 1 to 2 Gm/24 hr tetracycline orally for pregnant women,[89] if used at all. Toxic renal effects have been reported after the use of old (degraded) tetracyclines.[90,91] A potential for kidney damage should be considered even with tetracyclines that are not degraded. This is particularly true at high doses and with patients predisposed to kidney disease. The nephrotoxicity of tetracyclines will add to that of other drugs. Consequently, tetracyclines should not be used concomitantly with other drugs that are known to have a significant renal toxicity, such as methoxyflurane (Penthrane). Hematologic changes, such as hemolytic anemia, are infrequent but have occurred after tetracycline therapy.

Tetracyclines become incorporated in calcifying structures. If they are used during periods of enamel calcification, they may produce permanent discoloration of the teeth and enamel hypoplasia. Consequently, they should not be used during the last half of pregnancy or in children up to the age of 9 years. A decrease in the growth rate of bone has been demonstrated in infants given high dosages of tetracyclines.

Although serious reactions to tetracyclines are not frequently observed, troublesome side effects are often seen, including anorexia, nausea, vomiting, diarrhea, gastroenteritis, glossitis, stomatitis, xerostomia, and candidiasis (moniliasis). These side effects are largely related to local irritation and to alterations in oral, gastric, and enteric flora. They generally disappear rapidly when the tetracycline is discontinued. The specific member, tetracycline, has been said to be less likely to cause gastrointestinal upsets than do the other drugs of the group.[92]

Anaphylactic and various dermatologic reactions to the tetracyclines have occasionally occurred, but the overall allergenicity of these drugs is low. Some people exhibit an exaggerated sunburn reaction (photosensitivity) to tetracyclines, an effect that is probably allergic in nature. There is some indication that both allergic[93] and photosensitivity[94] reactions may occur more frequently with demethylchlortetracycline than with the other members. An individual who is allergic to one tetracycline is almost certain to be allergic to all tetracyclines.

Tetracyclines or any broad-spectrum antibiotic, especially at high doses or in long-term therapy, may reduce plasma prothrombin by killing intestinal bacteria that produce vitamin K. This is particularly significant in patients receiving anticoagulant therapy (for example, warfarin [Coumadin]) and may lead to bleeding.

Uses, preparations, and dosages. The tetracyclines are specifically useful in chronic bronchitis, shigellosis, anaerobe infections, psittacosis, lymphogranuloma venereum, rickettsial infections, mycoplasma pneumonia, and infections by gram-negative bacilli.[95] They are used only against other

Table 20-4. Tetracycline preparations (oral only)

Drug	Preparations
Tetracycline HCl* (Achromycin V, Panmycin HCl, Steclin, Sumycin, Tetrachel, Tetracyn HCl)	Capsules: 50, 125, and 250 mg Tablets: 250 mg
Tetracycline phosphate complex (Sumycin, Tetrex)	Capsules: 100 and 250 mg Syrup: 125 mg/5 ml Drops: 100 mg/ml
Chlortetracycline HCl (Aureomycin HCl)	Capsules: 250 mg
Oxytetracycline HCl* (Oxlopar, Oxy-Kesso Tetra, Oxy-Tetrachel, Terramycin HCl, Uri'Tet)	Capsules: 125 and 250 mg Tablets: 250 mg Suspension: 125 mg/ml Drops: 100 mg/ml
Demethylchlortetracycline HCl (Declomycin HCl, Demeclocycline HCl)	Capsules: 150 mg Tablets: 75, 150, and 300 mg Suspension: 75 mg/5 ml Drops: 60 mg/ml
Methacycline HCl (Rondomycin)	Capsules: 150 and 300 mg Suspension: 75 mg/5 ml
Doxycycline hyclate (Doxychel, Doxy-II, Vibramycin)	Capsules: 50 and 100 mg
Doxycycline monohydrate (Vibramycin)	Suspension: 25 mg/5 ml
Minocycline HCl (Minocin, Vectrin)	Capsules: 100 mg

*All preparations listed are not necessarily available in each trade name indicated. Most forms are available in both generic and trade name preparations.

infections when sensitivity tests indicate that more potent or more specific antibiotics are ineffective or cannot be used.

The tetracyclines are active against most organisms that cause dental infections. They have been reported to be effective against recurrent aphthous stomatitis[96] and acute necrotizing ulcerative gingivitis.[7] They are not effective for prophylaxis against subacute bacterial endocarditis. The tetracyclines may be useful against dental infections by sensitive organisms where a bacteriostatic effect is adequate. This may be particularly important in cases where the patient is allergic to penicillin or where a high predisposition to allergy exists.

If used in dental practice, the tetracyclines will be administered orally. Oral preparations are shown in Table 20-4 and oral dosages in Table 20-5. To obtain optimal absorption they should be administered 1 hour before or 2 hours after meals.

Chloramphenicol

Chloramphenicol (Chloromycetin) is a derivative of paranitrobenzene, was isolated from *Streptomyces venezuelae*, and is now produced synthetically. Chloramphenicol is rapidly absorbed orally and can also be administered IV, IM, and subcutaneously. It becomes well distributed throughout the body tissues including those of the central nervous system. It is rapidly metabolized by the liver, and the products, principally conjugates of glucuronic acid, are excreted in the urine.

Chloramphenicol is a broad-spectrum, principally bacteriostatic antibiotic. Its mechanism of action is by the inhibition of bacterial protein synthesis acting primarily on the 50 S ribosomal subunit like erythromycin, lincomycin, and clindamycin. It is active against a large number of gram-positive and gram-negative microorganisms, rickettsias, and some large viruses. It is particularly effective against *Salmonella typhi*.

Chloramphenicol is an extremely toxic drug. Serious and fatal blood dyscrasias (aplastic anemia, agranulocytosis, hypoplastic anemia, thrombocytopenia) have occurred even after short-term use. Bone marrow suppression has produced a pancytopenia,[97] which is not dose related. Although the incidence is low (1:40,000), it is almost always fatal. Other possible adverse effects include nausea, vomiting, glossitis, stomatitis, headache, depression, confusion, delirium, and allergic reactions including anaphylaxis. In view of the seriousness and frequency of adverse reactions to chloramphenicol, it must only be used against serious infections when less dangerous antibacterial agents are

Table 20-5. Usual oral dosages of tetracyclines*

Drug	Adult	Children
Tetracycline HCl, tetracycline phosphate complex, chlortetracycline HCl, and oxytetracycline HCl	250-500 mg/6 hr	10 mg/lb/24 hr in four divided doses
Demethylchlortetracycline HCl and methacycline HCl	600 mg/24 hr in two or four divided doses	3-6 mg/lb/24 hr in two or four divided doses
Doxycycline hyclate and doxycycline monohydrate	Day 1: 100 mg/12 hr Thereafter: 100 mg/24 hr in one or two divided doses	Day 1: 2 mg/lb in two divided doses Thereafter: 1 mg/lb/24 hr in one or two divided doses
Minocycline HCl	200 mg initially and 100 mg/12 hr thereafter (safety for use during pregnancy not established)	4 mg/kg initially, then 2 mg/kg/12 hr

*Higher dosages have been recommended for severe infections. In cases where higher dosages are necessary, the practitioner should monitor the patient's response and ensure that maximal doses as recommended by the manufacturer are not exceeded.

ineffective or cannot be used. Only in typhoid fever is chloramphenicol still the antibiotic of first choice.[98]

When chloramphenicol is used, it is imperative that blood studies be made frequently to detect early blood changes before they become irreversible. It is highly unlikely that any use for chloramphenicol in dentistry would be justified.

AMINOGLYCOSIDE ANTIBIOTICS

The aminoglycoside antibiotics include neomycin, streptomycin, kanamycin, gentamicin, tobramycin, and amikacin, which have many properties in common. They are poorly absorbed after oral administration, but after injection they are rapidly excreted by the normal kidney. Their primary use is in the treatment of gram-negative bacteria. Aminoglycosides act directly on the 30 S subunit of the ribosome inhibiting protein synthesis.

Resistance can be produced by mutation or by acquisition of a plasmid. One-way cross-resistance between different aminoglycosides occurs. The toxicity of the aminoglycosides severely limits their usefulness. The most important adverse reactions are ototoxicity, both auditory and vestibular, and nephrotoxicity. A neuromuscular blockade, resulting in a cessation of respiration, has been caused by the aminoglycosides, especially when they are given after the use of anesthesia or muscle relaxants.

Neomycin. Neomycin is now used only topically because of its toxicity. It will be discussed under the topical antibiotics.

Streptomycin. Streptomycin was one of the earliest antibiotics. It was isolated from *Streptomyces griseus* in 1944. Like all aminoglycosides it is poorly absorbed orally and is only used intramuscularly. Streptomycin becomes reasonably well distributed throughout the tissues, becomes concentrated in the kidney, and is excreted in the urine.

Streptomycin is a potent bactericidal antibiotic against many gram-negative and some gram-positive bacteria. The drug is particularly effective against gram-negative rods, along with *Pseudomonas aeruginosa* and *Mycobacterium tuberculosis*. Streptomycin is a toxic drug. Its most important adverse effect is on the eighth cranial nerve, causing tinnitus, vertigo, and deafness. Because of its toxicity and the rapid development of resistant strains of bacteria, the current use of streptomycin is principally in the treatment of tuberculosis. Therapy with streptomycin is not recommended in dental practice.[53]

Streptomycin is also discussed later in relationship to its use to treat tuberculosis.

Kanamycin. Kanamycin sulfate (Kantrex) is used orally for its local effect in reducing the bacterial population of the gastrointestinal tract. It is used systematically (intramuscularly and intravenously) for short-term treatment of serious infections caused by susceptible bacteria. It is a toxic drug and is of no particular importance in dental practice.

Gentamicin. Gentamicin sulfate (Garamycin) is a relatively new antibiotic whose chemical structure is similar to that of neomycin, streptomycin, and kanamycin. For several years gentamicin sulfate has been used topically against bacterial skin infections and is now available for intramuscular or intravenous injection. Peak blood levels are obtained within 1 hour, and principal excretion is in the urine. Gentamicin is bactericidal against a wide variety of gram-negative and gram-positive bacteria including *Staphylococcus aureus*, *Proteus*, and *Pseudomonas*.

Although topical gentamicin has been relatively free of significant adverse effects, parenteral use may cause damage to the eighth cranial nerve and kidney. Other reactions that have been observed to be associated with gentamicin include decreased hematocrit, depressed granulocytes, anemia, nausea, vomiting, urticaria, rash, drug fever, convulsions, and neuromuscular blockade. Since the principal route of excretion is the kidney, renal impairment may be expected to increase the toxicity. Safety of use in pregnancy has not been established.

In view of the potential toxicity of gentamicin, it should not be used against infections that can be treated with better known and less toxic agents. It should be reserved for use against serious gram-negative infections, such as *Proteus* and *Pseudomonas*, when less toxic drugs are ineffective. Its use in combination with carbenicillin may result in a synergism in the treatment of some *Pseudomonas*.[99] Sensitivity tests should demonstrate a need for its use. The usual adult intramuscular dose for patients with normal renal function is 3 mg/kg/24 hr in two, three, or four equally divided doses.

Tobramycin. Tobramycin (Nebcin) is a less active aminoglycoside antibiotic than gentamicin against most gram-negative bacteria, but it is more active against *Pseudomonas.* It is also used with carbenicillin to produce synergism. The toxicity and dosage are similar to those for gentamicin.

Amikacin. Amikacin (Amikin) is the most recently developed aminoglycoside. Many bacteria that are found to be resistant to the other aminoglycosides are susceptible to amikacin in vitro; otherwise, it is similar to the other aminoglycosides. The recommended dosage in a patient with normal renal function is 15 mg/kg/24 hr divided into two or three equal doses administered at equally spaced intervals. The dosage of all of the aminoglycosides must be altered in the presence of renal failure.

OTHER ANTIBIOTICS
Vancomycin

Vancomycin (Vancocin) is an antibiotic of unknown chemical structure and was isolated from *Streptomyces orientalis.* The absorption of vancomycin from the gastrointestinal tract is minimal; however, it has been used orally in the treatment of staphylococcic enterocolitis. It is too irritating to be used intramuscularly. When administered intravenously, bactericidal concentrations and wide tissue distribution are readily obtained. Vancomycin is excreted in the urine.

Vancomycin is a potent bactericidal agent against many gram-positive cocci, and it acts by inhibiting bacterial wall synthesis. Bacteria do not appear to develop resistance to vancomycin readily, and cross-resistance with other antibiotics is not believed to develop.

Except at high dosages significant toxic reactions to vancomycin are infrequent. High dosages, prolonged therapy, or administration to patients with renal impairment may cause some degree of hearing loss and depressed kidney function. Permanent deafness and fatal uremia have resulted.[55] Anaphylaxis and superinfection may occur but are rare. Prolonged or repeated use has caused thrombophlebitis. Occasionally, rash, urticaria, chills, fever, and nausea may be seen. Although hematopoietic and hepatic damage has not been reported during pro-

longed use, it is suggested that hematopoietic, liver, and renal function tests be performed. Vancomycin should not be administered to patients who have recently or are presently taking ototoxic or nephrotoxic agents. Safety for use in pregnant women and infants has not been established. Topical use, as in certain preliminary dental studies, has not presented a problem of adverse reactions.

Vancomycin has some current use in the treatment of serious staphylococcal infections that are resistant to less toxic antibiotics. Its usefulness against penicillinase-producing staphylococci is now limited to methacillin-resistant strains. However, vancomycin may be extremely important in serious cases of staphylococcal enterocolitis.[100]

Vancomycin is considered here in more detail than it ordinarily deserves in dentistry because of continued investigations concerning its topical use against oral lesions[101] and in preventing the formation of microbial plaque.[102]

Spectinomycin

Spectinomycin (Trobicin) is an antibiotic produced by *Streptomyces spectabilis.* It is somewhat active against a number of gram-negative bacteria, but other antibiotics are more effective. It readily inhibits the gonococci, and this effect has been used therapeutically. It is rapidly absorbed after intramuscular injection, producing a peak level in 1 hour. Urticaria, chills, fever, insomnia, and dizziness have been noted after one dose. The injection can be painful. The only indication for spectinomycin is in the treatment of acute genital and rectal gonorrhea. The recommended dosage is 2 to 4 Gm, depending on the clinical symptoms, in a single dose.

Novobiocin

There are no current indications for this drug because of its toxicity.

Colistin

Colistin (Coly-Mycin) is a synthetic antibiotic that is effective mainly against gram-negative bacteria. Since it is not absorbed from the gastrointestinal tract, it must be administered intramuscularly. As many as 20% of patients develop adverse reactions, including paresthesias, pruritus, dermatoses, visual and speech disturbances, drug fever, dizziness, and gastrointestinal effects. Superinfection, leukopenia, and granulocytopenia may also occur; renal toxicity and respiratory paralysis can be other adverse effects. It is used primarily in the treatment of certain *Pseudomonas* infections but has largely been replaced by less toxic antibiotics.

TOPICAL ANTIBIOTICS

Only antibiotics with a low degree of allergenicity and a limited value as systemic agents should be considered for topical use.[54] Bacitracin, polymyxin B (Aerosporin), neomycin (Mycifradin, Myciguent, Neobiotic), and gentamicin (Garamycin) are the most commonly used topical antibiotics. These drugs are poorly absorbed orally, and their toxicity has almost eliminated their systemic use except for gentamicin. Since they are poorly absorbed orally, some preparations have been used orally as intestinal antiseptics. Because gentamicin has proved to be a useful agent systemically, its topical use should be limited severely. The spectrum of activity and the nature of their systemic toxicity are shown in Table 20-6. Their principal use in dentistry has been the use of bacitracin in periodontal dressings.

ANTIFUNGAL AGENTS

Antifungal agents include nystatin (Mycostatin), amphotericin B (Fungizone), candicidin (Candeptin), griseofulvin (Fulvicin U/F, Grifulvin V, Grisactin), and flucytosine (Ancobon, 5-FC).

Nystatin. Nystatin is produced by *Streptomyces noursei*. It is active against fungi and yeasts, particularly *Candida albicans*. It is used topically against infections by *C. albicans* (candidiasis or moniliasis) of the skin and mucous membranes. It is taken orally to treat gastrointestinal candidiasis. Absorption after topical or oral administration is negligible. Allergic reactions have been reported, and nausea, vomiting, and diarrhea

may occur after oral use. Because nystatin has no effect on bacteria, superinfection is not a problem. Nystatin is bound by the yeasts and fungi membranes, which results in a change in permeability allowing small molecules to leak out.[103]

C. albicans is a usual inhabitant of the oral cavity. Oral candidiasis (thrush) is most likely to occur in debilitated patients and those taking broad-spectrum antibiotics or corticosteroids. Thrush has occurred during the use of tetracyclines in periodontal dressings,[104] but has not been associated with the similar use of bacitracin.[105] Thrush has also been related to the prolonged use of topical corticosteroids (triamcinolone acetonide) in the treatment of oral lesions.[106]

For the treatment of oral candidiasis, nystatin is available in an aqueous suspension containing 100,000 U/ml. It is dispensed in 60 ml bottles, each containing a dropper calibrated for 1 ml. The recommended adult dose for oral infections is 4 to 6 ml four times per 24 hours until 48 hours after signs of the infection have disappeared. The drug should be held in the mouth for 2 minutes before swallowing. It is also available as a vaginal tablet containing 100,000 units. In the treatment of oral candidiasis this tablet can be placed in the mouth and allowed to dissolve four times per 24 hours. This dosage form allows the drug to be in contact with the infection for a longer time. It is important that the patient understand exactly what to do with the medication dispensed. Some have recommended that treatment continue for at least 14 days and not be discontinued until two successive smears are negative.[107]

Amphotericin B. Amphotericin B is produced by *Streptomyces nodosus*. It is used intravenously in the treatment of systemic mycotic infections such as blastomycosis, histoplasmosis, coccidioidomycosis, cryptococcosis, and disseminated candidiasis. Fatal cases of the later have been reported after tooth extraction.[108] Amphotericin B is not ab-

Table 20-6. Topical antibiotics

Drug	Principal spectrum	Systemic toxicity
Bacitracin	Gram-positive spirochetes and amebas	Nephrotoxic
Polymyxin B	Gram-negative	Nephrotoxic
Neomycin	Gram-positive and gram-negative	Nephrotoxic and ototoxic
Gentamicin	Gram-positive, gram-negative, and *Pseudomonas*	Nephrotoxic and ototoxic

sorbed orally and is used topically against local candidal infections. Although it is combined with tetracycline in an oral preparation to suppress overgrowth of yeasts and fungi, there is no clinical evidence that this combination is necessary or effective. However, the currently available topical preparations are not recommended for oral use.[53] A 2% concentration of amphotericin B in an adhesive paste (Orabase) or an adhesive powder formulation (Orahesive) has been reported to be useful in the treatment of mucous membrane lesions infected with *C. albicans*.[109,110]

Amphotericin B is toxic. Its parenteral use should be justified by a definitely established need for the drug. Patients treated parenterally with this drug must be kept under close clinical supervision, particularly in regard to renal function. Severe allergic reactions, toxic irritative effects, and acute hepatic failure with jaundice have also occurred. Topical application may cause local irritation, but it is otherwise well tolerated topically.

Candicidin. Candicidin (Candeptin) is produced by *Streptomyces griseus*. It is used topically and only in the treatment of vaginal infections by *C. albicans*. It should not be used in oral candidiasis.

Griseofulvin. Griseofulvin (Fulvicin U/F, Grifulvin V, Grisactin) is produced by *Penicillium griseofulvum* and *P. patulum*. It is used orally against several dermatophytic infections.

Side effects include headache, peripheral neuritis, lethargy, mental confusion, fatigue, syncope, vertigo, and blurred vision. Nausea, vomiting, diarrhea, and hepatotoxicity have also been noted. Other untoward reactions include hematologic effects, renal effects, serum-sickness syndrome, and angioedema. It is used for long periods of treatment. It has no application in dental practice.

Flucytosine. Flucytosine (Ancobon) is a synthetic antifungal agent related structurally to fluorouracil, a cytotoxic agent. It inhibits the multiplication of susceptible strains of fungi. Resistance has developed during therapy.[111] It has been used successfully in the treatment of some cases of mucocutaneous candidiasis.[112] It is well absorbed from the gastrointestinal tract, with a peak level reached in 2 hours and a half-life of 3 to 4 hours.

Adverse reactions include bone marrow depression resulting in anemia, leukopenia, and thrombocytopenia and gastrointestinal irritation resulting in nausea, vomiting, and diarrhea.

SYNTHETIC ANTIBACTERIAL AGENTS
Sulfonamides

The demonstration that the antibacterial activity of the Prontosil molecule was para-aminobenzenesulfonamide (sulfanilamide) led to the synthesis of a large number of related antibacterial sulfonamides, principally by substitutions in the amide group of sulfanilamide. The earlier sulfonamides had very low urinary solubilities, and the danger of crystallization in the kidneys was particularly acute. Newer sulfonamides such as sulfisoxazole are more soluble and are less likely to precipitate in the kidney.

Structure and mechanism of action. The basis for most of the antibacterial activity of the sulfonamides is their structural similarity to para-aminobenzoic acid (PABA). Many bacteria are unable to use preformed folic acid, an essential component of several enzyme systems. They must synthesize folic acid using PABA. Because of their structural similarity, sulfonamides are accepted as PABA by bacterial enzymes for incorporation into folic acid. Thus, by competitive inhibition, adequate folic acid cannot be synthesized by the bacteria.

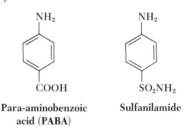

Para-aminobenzoic   Sulfanilamide
acid (**PABA**)

Activity and spectrum. The sulfonamides are bacteriostatic against many gram-positive and some gram-negative bacteria. They are ineffective against *Streptococcus viridans* but are active against some large viruses of trachoma and lymphogranuloma venereum.[113]

Administration, use, and body handling. The sulfonamides are generally used orally. The readily absorbable sulfonamides (sulfadiazine, sulfamerazine, and several others) are used for a systemic effect against susceptible organisms. Others that produce relatively low systemic blood levels but high concentrations in the urinary tract (sulfisoxazole, sulfathiazole, and several others) are used for infections of the urinary tract. Relatively insoluble sulfonamides (phthalylsulfathiazole, succinylsulfathiazole, and others) are used in ulcerative colitis and to reduce the gastrointestinal flora prior to certain surgical procedures.

Sulfonamide that is absorbed distributes throughout the body, including the cerebrospinal fluid. The drug is metabolized by acetylation or conjugation to glucuronides in the liver. Metabolites and some free drugs are excreted in urine.

Adverse reactions. The most common adverse effects of the sulfonamides are allergic reactions.[55] These may manifest as rashes, urticaria, pruritus, fever, a fatal exfoliative dermatitis, or periarteritis nodosa.[114] A patient who is allergic to one sulfonamide will be allergic to the others. Other relatively common side effects include nausea, vomiting, abdominal discomfort, headache, and dizziness. The following are seen less frequently: liver damage, depressed renal function, blood dyscrasias (agranulocytosis, thrombocytopenia, aplastic and hemolytic anemia), precipitation of lupus erythematosus and Stevens-Johnson syndrome (erythema multiforme exudativum). Stevens-Johnson syndrome, with a mortality of about 25%, is associated with the long-acting sulfonamides,[115,116] especially in children. The currently available long-acting sulfonamides include sulfadimethoxine (Madribon), sulfamethoxypyridazine (Kynex, Midicel), and acetyl sulfamethoxypyridazine (Kynex Acetyl). Since only convenience is served by long-acting sulfonamides, selecting them over other sulfonamides would appear questionable. The possibility of renal crystallization must always be kept in mind with the sulfonamides, particularly if the less soluble systemic agents are used or if renal function is not normal. Forcing fluids is generally advisable with these drugs.

Dental use. Sulfonamides have been reported to be effective in some dental infections.[117,118] However, antibiotics are almost without exception more effective and generally safer. Sulfonamides should be used against dental infections only in those rare instances where antibiotics are ineffective or cannot be used. Because of their relatively high allergenicity, they should *not* be used topically on oral lesions.

Trimethoprim-sulfamethoxazole

Trimethoprim was synthesized as an antibacterial agent and was later found to have antimalarial properties. This particular combination of drugs represents an application of theoretic considerations. The sulfonamides, like sulfamethoxazole, inhibit the utilization of PABA (incorporation into folic acid), and pyrimethamine inhibits the reduction of dihydrofolate to tetrahydrofolate. These two drugs then inhibit two steps in an essential metabolic pathway leading to a supra-additive effect.

Activity and spectrum. The antibacterial spectrum of trimethoprim alone is similar to that of sulfamethoxazole. In combination, trimethoprim and sulfamethoxazole are bacteriostatic against a wide variety of gram-positive and some gram-negative bacteria. Methicillin-resistant strains of *Staphylococcus aureus* are susceptible to the combination, even if they are not sensitive to either agent alone.

Administration, use, and body handling. The combination of trimethoprim and sulfamethoxazole is administered orally. The peak plasma level of these agents occurs in 2 hours for trimethoprim (half-life of 16 hours) and 4 hours for sulfamethoxazole (half-life of 10 hours). When a 5:1 ratio (sulfamethoxazole: trimethoprim) is given, an optimal ratio of 20:1 is obtained in the plasma.[119]

When used in combination, trimethoprim is rapidly distributed to body tissues and only slightly protein bound. The drug passes into the cerebrospinal fluid and the sputum easily.[120] About 65% of the sulfamethoxazole is plasma protein bound. The drug combination is available as trimethoprim-sulfamethoxazole (Bactrim, Septra) oral tablets containing 80 mg trimethoprim and 400 mg sulfamethoxazole. The usual adult dose is two tablets every 12 hours.

Adverse reactions. Over 75% of the adverse reactions involve the skin and they are similar to reactions of sulfonamides, including exfoliative dermatitis, Stevens-Johnson syndrome, and toxic epidermal necrolysis (Lyell's syndrome). Gastrointestinal reactions include nausea, vomiting, and diarrhea. Glossitis and stomatitis are not infrequent, and also reported have been jaundice, headache, depression, and hallucinations. Hematologic reactions noted include anemia, coagulation disorders, granulocytopenia, agranulocytosis, purpura, and sulfhemoglobinemia.[119]

Uses. The most common use of this combination is in the treatment of some selected urinary tract infections. It is also used occasionally in the management of acute gonococcal urethritis[121] or some pulmonary infections. This drug combination's main importance is in the application of theory to a practical situation.

Urinary tract antiseptics

Several antibacterial agents cannot be used to treat systemic infections, since therapeutic plasma concentrations are not reached in safe doses. But because they are concentrated in the kidney and urine, they can be used to treat urinary tract infections.

Methenamine. Methenamine is a urinary tract antiseptic that acts by the release of formaldehyde in an acid urine. It is orally absorbed and excreted in the urine. Since an acid pH (pH 5) promotes the production of formaldehyde, methenamine is administered with hippuric acid, mandelic acid, or cranberry juice. Gastrointestinal distress can occur with larger doses. Methenamine is available as methenamine mandelate (Mandelamine) or methenamine hippurate (Hiprex). Methenamine is useful for long-term suppressive therapy to prevent urinary tract infections in susceptible individuals.

Nitrofurantoin. Nitrofurantoin (Macrodantin) possesses a wide antibacterial spectrum including both gram-positive and gram-negative bacteria. It is active against many common urinary tract pathogens, including *Escherichia coli*, *Klebsiella*, *Enterobacter*, and staphylococci. It is rapidly absorbed from the gastrointestinal tract, but antibacterial plasma concentrations are not reached because the drug is rapidly excreted with a half-life of less than 1 hour.

The most common adverse reactions are nausea, vomiting, and diarrhea, but taking the drug with food decreases these effects. The administration of the drug in a larger crystal size may be less nauseating. Hypersensitivity reactions include chills, fever, leukopenia, granulocytopenia, hemolytic anemia, cholestatic jaundice, and hepatocellular damage. Other hypersensitivity reactions involving the lung include allergic pneumonitis and interstitial pulmonary fibrosis. Neurologic disorders observed include headache and a polyneuropathy with denervation and muscle atrophy. Nitrofurantoin's use is in the treatment or prevention of certain urinary tract infections, but is seldom as effective as antibiotics or sulfonamides for the treatment of these infections.

Nalidixic acid. Nalidixic acid (NegGram) is bactericidal to most of the gram-negative bacteria that cause urinary tract infections. Although resistance develops rapidly when tested, the population of resistant bacteria in the community does not seem to rise.[122] The compound is well absorbed orally, conjugated in the liver, and excreted with a half-life of 8 hours.

Nalidixic acid, taken orally, may cause nausea, vomiting, and diarrhea. Allergic reactions reported include pruritus, urticaria, rashes, photosensitivity, eosinophilia, and fever. Central nervous system effects include headache, drowsiness, vertigo, visual disturbances, and myalgia.

This drug is useful in the treatment of certain urinary tract infections, especially those caused by susceptible *Proteus* organisms.

AGENTS USED IN THE TREATMENT OF TUBERCULOSIS

The treatment of tuberculosis, a disease caused by the acid-fast bacteria *Mycobacterium tuberculosis*, is difficult for several reasons. First, patients with tuberculosis often have inadequate defense mechanisms. Second, the microorganisms develop resistant strains easily and have unusual metabolic characteristics. Finally, the drugs available are not bactericidal and because of toxicity cannot often be used in sufficient doses.

The treatment of tuberculosis relies almost entirely on chemotherapy. Because of the problem of resistance, at least two drugs are administered concurrently in all active cases. For the treatment of mild pulmonary tuberculosis, isoniazid, ethambutol, and pyridoxine are combined. When the pulmonary tuberculosis is severe, streptomycin is added. These therapeutic regimens are continued for 1½ years. The following types of patients are given isoniazid 300 mg/24 hr for 1 year: tuberculin converters and reactors exposed to tuberculosis, patients with inactive tuberculosis who have no history of adequate treatment, tuberculin reactors with pulmonary scars, and patients with diabetes mellitus or who are taking corticosteroids.

Isoniazid

Isoniazid (INH, Nydrazid) is the hydrazide of isonicotinic acid. Even though INH is both bacteriostatic and bactericidal in vitro, its action in vivo is only against actively growing tubercle bacilli. Those resting bacilli exposed to the drug are able to resume normal growth when the drug is removed. Resistant strains develop within a few weeks after the beginning of therapy. INH is readily absorbed and its metabolic rate is genetically determined. It is available as 50, 100, and 300 mg tablets, a syrup (10 mg/ml), an injection, and a powder. The usual dose is 5 mg/kg up to a maximum of 300 mg/24 hr.

The most important side effects of this drug relate to its effect on the peripheral and central nervous system. Peripheral neuritis, a common reaction, can be prevented by the administration of pyridoxine daily. Convulsions may result. Optic neuritis requires that vision be monitored. Other adverse reactions include mental abnormalities, excessive sedation, and incoordination. The incidence of severe hepatic injury with jaundice increases with age. Hypersensitivity reactions including skin eruptions, fever, hematologic reactions, and arthritic symptoms have been noted. Dryness of the mouth, epigastric distress, urinary retention in men, methemoglobinemia, and tinnitus have also been reported.

INH is used alone for prophylaxis of tuberculosis and in combination with other agents in the treatment of tuberculosis.

Ethambutol

Ethambutol (Myambutol) is a synthetic tuberculostatic agent. About 75% of *Mycobacterium tuberculosis* are sensitive to the usual dose of ethambutol. When given orally, it is 80% absorbed, reaching a maximum serum concentration in 2 to 4 hours. It is available as 100 and 400 mg tablets, and the usual dose is 15 to 25 mg/kg/24 hr. The usual daily doses are minimally toxic. The most important side effect is optic neuritis, resulting in a decrease of visual acuity and loss of ability to perceive the color green. It is used in combination with INH. It has replaced aminosalicylic acid because of fewer side effects and better patient acceptance.

Streptomycin

Streptomycin is both bacteriostatic and bactericidal for the tubercle bacillus in vitro, but in vivo it is merely suppressive. Random mutations result in some bacilli that are highly resistant to streptomycin. The longer that therapy is continued the more resistant strains will develop. Within 1 month resistance is a problem in some patients. Mixing streptomycin with another drug will delay, but not prevent, the development of resistant strains. This aminoglycoside antibiotic's primary use is in combination with other agents in the treatment of pulmonary tuberculosis.

Aminosalicylic acid

Aminosalicylic acid (para-aminosalicylic acid, PAS) is bacteriostatic, and large doses are required. The development of resistant strains requires at least 4 months. An irritation of the gastrointestinal tract producing anorexia, nausea, and diarrhea is produced in from 2% to 4% of patients. The advent of ethambutol has decreased the importance of this drug in the treatment of tuberculosis.

Rifampin

Rifampin (Rifadin, Rimactane) inhibits the growth of most gram-positive and some gram-negative bacteria. It is inhibitory to the tubercle bacilli. Since the mycobacteria develop resistance to rifampin in a one-step process, it should not be used alone. It is orally absorbed, reaching a peak blood level in 2 to 4 hours. It is distributed throughout the body, producing an orange-red color in the urine, feces, saliva, sputum, tears, and sweat. Adverse reactions include jaundice, hepatorenal syndrome, and gastrointestinal disturbances. It is available in 300 mg capsules, and the dosage is usually 600 mg/24 hr. It is used in combination with other agents in the treatment of tuberculosis or reserved for treatment failures.

ANTIVIRAL AGENTS

The development of agents useful in the treatment of viral infections is difficult because viruses are obligate intracellular parasites. Since the clinical symptoms of a viral infection often signal the last stage in the disease, eradication of the offending agent at that point would change the disease process little.

Idoxuridine

Idoxuridine (Dendrid, Herplex, IDU, Stoxil) exerts its activity on pyrimidine synthesis, nucleotide interconversion, and deoxyribonucleic acid (DNA) synthesis. After incorporation into the viral DNA, that DNA is more likely to break or transcribe inaccurately.[123] Thus its activity is largely limited to DNA viruses, primarily the herpesvirus group. The development of resistance is common. Because idoxuridine is rapidly inactivated by nucleotidases, it can only be used topically or intravenously. The main clinical use of idoxuridine has been in the treatment of herpes simplex keratitis.[124] Herpes genitalis may respond favorably to the local application of the drug, and herpetic stomatitis has been successfully treated with it.[125]

Amantadine

Amantadine (Symmetrel) is a synthetic antiviral agent structurally unrelated to any other antimicrobial agent. It is well absorbed orally and excreted in the urine unchanged. Studies have documented its effectiveness in prevention of infection with different strains of Asian (A_2) influenza.[126] This drug has the ability to prevent viral penetration of the host cell. It can also ameliorate clinical symptoms if given within 20 hours after the onset of illness.[126-128] It must be kept in mind that this drug is prophylactic only against *one* type of virus—the A_2 virus (Asian). It may prove useful in high-risk patients during a documented A_2 epidemic.[129] It is also effective in the treatment of parkinsonism.

REFERENCES

1. Dorland's illustrated medical dictionary, ed. 25, Philadelphia, 1974, W. B. Saunders Co.
2. Burnett, G. W.: The microbiology of dental infections, Dent. Clin. North Am. 14:681, 1970.
3. Goldberg, M. H.: The changing biologic nature of acute dental infection, J.A.D.A. 80:1048, 1970.
4. Pogrel, M. A., and Welsby, P. D.: The dentist and prevention of infective endocarditis, Br. Dent. J. 139:12, 1975.
5. Rubin, R., Salvati, E. A., and Lewis, R.: Infected total hip replacement after dental procedures, Oral Surg. 41:18, 1976.
6. Zallen, R. D., and Curry, J. T.: A study of antibiotic usage in compound mandibular fractures, J. Oral Surg. 33:431, 1975.
7. Holroyd, S. V.: Antibiotics in the practice of periodontics, J. Periodontol. 42:584, 1971.
8. Karl, R. C., Mertz, J. J., Veith, F. J., and Dineen, P.: Prophylactic antimicrobial drugs in surgery, N. Engl. J. Med. 275:305, 1966.
9. Johnstone, F. R. C.: An assessment of prophylactic antibiotics in general surgery, Surg. Gynecol. Obstet. 116:1, 1963.
10. King, G. C.: The case against antibiotic prophylaxis in major head and neck surgery, Laryngoscope 71:647, 1961.
11. Hogman, C. F., and Sahlin, O.: Infections complicating gastric surgery, Acta Chir. Scand. 112:271, 1957.
12. Pulaski, E. J.: Antibiotics in surgical cases, Arch. Surg. 82:454, 1961.
13. McKittrick, L. S., and Wheelock, F. C.: The routine use of antibiotics in elective abdominal surgery, Surg. Gynecol. Obstet. 99:376, 1954.
14. Marshall, A.: Prophylactic antimicrobial therapy in retropubic prostatectomy, Br. J. Urol. 31:431, 1959.
15. Editorial: N. Engl. J. Med. 275:335, 1966.
16. Petersdorf, R. G., Curtin, J. S., Hoeprick, P. D., Peeler, R. N., and Bennett, I. L.: Study of antibiotic prophylaxis in unconscious patients, N. Engl. J. Med. 257:1001, 1957.
17. Petersdorf, R. G., and Merchant, R. K.: A study of antibiotic prophylaxis in patients with acute heart failure, N. Engl. J. Med. 265:565, 1959.
18. Lachdjiam, M. O., and Compere, E. C.: Postoperative wound infections in orthopedic surgery, J. Int. Coll. Surg. 28:797, 1957.
19. Taylor, G. W.: Preventive use of antibiotics in surgery. Br. Med. Bull. 16:51, 1960.
20. Weinstein, L.: Chemoprophylaxis of infection, Ann. Intern. Med. 43:287, 1955.
21. Cole, W. R., and Bernard, H. R.: A reappraisal of the effects of antimicrobial therapy during the course of appendicitis in children, Am. Surg. 27:29, 1961.
22. Stahl, S. S.: The healing of a gingival wound in protein-deprived, antibiotic-supplemented adult rats, Oral Surg. 17:993, 1964.
23. Schaefer, T. J., Collings, C. K., Bishop, J. G., and Dorman, H. L.: The effect of antibiotics on healing following osseous contouring in dogs, Periodontics 2:243, 1964.
24. Stahl, S. S., Soberman, A., and DeCesare, A.: Gingival healing. V. The effect of antibiotics administered during the early stages of repair, J. Periodontol. 40:521, 1969.
25. Ariaudo, A. A.: The efficacy of antibiotics in periodontal surgery: a controlled study with lincomycin and placebo in 68 patients, J. Periodontol. 40:150, 1969.
26. Med. Lett. Drug Ther. 9:104, 1967.
27. Gabrielson, M. L., and Stroh, E.: Antibiotic efficacy in odontogenic infections, J. Oral Surg. 33:607, 1975.
28. Chain, E., Florey, H. W., Jennings, M. A., and Williams, T. I.: Penicillin as chemotherapeutic agent, Lancet 2:226, 1940.

29. Krantz, J. C., Jr., and Carr, C. J.: The pharmacologic principles of medical practice, ed. 7, Baltimore, 1969, The Williams & Wilkins Co.
30. Oldstone, M. B. A., and Nelson, E.: Central nervous system manifestations of penicillin toxicity in man, Neurology 16:693, 1966.
31. Lerner, P. I., Smith, H., and Weinstein, L.: Penicillin neurotoxicity, Ann. N.Y. Acad. Sci. 145:310, 1967.
32. Schrier, R. W., Bulger, R. J., and van Arsdel, P. P., Jr.: Nephropathy associated with penicillin and homologues, Ann. Intern. Med. 64:116, 1966.
33. Baldwin, D. S., Levine, B. B., McCluskey, R. T., and Gallo, G. R.: Renal failure and interstitial nephritis due to penicillin and methicillin, N. Engl. J. Med. 279:1245, 1968.
34. White J. M., Brown, D. L., Hepner, B. W., and Worlledge, S. M.: Penicillin-induced haemolytic anaemia, Br. Med. J. 3:26, 1968.
35. Penicillin-induced haemolytic anaemia, Br. Med. J. 3:4, 1968.
36. Feigin, R. D., and Fiascone, A.: Hematuria and proteinuria associated with methicillin administration, N. Engl. J. Med. 272:903, 1965.
37. Feinberg, S. M.: Allergy from therapeutics products: incidence, importance, recognition, and prevention, J.A.M.A. 178:815, 1961.
38. Westerman, G., Corman, A., Stelos, P., and Nodine, J. H.: Adverse reactions to penicillin, J.A.M.A. 198(2):173, 1966.
39. Smith, J. W., Johnson, J. E., and Cluff, L. E.: Studies on the epidemiology of adverse drug reactions, N. Engl. J. Med. 274:998, 1966.
40. Isbister, J. P.: Penicillin allergy: a review of the immunological and clinical aspects, Med. J. Aust. 1:1067, 1971.
41. Idsoe, O., Guthe, T., Willcox, R. R., and deWeck, A. L.: Nature and extent of penicillin side reactions, with particular reference to fatalities from anaphylactic shock, Bull. W.H.O. 38:159, 1968.
42. Rudolph, A. H., and Price, E. V.: Penicillin reactions among patients in venereal disease clinics, J.A.M.A. 223:499, 1973.
43. Johnson, A.: Hypersensitivity to penicillin: a short review, Med. J. Aust. 2:432, 1962.
44. Welch, H., Lewis, C. N., Weinstein, H. F., and Boeckman, B. B.: Severe reactions to antibiotics, Antibiot. Med. 4:800, 1957.
45. Feinberg, S. M., and Feinberg, A. R.: Allergy to penicillin, J.A.M.A. 160:778, 1956.
46. Welch, H., Lewis, C. N., and Putnam, L. E.: Acute anaphylactoid reactions attributable to penicillin, Antibiot. Chemother. 3:891, 1953.
47. Cohen, S. B.: Brain damage due to penicillin, J.A.M.A. 186:899, 1963.
48. Batson, J. M.: Anaphylactoid reactions to oral administration of penicillin, N. Engl. J. Med. 262:590, 1960.
49. Coates, W. H.: A case of anaphylactic shock following the administration of oral penicillin, Aust. Dent. J. 8:189, 1963.
50. Dunn, J. H.: Oral penicillin and anaphylactoid reactions, J.A.M.A. 202:552, 1967.
51. Spark, R. P.: Fatal anaphylaxis due to oral penicillin, Am. J. Clin. Pathol. 56:407, 1971.
52. Glauda, N. M., Henefer, E. P., and Super, S.: Nonfatal anaphylaxis caused by oral penicillin: report of case, J.A.D.A. 90:159, 1975.
53. American Dental Association Council on Dental Therapeutics: Accepted dental therapeutics, ed. 35, Chicago, 1975, American Dental Association.
54. Pharmacotherapeutics in dental practice (NAV PERS 10486), Washington, D.C., 1969, Bureau of Naval Personel.
55. American Medical Association Department of Drugs: AMA drug evaluations, ed. 2, Chicago, 1973, American Medical Association.
56. Yet another penicillin, Br. Med. J. 4:466, 1970.
57. Shapiro, S., Siskind, V., Slone, D., Lewis, G. P., and Jick, H.: Drug rash with ampicillin and other penicillins, Lancet 2:969, 1969.
58. Skin reactions to ampicillin, Br. Med. J. 1:195, 1972.
59. Bass, J. W., Crowley, D. M., Steele, R. W., Young, F. S. H., and Harden, L. B.: Adverse effects of orally administered ampicillin, J. Pediatr. 83:106, 1973.
60. Report of a Collaborative Study Group: prospective study of ampicillin rash, Br. Med. J. 1:7, 1973.
61. Annotation: Ampicillin rashes, Lancet 2:993, 1969.
62. Pullen, H., Wright, N., and Murdoch, J. M.: Hypersensitivity reactions to antibacterial drugs in infectious mononucleosis, Lancet 2:1176, 1967.
63. Brown, G. L., and Kanwar, B. S.: Drug rashes in glandular fever, Lancet 2:1418, 1967.
64. Med. Lett. Drug Ther. 13:49, 1971.
65. Med. Lett. Drug Ther. 12:101, 1970.
66. Billow. B. W., Thompson, E. A., Stern, A., and Florio, A.: A clinical study of erythromycin: a comparative evaluation of several salts, Curr. Ther. Res. 6:381, 1964.
67. Clapper, W. E., Mostyn, M., and Meade, G. H.: An evaluation of erythromycin stearate and propionyl in normal and hospitalized subjects, Antibiot. Med. 7:91, 1960.
68. Sprunt, K., Leidy, G., and Redman, W.: Cross resistance between lincomycin and erythromycin in *viridans* streptococci, Pediatrics 46:84, 1970.
69. Kunin, C. M., and Atuk, N.: Excretion of cephaloridine and cephalothin in patients with renal impairment, N. Engl. J. Med. 274:654, 1966.
70. Benner, E. J.: Renal damage associated with prolonged administration of ampicillin, cephaloridine and cephalothin, Antimicrob. Agents Chemother. 9:417, 1969.
71. Med. Lett. Drugs Ther. 10:45, 1968.
72. Kagan, B. M.: Antimicrobial therapy, ed. 2, Philadelphia, 1974, W. B. Saunders Co.
73. Mohr, J. A., Rhoades, E. R., and Muchmore, H. G.: Actinomycosis treated with lincomycin, J.A.M.A. 21:2260, 1970.
74. Med. Lett. Drug Ther. 11:107, 1969.
75. Davis, W. M., and Balcom, J. H.: Lincomycin studies of drug absorption and efficacy, Oral Surg. 27:688, 1969.
76. Khosla, V. M.: Lincomycin in oral surgery, Oral Surg. 29:485, 1970.
77. Phillips, I., Fernandes, R., and Warren, C.: In vitro comparison of erythromycin, lincomycin, and clindamycin, Br. Med. J. 2:89, 1970.
78. Geddes, A. M., Bridgwater, F. A., Williams, D. N., Oon, J., and Grimshaw, G. J.: Clinical and

bacteriological studies with clindamycin, Br. Med. J. 2:703, 1970.

79. Sanders, E.: Lincomycin: fact, fancy, and future, Med. Clin. North Am. 54:1295, 1970.

80. Swartzberg, K. E., Maresca, R. M., and Remington, J. S.: Gastro-intestinal side effects associated with clindamycin, Arch. Intern. Med. 136:876, 1976.

81. Cohen, L. E., McNeill, C. J., and Wells, R. F.: Clindamycin associated colitis, J.A.M.A. 223:1379, 1973.

82. Wells, R. F., Cohen, L. E., and McNeill, C. J.: Clindamycin and pseudomembranous colitis, Lancet 1:66, 1974.

83. Tedesco, F. J., Stanley, R. J., and Alpers, D. H.: Diagnostic features of clindamycin—associated pseudomembranous colitis, N. Engl. J. Med. 290: 841, 1974.

84. Any questions? Tetracycline in breast milk, Br. Med. J. 4:5686, 1969.

85. Barr, W. H., Adir, J., and Barnetson, L.: Decrease of tetracycline absorption in man by sodium bicarbonate, Clin. Pharmacol. Ther. 12:779, 1971.

86. Wruble, L. D., Lodman. A. J., Britt, L. G., and Cummins, A. J.: Hepatotoxicity produced by tetracycline overdosage, J.A.M.A. 192:6, 1965.

87. Peters, R. L.: Tetracycline induced fatty liver in nonpregnant patients: a report of 6 cases, Am. J. Surg. 113:622, 1967.

88. Dowling, H. F., and Lepper, M. H.: Hepatic reactions to tetracycline, J.A.M.A. 188:307, 1964.

89. Whalley, P. J., Odoms, R. H., and Combes, B.: Tetracycline toxicity in pregnancy, J.A.M.A. 189: 357, 1964.

90. Sulkowski, S. R., and Haserick, J. R.: Simulated systemic lupus erythematosus from degraded tetracycline, J.A.M.A. 189:152, 1964.

91. Primpter, G. W., Timpanelli, A. E., Eisenmunger, W. J., Stein, H. S., and Ehrlich, L. F.: Reversible "Fanconi syndrome" caused by degraded tetracycline, J.A.M.A. 184:111, 1963.

92. Goth, A.: Medical pharmacology: principles and concepts, ed. 5, St. Louis, 1976, The C. V. Mosby Co.

93. Pollen, R. H.: Anaphylactoid reaction to orally administered dimethylchlortetracycline, N. Engl. J. Med. 271:673, 1964.

94. Med. Lett. Drug Ther. 7:72, 1965.

95. Med. Lett. Drug Ther. 6:85, 1964.

96. Graykowski, E. A., Barile, M. F., Lee, W. B., and Stanley, H. R., Jr.: Recurrent aphthous stomatitis: clinical, therapeutic, histopathologic, and hypersensitivity aspects, J.A.M.A. 196:637, 1966.

97. Polak, B. C. P., Wesseling, H., Herxheimer, A., and Meyler, L.: Blood dyscrasias attributed to chloramphenicol, Acta Med. Scand. 192:409, 1972.

98. Med. Lett. Drug Ther. 10:50, 1968.

99. Rodriguez, V., Whitecar, J. P., Jr., and Bodey, G. P.: Therapy of infections with the combination of carbinicillin and gentamicin, Antimicrob. Agents Chemother. 9:386, 1969.

100. Khan, M. Y., and Hall, W. H.: Staphylococcic enterocolitis treated with oral vancomycin, Ann. Intern. Med. 65:1, 1966.

101. Scopp, I. W., Gillette, W., Kumar, V., and Larato, D.: Treatment of oral lesions with topically applied vancomycin hydrochloride, Oral Surg. 24:703, 1967.

102. Mitchell, D. F., and Holmes, L. A.: Topical antibiotic control of dentogingival plaque, J. Periodontol. 36:202, 1965.

103. Kinsky, S. C.: Nystatin binding by protoplasts and a particulate fraction of *Neurospora crassa*, and a basis for the selective toxicity of polyene antifungal antibiotics, Proc. Natl. Acad. Sci. USA 48:1049, 1962.

104. Fraleigh, C. M.: An evaluation of topical Terramycin in post-gingivectomy pack, J. Periodontol. 27: 201, 1956.

105. Baer, P. N., Goldman. H. M., and Seigliano, J.: Studies on a bacitracin periodontal dressing, Oral Surg. 11:712, 1958.

106. Zegarelli, E. V., and Kutscher, A. H.: Oral moniliasis following intraoral topical corticosteroid therapy, J. Oral Ther. Pharm. 1:304, 1964.

107. Med. Lett. Drug Ther. 12:29, 1970.

108. Lehner, T.: Candidal fungaemia following extraction of teeth and its relationship to systemic candidiasis, Br. Dent. J. 117:253, 1964.

109. Kutscher, A. H., Zegarelli, E. V., Herlands, R. E., and Silvers, H. F.: Amphotericin B in the treatment of oral monilial infections, Oral Surg. 17:31, 1964.

110. Alban, J., and Grael, J.: Amphotericin B oral suspension in the treatment, Curr. Ther. Res. 12:479, 1970.

111. Normark, S., and Schonebeck, J.: In vitro studies of 5-fluorocytosine resistance in *Candida albicans* and *Torulopsis glabrata*, Antimicrob. Agents Chemother. 2:114, 1972.

112. Weissmann, G., and Sessa, G.: The action of polyene antibiotics on phospholipid-cholesterol structures, J. Biol. Chem. 242:616, 1967.

113. Cutting, W.: Handbook of pharmacology, ed. 3, New York, 1967, The Meredith Publishing Co.

114. Sutherland, V. C.: A synopsis of pharmacology, ed. 2, Philadelphia, 1970, W. B. Saunders Co.

115. Med. Lett. Drug Ther. 8:13, 1966.

116. Cohlan, S. Q.: Erythema multiforme exudativum associated with the use of sulfomethoxypyridazine, J.A.M.A. 173:799, 1960.

117. Cappuccio, J. P., and Dobbs, E. C.: Clinical evaluation of sulfodimethoxine, a long acting antibacterial sulfonamide, in oral infections, J. Oral Surg. 18:230, 1960.

118. Norris, J. P., and Becker, E. F.: A clinical comparison of sulfodimethoxine and penicillin in the endodontic management of acute dentoalveolar infection, J. Oral Ther. Pharm. 1:376, 1955.

119. Symposium: Trimethoprim-sulfamethoxazole, J. Infect. Dis. 128:(supp.)425, 1973.

120. Nolte, H., and Büttner, H.: Pharmacokinetics of trimethoprim and its combinations with sulfamethoxazole in man after single and chronic oral administration, Chemotherapy 18:274, 1973.

121. Svindland, H. B.: Treatment of gonorrhea with sulphamethoxazole-trimethoprim: lack of effect on concomitant syphilis, Br. J. Vener. Dis. 49:50, 1973.

122. Brumfitt, W., and Pursell, R.: Observations on bacterial sensitivities to nalidixic acid and critical

comments on 6-centre survey, Postgrad. Med. J. **47**:16, 1971.

123. Pratt, W. B.: Fundamentals of chemotherapy, New York, 1973, Oxford University Press.
124. Maxwell, E.: Treatment of herpes keratitis with 5-iodo-2-deoxyuridine (IDU): a clinical evaluation of 1500 cases, Am. J. Ophthalmol. **56**:571, 1963.
125. Jaffe, E. C., and Lehner, T.: Treatment of herpetic stomatitis with idoxuridine, Br. Dent. J. **125**:392, 1968.
126. Nafta, I., Turcanu, A. G., Braun, I., Companetz, W., Simionescu, A. B. E., and Florea, V.: Administration of amatandine for the prevention of Hong Kong influenza, Bull. W.H.O. **42**:423, 1970.

127. Togo, Y., Hornick, R. B., and Dawkins, A. T.: Studies on induced influenza in man. I. Double-blind studies designed to assess prophylactic efficacy of amantadine hydrochloride against A2/Rockville/1/65 strain, J.A.M.A. **203**:1089, 1968.
128. Wingfield, W. L., Pollack, D., and Grunert, R. R.: Therapeutic efficacy of amantadine HCl and rimantadine HCl in naturally occurring influenza A2 respiratory illness in man, N. Engl. J. Med. **281**:579, 1969.
129. American Medical Association Council on Drugs: The amantadine controversy, J.A.M.A. **201**:372, 1967.

21

Antiseptics and disinfectants

GEORGE B. PELLEU, Jr.

The application of antimicrobial measures in dentistry began with the realization that many diseases could be transmitted from one patient to another by contaminated dental instruments. Over the years, many physical and chemical methods for removing or destroying microorganisms have been tested. This chapter provides a review and evaluation of various methods of sterilization and disinfection with an emphasis on chemical means. However, prior to discussions of specific methods and agents, certain terms must be clearly defined.

Sterilization is the process by which all forms of life within a particular environment are totally destroyed. *Disinfection* is the process of reducing microbial populations in an environment with particular emphasis on the killing of pathogenic microorganisms. A disinfectant is an agent capable of accomplishing this result. Disinfection, like sterilization, may be achieved with the use of chemical agents or from the application of physical means, for example, boiling water. The levels of disinfection accomplished by chemical agents are discussed under the subject of chemical methods.

Antiseptic is the term ordinarily used to denote a compound that can be applied to living tissue to disinfect or to kill pathogenic microorganisms. Most disinfectants are destructive to tissue and cannot be used as antiseptics. In some special cases, however, a disinfectant may be used as an antiseptic. For example, disinfectants have been used as antiseptics in root canal treatment. In cases like this the solution strength and exposure time will usually differ for the type of disinfectant or antiseptic used.

☐ The opinions or assertions contained herein are the private ones of the writer and are not to be construed as official or as reflecting the views of the Navy Department or the naval service at large.

Antimicrobial agents may affect microorganisms by killing (*-cidal* agents) or by inhibiting growth (*-static* agents). A *bactericidal* agent is one capable of killing bacteria, whereas a *bacteriostatic* agent is one that inhibits or prevents multiplication of bacteria. There is no clear distinction between these activities. An agent that is bactericidal under certain conditions may be only bacteriostatic when used in lower concentrations or for shorter times of exposure.

PHYSICAL METHODS OF STERILIZATION

Physical methods are the most practical and dependable means of achieving sterilization. A physical method should always be considered before resorting to a chemical method. For this reason a brief discussion of physical methods is presented.

Steam under pressure

The use of heat is usually the most certain method of killing microorganisms. Heat is used in many forms, but generally the more moisture present the more rapid will be the lethal effect.

Steam under pressure is the most effective and quickest medium for sterilization. At 15 pounds' pressure, steam reaches a temperature of 121° C (250° F) in an autoclave and kills all forms of life in about 15 minutes. Some materials, like anhydrous oils, greases, and powders, cannot be sterilized in the autoclave because they are impervious to steam.

A variety of autoclaves with automatic controls to ensure proper operation are available. The operator of an autoclave should be aware of the precautions to be observed and limitations inherent in the use of the equipment. A sterilizing cycle must be timed by the reading on the temperature gauge and *not* the reading on the pressure gauge. The air within the autoclave must always be

221

completely replaced with free-flowing steam before the sterilizing cycle begins. A minimum time of 15 minutes is usually adequate, but about 30 minutes is needed if the autoclave is fully loaded or the materials are only slightly porous to steam. Wrappings for materials to be sterilized should be porous to steam but must also offer protection against outside contamination during storage.

Boiling water

Boiling water seldom accomplishes sterilization because the temperature can never be high enough to destroy viruses or bacterial spores. A boiling time of 10 to 20 minutes will usually destroy most vegetative forms, but spores and viruses are known to survive boiling for several hours. A small amount of sodium carbonate added to the water will reduce the possibility of damage to metal instruments and accelerate the death rate of microorganisms.

Dry heat

Dry heat, in an enclosed space, is another medium by which sterilization can be achieved. Dentists use this method of sterilization less frequently than other conventional methods because it is slow and limited in application to only a few types of materials. Wider application of dry heat could be made in dentistry, particularly for sterilizing materials like glassware, sharp instruments, petrolatum, oils, and powders. The main advantage of dry heat sterilization is in its penetrating power and its lack of deleterious effects on metals and glass surfaces.

The following temperature-time relationships are recommended for sterilizing materials in an oven:

170° C (338° F)	60 minutes
160° C (320° F)	120 minutes

Higher temperatures may be used for shorter times, but most paper materials and cotton textiles begin to scorch above 170° C.

Hot materials

A well sterilizer containing glass or metal beads, or common table salt crystals, can be used at chair side to quickly sterilize small instruments. The instruments are plunged deep within the material, which is maintained at temperatures above 232° C (450° F), for times of no less than 10 seconds. The difficulty with this method is in the temperature variation at different sites within the well.

Hot oils, including liquid petrolatum and silicone fluids, can be used to sterilize instruments with movable parts such as handpieces. Although exposures at temperatures of 160° C for 1 hour are used, the efficacy of hot oils for sterilization is questionable. Furthermore, silicone fluids must be removed from instruments after the procedure because many are toxic to tissues.

Incineration

Incineration by gas or alcohol flaming is another method of sterilization, but to be effective, instruments must be heated to redness, which destroys the temper of the metal. Dipping instruments in 70% to 90% alcohol and burning it off is not an effective means of sterilization.

Radiation

Practical application of radiation types of energy for sterilization and disinfection has been limited to two forms of electromagnetic radiation: (1) ultraviolet light, which is of relatively long wavelength, and (2) ionizing short-wave radiations (gamma rays and x rays).

The bactericidal effect of sunlight and rays in the ultraviolet wavelengths has been known for many years. Artificially produced ultraviolet light is used for sterilization and disinfection of flat surfaces and moving air. However, ultraviolet waves have little penetrating power so that their application is limited.

In practice, mercury vapor lamps generating wavelengths of 2537 Ångström units (Å) are used as sources of ultraviolet light. Killing of microorganisms is dependent on the amount of energy absorbed from the beam of light, the intensity of the light, the distance of the source of light, and the availability of the cell for exposure. Care must be taken by the user to avoid direct contact with skin and eyes.

Ionizing radiations are used routinely in sterilizing foods, plastic materials, and pharmaceuticals. The application of this form of radiation will undoubtedly be expanded, but its use is limited because of high costs and the deleterious effect of large doses of radiation on materials.

Ultrasonic vibration

Ultrasonic vibration is used principally in breaking up bacterial cell walls for the release of cell contents, but it is not a practical method of sterilization because most microorganisms are resistant to intense sonic and ultrasonic vibrations. Death of microorganisms occurs only in liquid suspensions, where physical destruction is brought about by cavitation, which is the rhythmic forming and collapsing of gas bubbles that occurs within the cell. The uses for ultrasonics have not been fully explored, but in dentistry ultrasonics are effectively used in scaling teeth and in cleaning dental instruments.

Filtration

Filtration, such as that obtained with Millipore units, involves the separation of solid particles from liquids or gases. This is a practical method of sterilizing many liquids, particularly those which are heat labile. There are available relatively inexpensive high efficiency particulate air (HEPA) filters and electrostatic precipitation air cleaners that can effectively reduce concentrations of viable airborne microorganisms in dental operating rooms.

Pressure, desiccation, and freezing

Pressure, desiccation, and freezing should not be relied on for sterilization, but they will produce various levels of disinfection. Pressures as high as several thousand atmospheres will kill some but not all bacteria. Vegetative forms of most bacteria are sensitive to drying. Resistance to drying varies among species; for example, the tubercle bacillus and spores of certain bacteria are highly resistant to drying. Low temperatures arrest growth but are not bactericidal. Temperatures below 0° C in general have a preservative effect on microorganisms. Microorganisms are known to survive the extremely low temperatures of liquid hydrogen ($-250°$ C). Although freeze-dry procedures have been used to preserve microorganisms for many years, repeated freeze-thaw procedures do exert a lethal effect on bacteria.

CHEMICAL METHODS

Chemical disinfection was primarily popularized by Lord Lister, who, in the 1860s, experimented with the use of carbolic acid (phenol) to achieve aseptic surgery. He disinfected surgical instruments by soaking them in a 5% phenol solution. Since that time, chemists have produced a variety of disinfectants for this purpose. The chemical compounds are convenient to use, and there is a need for them because many materials that must be disinfected are destroyed by heat. Chemical disinfection is a controversial subject, however, primarily because of the contradictory statements made about its value. There is no general agreement as to the best product to use, and practitioners are faced with an array of "all purpose disinfectants."

No one disinfectant can qualify as the ideal agent for all situations. These questions must be asked: What should a disinfectant solution be required to do? Should it destroy vegetative bacteria only? Or should it also destroy the tubercle bacillus, fungi, lipid and nonlipid viruses, and spores? Most of the latter microorganisms are more resistant than vegetative forms of bacteria, and a more powerful disinfectant is required to destroy them.

Spaulding[1] classifies the disinfectant action of chemical agents on three levels: First-level disinfection produces sterility if time of contact is adequate. Second-level disinfection kills vegetative forms of bacteria, fungi, lipid and nonlipid viruses, and tubercle bacilli, but *not* spores. Third-level disinfection kills only vegetative forms of bacteria, fungi, and lipid-containing viruses.

Another factor that must be considered is the risk of infection through direct contact with the particular item or material requiring sterilization or disinfection. Spaulding[1] divides items into three categories on this basis and relates the categories to the level of disinfection required:

1. Critical items carry the greatest risk of infection because they are introduced beneath the surface of the body. Sterility, or first-level disinfection, is required.
2. Semicritical items make direct contact with mucous membranes, which act as a barrier to infection. Second-level disinfection is usually sufficient for these items.

3. Noncritical items that do not come in direct contact with the patient need only third-level disinfection. They would be treated in the same manner as furniture and similar articles within the dental operatory.

One must also decide what is practical for a given situation. The level of disinfection achieved depends on many factors, for example, types and numbers of microorganisms present, the nature and cleanliness of the materials to be disinfected, the nature and concentration of the disinfectant used, and the time of contact.

The principal disinfectants in current use, the level of disinfection achieved with them, and the advantages and disadvantages they present are discussed in the following paragraphs.

First-level disinfection

There are three chemical disinfectants that can be used to sterilize critical items. These are gaseous ethylene oxide, aqueous solutions of glutaraldehyde, and aqueous solutions of formaldehyde. It should be emphasized that whenever spores are present, several hours of contact with liquid disinfectants may be needed to sterilize critical items.

Ethylene oxide

Ethylene oxide is used as a gaseous agent. Although the bactericidal properties of ethylene oxide were known as early as 1929, its use for this purpose did not begin until 1949. For the dental profession it is still a relatively new medium that has unlimited possibilities for successful application. Ethylene oxide is a gas at ordinary temperatures, liquefies at 10.8° C, and freezes at −111.3° C. It can be obtained either in the pure state as a liquid under pressure or mixed with carbon dioxide or fluorinated hydrocarbons to produce a nonflammable mixture. Each preparation has special advantages for the particular situation. Ethylene oxide is the most reliable substance available for gaseous sterilization. Among its advantages are that in a gaseous state it is seldom damaging to materials, it is effective at room temperature, it is effective at low humidities, it leaves no residual chemical, it is microbicidal, and it is highly penetrative. The primary disadvantage is its slowness in action, but the time required for

sterilization can be reduced to about 1 hour by increasing the temperature to 130° F (54° C) or by using higher concentrations of gas. Proper ventilation should be employed to avoid direct inhalation of vapors. A gas sterilizer can be any airtight container, ranging from a complex autoclave to a simple heavy plastic bag. Other chemicals used as gaseous agents are propylene oxide, propiolactone, methyl bromide, ethylene glycol, formaldehyde, and ozone. The application of these agents in dentistry has not been fully explored.

Formaldehyde

An 8% aqueous solution of formaldehyde (20% formalin) will kill vegetative bacteria, the tubercle bacillus, spores, and viruses. A combination of 20% formalin and 70% isopropyl alcohol is more effective and requires less time to produce sterility. The primary disadvantages of formaldehyde solutions are the noxious fumes given off and the solutions' toxicity to the tissues. All items disinfected in formaldehyde solution must be thoroughly rinsed before use.

As a gaseous agent, formaldehyde has for many years been widely used for disinfecting vertical and horizontal surfaces in enclosed areas. It vaporizes at and above room temperature, and in this gaseous state diffuses to surfaces, where it condenses to form either formaldehyde solution (formalin) or paraformaldehyde, an ineffective reversible polymer. A high relative humidity is required for the production of formalin and effective sterilization. Gaseous formaldehyde is most useful for surface disinfection because it has poor penetrating power; it also leaves irritating residues, which require that materials be well aired or washed before use.

Glutaraldehyde

Glutaraldehyde is a promising disinfectant for use in dentistry. It does not harm lensed instruments or materials that would be damaged by alcohol, and it is said to have a relatively low order of toxicity. A 2% alkalinized aqueous solution of glutaraldehyde (CIDEX) is about equal in activity to 8% aqueous formaldehyde. To be effective the disinfectant must be alkalinized from pH 7.5 to 8.5 with a base like sodium bicarbonate. Solutions lose activity in about 2 weeks at room temperature and must be replaced.

Second- and third-level disinfection

The following disinfectants are used under semicritical and noncritical conditions.

Alcohols

The germicidal action of ethanol and isopropyl alcohol is generally underrated. Although ethanol (CH_3CH_2OH) is used most commonly, isopropyl alcohol ($CH_3CHOH-CH_3$) is a less volatile and slightly more active disinfectant. At a concentration of 70%, aqueous solutions act as protein coagulants. In addition to being good second level disinfectants for semicritical and noncritical items, alcohols remove the protective lipid layers on skin that act as a barrier to microorganisms, and they leave no residue after evaporating on surfaces.

Phenol

Phenol and phenolic compounds are strong antibacterial agents. Phenol (carbolic acid) kills most vegetative bacteria at a 1:100 dilution. A 5% solution has been used to disinfect surgical instruments. Phenol is seldom used currently as a disinfectant, but many compounds derived from it are commonly employed in housekeeping procedures for noncritical medical and surgical items. Cresols, for example, used in a mixture known as tricresol, are considerably more effective than is phenol. The phenolics are not readily inactivated by organic compounds and remain effective for long periods of time; they are also extremely toxic to tissues.

Mercury

At high concentrations the soluble forms of mercury are bactericidal, but they are too injurious for use on tissues. Organic compounds of mercury are used as skin disinfectants, but they are of doubtful practical value. Except for the lethal effect on some nonlipid viruses, the mercurials have little application in modern disinfection.

Detergents

Chemical agents in this group are low level disinfectants with the ability to destroy certain vegetative cells only. There are two general types of detergents: anionic and cationic. The detergent action concentrates at the surface of the bacterial cell wall by first dissolving the lipid film around bacteria and then disrupting the normal function of the cell membrane. Quaternary ammonium compounds, called "quats," are the most commonly used agents of this group. They are cationic detergents active against all types of bacteria. One of these cationic agents, benzalkonium chloride (Zephiran Chloride), is nonirritating to tissues and widely used in dentistry for disinfecting materials and instruments. It is normally used in a dilution of 1:1000, but a 1:500 dilution has been recommended in the interest of public safety. Benzalkonium chloride is bactericidal to staphylococci in dilutions as high as 1:400,000. The major disadvantage of this group of disinfectants is that they are readily inactivated by many materials, and fresh solutions must be prepared frequently.

Oxidizing agents

Among the principal oxidizing agents are the halogens, hydrogen peroxide, potassium permanganate, and ozone. These compounds exert their "-cidal" or "-static" effect by oxidizing chemical groups essential for microbial enzyme activity. The reaction may be reversible or irreversible depending on the strength of the agent.

Halogens. Chlorine, bromine, iodine, and fluorine compounds are all bactericides, with chlorine being the most active and fluorine the least active of the group.

Chlorine. Chlorine has been used for many years in the purification of water and disinfection of hospital areas. Chlorine will kill vegetative cells, is tuberculocidal and virucidal, and has some sporicidal activity in 5% solution. It is an excellent disinfectant for semicritical and noncritical items. Chlorine is most effective in acid solutions and is available commercially as 5% or 0.5% sodium hypochlorite solution, which is still the most practical disinfectant for general use. The major disadvantages of chlorine are that it is corrosive to surgical instruments and is rapidly inactivated by organic material.

Iodine. Iodine is a second-level disinfectant for use with semicritical and noncritical items. Iodine, like chlorine, is unstable and is readily inactivated when organic materials are present in a solution. In 2% to 7% tincture form, iodine is an effective antiseptic for use on the skin, being strongly bactericidal against many kinds of microorganisms including the tubercle bacillus and bacterial spores. The stronger, 7% solution of iodine, however, is destructive to exposed tissue, and for this reason the milder tincture is more widely used.

The mixing of iodine with surface active agents to produce *iodophors* brings about a slow release of iodine. Unlike tinctures of iodine, iodophors are nonirritating and non-staining. These compounds change from the normal brown to pale yellow when they lose their effectiveness.

Bromine and fluorine. Although bromine and fluorine are microbicidal, they are seldom used as disinfectants because of their irritating properties.

Hydrogen peroxide. Hydrogen peroxide (H_2O_2) in a 3% solution is a harmless but relatively ineffective antiseptic because it is rapidly destroyed by catalase produced by tissues and bacteria.

Potassium permanganate. Potassium permanganate is a strong oxidizing solution used primarily in urethral infections at a concentration of 1:1000. For general use, however, the solution stains and is easily inactivated by inert organic materials.

Ozone. Ozone is a strong but unstable oxidizing substance. It rapidly kills bacteria, viruses, and cysts of protozoa in water and has been extensively used for many years in the purification of water. It is too expensive, however, to compete with chlorine for water treatment. Ozone has also been advocated for use in disinfection of air, but ozone concentrations needed for this purpose are well above the threshold limit value of 0.1 ppm established by the American Conference of Governmental Industrial Hygienists.

DISINFECTION OF INANIMATE OBJECTS

Proper cleansing of dental items is essential before sterilization and disinfection procedures are undertaken. Coagulated protein such as blood and other debris, which may protect microorganisms or inactivate disinfecting solutions, must be removed by thorough cleansing. Another factor that must be considered is the construction of instruments. Many items are constructed for easy cleansing, but others contain crevices or areas inaccessible to scrubbing. Ultrasonic cleaners of multifrequency wavelengths can be used with highly satisfactory results.

The method of disinfection used for dental equipment, instruments, and materials depends on the level of disinfection desired and the item to be treated. If *sterility* is needed, the autoclave is the most reliable and practical means available. Heat in any form is more effective than chemicals and should be used in preference to them. Some items are destroyed by heat, however, and chemical methods must be considered. *Dental instruments* made of stainless steel can be sterilized in the autoclave without appreciable harm, but sharp cutting edges are best preserved by sterilizing instruments with ethylene oxide gas or by dry heat. Oil suspensions or emulsions used to coat instruments before autoclaving to prevent corrosion may inhibit sterilization by placing a protective barrier around microorganisms.

Dental handpieces that cannot be sterilized in the autoclave present a special problem. If sterilization is required, ethylene oxide gas is the best medium. If a lower level of disinfection is acceptable, ethyl alcohol or some other chemical disinfectant wipe may be used. *Cloth* materials and cotton should be sterilized in the autoclave and not in the hot air oven because temperatures above 170° C may scorch them. *Rubber* articles such as gloves and the rubber dam may be sterilized in the autoclave or with ethylene oxide gas. Repeated exposure to autoclaving will eventually deteriorate rubber products. *Glassware* may be sterilized in the autoclave, but for items that must be dried the hot air oven is best. *Oils, greases,* and *powders* should be sterilized in the hot air oven because steam in an autoclave does not permeate these substances. *Endodontic instruments* can be sterilized at chair side in a well containing molten metal, table salt, steel balls, or glass beads heated to very high temperatures. The major difficulties of this method lie in the application of proper times needed for sterilization and in the deleterious effect of the high temperatures on the metal. It is preferable to sterilize endodontic instruments with steam under pressure, dry heat, or ethylene oxide.

TISSUE ANTISEPSIS

The microbicidal effectiveness of antiseptics in contact with tissues is questionable. In vitro testing for disinfection does not accurately indicate effectiveness under conditions of actual use. Many factors in tissues act to inhibit the effectiveness of antiseptics.

Furthermore, chemical agents must be in contact with tissues for adequate times before a lethal reaction can take place. This means that sterilization of tissues by the use of chemical agents is difficult without tissue damage.

The complete elimination of all forms of microorganisms on skin is impractical, but effective reductions in number can be achieved with a program of combined scrubbing and antiseptic treatment. Alcohol, particularly of the isopropyl type, is the most popular compound and is a highly effective skin antiseptic. Other antiseptics used for this purpose include benzalkonium chloride and iodine.

INTRACANAL ANTISEPSIS

Another area of controversy is the efficacy of antimicrobial agents (medicaments) for disinfecting root canals in endodontic therapy. Although classified as antiseptics by virtue of their use in tissues, many are actually disinfectants and toxic to tissues. The more effective an antimicrobial agent is the more toxic it will be to tooth tissues. Sodium hypochlorite is probably the most popular medicament employed as an irrigating solution. The two most widely used intracanal dressings are camphorated parachlorophenol and meta-cresyl-acetate (Cresatin). These agents will provide only second- or third-level disinfection. Camphorated parachlorophenol is a phenol derivative that has been used since 1891 as a root canal disinfectant.[2] The camphor in the compound serves as a diluent and is said to reduce the irritating and caustic effect of pur chlorophenol. Meta-cresyl-acetate is the acetic acid ester of meta-cresol with fungicidal properties.

REFERENCES

1. Spaulding, E. H.: In Lawrence, C. A., and Block, S. S., editors: Disinfection, sterilization, and preservation, Philadelphia, 1968, Lea & Febiger.
2. Penick, E. C., and Osetek, E. M.: Intracanal drugs and chemicals in endodontic therapy, Dent. Clin. North Am. 14:743-756, Oct., 1970.

BIBLIOGRAPHY

Appleton, J. L. T.: Bacterial infection in dental practice, ed. 4, Philadelphia, 1950, Lea & Febiger.

Benarde, M. A., editor: Disinfection, New York, 1970, Marcell Dekker, Inc.

Burnett, G. W., and Scherp, H. W.: Oral microbiology and infectious disease, ed. 3, Baltimore, 1968, The Williams & Wilkins Co.

Burrows, W., editor: Textbook of microbiology, ed. 18, Philadelphia, 1963, W. B. Saunders Co.

Carpenter, P. L.: Microbiology, Philadelphia, 1972, W. B. Saunders Co.

Schilder, H., editor: Symposium on endodontics, The Dental Clinics of North America, Philadelphia, November, 1967, W. B. Saunders Co.

Grossman, L. I.: Endodontic practice, ed. 7, Philadelphia, 1970, Lea & Febiger.

Jawetz, E., Melnick, J. L., and Adelberg, E. A.: Review of medical microbiology, ed. 10, Los Altos, Calif., 1972, Lange Medical Publications.

Lawrence, C. A., and Block, S. S.: Disinfection, sterilization, and preservation, Philadelphia, 1968, Lea & Febiger.

Reddish, G. F., editor: Antiseptics, disinfectants, fungicides, and chemical and physical sterilization, Philadelphia, 1954, Lea & Febiger.

Smith, D. T., Conant, N. F., and Willett, H. P.: Zinsser microbiology, ed. 14, New York, 1968, Appleton-Century-Crofts.

Sykes, G., editor: Disinfection and sterilization, Princeton, N.J., 1958, D. Van Nostrand Co., Inc.

Wilson, G. S., and Miles, A. A.: Topley and Wilson's principles of bacteriology and immunity, Baltimore, 1964, The Williams & Wilkins Co.

22

Fluorides

R. C. TERHUNE

The effects of fluorides on biologic systems have been the subject of an ever-increasing amount of investigation since the fact was determined in the 1930s that small amounts of fluoride had a remarkable effect on the human dentition. There are presently enough textbooks, periodicals, and reports of clinical and laboratory research about the subject to fill a library. Nevertheless, despite all the accumulation of knowledge about fluorides, there is much remaining to be learned about their chemistry and mechanisms of action in biologic systems. Because of widely disseminated misinformation about fluorides, their effects on humans are still a subject of considerable controversy among many laymen. Although the beneficial effects of fluorides are widely recognized by scientists knowledgeable in the field, there is still disagreement about precise mechanisms of action and the value of various fluoride compounds.

It is extremely important for the dentist to have a good understanding of the action of fluorides on both the dentition and the remainder of the body. In addition to helping him provide his patients with the best possible preventive dental care, this information will enable the dentist to answer convincingly the inevitable questions posed by patients regarding the action and value of fluorides. Only by being highly knowledgeable on the subject of fluorides can the dentist properly evaluate and reply to the misinformation about their use and effects and be an effective spokesman for community fluoridation measures.

After a brief overall review of the occur-

rence, metabolism and toxicity of fluorides, the bulk of the material in this chapter is devoted to the current status of fluoride therapy for dental diseases. Fluoridation of communal water supplies and some other methods of systemic application are examined first, followed by a discussion of the major approaches to topical fluoride therapy.

OCCURRENCE OF FLUORIDE

Fluorine (F) is the most electronegative chemical element and is so reactive that it is rarely, if ever, encountered in nature as elemental fluorine. Chemically combined in the form of fluoride, it is one of the most ubiquitous of all elements, being the seventeenth most common in the earth's crust.[1] Although the two principal sources of fluoride available to humans are the water they drink and the foods and drugs they consume, it is even present in the air they breathe. In short, fluoride, is everywhere and in everything humans take into their bodies.

Water derives its fluoride content primarily from its solvent action on the rocks and soil of the earth's crust. The fluoride content of soil tends to increase with depth. Fluoride occurs most commonly as fluorspar (CaF_2) but is also found in a wide variety of minerals such as apatite, the micas, hornblende, topaz, and cryolite, to name only a few. The amount of fluoride present in the water washing over these minerals depends on the solubility of the particular mineral present. In most cases the solubility is low. When fluoride compounds are dissolved in water, fluorine is mainly present as the fluoride ion F^-. Fluoride levels tend to be high in alkaline waters and in water with a relatively high temperature such as is associated with volcanic activity. Surface waters are generally low in fluoride, whereas underground waters may contain appreciable amounts because of

□ The opinions or assertions contained herein are the private ones of the writer and are not to be construed as official or as reflecting the views of the Navy Department or the naval service at large.

their greater opportunity to contact fluoride-containing minerals.

Virtually every food consumed by humans contains fluoride in at least trace amounts. Some foods such as tea and some varieties of fish have very high levels of fluoride. Plants used as food derive fluoride from soil and water, whereas animals used as food derive fluoride from plants and other animals they eat as well as from the water they consume. The fluoride content of food will also be influenced by the fluoride content of the water in which it is prepared. With the exception of drugs administered as anticariogenic agents and for treatment of skeletal disorders, most fluorides contained in drugs are in biologically inert forms and are thus unavailable for metabolism.

Considerable amounts of fluoride may enter the human environment as dusts and vapors. The dusts may be from surface soil containing large quantities of fluoride or from industrial processes. Vapors are entirely of industrial origin. The physiologic effects of these fluoride-containing dusts and vapors may result from swallowing as well as from inhalation. Deposition of dusts on plants and in water supplies will also increase human fluoride consumption.

Total consumption of fluoride will vary considerably in accordance with the fluoride content of the food and water an individual consumes, as previously discussed, and with the volume consumed. The average 1- to 3-year-old child consumes approximately 500 ml water a day and the adult, approximately 1 liter. If the water contains 1 ppm of fluoride, they will consume 0.5 and 1 mg fluoride a day, respectively, from their drinking water. Fluoride intake by adults from food exclusive of drinking water in some communities in the United States ranges from 0.34 mg to as high as 3.13 mg.[1]

FLUORIDE METABOLISM

As has been explained, fluoride ions may be ingested by means of food and water or inhaled as vapors or particulate matter in the air. Inhaled fluorides from dust or vapors are rapidly and almost completely absorbed into the bloodstream through the respiratory tract. Fluoride ingested in the dust is rapidly absorbed into the bloodstream from the alimentary tract, primarily from the stomach. The mechanism of fluoride absorption is one of simple diffusion across a semipermeable membrane. The fluoride that is in insoluble compounds or is not absorbed is eliminated in the feces. The presence of calcium, magnesium, or aluminum ions interferes with the absorption of fluoride in that they form insoluble compounds with it.

The mean plasma fluoride level in normal humans ranges from 0.14 to 0.19 ppm and is not elevated above this range in persons consuming water with up to 2.5 ppm fluoride.[2] Higher mean plasma levels are found when drinking water levels of fluoride are above 2.5 ppm. These water levels will also be reflected in a higher concentration of fluoride retained in hard tissues.

The fluoride content of soft tissue is approximately the same as that found in plasma. Fluoride is probably not incorporated into soft tissue structure itself (except perhaps for ectopic calcifications) but is present in the interstitial fluid. Fluoride is present in the hard tissues in the following descending order of concentration: cementum, bone, dentin, and enamel. It is incorporated in the mineral lattice of bones and teeth and may also be found at the hydroxyapatite crystal surfaces.

Fluoride is deposited in calcified tissues by the circulating blood and tissue fluids. Since bone is continually in a dynamic state of remodeling, fluoride will be released back into the blood by decalcification. As long as decalcification and recalcification stay in equilibrium, a state of fluoride equilibrium will exist. This will be manifested by the excretion of approximately the same amount of fluoride that is ingested. In children, who are undergoing bodily growth and the calcification of bones and teeth, less fluoride will be excreted than is ingested. If a person who has been ingesting water with a high level of fluoride moves to an area with water containing less fluoride, excess fluoride will be excreted because the plasma fluoride will decrease somewhat and exchangeable fluoride on the bone surface will be replaced by hydroxyl ions. The fluoride thus freed will be lost. On the other hand, the reverse process will be in effect for a person moving from an area with low amounts of fluoride in the water to an area with high amounts. He will excrete less fluoride than he ingests. In both cases equilibrium will eventually be reached.

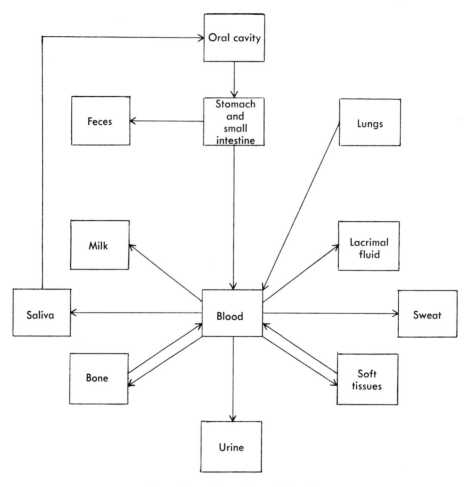

Fig. 14. Metabolic pathway of fluoride.

Most fluoride is excreted in the urine. Appreciable amounts are also excreted by sweat, with trace amounts being found in milk, saliva, and lacrimal fluid. The metabolic pathway of fluoride may be summarized briefly in Fig. 14.

FLUORIDE TOXICITY

Before the recognition of the importance of fluorides in relation to dental disease, the ion was well known in the form of hydrofluoric acid, an agent used for etching glass, and as sodium fluoride, a common household insecticide and rodenticide. Unfortunately, its effect as a potent protoplasmic poison has colored its biologic appraisal over the years. A clear distinction must be made between the acute toxic effects resulting from a single massive dose of fluoride and the chronic toxic effects of small doses spread over an interval of time.

Acute fluoride poisoning is very rare, with only 435 cases being recorded worldwide in medical reports covering a period of 85 years.[3] These cases were primarily suicides, or accidents where fluoride compounds were mistakenly ingested. Sodium fluoride crystals are usually artificially colored blue so that they will not be mistaken for table salt. An acute lethal dose for a human being is approximately 5 Gm fluoride as sodium fluoride.[3] The effects of large doses of fluoride are first manifested as irritation of the alimentary tract with nausea, vomiting, abdominal pain, and diarrhea. Excessive salivation, thirst, perspiration, and muscular spasms are also seen. Later, there may be depression of the respiratory, circulatory, and nervous systems, with such cases commonly having a fatal outcome in 2 or 3 days.[3] If large doses of fluoride are ingested, the stomach should be emptied as rapidly as possible and measures taken to reduce fluoride absorption. This can be accomplished by induced emesis and ingestion of milk or calcium salts, which will react with the fluoride ion to form relatively insoluble calcium fluoride.

Chronic fluoride toxicity may, depending on the dosage, be confined to minor physiologic alterations such as mottled enamel or result in a major crippling disease. It has been estimated that 10% to 15% of persons consuming water with 8 ppm fluoride will develop radiographically detectable osteosclerosis. To develop the crippling fluorosis found among some workers in the cryolite industry and in some areas of India, 20 to 80 mg fluoride must be ingested daily over a period of 10 to 20 years.[2] This would require a water fluoride level of 10 ppm or greater coupled with high water consumption. Excessive levels of fluoride are deposited in the skeleton over the years. The bones become heavy and irregular with multiple exostoses. There is often a reduced diameter of the spinal canal with compression of the cord. The vertebrae may become fused in numerous places, resulting in a so-called "poker back." Irregular bony deposits limit the movement of many other joints as well. Radiologically, affected bones appear very radiopaque with thickened cortexes and diminished medullary cavities.[3]

SYSTEMIC FLUORIDES AND DENTAL DISEASE
Chronic endemic dental fluorosis

The first relationship between fluoride and the dentition was established when the substance was discovered to be the cause of chronic endemic fluorosis, or mottled enamel. Although this condition was first described at the beginning of the twentieth century,[4] it was not until 1931 that the causative factor was determined to be fluoride.[5,6]

The mottling and staining of the enamel associated with chronic endemic dental fluorosis has been shown to be a hypoplastic defect resulting from a disturbance in the functioning of the ameloblasts during tooth development. Depending on the fluoride concentration in the drinking water, the condition has a wide variety of manifestations. These range from white spots or flecking of the enamel at concentrations up to 1.5 ppm to moderate and severe pitting and brownish staining of enamel at higher concentrations. It is commonly, but mistakenly, believed that erupted teeth can develop mottling when exposed to fluoride. The fact is that excessive fluoride affects the ameloblasts and therefore can cause mottling of the enamel *only* while the enamel is forming. Fluoride absorbed from topical contact or ingestion after eruption will not cause mottling.

Dental caries

Even before fluoride was discovered to be the causative agent for chronic endemic dental fluorosis, children with this defect were observed to have a lower than average caries prevalence.[7] In 1938, H. Trendley Dean established that there was a greater percentage of caries-free children in areas with high levels of fluoride in the water than in areas with low amounts of fluoride.[8] These findings suggested the possibility of reducing the prevalence of dental caries through adjustment of the fluoride content of public water supplies.

These findings and others[9] demonstrated a generally inverse relationship between the amount of fluoride in a water supply and the dental caries experience of the children, with the amount of caries being as much as two or three times greater among children in some areas than in others. A strikingly low caries prevalence was found in communities with water containing as little as 1 ppm fluoride. This concentration produced only sporadic findings of the mildest form of chronic endemic dental fluorosis. Thus it was concluded that significant inhibition of dental caries could be expected at fluoride concentrations not causing unesthetic enamel mottling.

Optimum fluoride level. The optimum fluoride level in a water supply should be one that will provide maximal protection against dental caries without producing adverse effects. This concentration has been established as approximately 1 ppm fluoride. The amount of fluoride consumed is a function not only of the amount of fluoride in the water supply but also of the mean annual air temperature. A high mean annual tem-

Table 22-1. Temperature ranges and recommended fluoride concentrations*

Annual average of maximum daily temperatures (° F)	Fluoride concentrations (ppm)	
	Optimum	Acceptable range
50.0-53.7	1.2	0.9-1.7
53.8-58.3	1.1	0.8-1.5
58.4-63.8	1.0	0.8-1.3
63.9-70.6	0.9	0.7-1.2
70.7-79.2	0.8	0.7-1.0
79.3-90.5	0.7	0.6-0.8

*Modified from U.S. Department of Health, Education, and Welfare, Public Health Service: Public Health Service drinking water standards, 1962, PHS Publication no. 956, Washington, D.C., 1962, U.S. Government Printing Office.

perature will lead to a high fluoride intake because of the relatively large quantities of water consumed. Optimum fluoride levels therefore depend on climatic conditions. Based on safety standards and water consumption estimates, the U.S. Public Health Service has established recommended levels for fluoride concentrations in water supplies for various mean annual air temperatures.[10] These levels are shown in Table 22-1. All water supplies whose fluoride levels have been adjusted should conform to these standards.

Mechanisms of protection. The mechanism by which fluoride imparts its protection against dental caries is not fully understood. It has been known for some time that the fluoride ion can replace the hydroxyl ion in the hydroxyapatite lattice in the inorganic portion of all calcified body tissues. This includes tooth enamel, dentin, and cementum, as well as bone and ectopic calcifications.[11] Because of its crystalline configuration, the fluoroapatite thus formed is less susceptible than hydroxyapatite to the attack of weak organic acids. Only a small portion of the hydroxyapatite is converted to fluoroapatite. The highest concentrations of 3000 to 4000 ppm fluoride are found at the crystal surface, whereas pure fluoroapatite has 38,000 ppm fluoride.[12]

In hard tissues, fluoride accumulates in proximity to circulating fluids; thus the fluoride level is greater in periosteal tissue than underlying bone, in dentin nearer the pulp, and in enamel near the surface.[12] The amount of these surface concentrations is directly proportional to the concentration of fluoride in the drinking water and the length of time the water was consumed. During the pre-

eruptive maturation phase of tooth development, surface enamel continues to be bathed in fluoride-containing tissue fluid, thus accounting for the higher fluoride level found in surface enamel. The concentration of ionic fluoride in the tissue fluid is closely related to the concentration found in the drinking water.[13] Only when there are very high concentrations in the water is the amount of fluoride in the deeper layers of enamel raised appreciably because the bulk of enamel mineralized quickly. The critical times for fluoride incorporation are from shortly after birth until 2½ years of age for deciduous teeth and from 3 until 12 years for permanent teeth.

Since greater resistance to acid dissolution is one of the characteristics of fluoroapatite-rich enamel and the surface enamel has the highest concentration, subsurface enamel would be more susceptible to initial demineralization. The commonly observed "white spot lesion" is subsurface enamel demineralization.

It has also been suggested that fluoride may inhibit caries by enzyme-inhibitory properties.[11,14,15] The inhibition of acidogenic bacterial enzyme systems can considerably reduce their acid production, but much higher concentrations of fluoride are required than are present in the saliva of persons drinking fluoridated water. It has been found, however, that the fluoride ion is concentrated in bacterial plaque. The degree of concentration may be of such magnitude as to inhibit acid production by many of the organisms in plaque. It has been demonstrated that the plaque taken from individuals consuming optimally fluoridated water undergoes a significantly smaller drop in pH when incubated with sucrose than does plaque

Table 22-2. Results of controlled fluoridation among 16- and 17-year-olds in three communities in Ontario

	Brantford 1.00 ppm F (adjusted)	Stratford 1.0 ppm F (natural)	Sarnia negligible F
Percentage of individuals with caries-free teeth	11.8	12.8	0.41
Number of DMF teeth per individual	4.74	4.19	10.44

from individuals consuming water with negligible concentrations of fluoride.[16] The increased fluoride levels found in plaque are thought to be from exogenous sources such as saliva, drinking water, or topical applications rather than from fluoride released from the enamel surface.[17,18]

It has been proposed that the presence of fluoride in a supersaturated calcifying solution increases the precipitation of hydroxyapatite from the solution.[19] Thus the fluoride liberated by acid from enamel would favor remineralization of the enamel and be antagonistic to demineralization.

It may be that the combined effects of decreased enamel solubility, bacterial enzyme inhibition, and enhanced remineralization give fluoride its importance in preventive dentistry.

Fluoridation studies. Whatever the exact mechanism may be, the action of fluoride in caries reduction is well documented, both in areas where the substance is naturally present in the water at optimum or higher levels and in communities that have adjusted their water supplies to optimum levels. In January, 1945, Grand Rapids, Michigan, became one of the first cities to adjust its water supply to an optimum fluoride level.[20] Fifteen years later the number of decayed, missing, and filled teeth among 12- through 16-year-olds was from 47.9% to 63.2% lower than was found among the same age group at the beginning of the program. Seventeen and one-half years after controlled fluoridation had been instituted in Brantford, Ontario,[21] the relationships shown in Table 22-2 were found among 16- and 17-year-olds residing there and in the neighboring cities of Stratford and Sarnia.

Although most studies have been devoted to the effects of waterborne fluorides on children's permanent teeth, the benefits have been found to carry over into adults.

Lifelong adult residents of communities with fluoridated water have been shown to have 50% to 60% fewer decayed, missing, and filled teeth than do their counterparts in communities with negligible amounts of fluoride in the water.[22,23]

It was generally accepted in the past that the protection imparted to the enamel by fluoride during tooth formation is not lost, regardless of whether fluoridated water is consumed after eruption. Investigators have observed, however, that with the cessation of fluoridation there is an increase in the caries experience in children who had previously consumed fluoridated water.[24] It has also been shown that fluoride levels of surface enamel increase throughout life in individuals who drink water containing 1 ppm or more fluoride.[11] Since the caries-protective effect of fluoride is exerted at the enamel suface, it would be logical to conclude that fluoride is beneficial not only during tooth formation but throughout life.

Malocclusion

Although the benefits of optimally fluoridated water supplies are well established in relationship to dental caries, their relationship to the prevalence of malocclusion is not so clear cut. The hypothesis has been advanced that the loss of tooth substance either through extraction or through destruction of mesiodistal contour because of caries results in loss of continuity of the dental arches, abnormal arch relationships, and subsequent malocclusion.[25] Malocclusion resulting from premature loss of deciduous teeth from caries is well documented. It would logically follow that the reduction in caries and tooth loss attendant on fluoridation would in turn reduce the prevalence of malocclusion. Some clinical studies have lent support to this hypothesis,[26-28] whereas others have detected no differences in the prevalence of malocclusion among children in fluoridated and nonfluoridated communities.[29-31]

Periodontal disease

Several studies have been undertaken to investigate a possible relationship between water fluoride levels and periodontal health.[32-35] From the results of these investigations, it is generally conceded that neither the incidence nor the severity of gingivitis and periodontal disease in a community is influenced by the fluoride level of its water supply.

Dental care requirements and cost

A time and cost analysis of dental care was performed in a fluoridated and a nonfluoridated community where a program of complete dental care for poor children had been instituted.[36] Initial care cost $40.78 per child in the nonfluoridated city as opposed to $16.93 per child in the fluoridated city. Subsequent incremental care also cost significantly less in the fluoridated city. These findings would certainly support the hypothesis that a community water fluoridation program will reduce the cost of dental care for children. This becomes an extremely important consideration in light of the present trend toward government- and labor union–sponsored prepaid dental care programs. Fluoridation is also taken into account when premiums are calculated by dental care insurance underwriters.

ALTERNATIVE METHODS OF SUPPLYING SYSTEMIC FLUORIDE

The value of optimum fluoride levels in the water supply is unquestioned by knowledgeable workers in the health professions. Nevertheless, there have been a vocal few who have opposed this well-tested public health measure because of misinformation about its safety and effectiveness or through political and moral convictions. Unfortunately, this group has exerted an influence vastly disproportionate to its numbers and has seriously impeded the universal fluoridation of communal water supplies.

Even when all public water supplies are fluoridated, the significant proportion of the population who do not receive their water from public supplies will not directly benefit. It is obvious that other means must be utilized to provide the protective effects of systemic fluorides for those who are either (1) using public water supplies that are not fluoridated, or (2) are not using public water supplies and do not have their own source of naturally fluoridated water.

Many different methods of fluoride supplementation have been proposed and studied. Only a few of the more widely used and documented methods are discussed here. An extensive review of fluoride supplements has been made by Stookey,[14] and parts of his review are cited in this section.

Home fluoridators and bottled water

Home fluoridating units provide an optimally fluoridated water supply, but their very high cost severely limits their widespread use. Fluoridated bottled water contains a similar level of fluoride as a fluoridated water supply. The use of bottled water for drinking and cooking is increasing rapidly throughout the nation for reasons of taste and purity. The cost of fluoridated bottled water is nominal, being no more than that of plain bottled water. Therefore this is a highly effective home fluoridation method to recommend. The primary objection to both home fluoridators and bottled water other than cost is that only water consumed in the home will be fluoridated. If the children consume a large proportion of their daily water intake at school or elsewhere, they may not ingest enough fluoride for optimal benefit.

Fluoridated school water supplies

Lack of a central water supply makes water fluoridation impractical for 23% of the United States population.[37] The proportion of the population not served by centralized water supplies is even higher in foreign countries. In some areas where fluoridation of the main water supply is not feasible, fluoridation of school water supplies has reduced the DMFT (decayed, missing, and filled teeth) of the children by as much as 39%.[38]

Although maximum benefits are derived from fluoridated water when it is consumed from birth, a significant amount of tooth calcification takes place after the child reaches school age. As discussed previously, there is also evidence to indicate a topical action of fluoridated water.

A limitation of school water fluoridation is that the children's consumption of water is intermittent. They attend school for only part of the day, 5 days a week, 9 to 10 months each year. To compensate for lack of continuous consumption, school water supplies have been adjusted to higher levels than those normally recommended. Water fluoride levels of up to 6.30 ppm have been used with little or no evidence of fluorosis resulting.[39]

Fluoride tablets

In areas where the public water supplies are sometimes not potable, a great deal of attention has been focused on fluoride tablets. Benefits equivalent to or greater than having the water fluoridated have been reported, with maximum caries reductions of up to 80% being found in both permanent and deciduous teeth.[40] In a review of twenty-seven studies,[14] only five showed a partially or entirely negative caries-reducing effect for fluoride tablets.

Before fluoride supplements are prescribed, the fluoride content of the water supply should be known. The Council on Dental Therapeutics of the American Dental Association suggests the following daily allowances for children 3 years of age and older.[41]

For children 2 to 3 years of age, the dosage should be cut in half. For those under 2 years, no specific allowance is suggested; instead, 2.2 mg sodium fluoride may be dissolved in 1 quart of water for use in drinking, cooking, and formula preparation.[41]

As a safety precaution, no more than 264 tablets (264 mg fluoride) should be prescribed at one time. Each package should bear the warning: CAUTION—*Store out of reach of children.*

Much more information is needed about the metabolism of fluoride ingested in the form of tablets in relation to its effects on the dentition. Fluoride ingested in a single dose is rapidly absorbed and excreted in the urine with a very brief rise in the blood and tissue fluid level.[42,43] When the same amount of fluoride is given in three doses rather than a single large dose, about 50% less is excreted in the urine and much more is thus retained.[43] If much of the value of systemic fluoride is derived from bathing the developing tooth in tissue fluids containing elevated amounts of fluoride, a large number of small doses would appear to be more valuable than a single large dose.

The concentration of fluoride in human saliva is greatly increased after the administration of sodium fluoride tablets. Significantly higher salivary fluoride levels persist even after 24 hours.[44] These elevated salivary fluoride levels may contribute to the anticaries effect of fluoride tablets.

A number of other problems are inherent in the use of fluoride tablets. Although there is evidence to indicate the need for lifetime fluoride ingestion to obtain its optimum effects, it is unlikely that many individuals can be motivated to take tablets daily for their entire lives. Only the most highly motivated parents will see that their children take a tablet each day. A possible way of overcoming this problem is to use the tablets to fluoridate the water used in the home for cooking and drinking. (Dissolve 1 tablet, that is, 2.2 mg sodium fluoride, in 1 quart water.) The inconvenience of even this measure limits its use to those highly motivated toward good dental health.

Although fluoride tablets seem to be of value, evidence available to date would indicate that they are not an adequate substitute for water fluoridation.

Fluoride vitamins

The addition of sodium fluoride in therapeutic quantities does not appear to have any effect on the action of vitamin preparations and vice versa.[14] Fluoride-vitamin preparations have been shown to be highly effective in reducing dental caries attack in both deciduous and permanent teeth of children. For children whose water supply contains less than 0.7 ppm fluoride, the dosage is as follows.[45]

Under 2 years of age: 0.5 mg fluoride as sodium fluoride daily with vitamin drops

2 years of age and over: 1 mg fluoride as sodium fluoride daily with a chewable vitamin

Table 22-3. Daily fluoride allowances for children 3 years of age and older

Amount of fluoride in water	Sodium fluoride (mg)	Fluoride (mg)
Negligible	2.2	1.0
0.2 ppm	1.8	0.8
0.4 ppm	1.3	0.6
0.6 ppm	0.9	0.4

A portion of the caries reductions may result from the topical effect of the chewable vitamins. An advantage of giving fluoride supplements combined with vitamins is the greater acceptability of these products. Parents are more likely to see that their children take vitamins prescribed for them than a fluoride tablet alone. This also points to the great disadvantage of this method of fluoride supplementation. Vitamins should never be prescribed indiscriminately. Therefore only the small group of children who require vitamin supplementation should receive fluoride in this manner.

Prenatal fluoride

Since the deciduous dentition and the permanent first molars undergo partial or complete calcification in utero, it could be reasoned that increased fluoride levels in the fetal circulation would be beneficial in reducing caries susceptibility in these teeth. Therefore increased fluoride ingestion by the mother, either from fluoridated water or prenatal fluoride supplements, would be thought to be of value.

The placenta acts as a barrier, protecting the fetus from sharp increases of fluoride concentration in the maternal circulation. However, there is evidence to indicate that some additional fluoride does pass the placenta because increasing the amount in water supplies leads to higher fluoride levels in fetal hard structures.[1] It is not known what levels of fluoride in the water are required to supply sufficient fluoride to the teeth in utero for significant caries protection. Clinical studies of fluoride's effects on the deciduous dentition calcified in utero have yielded conflicting evidence.[46,47] The currently available prenatal preparations that contain fluoride also contain minerals that, in animals, have been shown to interfere with the metabolic activity of fluorides, thus reducing the amount available to the fetus.[48]

Much further study of prenatal fluoride supplements is required before they should be routinely prescribed for expectant mothers residing in areas without appreciable fluoride in the water.

Fluoridated milk and salt

Fluoridated table salt and milk have been shown to be effective in lowering the incidence of dental caries in areas where the water is fluoride deficient, but to a lesser degree than fluoridated water.[14,49] These measures have aroused the greatest interest for use in areas lacking in communal water supplies and with low socioeconomic levels.

There are major problems attendant on both milk and salt fluoridation. For example, it is difficult to monitor all commercial milk processing plants to ensure a safe and effective fluoride level. The consumption of milk also varies greatly among children so that some would be likely to receive ineffectual amounts of fluoride, whereas others would receive too much. Since adults generally drink little milk, any posteruptive topical effect would be unavailable to them.

Much additional information is needed about the body's handling of fluoridated milk after ingestion before proper dosage levels can be determined. A similar problem exists with salt. Children ingest variable amounts of salt, usually not a great deal, and therefore it is difficult to regulate the intake. A program of supplementing table salt with 552.6 mg sodium fluoride per kilogram of salt (250 ppm fluoride) has yielded 40% reductions in the caries experience of 2- to 6-year-old children.[50]

Since it is believed that fluoride supplementation should be continued throughout life, a program of both salt and milk fluoridation has been proposed.[49] With this regimen children would be receiving the bulk of their fluoride through milk, and adults through salt. A great deal of additional information will be required before either part of this regimen should be instituted as a public health measure.

TOPICAL FLUORIDES

In addition to having anticariogenic properties when ingested during tooth formation, fluoride has been shown to exert an anticariogenic effect when applied topically to the erupted dentition. It is reasonable to assume that the mechanism by which topically applied fluorides inhibits caries is the same as for systemically applied fluorides, although it is incompletely understood.

A primary objective of topical fluoride therapy is to deposit maximal amounts of fluoride in the enamel as fluoroapatite, which is generally believed to impart caries resistance to the tooth. This may be in the form of a simple ionic exchange as represented by the following chemical reaction[51]:

$$Ca_{10}(PO_4)_6(OH)_2 \xrightarrow[\text{concentration}]{F^- \text{ in low}} Ca_{10}(PO_4)_6F_2 + 2(OH)^-$$
Hydroxyapatite   **Fluoroapatite**

When high concentrations of fluoride are applied to enamel surfaces, the primary product is calcium fluoride.[51]

$$Ca_{10}(PO_4)_6(OH)_2 \xrightarrow[\text{concentration}]{F^- \text{ in high}} CaF_2 + 6(PO_4)^{3-} + 2(OH)^-$$

After topical application the initially high surface fluoride levels are rapidly lost. First to go are unreacted fluoride ions, followed by calcium fluoride. Calcium fluoride is soluble in saliva so that surface deposits tend to dissolve or wash away. When calcium fluoride is deposited within enamel defects and fissures, it may remain for some time. This residual calcium fluoride may yield fluoride ions, which are then incorporated into the apatite crystal by direct replacement of the hydroxyl ions or by recrystallization (dissolution and reprecipitation of the apatite crystal incorporating fluoride rather than hydroxyl ions).[12]

In addition to the formation of fluoroapatite, the fluoride ions originating from the topical agent or released from calcium fluoride may serve as enzyme inhibitors in the plaque and aid in remineralization of early carious lesions.[52,53] Fluoride ions in low concentrations may also desorb both pellicle protein and bacteria from the enamel surface.[54]

Many different fluoride compounds have been evaluated with various methods of application. Some of the studies have yielded directly conflicting results, giving rise to considerable controversy among workers in the field as to the efficacy of some of the various compounds and techniques of application. The current status of only the more commonly used compounds and techniques of application are reviewed in this chapter.

Fluoride solutions

Sodium fluoride. The application of aqueous solutions of sodium fluoride is the oldest and probably the most widely tested and accepted method of topical fluoride therapy. Although various application techniques and solution concentrations have been used, the procedure adopted by the Council on Dental Therapeutics of the American Dental Association[41] has produced the most consistently

beneficial results. It will reduce by 30% to 40% the incidence of new carious permanent teeth in children living in an area where the water supply is fluoride deficient.[14]

With the accepted procedure a series of four applications of a 2% sodium fluoride solution are made at 1-week intervals at 3, 7, 11, and 13 years of age. These ages were selected so that fluoride would be applied shortly after eruption of groups of teeth. The ages should be varied according to the eruption pattern of each individual patient. A prophylaxis is given prior to the first application in each series. The teeth are isolated and thoroughly wetted with the solution, which is allowed to dry for 4 minutes. No prophylaxis is given before the second, third, and fourth applications; however, its omission prior to the first application lessens the effectiveness of the treatment by one half.

The effectiveness of sodium fluoride in preventing caries in deciduous teeth, permanent teeth of children reared in fluoridated areas, and adult dentitions has not been investigated extensively. There is evidence to indicate that a 25% to 30% reduction in caries of deciduous teeth of children raised in a nonfluoridated area will result from sodium fluoride application.[14] Limited data do not indicate any benefits for the permanent teeth of children reared in a fluoridated area or for adults.[14]

The taste of sodium fluoride is not unpleasant, and since this compound is stable in solution, it does not have to be mixed for each patient.

Stannous fluoride. The stannous fluoride application procedure, as originally developed,[55] calls for a single annual application of a freshly prepared 8% solution. This is preceded by a thorough prophylaxis, which includes carrying the pumice between the teeth with floss. The solution is applied to the teeth, which have been air dried and isolated, a quadrant or a half mouth at a time. The teeth are continually wetted for a period of 4 minutes. In patients whose caries susceptibility is high, applications of stannous fluoride every 6 months or even more frequently are recommended.

Stannous fluoride applied in the manner just described to the permanent teeth of children reared in nonfluoride areas has generally been shown to be more beneficial than sodium fluoride in reducing dental caries increments. It is also effective in reducing the caries increment in deciduous teeth of children reared in a nonfluoride area and in permanent teeth of children reared in fluoride areas. When applied in a 10% concentration, stannous fluoride has been shown to reduce the caries increment in adults.[14] The application of a 10% stannous fluoride solution for 15 or 30 seconds has yielded conflicting clinical results.[56-58]

Large amounts of calcium fluoride are formed when stannous fluoride is applied to sound enamel surfaces. Phosphate ions released by the calcium fluoride formation combine with the stannous tin to form insoluble tin-phosphate complexes.[59] Insoluble tin-phosphate complexes may also be formed when stannous fluoride is applied to pre-carious or carious enamel, which would give a caries-arrestment property in addition to a caries-preventive property.[60,61] This may account for the greater anticaries effect of stannous fluoride when compared with sodium fluoride.

The tin-phosphate complex imparts a light brown pigmentation to the carious or pre-carious areas that has caused objections from some patients and practitioners. This pigmentation is probably desirable, since it indicates the arrestment of a pre-carious or frankly carious lesion. The incidence and severity of this pigmentation is directly related to the caries activity and oral hygiene habits of the individual, with those exhibiting a high degree of caries activity and poor oral hygiene having the most pigmentation.[62] Very dark, objectionable stains, which are sometimes observed, result from the tin's forming a sulfide complex with the products of bacterial plaque.[60]

Although topical application of stannous fluoride will slow the progress of existing carious lesions,[63,64] the pigmented tin-phosphate complex is lost through washing and abrasion over a period of time, which indicates the necessity for repeated replacement of the stannous ion. The frequency of application of stannous fluoride therefore depends on the caries activity of the individual. Some may require treatment as often as every 3 or 4 months, whereas annual or semiannual treatment will suffice for others.

Stannous fluoride in a 10% solution has been successfully used as an indirect pulp-capping agent in both permanent and deciduous teeth. After a 3-month interval carious dentin treated with stannous fluoride has been found to be more radiopaque and harder than carious dentin treated with calcium hydroxide compounds.[65]

Stannous fluoride solutions have a highly unpleasant taste resulting from the presence of the tin ion. This taste is difficult to mask by flavoring agents. The solutions are unstable and should be freshly prepared for each patient.

Acidulated phosphate fluoride. Acidulated phosphate fluoride (APF) is currently available in solution or gel form with various flavors added. The solution is applied in the same manner as 8% stannous fluoride (4 minutes to dried and isolated teeth), whereas the gels are applied in either wax trays or custom-made mouthguard type of applicators.

In vitro and in vivo studies have shown that there is increased uptake of fluoride by the enamel when the fluoride solution has a low pH. The acidic solution dissolves the surface hydroxyapatite crystals of the enamel, thus freeing more calcium ions for reaction to calcium fluoride and subsequent recrystallization as fluoroapatite.[51] Unfortunately, the dissolution of the surface enamel may overshadow the beneficial effects of increased fluoride uptake. The addition of phosphates to the acidulated fluoride solutions allows a high fluoride uptake without objectionable dissolution of the surface enamel.[66]

Acidulated phosphate fluorides have been shown to be effective in reducing new caries in the permanent teeth of children residing in a nonfluoride area. The more frequent the applications the larger are the caries reductions that result.[14,67] Daily applications of acidulated or neutral sodium fluoride gels by mouthguards have achieved caries reductions as high as 89% over a 21-month period.[68] Caries reductions of up to 63% were still evident 2 years after cessation of this treatment.[69] A thrice weekly application of APF gel to children residing in an area with optimally fluoridated water reduced the caries increment of their permanent teeth by 29%.[70]

Fluoride uptake by the enamel surface is much higher and the fluoride penetrates the enamel much more deeply with APF solutions than with either sodium or stannous fluoride. There is also a significant reduction in the number of *Streptococcus mutans* from occlusal plaque samples after eight to ten daily applications of APF.[71] Although increased fluoride levels in enamel are undoubtedly beneficial in protecting against dental caries, it does not necessarily follow that higher and higher levels of fluoride in enamel will give correspondingly higher levels of caries protection, as evidenced by the similar caries reductions resulting from daily applications of both neutral and acidulated sodium fluoride.[68]

Acidulated phosphate fluorides taste acidic, but not disagreeably so. The addition of flavoring agents, although not affecting the clinical effectiveness of APF solutions, makes them pleasant tasting and highly acceptable to children. The solutions are stable and have a long shelf life so that they can be made up in bulk and not prepared for each patient.

The properties of the three best known fluoride compounds are summarized in Table 22-4.

A topical application of APF followed by a topical application of stannous fluoride yields an enamel surface that is less porous and soluble than when either agent is used alone.[72,73]

Other fluoride compounds. Numerous other fluoride compounds, such as aluminum fluoride, ammonium fluoride, and stannous hexafluorozirconate, have been developed and tested both clinically and in the laboratory. Although some of these compounds have shown considerable promise as anticariogenic agents, there is insufficient evidence to indicate their use in either dental practice or public health programs.

One of the more recently developed and promising fluoride compounds is titanium tetrafluoride. Under the scanning electron microscope it appears to form an acid-resistant coating over the enamel surface.[74] Among children an annual 1-minute application of 1% titanium tetrafluoride has been found to be significantly more effective than a similar 4-minute treatment regimen with APF.[75]

Fluoride dentifrices

Numerous fluoride compounds have been incorporated in dentifrices with widely varying clinical effectiveness. The earliest fluoride dentifrices contained sodium fluoride. They proved to be of little value because the calcium carbonate or calcium phosphate in their abrasive systems yielded enough free calcium to inactivate the fluoride. Subsequently, many other fluoride compounds and abrasive systems have been used and manufacturers have made many claims, mostly unsubstantiated. There are currently two types of fluoride dentifrices that have undergone sufficient laboratory and clinical testing to be accepted by the Council on Dental Therapeutics of the American Dental Association as being effective in reducing the incidence of new dental caries.[41,76] These are a stannous fluoride dentifrice and two sodium monofluorophosphate dentrifices (MFP).

Many dentifrices have added fluoride to their formulation, but this does not mean that they are effective cariostatic agents. Other substances in the dentifrice may inactivate the fluoride or stannous ion. Results of carefully designed, long-term clinical testing should be required before any dentifrice is recommended to the patient as an effective caries-preventive agent.

Stannous fluoride dentifrice. The only stannous fluoride dentifrice currently accepted by the Council on Dental Therapeutics of the American Dental Association contains 0.4% stannous fluoride with a calcium pyrophosphate abrasive system. Caries reductions brought about by this dentifrice range from 23% to 34% in both fluoride and nonfluoride areas. The higher caries reductions are found when the teeth are brushed with greater frequency and when the brushing is done under supervision.[41]

Sodium monofluorophosphate dentifrices. Monofluorophosphate is different from other fluorides in that the fluoride is covalently bound rather than in ionic form. The fluoride

Table 22-4. Properties of three best known fluoride compounds

Properties	NaF	SnF$_2$	APF
Is effective in permanent teeth of children in nonfluoride areas?	Yes	Yes	Yes
Is effective in deciduous teeth in nonfluoride areas?	Yes	Yes	?
Is effective in fluoride areas?	No	Yes	?
Is effective in adults?	No	Yes	?
Requires a simple, one-appointment procedure?	No	Yes	Yes
Is stable in solution?	Yes	No	Yes
Has a pleasant taste?	Yes	No	Yes
Stains teeth?	No	Yes	No
Can arrest existing caries?	No	Yes	No

ion is released in the mouth by hydrolysis and tends to form fluoroapatite.[77,78] Controlled clinical studies have shown that brushing with a sodium monofluorophosphate dentifrice reduces new caries in the range of 17% to 34% in both fluoridated and nonfluoridated communities. Both of the dentifrices accepted by the Council on Dental Therapeutics contain 0.76% monofluorophosphate but have different abrasive systems (sodium metaphosphate and calcium carbonate).[41,76] The effectiveness of both is in the same general range that has been reported for the stannous fluoride dentifrice.

Fluoride prophylaxis pastes

The caries-inhibitory effects produced by incorporating fluorides into dentifrices have suggested the value of adding them to prophylaxis pastes. Much higher concentrations of fluoride can be added to prophylaxis pastes than to dentrifrices because these pastes are used so infrequently. As in the case of dentifrices, the ingredients of the prophylaxis pastes must be compatible with the fluoride used, or the fluoride will be inactivated and of no value.

All commonly used prophylaxis pastes are abrasive and remove significant amounts of enamel. This surface enamel is high in fluoride and gives caries protection to the tooth. The fluoride in a prophylaxis paste not only replaces the surface fluoride lost but raises the surface level slightly.[79] A nonfluoride prophylaxis, on the other hand, is of questionable cariostatic value to the patient.

Sodium fluoride prophylaxis paste. In the 1940s and 1950s sodium fluoride was added to prophylaxis pastes and clinically tested. The results, although generally encouraging, were highly inconsistent.[11] Little attention is presently being devoted to using this compound in a prophylaxis paste.

Stannous fluoride prophylaxis pastes. Semiannual prophylaxis with an 8.9% stannous fluoride–lava pumice paste has been shown to reduce the caries increment in permanent teeth of children in a nonfluoride community by 34%.[80] A similar caries reduction among children resulted from the same treatment in a natural fluoride area.[81] A 12% reduction in new carious surfaces was noted among United States naval personnel treated without regard to previous fluoridated water intake.[57] Another study has shown no caries-

reducing effect from annual prophylaxis with a stannous fluoride–lava pumice paste.[82]

Acidulated phosphate fluoride prophylaxis pastes. Although acidulated sodium fluoride phosphate has been incorporated with various abrasives into pastes that are commercially marketed, there is meager clinical evidence to indicate their effectiveness as anticariogenic agents.

Multiple fluoride treatment

Although many of the previously described fluoride compounds and treatment techniques have been shown to have anticariogenic value, the stannous fluoride compounds have been used primarily in multiple treatment approaches. The anticariogenic effect of a stannous fluoride prophylaxis and topical application in children in fluoride and nonfluoride areas[80,81] as well as in adults[57] has been discussed. The inclusion of a topical application of stannous fluoride and daily use of a stannous fluoride dentifrice accepted by the American Dental Association have demonstrated an additive effect for each element in reducing the increment of dental caries attack.[57,80,81] In addition to reducing the initiation of new carious lesions, multiple stannous fluoride therapy has been shown to slow the progression of already existing carious lesions.[64]

Self-treatment with topical fluorides

Traditionally, topical fluorides have been applied in a dental office by either dentists or trained auxiliary personnel. The cost of such a procedure, because of the professional man-hours required and the need for dental treatment facilities, severely restricts the use of topical fluoride treatment in any public health program. To bring the benefits of topical fluoride treatment to more people at minimal cost, various methods in which the patients themselves apply the fluoride without special treatment facilities have been proposed and investigated.

Self-application of topical fluoride gel. The daily self-administration of a topical fluoride gel by means of a mouthguard type of applicator[68] has been discussed. Although the technique is of great value in a private dental practice, providing remarkable caries reductions, it is impractical for mass treatment programs. The initial cost of constructing mouthguards is considerable, and they would have to be replaced periodically because of loss, breakage, and changes in the dentition, especially in children.

Brushing the teeth with an APF gel alone has not been shown to reduce caries significantly. However, if the teeth are brushed with a nonfluoride prophylaxis paste prior to brushing with the gel, the caries increment has been reduced over 30%.[83]

Brushing with fluoride solution. Supervised brushing five times a year with various fluoride solutions such as acidulated fluoride phosphate, sodium fluoride, and ferric fluoride has yielded mixed results, with caries reductions ranging from nonsignificant to over 30%.[83-86] Daily home brushing with 6% sodium monofluorophosphate has resulted in a reduction of decay in children's teeth of up to 50%.[87]

Brushing with fluoride prophylaxis paste. In the three-phase stannous fluoride treatment previously discussed, the most time-consuming portion of the procedure is the prophylaxis. By having the patients perform their own prophylaxis in groups by means of supervised brushing with a fluoride prophylaxis paste, a great deal of time is saved and the requirement for a dental operatory is eliminated. The cariostatic effectiveness of this treatment technique using a lava pumice paste in conjunction with a topical application of aqueous stannous fluoride and daily use of a stannous fluoride dentifrice has been demonstrated among United States naval personnel.[88] Among children from both fluoride and nonfluoride areas, a self-prophylaxis alone with a zirconium silicate paste has yielded significant, although lesser, anticariogenic benefits than when all elements were included in the program.[89,90] Self-brushing with APF prophylaxis pastes has not proved to be a particularly effective caries-inhibitory measure. Results of clinical studies have varied from no significant caries reductions to slightly over 20%.[41,91]

Fluoride mouthwashes. The frequent use of fluoride mouthwashes has yielded highly promising results in reducing dental caries. Most studies have been conducted using either neutral sodium fluoride or an APF solution. The procedures most often followed have been either 0.02% fluoride used daily or 0.1% fluoride used weekly. Caries reductions have ranged from negligible to over 40%. Although most of these studies were conducted in nonfluoride areas, significant benefits also resulted in fluoride areas.[92]

Daily use of a 0.1% stannous fluoride solution has also been shown to be a highly effective anticaries procedure, with caries reductions as high as 43% resulting in areas where the water was optimally fluoridated.[93] Part of a stannous fluoride mouthrinse's effectiveness in reducing caries may stem from its antibacterial properties. When mouthrinses with equivalent fluoride ion concentrations of sodium fluoride and stannous fluoride were tested, the stannous fluoride had a significant antibacterial effect, but the sodium fluoride did not. These bactericidal properties have been attributed to the tin ion.[94]

Daily or periodic rinsing with a fluoride solution is a valuable adjunct to any caries prevention program. This treatment requires no professional supervision or facilities and is inexpensive. However, the presence in the home of mouthwashes with high fluoride concentrations may represent a potential hazard from a toxicity viewpoint. It is for this reason that the Council on Dental Therapeutics of the American Dental Association limits its acceptance of sodium fluoride mouthrinses to those packaged to contain a maximum of 300 mg sodium fluoride.[92] Proper indoctrination of the patients and parents is mandatory for such a program.

Other fluoride vehicles

After all topical fluoride treatments the initially high fluoride levels of the surface enamel are rapidly lost. Applying fluoride in a urethane lacquer preserves the high fluoride levels indefinitely in vitro. The adherent lacquer prolongs the time the fluoride ion is in contact with hydroxyapatite and thus leads to fluoroapatite formation. It also serves as a fluoride reservoir.[95] Application of a commercially available varnish containing 50 mg/ml sodium fluoride has greatly increased the surface fluoride levels of children's teeth and reduced caries by 75%. In contrast with other topical fluoride treatments, caries were greatly reduced in pits and fissures as well as on smooth and interproximal surfaces.[96,97]

A prophylaxis cup impregnated with either stannous fluoride or sodium fluoride increases the fluoride uptake of enamel when used in conjunction with fluoride-containing pastes at low pH.[98] The fluoride content of interproximal enamel has been increased by using fluoride-impregnated dental floss.[99]

Fluorides in restorative materials

Fluoride has been added to the flux of silicate cements to reduce enamel solubility at the margin of silicate restorations. The positive effect is well documented. In the hope of eliciting a similar effect from amalgam restorations, both sodium fluoride and stannous fluoride have been added to commercially available silver amalgam. Studies have shown that a concentration of 0.1% of either sodium or stannous fluoride does not significantly alter the amalgam's compressive strength, but higher concentrations decrease the strength. Sodium fluoride provides twice as much available fluoride as stannous fluoride does.[100] After placement of amalgam restorations containing stannous fluoride, the fluoride concentration of the adjacent tooth structure increased nearly twofold, with a sharp accompanying decrease in demineralization.[101]

Sodium and stannous fluorides have been added to zinc oxide and eugenol cements in the hope of giving an anticariogenic effect to temporary restorations and cemented crowns and inlays. The increased fluoride uptake and decreased solubility of enamel adjacent to zinc oxide and eugenol cements with fluoride compare with that adjacent to silicate cements.[102] The microhardness and fluoride content of underlying dentin are also increased.[103]

Because of the low pH of the liquid used in mixing zinc oxyphosphate cements, these cements have a tendency to decalcify the tooth structure next to which they are placed. By addition of an equal amount of a 30% solution of stannous fluoride to a dehydrated cement liquid, a pronounced degree of solubility protection is imparted without any adverse effect on the compressive strength or setting time of the cement.[104] This solubility protection decreases after a period of time, however.

Various other dental materials, such as cavity liners, are available with fluorides added, but there are currently no clinical data available regarding their benefits, if any.

REFERENCES

1. Bell, M. E., Largent, E. J., Ludwig, T. G., Muhler, J. C., and Stookey, G. K.: The supply of fluorine to man. In Fluorides and human health, Geneva, 1970, World Health Organization, pp. 17-74.
2. Armstrong, W. D., Gedalia, I., Singer, L., Weatherell, J. A., and Weidmann, S. M.: Distribution of fluorides. In Fluorides and human health, Geneva, 1970, World Health Organization, pp. 93-139.
3. Bhussry, B. R., DeMole, V., Hodge, C., Jolly, S. S., Singh, A., and Taves, D. R.: Toxic effects of larger doses of fluoride. In Fluorides and human health, Geneva, 1970, World Health Organization, pp. 225-271.
4. Eager, J M.: Denti di chiaie (Chiaie teeth), Public Health Rep. 16:2576-2577, 1901.
5. Churchill, H. V.: The occurrence of fluoride in some waters of the United States, J. Indust. Engin. Chem. 23:996-998, 1931.
6. Smith, M. C., Lantz, E. M., and Smith, H. V.: The cause of mottled enamel, Science 74:244, 1931.
7. McKay, F. S.: The establishment of a definite relation between enamel that is defective in its structure as mottled enamel, and the liability to decay, Dent. Cosmos 71:747-755, 1929.
8. Dean, H. T.: Endemic fluorosis and its relations to dental caries, Public Health Rep. 53:1443-1452, 1938.
9. Dean, H. T., Arnold, F. A., and Elvove, E.: Domestic water and dental caries. V. Additional studies of the relation of fluoride domestic waters to dental caries experience in 4,425 white children aged 12 to 14 years, of 13 cities in 4 states, Public Health Rep. 57:1155-1179, 1942.
10. U.S. Department of Health, Education, and Welfare, Public Health Service: Public Health Service drinking water standards, 1962, PHS Publication no. 956, Washington, D.C., 1962, U.S. Government Printing Office.
11. Hodge, H. C., and Smith, F. A.: Biological effects of organic fluorides. In Simons, J. H., editor: Fluorine chemistry, New York, 1964, Academic Press Inc., vol. 4, pp. 458-516.
12. Brudevold, F.: Fluoride therapy. In Bernier, J. L., and Muhler, J. C., editors: Improving dental practice through preventive measures, ed. 3, St. Louis, 1976, The C. V. Mosby Co., pp. 77-103.
13. Gay, W. S., and Taves, D. R.: Relation between (F⁻) in drinking water and human plasma, International Association for Dental Research Program and Abstracts, no. 718, 1973.
14. Stookey, G. K.: Fluoride therapy. In Bernier, J. L., and Muhler, J. C., editors: Improving dental practice through preventive measures, ed. 2, St. Louis, 1970, The C. V. Mosby Co., pp. 92-156.
15. Jenkins, G. N.: In vitro studies using chemicals. In Harris, R. S., editor: Art and science of dental caries research, New York, 1968, Academic Press Inc., pp. 331-354.
16. Edgar, W. M., Jenkins, G. N., and Tatevossian, A.: The inhibitory action of fluoride on plaque bacteria, Br. Dent. J. 128:129-132, 1970.
17. Gron, P., Yao, K., and Spinelli, M.: A study of inorganic constituents in dental plaque, J. Dent. Res. 48:799-805, 1969.
18. Fitzgerald, D. B., and Fitzgerald, R. J.: Plaque acid production in hamsters pre-treated with fluoride, J. Dent. Res. 52:111-115, 1973.
19. Koulourides, T.: Experimental changes of enamel mineral density, In Harris, R. S., editor: Art and science of dental caries research, New York, 1968, Academic Press, Inc., pp. 355-378.

20. Arnold, F. A., Likins, R. C., Russell, A. L., and Scott, D. B.: Fifteenth year of the Grand Rapids fluoridation study, J.A.D.A. **65**:780-785, 1962.

21. Brown, H. K., and Poplove, M.: Brantford-Sarnia-Stratford fluoridation caries study: final survey, 1963, J. Can. Dent. Assoc. **31**:505, 1965.

22. Englander, H. R., and Wallace, D. A.: Effects of naturally fluoridated water on dental caries in adults, Public Health Rep. **77**:887-893, 1962.

23. Russell, A. L., and Elvove, E.: Domestic water and dental caries. VII. A study of the fluoride–dental caries relationship in an adult population, Public Health Rep. **66**:1389-1401, 1951.

24. Way, R. M.: The effect on dental caries of a change from a naturally fluoridated to a fluoride-free communal water, J. Dent. Child. **31**:151-157, 1964.

25. Salzmann, J. A.: The effects of fluoride on the prevalence of malocclusion, J. Am. Coll. Dent. **35**:82-91, 1968.

26. Ast, D. B., Allaway, V., and Draker, H. L.: The prevalence of malocclusion, related to dental caries and lost first permanent molars, in a fluoridated city and a fluoride-deficient city, Am. J. Orthod. **48**:106-113, 1962.

27. Tank, G., and Storvick, C. A.: Caries experience of children one to six years old in two Oregon communities (Corvallis and Albany). II. Relation of fluoride to hypoplasia, malocclusion, and gingivitis, J.A.D.A. **70**:100-104, 1965.

28. Erickson, D. M., and Graziano, F. W.: Prevalence of malocclusion in seventh grade children in two North Carolina cities, J.A.D.A. **73**:124-127, 1966.

29. Pelton, W. J., and Elsasser, W. A.: Studies of dento-facial morphology. III. The role of dental caries in the etiology of malocclusion, J.A.D.A. **46**:648-657, 1957.

30. Hill, I. N., Blayney, J. R., and Wolf, W.: The Evanston dental caries study. XIX. Prevalence of malocclusion of children in a fluoridated and control area, J. Dent. Res. **38**:782-794, 1959.

31. Davis, W. R., McDonald, R. E., and Muhler, J. C.: The occlusion of children as related to water fluoride concentration and socioeconomic status, J. Dent. Res. (Abst.) **43**:783-784, 1964.

32. Russell, A. L., and White, C. L.: Fluorides and periodontal health. In Muhler, J. C., and Hines, M. K., editors: Fluoride and dental health, Bloomington, Ind., 1959, Indiana University Press, pp. 115-127.

33. Englander, H. R., Kesel, R. G., and Gupta, O. P.: Effect of natural fluoridation on the periodontal health of adults: the Aurora-Rockford Illinois Study, II, Am. J. Public Health **35**:1233-1242, 1963.

34. Englander, H. R., and White, C. L.: Periodontal and oral hygiene status of teenagers in optimum and fluoride-deficient cities, J.A.D.A. **68**:173-177, 1964.

35. Murray, J. J.: Gingivitis in 15-year-old children from high fluoride and low fluoride areas, Arch. Oral Biol. **14**:951, 1969.

36. Ast, D. B., Cons, N. C., Pollard, S. T., and Garfinkel, J.: Time and cost factors to provide regular, periodic dental care for children in a fluoridated and non-fluoridated area: final report, J.A.D.A. **80**:770-776, 1970.

37. U.S. Department of Health, Education, and Welfare: Fluoridation census, 1969, Washington, D.C., 1970, U.S. Government Printing Office.

38. Horowitz, H. S., Heifetz, S. B., and Law, F. E.: Effect of school water fluoridation on dental caries: final results in Elk Lake, Pa., after 12 years, J.A.D.A. **84**:832, 1972.

39. Heifetz, S. B., and Horowitz, H. S.: Effect of school water fluoridation on dental caries: interim results in Seagrove, N.C., after four years, J.A.D.A. **88**:352-355, 1974.

40. Aasenden, R., and Peebles, T. C.: Effects of fluoride supplementation from birth on deciduous and permanent teeth, Arch. Oral Biol. **19**:321-326, 1974.

41. American Dental Association Council on Dental Therapeutics: Accepted dental therapeutics, ed. 35, Chicago, 1973, American Dental Association, pp. 237-252.

42. Stookey, G. K., and Muhler, J. C.: Laboratory studies concerning fluoride metabolism using two different types of fluoride tablets, J. Dent. Child. **33**:90-100, 1966.

43. Muhler, J. C., Stookey, G. K., Spear, L. B., and Bixler, D.: Blood and urinary fluoride studies following the ingestion of single doses of fluoride, J. Oral Ther. Pharm. **2**:241-260, 1966.

44. Shannon, I. L., Feller, R. P., and Chauncey, H. H.: Fluoride in human parotid saliva, J. Dent. Res. **55**:506-509, 1976.

45. Hennon, D. K., Stookey, G. K., and Muhler, J. C.: The clinical anticariogenic effectiveness of supplementary fluoride-vitamin preparations—results at the end of four years, J. Dent. Child. **34**:439-443, 1967.

46. Blayney, J. R., and Hill, I. N.: Evanston dental caries study. XXIV. Prenatal fluorides—value of waterborne fluorides during pregnancy, J.A.D.A. **69**:291-294, 1964.

47. Katz, S., and Muhler, J. C.: Pre-natal and post-natal fluoride and dental caries experience in deciduous teeth, J.A.D.A. **76**:305-311, 1968.

48. Stookey, G. K., Hennon, D. K., and Muhler, J. C.: Skeletal retention and anticariogenic efficacy of fluoride when administered in the presence of a prenatal vitamin-mineral supplement, J. Dent. Res. **48**:1224-1230, 1969.

49. Marthaler, J. M.: The value in caries prevention of other methods of increasing fluoride ingestion, apart from fluoridated water, Int. Dent. J. **17**:606, 1967.

50. Toth, K.: Caries prevention in deciduous dentition using table salt fluoridation, J. Dent. Res. **52**:533-534, 1973.

51. Brudevold, F.: Interaction of fluoride with human enamel. In Symposium on Chemistry and Physiology of Enamel, Ann Arbor, Mich., 1971, University of Michigan Press, pp. 73-89.

52. Hardwick, J. L.: The mechanism of fluorides in lessening susceptibility to dental caries, Br. Dent. J. **114**:222-228, 1963.

53. Mühlemann, H. R.: Post-eruptive fluoridation, Br. Dent. J. **114**:216-221, 1963.

54. Rolla, G., and Melsen, B.: Desorption of protein and bacteria from hydroxyapatite by fluoride and monofluorophosphate, Caries Res. **9**:66-73, 1975.

55. Muhler, J. C.: Topical treatment of the teeth with stannous fluoride—single application technique, J. Dent. Child. **25**:306-309, 1958.

56. Mercer, V. N., and Muhler, J. C.: The effect of a

30 second topical SnF$_2$ treatment on dental caries reduction in children, J. Oral Ther. **1**:141-146, 1964.

57. Scola, F. P., and Ostrom, C. A.: Clinical evaluation of stannous fluoride when used as a constituent of a compatible prophylaxis paste, as a topical solution, and in a dentifrice in naval personnel. II. Report of findings after two years, J.A.D.A. **77**:594-597, 1968.

58. Horowitz, H. S., and Heifetz, S. B.: Evaluation of topical applications of stannous fluoride to teeth of children born and reared in a fluoridated community: final report, J. Dent. Child. **34**:355-361, 1969.

59. Wei, S. H. Y., and Forbes, W. C.: Electron microprobe investigations of stannous fluoride reactions with enamel surfaces, J. Dent. Res. **53**:51-56, 1974.

60. Muhler, J. C.: Stannous fluoride enamel pigmentation—evidence of a caries arrestment, J. Dent. Child. **27**:157-161, 1960.

61. Myers, H. M.: A hypothesis concerning the caries preventive mechanism of tin, J.A.D.A. **77**:1308, 1968.

62. Hyde, E. J., and Muhler, J. C.: Pigmentation of teeth treated with stannous fluoride and association with caries incidence and oral hygiene, J. Can. Dent. Assoc. **29**:514-520, 1963.

63. Mercer, V. N., and Muhler, J. C.: The clinical demonstration of caries arrestment following topical stannous fluoride treatment, J. Dent. Child. **32**:65-72, 1965.

64. Muhler, J. C., Spear, L. B., Bixler, D., and Stookey, G. K.: The arrestment of incipient dental caries in adults after the use of three different forms of SnF$_2$ therapy: results after 30 months, J.A.D.A. **75**:1402-1406, 1967.

65. Nordstrom, D. O., Wei, S. H. Y., and Johnson, R.: Use of stannous fluoride for indirect pulp capping, J.A.D.A. **88**:997-1003, 1974.

66. Brudevold, F., Savory, A., Gardner, D. E., Spinelli, M., and Speirs, R.: A study of acidulated fluoride solutions. I. In vitro effects on enamel, Arch. Oral Biol. **8**:167-177, 1963.

67. Horowitz, H. S., and Doyle, J.: The effect on dental caries of topically applied acidulated phosphate-fluoride: results after three years, J.A.D.A. **82**:359-365, 1971.

68. Englander, H. R., Keyes, P. H., Gestwicki, M., and Sultz, H. A.: Clinical anticaries effect of repeated topical sodium fluoride applications by mouthpiece, J.A.D.A. **75**:638-644, 1967.

69. Englander, H. R., Carlos, J. P., Senning, R. S., and Mellberg, J. R.: Residual anticaries effect of repeated sodium fluoride applications by mouthpieces, J.A.D.A. **78**:783-787, 1969.

70. Englander, H. R., Sherrill, L. T., Miller, B. G., Carlos, J. P., Mellberg, J. R., and Senning, R. S.: Incremental rates of dental caries after repeated topical sodium fluoride applications in children with lifelong consumption of fluoridated water, J.A.D.A. **82**:354-358, 1971.

71. Loesche, W. J., Syed, S. A., Murray, R. J., and Mellber, J. R.: Effect of topical acidulated phosphate fluoride on percentage of *Streptococcus mutans* and *Streptococcus sanguis* in plaque, Caries Res. **9**:139-155, 1975.

72. Shannon, I. L., and Edmonds, E. J.: Chemical alterations of enamel surfaces by single and sequential treatment with fluorides, J. Irish Dent. Assoc. **19**:135-139, 1973.

73. Wei, S. H. Y.: Effect of topical fluoride solutions on the enamel surface as studied by scanning electron microscopy, Caries Res. **9**:445-458, 1975.

74. Wei, S. H. Y., Sabaroff, D. M., and Wefel, J. S.: Effects of titanium tetrafluoride on human enamel, J. Dent. Res. **55**:426-431, 1976.

75. Reed, A. J., and Bibby, B. G.: Preliminary report on effect of topical applications of titanium tetrafluoride on dental caries, J. Dent. Res. **55**:357-358, 1976.

76. American Dental Association Council of Dental Therapeutics: Council accepts Macleans fluoride dentifrice, J.A.D.A. **92**:966-967, 1976.

77. Gron, P., Brudevold, F., and Aasenden, R.: Monofluorophosphate interaction with hydroxyapatite and intact enamel, Caries Res. **5**:202-214, 1971.

78. Duff, E. J.: Orthophosphates. XV. A suggested mechanism for the inhibition of dental caries by monofluorophosphates, Caries Res. **7**:79-84, 1973.

79. Stearns, R. I.: Incorporation of fluoride by human enamel. III. In vivo effects of nonfluoride and fluoride prophylactic pastes and APF gels, J. Dent. Res. **52**:30-35, 1973.

80. Bixler, D., and Muhler, J. C.: Effect on dental caries in children in a non-fluoride area of combined use of three agents containing stannous fluoride: a prophylactic paste, a solution, and a dentifrice. II. Results at the end of 24 and 36 months, J.A.D.A. **72**:392-396, 1966.

81. Gish, C. W., and Muhler, J. C.: Effect on dental caries in children in a natural fluoride area of combined use of three agents containing stannous fluoride: a prophylactic paste, a solution, and a dentifrice, J.A.D.A. **70**:914-920, 1965.

82. Horowitz, H. S., and Lucye, H. S.: A clinical study of stannous fluoride in a prophylaxis paste and as a solution, J. Oral Ther. Pharm. **3**:17, 1966.

83. Horowitz, H. S., Heifetz, S. B., McClendon, J., Uregas, A. R., Guimaraes, L. O. C., and Lopes, E. S.: Evaluation of self-administered prophylaxis and supervised toothbrushing with acidulated phosphate fluoride, Caries Res. **8**:39-51, 1974.

84. Bullen, D. C. T.: Two year effect of supervised tooth brushing with an acidulated fluoride-phosphate solution, J. Can. Dent. Assoc. **32**:89-93, 1966.

85. Berggren, H., and Welander, E.: The caries-inhibiting effect of sodium, ferric and zirconium fluorides, Acta Odontol. Scand. **22**:401-413, 1964.

86. Gallagher, S. J., Maclean, M. W., Castanzo, B., and Caldwell, R.: Self-application in a phospho-fluoride brushing study, J. Can. Dent. Assoc. **41**:505-510, 1975.

87. Goaz, P. W., McElwaine, L. P., Biswell, H. A., and White, W. E.: Effect of daily applications of sodium monofluorophosphate solution on caries rate in children, J. Dent. Res. **42**:965-972, 1963.

88. Scola, F. P.: Self-preparation stannous fluoride prophylactic technique in preventive dentistry: report after two years, J.A.D.A. **81**:1369, 1970.

89. Gish, C. W., Mercer, V. H., Stookey, G. K., and Dahly, L. O.: Self-application of fluoride as a community preventive measure: rationale, procedures, and three-year results, J.A.D.A. **90**:388-397, 1975.

90. Horowitz, H. S., and Bixler, D.: The effect of self-applied SnF$_2$–ZrSiO$_4$ prophylactic paste on dental

caries: Santa Clara County, Calif., J.A.D.A. **92:** 369-373, 1976.

91. Mellberg, J. R., Peterson, J. K., and Nicholson, C. R.: Fluoride uptake and caries inhibition from self-application of acidulated phosphate–fluoride prophylaxis paste, Caries Res. **8:**52-60, 1974.
92. American Dental Association Council on Dental Therapeutics: Council classifies fluoride mouthrinses, J.A.D.A. **9:**1250-1251, 1975.
93. Radike, A. W., Gish, C. W., Peterson, J. K., King, J. D., and Segreto, V. A.: Clinical evaluation of stannous fluoride as an anticaries mouthrinse, J.A.D.A. **86:**404-408, 1973.
94. Andres, C. J., Shaeffer, J. C., and Windeler, A. S., Jr.: Comparison of antibacterial properties of stannous fluoride and sodium fluoride mouthwashes, J. Dent. Res. **53:**457-460, 1974.
95. Arends, J., and Schuthof, J.: Fluoride content in human enamel after fluoride application and washing—an in vitro study, Caries Res. **9:**363-372, 1975.
96. Stamm, J. W.: Fluoride uptake from topical sodium fluoride varnish measured by an in vivo enamel biopsy, J. Can. Dent. Assoc. **40:**501-505, 1974.
97. Kock, G., and Petersson, L. G.: Caries preventive effect of a fluoride containing varnish (Duraphat)

after 1 year's study, Community Dent. Oral Epidemiol. **3:**262-266, 1975.
98. Stookey, G. K., and Stahlman, D. B.: Enhanced fluoride uptake in enamel with a fluoride-impregnated prophylactic cup, J. Dent. Res. **55:**333-341, 1976.
99. Chaet, R., and Wei, S. H. Y.: Enamel fluoride uptake from fluoride impregnated dental floss, International Association for Dental Research Program and Abstracts, No. 98, 1976.
100. Custer, F., and Cayle, T.: Mixed, spherical filling alloy amalgams, J. Mich. Dent. Assoc. **52:**93, 1970.
101. Jerman, A. C.: Silver amalgam restorative material with stannous fluoride, J.A.D.A. **80:**787-791, 1970.
102. Swartz, M. L., Phillips, R. W., and Norman, R. D.: The effect of fluoride-containing zinc oxide–eugenol cements on solubility of enamel, J. Dent. Res. **49:**576-580, 1970.
103. Wolf, O., Gedalia, I., Reisstein, I., Goldman, J., and Stieglitz, H.: Effect of addition of $CaFPO_3$ to a zinc oxide–eugenol base liner on the microhardness and fluoride content of dentin, J. Dent. Res. **52:**467-471, 1973.
104. Gursin, H. V.: A study of the effect of stannous fluoride incorporated in dental cement, J. Oral Ther. **1:**630, 1965.

23
Vitamins

RICHARD L. WYNN

The importance of nutrition in both general and dental health is well known. Dental practitioners must be concerned with the diagnosis and correction of deficiency states and should be aware of the relationships between nutrition and the growth and development of teeth, the prevention of dental caries, and the prevention and treatment of periodontal disease. For a discussion of general nutrition and its relationship to dental practice the reader is referred to the work of Nizel.[1] This chapter will deal with the more pharmacologic aspects of nutrition—the vitamins.

The vitamins are a group of small molecular weight organic compounds that are essential in small quantities for the maintenance of normal cellular metabolism and cell structure. Vitamins are classified into two large groups, *water-soluble* and *fat-soluble* vitamins. The water-soluble vitamins, except for vitamin C, function as components of coenzymes to aid in catalysis in a variety of enzyme reactions and are essential for the activity of a given enzyme. On a functional basis the water-soluble vitamins, except for vitamin C, may be subdivided into three classes: (1) those which primarily release energy from carbohydrates and fats (thiamine, pyridoxine, niacin, riboflavin, pantothenic acid, biotin), (2) those which among many other functions catalyze the formation of red blood cells (folic acid, vitamin B_{12}), and (3) those which have not been shown to be required in human nutrition (choline, inositol). Vitamin C does not function as a component of coenzymes but, rather, plays a role in biologic oxidation and reduction in cellular respirations.

In contrast to the water-soluble vitamins, the functions of the fat-soluble vitamins remain rather obscure. The fat-soluble vitamins are found in nature in association with lipid substances (vegetable oils, etc.) and include vitamins, A, D, E, and K. They do not appear to serve as components of coenzymes but function in other ways, requiring only trace amounts.

The water-soluble vitamins, except for vitamin C, are known as the *B complex vitamins* and a close interrelationship among these vitamins exists so that the deficiency of one will impair the utilization of the others. Also, there are many similarities in the signs and symptoms of deficiencies between individual B vitamins. This is probably because a deficiency of a particular member of the B complex is seldom produced. Rather, a diet deficient in one B vitamin is usually lacking in other B vitamins.

The vitamins are discussed individually with respect to their sources, chemical structures, requirements, physiologic and biochemical roles, and signs and symptoms of deficiencies. In addition, clinical considerations of the individual vitamins in dentistry and medicine are discussed.

WATER-SOLUBLE VITAMINS
Pyridoxine (vitamin B_6)

Pyridoxine is one of three different pyridine derivatives known as vitamin B_6, and its structure is shown below. The other two derivatives *pyridoxal* and *pyridoxamine* have similar chemical structures.

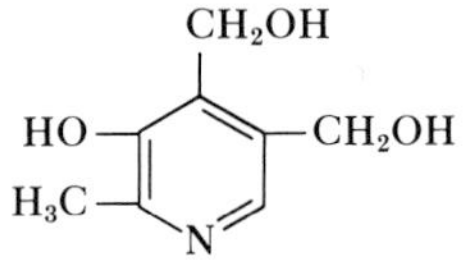

Pyridoxine

Vitamin B_6 is present in most foods of both plant and animal origin. Good sources of this vitamin include cereal grains, milk, meat, and certain vegetables. The recommended

Table 23-1. Recommended daily vitamin allowances*

	Age (years)	Water-soluble vitamins							Fat-soluble vitamins		
		Pyridoxine (vit. B_6) mg	Thiamine (vit. B_1) mg	Riboflavin (vit. B_2) mg	Niacin mg	Vit. B_{12} ng	Folic acid μg	Ascorbic acid mg	Vit. A IU	Vit. D IU	Vit. E IU
Children	1-3	0.6	0.7	0.8	9	1.0	100	40	2000	400	7
	4-6	0.9	0.9	1.1	12	1.5	200	40	2500	400	9
	7-10	1.2	1.2	1.2	16	2.0	300	40	3300	400	10
Men	11-14	1.6	1.4	1.5	18	3.0	400	45	5000	400	12
	15-18	2.0	1.5	1.8	20	3.0	400	45	5000	400	15
	19-22	2.0	1.5	1.8	20	3.0	400	45	5000		
	23-50	2.0	1.4	1.6	18	3.0	400	45	5000	400	15
	51+	2.0	1.2	1.5	16	3.0	400	45	5000	400	15
Women	11-14	1.6	1.2	1.3	16	3.0	400	45	4000	400	12
	15-18	2.0	1.1	1.4	14	3.0	400	45	4000	400	12
	19-22	2.0	1.1	1.4	14	3.0	400	45	4000	400	12
	23-50	2.0	1.0	1.2	13	3.0	400	45	4000	400	12
	51+	2.0	1.0	1.1	12	3.0	400	45	4000	400	12
Pregnant women		2.5	+0.3	+0.3	+2	4.0	800	60	5000	400	15
Lactating women		2.5	+0.3	+0.5	+4	4.0	600	80	6000	400	15

* Modified from Food and Nutrition Board, National Research Council: Recommended dietary allowances, ed. 8, Publication no. 2216, Washington, D.C., 1974, National Academy of Sciences.

allowances for this vitamin are shown in Table 23-1, and approximately 2 mg daily are recommended for adults, with an additional 0.5 mg during pregnancy and lactation. To exert physiologic activity, all three forms of vitamin B_6 are converted to pyridoxal phosphate in the body. Pyridoxal phosphate is the active coenzyme form of vitamin B_6 and participates in all metabolic reactions that require the vitamin.

The tuberculostatic drug isoniazid (isonicotinic acid hydrazide) inhibits the actions of vitamin B_6, and isoniazid-induced vitamin B_6 deficiency can be prevented by the administration of pyridoxine.[2]

Physiologic and biochemical role. Pyridoxal phosphate acts as a coenzyme for en-

zymes in a variety of metabolic transformations of amino acids, including transaminations and decarboxylations. An example of transamination involving pyridoxal phosphate is the conversion of alpha-ketoglutaric acid to L-glutamic acid, illustrated below. The pyridoxal phosphate is aminated to pyridoxamine phosphate by the donor amino acid and the pyridoxamine phosphate is subsequently deaminated by the acceptor alpha-ketoglutaric acid.

Decarboxylations requiring pyridoxal phosphate as a coenzyme include the decarboxylations of the amino acids tyrosine, arginine, and glutamine.

Clinical considerations. Vitamin B_6 deficiency is rare because of the widespread dis-

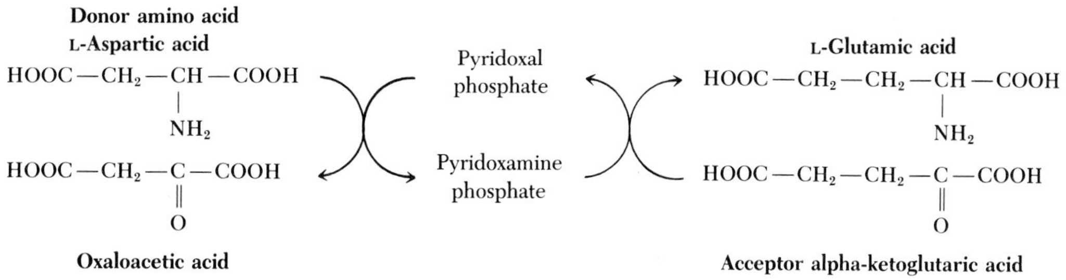

Donor amino acid
L-Aspartic acid
$HOOC-CH_2-CH-COOH$
$\quad\quad\quad\quad\quad NH_2$

$HOOC-CH_2-C-COOH$
$\quad\quad\quad\quad\quad \|$
$\quad\quad\quad\quad\quad O$

Oxaloacetic acid

Pyridoxal phosphate

Pyridoxamine phosphate

L-Glutamic acid
$HOOC-CH_2-CH_2-CH-COOH$
$\quad\quad\quad\quad\quad\quad\quad NH_2$

$HOOC-CH_2-CH_2-C-COOH$
$\quad\quad\quad\quad\quad\quad\quad \|$
$\quad\quad\quad\quad\quad\quad\quad O$

Acceptor alpha-ketoglutaric acid

tribution of this vitamin in food. However, skin lesions about the eyes, nose, and mouth accompanied by stomatitis and glossitis can be produced by feeding a diet poor in vitamin B complex plus a vitamin B_6 antagonist 4-deoxypyridoxine. These lesions will clear rapidly after the administration of pyridoxine. The characteristics of vitamin B_6 deficiency resemble those of riboflavin, niacin, and thiamine deficiencies. These include angular cheilosis, stomatitis, dermatitis, and erythema of the nasolabial folds. The dorsal mucosa of the tongue seems to be unusually sensitive to single or mixed deficiencies of B vitamins. Specifically, a glossitis has been described resulting from pyridoxine deficiency in which the tongue surface was smooth, slightly edematous, painful, and purplish.[3]

A cariostatic effect of vitamin B_6 has been observed in rhesus monkeys, and it was attributed to the influence of the vitamin on protein metabolism of the microorganisms on the tooth.[4] Also, a higher incidence of caries in vitamin B_6–deficient rats has been observed.[5]

Vitamin B_6 can alter the therapeutic effectiveness of some selected drugs. For example, the administration of vitamin B_6 cancels the therapeutic and side effects of levodopa in the treatment of Parkinson's disease.[6,7] Industry, however, has produced and marketed a pyridoxine-free vitamin preparation (Larobec), which can be used to cover the needs of vitamins in patients receiving levodopa. The administration of vitamin B_6 enhances the therapeutic effectiveness of nicotinic acid in the treatment of schizophrenia.[8]

Estrogenic steroids can produce a state of vitamin B_6 deficiency in women. Specifically, 50% of women taking oral contraceptive agents containing estrogens experienced a deficiency in vitamin B_6.[9] The administration of 20 mg pyridoxine hydrochloride daily appeared necessary to prevent this deficiency. It is suggested that pyridoxine supplements be routinely taken by women who use oral contraceptive agents.

Preparations. Pyridoxine hydrochloride tablets, USP, are available in 10, 25, 50, and 100 mg amounts. *Pyridoxine hydrochloride injection*, USP, is a sterile solution of pyridoxine hydrochloride in water containing 50 to 100 mg/ml.

Thiamine (vitamin B_1)

Thiamine, or vitamin B_1, is an essential water-soluble vitamin in humans. It is converted in the liver to its active coenzyme form, thiamine pyrophosphate (TPP). The chemical structure of TPP is as follows:

Thiamine pyrophosphate

Thiamine is present in foods of both animal and vegetable origin such as green vegetables, fish, meat, fruit, and milk. The highest levels are found in pork, whole grain, enriched cereal grains, and seeds of legumes such as peas. The vitamin tends to be destroyed if heated above 100° C. Thus significant amounts of the vitamin may be lost in foods by cooking too long above this temperature. The vitamin can also be leached out of foodstuffs being washed or boiled.

The requirement for thiamin is related to caloric intake. The recommended daily allowance is 0.4 mg/1000 cal with an additional 0.3 mg daily during the last two trimesters of pregnancy and during lactation. It is suggested that the average adult have an intake of approximately 1 mg thiamine daily.

Physiologic and biochemical role. Thiamine pyrophosphate (TPP) plays a principal role in intermediary metabolism. It is a coenzyme required for the oxidative decarboxylation of alpha-keto acids. For example, TPP is required for the oxidative decarboxylation of pyruvate to eventually form acetylcoenzyme A (acetyl-CoA); and in the oxidative decarboxylation of alpha-ketoglutarate to form succinylcoenzyme A. In this role TPP is sometimes referred to as *cocarboxylase.* TPP is also a coenzyme in the transketolation reactions that occur in the direct oxidative pathway of glucose metabolism (hexose monophosphate pathway). In these transketolation reactions two-carbon fragments are transferred from one sugar to another. An illustration of a transketolation reaction is shown at the top of p. 249.

Clinical considerations. A severe deficiency of thiamine leads to a condition known as beriberi. Characteristics of beriberi are

$$\text{D-Xylulose 5-phosphate} + \text{D-Ribose 5-phosphate} \underset{\text{(TPP) Mg}^{++}}{\overset{\text{Transketolase}}{\rightleftarrows}}$$

(5 carbon)   (5 carbon)

D-Sedoheptulose 7-phosphate + Glyceraldehyde 3-phosphate

(7 carbon)   (3 carbon)

peripheral neuritis, muscular weakness, paralysis of the limbs, enlargement of the heart, tachycardia, and edema. Gastrointestinal tract effects may also be present, including loss of appetite, intestinal atony, and constipation. The symptoms of mild thiamine deficiency are not nearly as characteristic as the preceding symptoms. They include tiredness and apathy, loss of appetite, moodiness and irritability, pain and paresthesias in the extremities, slight edema, decreased blood pressure, and a lowered body temperature. Possible oral manifestations of thiamine deficiency are burning tongue, loss of taste, and hyperesthesia of the oral mucosa. Thiamine deficiency is common in the more economically deprived areas of the world but uncommon in the United States and Europe.

Thiamine and other B vitamins may be effective in inhibiting bacterial growth in human saliva. One study has reported a significant reduction of *Staphylococcus aureus*, *S. albus*, and nonhemolytic group A *Streptococcus* when cultured from saliva that contained thiamine, riboflavin, and vitamin B_6.[10] Thiamine has also been shown to increase the fluoride retention effectively in rats exposed to daily fluoride supplements.[11]

Preparations. *Thiamine hydrochloride tablets*, USP, are available in sizes ranging from 5 to 250 mg. *Thiamine hydrochloride injection*, USP, is a sterile aqueous solution of the vitamin available in 50, 100, or 200 mg/ml. Thiamine hydrochloride is also available as an elixir containing 2.25 mg/5 ml.

Pantothenic acid

Pantothenic acid is another essential compound in addition to thiamine that is required for the oxidative decarboxylation of pyruvate to form acetyl-CoA. The structure of pantothenic acid is as follows:

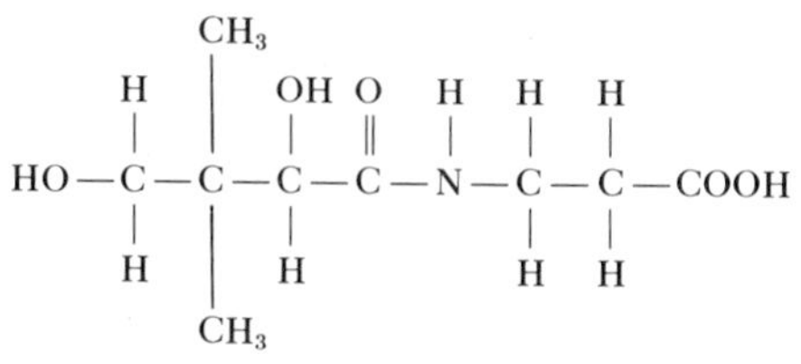

Pantothenic acid

The active form of pantothenic acid is as a component of the more complex compound *coenzyme A*.

Pantothenic acid is a component of all living material, and egg yolk, liver, and yeast are excellent sources. Pantothenic acid is required by humans, other vertebrates, some bacteria, and some plants. No quantitative requirement has been established in humans for this substance. The Food and Nutrition Board of the National Research Council, however, has suggested that a daily intake of 5 to 10 mg pantothenic acid is likely to satisfy human requirements.[12]

Physiologic and biochemical role. Pantothenic acid is a constituent of coenzyme A, which is a required coenzyme in various metabolic reactions, some of which involve the transfer of acetyl (two carbon) groups. As mentioned earlier, one of these reactions is catalyzed by the pyruvate dehydrogenase complex, which converts pyruvate to acetyl-CoA. Acetyl-CoA in turn serves as a central intermediate in the oxidation of carbohydrates, lipids, and some amino acids. Acetyl-CoA also serves as the biosynthetic building block in steroid biosynthesis (adrenal steroids, testosterone, estrogen) and fatty acid biosynthesis.

Coenzyme A is also involved in the decarboxylation of alpha-ketoglutarate to succinate in the Krebs tricarboxylic acid cycle (TCA cycle). This reaction produces succinyl-CoA as an intermediate. Finally, coenzyme A has an essential function in the metabolism of fatty acids.

Clinical considerations. Clinical deficiencies of pantothenic acid are extremely rare in humans. Deficiencies have been produced experimentally in humans using a pantothenic acid antagonist, however, which were characterized by fatigue, headache, malaise, nausea, abdominal pain, "burning" of hands and feet, and cramping of leg muscles.[13]

Preparations. *Calcium pantothenate*, USP, is available as tablets containing 10 or 30 mg and as an injectable preparation containing 50 mg/ml.

Riboflavin (vitamin B$_2$)

Riboflavin (vitamin B$_2$) is a water-soluble vitamin composed of flavin and D-ribitol. It has the following structure:

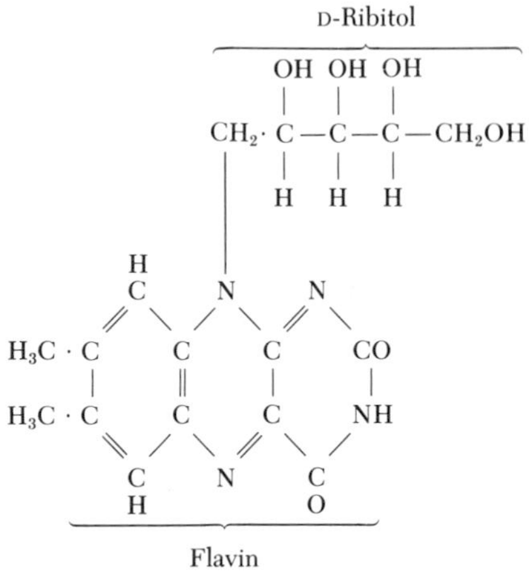

D-Ribitol

$$CH_2 \cdot \overset{\overset{\displaystyle OH}{|}}{C} - \overset{\overset{\displaystyle OH}{|}}{\underset{\underset{\displaystyle H}{|}}{C}} - \overset{\overset{\displaystyle OH}{|}}{\underset{\underset{\displaystyle H}{|}}{C}} - CH_2OH$$

Flavin

Riboflavin

Riboflavin occurs abundantly in both plants and animals. However, dairy products and meats serve as the best source for this vitamin. Riboflavin is relatively stable to heat, and cooking will not cause appreciable loss of the vitamin from foodstuffs. It is destroyed by ultraviolet irradiation.

The requirements for this vitamin are related to energy expenditure with a minimum daily requirement established at 0.3 mg/1000 Kcal. The Food and Drug Administration has set the adult daily minimum requirement of vitamin B$_2$ at 1.2 mg. The Food and Nutrition Board of the National Research Council, however, recommends a somewhat higher adult riboflavin allowance (Table 23-1).

Physiologic and biochemical role. Riboflavin carries out its functions in the body as a component of two flavoprotein coenzymes, riboflavin phosphate (flavin mononucleotide, FMN) and flavin adenine dinucleotide (FAD). Flavoprotein coenzymes in turn are proteins that act as electron acceptors and are involved in a variety of oxidation-reduction reactions. These reactions include those within the electron transport chain of the mitochondria which produce much of the cellular energy and also certain dehydrogenase reactions. In the mitochondrial electron transport chain, flavoproteins act as electron acceptors from the nicotinamide-containing electron carrier NADH. In other dehydrogenase reactions, flavoprotein dehydrogenases transfer electrons directly from a substrate to the electron transport chain. An example is succinate dehydrogenase in the TCA cycle.

The riboflavin-containing coenzyme FAD is also involved in the reduction of dihydrolipoic acid, which participates in the pyruvate decarboxylase complex mentioned previously. Thus riboflavin, as a constituent of FMN or FAD, has a fundamental role in metabolism by participating in various oxidation-reduction reactions involving carbohydrates, lipids, and electron transfer reactions.

Clinical considerations. Symptoms of riboflavin deficiency usually involve the lips, tongue, eyes, and skin. Angular stomatitis is an early and frequent finding. The lips may be either redder than usual or whitish because of desquamation. Ulceration may occur along with painful fissuring at the corners of the mouth. Glossitis generally occurs, with the dorsum of the tongue becoming pebbly or granular; contact with food or drink may produce pain or a burning sensation on the tongue. In some instances the tongue may become magenta colored or purplish red. Vascularization of the cornea frequently occurs. In advanced cases capillaries may invade the entire cornea, and there may be ulceration. Skin manifestations comprise a greasy, scaling inflammation about the nose, cheeks, and chin. Involvement of the scrotum and vulva is frequent. Other manifestations of riboflavin deficiency include anemia and neuropathy.

Riboflavin deficiency is most likely to be seen in alcoholics, economically deprived individuals, or in patients with severe gastrointestinal disease which cause loss of appetite, vomiting, and malabsorption syndromes. The manifestations of riboflavin deficiency are difficult to distinguish from other B vitamin deficiencies because of the similarities in syndromes.

Preparations. Riboflavin tablets, USP, are usually available in sizes ranging from 3 to 100 mg. *Riboflavin injection,* USP, contains 35 mg/ml.

Niacin (nicotinic acid) and niacinamide (nicotinamide)

Niacin (nicotinic acid) and niacinamide (nicotinamide) are water-soluble organic compounds that have the ability to alleviate a deficiency syndrome known as pellagra (*pelle*, skin; *agra*, rough). The chemical structures of these compounds are as follows:

Niacin
(nicotinic acid)

Niacinamide
(nicotinamide)

Niacin, in the form of niacinamide is a component of two coenzymes that participate in biologic oxidation-reduction reactions. These coenzymes are nicotinamide adenine dinucleotide (NAD) and nicotinamide adenine dinucleotide phosphate (NADP).

Good sources of this vitamin are lean meats, liver, and poultry. The requirement for niacin in the diet is somewhat dependent on caloric intake. It also probably depends on the amount of protein in the diet because tryptophan, an amino acid found in dietary protein, is metabolized to niacin in the body. It is estimated that approximately 60 mg tryptophan is converted to 1 mg niacin. Pellagra at one time was a common disease in the southeastern United States among individuals subsisting on a diet exclusively of corn products because the protein in corn is extremely low in tryptophan. The minimal requirement of niacin, including that formed from tryptophan to prevent pellagra, is approximately 4.4 mg/1000 Kcal. According to the Food and Nutrition Board of the National Research Council, the minimum daily requirement for niacin in the adult male is as great as 20 mg (Table 23-1).

Physiologic and biochemical role. The role of niacin is similar to that of riboflavin in that it plays a key role in metabolism by participating in a variety of oxidation-reduction reactions (the transfer of electrons). As a component of NAD and NADP, niacin is involved in the metabolism of carbohydrates and lipids as well as being involved in mitochondrial electron transport. The nicotinamide portion of NAD and NADP participates directly in these oxidation-reduction reactions because it has the ability to accept electrons as follows:

Oxidation-reduction of nicotinamide portion of NAD⁺ or NADP⁺

The lactate dehydrogenase reaction in which lactic acid is oxidized to pyruvic acid is an important reaction of carbohydrate metabolism, requiring NAD as a coenzyme. The lactate dehydrogenase reaction is a part of the anaerobic catabolism of glucose, and the reverse of this reaction (the conversion of lactic acid from pyruvate) is of primary significance in the production of lactic acid by oral microorganisms in that this will eventually cause demineralization of the tooth.

An important reaction in carbohydrate metabolism involving NADP is the glucose-6-phosphate dehydrogenase reaction, in which glucose-6-phosphate is converted to 6-phosphogluconate. These reactions are only two of the numerous reactions in which either NAD or NADP serve as coenzymes.

Clinical considerations. The clinical syndrome produced by niacin deficiency is called pellagra. Early symptoms appear as an erythematous cutaneous eruption on the back of the hands, glossitis, and stomatitis. In advanced stages pellagra can be diagnosed by the classic "three D's"—dermatitis, diarrhea, and dementia. The dermatitis consists of redness, thickening, and roughening of the skin followed by scaling desquamation and depigmentation. Diarrhea is caused by atrophy of the gastrointestinal tract mucosal epithelium, followed by inflammation of the mucosal lining of the esophagus, stomach, and colon. The dementia results from regressive changes in the ganglion cells of the brain and tracts of the spinal cord.

Throughout the course of pellagra, symptoms are extremely evident in the oral cavity. A burning sensation occurs throughout the oral mucosa. The lip and lateral margins of the tongue are initially reddened and swollen. In the later stages the entire dorsum becomes red and swollen. In acute stages vascular hyperemia, proliferation, hypertrophy, atrophy, and extinction occur successively in the papillae.[2] Papillary loss may ultimately become complete, with the tongue surface becoming beefy red. Deep penetrating ulcers may appear on the tongue surface. In the gingiva desquamative epithelial degeneration may occur, exposing the tissue to infection, inflammation, and fibrinous exudation. Gingivitis due to pellagra is characterized by ulcers in the interdental papillae and marginal gingiva. There is also excessive salivary secretion with enlargement of the salivary glands.[2]

Niacin deficiency most likely occurs in the poverty-stricken areas of the world because of inadequate intake. Deficiency may also arise from chronic alcoholism, gastrointestinal disturbances, pregnancy, hyperthyroidism, and infections.

Preparations. Niacin tablets, NF (nicotinic acid), are available in 20, 25, 50, 100, and 500 mg amounts. Niacin injection, NF, is available in 10, 50, or 100 mg/ml. Niacinamide tablets, USP (nicotinamide), are available in 25, 50, 100, and 500 mg amounts. Niacinamide injection is available in concentrations of 100 or 200 mg/ml.

Biotin

Biotin was initially demonstrated to be an essential growth factor for yeast, and it was later shown that this substance could be isolated from both yeast and egg yolk. Its chemical structure was established in 1942, and shortly thereafter the vitamin was synthesized. Its chemical structure is as follows:

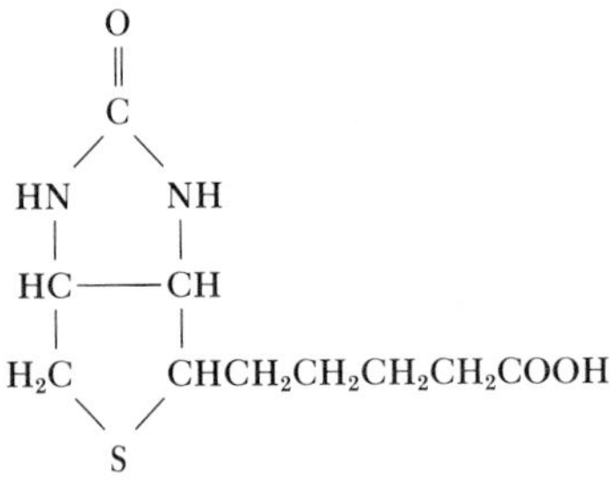

Biotin

A deficiency of biotin can be induced by the feeding of large quantities of raw egg whites. Avidin, a glycoprotein component of egg white, has the ability to combine with biotin in the gastrointestinal tract to prevent its absorption. The avidin is denatured when the egg white is cooked, and the binding to biotin does not occur. Biotin is synthesized by the microflora of the intestinal tract. In fact, it has been demonstrated that the excretion of biotin in the feces exceeds its intake and is probably due to the synthesis of the vitamin by the intestinal flora.

A deficiency in biotin is extremely rare but probably can be produced by concurrent administration of large amounts of raw egg white. A minimum daily requirement for this vitamin has yet to be established.

Physiologic and biochemical role. Biotin is a coenzyme required in metabolism in carbon dioxide fixation reactions (carboxylations). An important carboxylation reaction requiring biotin is the acetyl-CoA carboxylase reaction in which acetyl-CoA is carboxylated to form malonyl-CoA. This reaction is the first in a sequence of reactions giving rise to fatty acid biosynthesis.

Clinical considerations. A deficiency of biotin is extremely rare in humans. Experimentally induced biotin deficiency has produced a variety of symptoms. These include loss of appetite, mental depression, hyperesthesia of the skin, nausea, and malaise.

Preparations. There is no official preparation of biotin marketed in the United States.

Vitamin B$_{12}$ (cyanocobalamin)

Vitamin B$_{12}$, or cyanocobalamin, is a chemically complex substance that contains an extensively substituted pyrole ring system surrounding an atom of cobalt. The structure of this water-soluble vitamin is so complex as to be beyond the scope of this discussion. The structural formula of vitamin B$_{12}$ was elucidated by Hodgkin,[14] a work of such importance as to warrant her receiving the Nobel prize in chemistry. Vitamin B$_{12}$ contains a cyanide molecule attached to the cobalt, hence the name *cyano*cobalamin. There exists a chemical family of cobalamins, depending on what group replaces cyanide. The hydroxyl derivative is *hydroxocobalamin* (vitamin B$_{12a}$), the H$_2$O derivative is *aquocobalamin* (vitamin B$_{12b}$), the nitro derivative is *nitritocobalamin* (vitamin B$_{12c}$), the 5'-deoxyadenosyl derivative is *coenzyme B*$_{12}$, and the methyl derivative is methyl B$_{12}$. Vitamin B$_{12}$ is stable to heat at neutral pH but is readily destroyed by heat at an alkaline pH.

Foods of animal origin are good sources of the vitamin, with liver and kidney serving as the best sources and milk, cheese, and eggs serving as adequate sources.

Vitamin B$_{12}$ is not adequately absorbed from the gastrointestinal tract without the presence of a protein-binding factor (intrinsic factor) secreted by the gastric mucosa. The intrinsic factor is a glycoprotein formed and secreted by the parietal cells of the stomach, and it aids the mucosal absorption of B$_{12}$ through a binding mechanism with the vitamin. Pernicious anemia is a conditional vitamin B$_{12}$ deficiency disease caused by a lack of intrinsic factor in the gastric mucosa. Pernicious anemia can be treated by intramuscular injection of vitamin B_{12}, since adequate amounts of the vitamin are absorbed into the plasma by this route without the requirement of intrinsic factor.

A daily intake of 0.6 to 1.2 μg will sustain modest body stores of vitamin B_{12} in normal adults. The World Health Organization recommends a daily dietary intake for adults of 2 μg, after allowing for 60% to 80% absorption from food.[15] The Food and Nutrition Board of the National Research Council recommends a daily adult allowance of 3 μg vitamin B_{12} with an additional 1 μg during pregnancy and lactation (Table 23-1).

Physiologic and biochemical role. Vitamin B_{12} serves as a coenzyme for the hydrogen transfer and isomerization process required in the conversion of methylmalonyl-CoA to succinyl-CoA. Thus vitamin B_{12} is an important requirement for fat and carbohydrate metabolism, a reaction that occurs as follows:

$$CH_3-CH-\overset{\overset{\displaystyle O}{\|}}{C}\sim S-CoA \quad \underset{\underset{\displaystyle \longleftarrow}{\longrightarrow}}{\overset{\text{Methylmalonyl-CoA}}{\overset{\text{mutase}}{}}}$$

$$\underset{\text{COOH}}{|}$$

Methylmalonyl-CoA   **Coenzyme B_{12}**

$$HOOC-CH_2CH_2\overset{\overset{\displaystyle O}{\|}}{C}\sim S-CoA$$

Succinyl-CoA

Vitamin B_{12} functions in this reaction in the form of the 5'-deoxyadenosyl derivative known as *coenzyme B_{12}*, or the *cobamide* coenzyme. Other reactions thought to require vitamin B_{12} as a coenzyme include the metabolism of the one-carbon group required in the synthesis of the bases for nucleic acids (for example, the methylation of uridine to form thymidine); transmethylation reactions, as in the biosynthesis of methionine; the synthesis of proteins in the microsomal system; and the synthesis of deoxyribonucleotides from ribonucleotides. The foregoing reactions have been suggested to require vitamin B_{12} to account for the clinical signs of deficiency. The involvement of the vitamin in these reactions has yet to be definitely established, however.

Clinical considerations. The symptoms of vitamin B_{12} deficiency include inadequate hematopoiesis, gastrointestinal tract disturbances, inadequate myelin synthesis, and generalized debility. The lack of this vitamin affects those cells that are most actively dividing, such as those in the marrow and gastrointestinal tract. The erythroblasts do not undergo proper division and thus become megaloblasts. This results in a failure to maintain a normal level of red blood cells, resulting in anemia. Atropic changes occur in the alimentary canal. There is also myelin degeneration of the spinal cord. The patient suffers from weakness, numbness, and difficulty in walking, symptoms that fluctuate with remission and relapses. A distinctive lemon-yellow hue of the skin may occur.

The most common cause of vitamin B_{12} deficiency is pernicious anemia. This condition is thought to result from a defect in the stomach characterized by atrophic gastritis. As a result of the gastritis, intrinsic factor is not produced by the mucosal cells and thus vitamin B_{12} is not absorbed. Other causes of B_{12} deficiency include inadequate dietary intake and malabsorption syndromes due to structural or functional damage to the stomach, where intrinsic factor is secreted, or to the ileum, where intrinsic factor functions to enhance vitamin B_{12} absorption.

Pernicious anemia results in a number of oral manifestations. Recurrent attacks of soreness and burning of the tongue occur prior to glossitis, at the peak of which the tongue is extremely painful and red. Atrophy of the filiform and fungiform papillae is a common occurrence. Involvement of the circumvallate papillae may cause diminution of taste. Painful, bright red lesions may occur in the buccal and pharyngeal mucosa and undersurface of the tongue.

Preparations. Cyanocobalamin injection, USP (Rubramin), is an isotonic saline solution available in 1, 5, 10, and 30 ml vials for intramuscular injection containing 30, 50, 60, 100, or 1000 μg/ml. *Vitamin B with intrinsic factor concentrate* is marketed for oral use in patients who lack adequate intrinsic factor and who refuse parenteral therapy.

Folic acid (pteroylglutamic acid)

Folic acid is a complex molecule consisting of glutamic acid, para-aminobenzoic acid (PABA), and pteridine and has the following chemical structure.

Glutamic acid | Para-aminobenzoic acid | Pteridine

Folic acid

Folic acid is sparingly soluble in water and is destroyed on heating in neutral or alkaline solutions.

Sources of folic acid include glandular meats such as liver, leafy vegetables (folic acid from Latin *folium*, leafy), and yeasts. The intestinal flora probably supplies some of the requirements for this vitamin. Protracted cooking or canning may destroy 50% to 95% of the folic acid content in foods.

The minimum daily human requirement of folic acid is approximately 5 μg in adults.[16] The World Health Organization recommends a dietary intake of 200 μg for adults, 50 μg for infants, 100 μg for children, and 400 μg during pregnancy and lactation. The Food and Nutrition Board of the National Research Council recommends a daily intake of 400 μg in adults (Table 23-1).

Para-aminobenzoic acid (PABA), a component of the folic acid molecule, is essential in itself for certain microorganisms because of its incorporation into folic acid. The bacteriostatic agents, the sulfonamides, exert their mechanism of action by acting as antagonists to PABA and thus interfere with the folic acid biosynthesis in these microorganisms.

Physiologic and biochemical role. The biologically active form of folic acid is the reduced derivative tetrahydrofolic acid (THFA), formed enzymatically in the body. THFA functions primarily in the transfer and utilization of one-carbon groups, such as formyl ($-CHO$), formate ($-COOH$), hydroxymethyl ($-CH_2OH$), and methyl (CH_3). The transfer and utilization of one-carbon groups are important in relation to the metabolism of amino acids and nucleic acids and also in the formation of purine and pyrimidine bases. With the lack of folic acid, cells fail to complete mitosis and do not progress from metaphase to anaphase because of the absence of the biosynthesis of nucleoprotein.

Clinical considerations. Folic acid deficiency results in megaloblastic anemia, which is indistinguishable from that due to vitamin B$_{12}$ deficiency. Other symptoms include weakness, weight loss, loss of skin pigmentation, and mental irritability. Oral manifestations include glossitis, angular chilosis, and gingivitis. The glossitis begins with swelling and pallor of the tongue, followed by desquamation of the papillae and accompanied by minute ulcers with fiery red borders. The angular chilosis and gingivitis resemble that seen with a deficiency of riboflavin.

Some of the causes of folic acid deficiency include inadequate diet, pregnancy, malabsorption syndromes, and chronic alcoholism. Folic acid deficiencies have been reported in association with anticonvulsant drug therapy.[17]

The administration of folic acid will cause a remission of the hematologic effects of pernicious anemia. Folic acid will not prevent the neurologic effects of vitamin B$_{12}$ deficiency.

Preparations. Folic acid tablets, USP, are available in strengths of 0.1, 0.4, 5, 10, and 20 mg. *Folic acid injection*, USP, is an aqueous solution of the sodium salt of folic acid available in 1, 2, and 10 ml ampules containing 5 mg/ml.

Choline and inositol

The presence of choline and inositol in foods such as meat, eggs, fish, and cereals led to their consideration as members of the B complex vitamins. However, neither choline nor inositol has been demonstrated to be required in the human diet. The chemical structures of choline and inositol (*myo*-inositol) are as follows:

Choline   *myo*-Inositol

Inositol is an isomer of glucose. Of several optically active forms of inositol, possibly only one, *myo*-inositol, is nutritionally active. It is estimated that the normal daily intake of choline is 250 to 600 mg and of inositol, about 1 Gm.

Physiologic and biochemical role. Choline and inositol serve as lipotropic agents. These are agents that are necessary in the diet to prevent or correct fatty infiltration of the liver. In addition, choline serves as the precursor in the formation of acetylcholine, an important chemical mediator in the parasympathetic nervous system. Choline can also serve as a methyl donor in intermediary metabolism.

Clinical considerations. No deficiency symptoms for choline or inositol have been described for humans. A deficiency of choline in the rat results in both hemorrhagic kidney and fatty livers. Inositol deficiency in mice is characterized by spectacled eyes, alopecia, failure of lactation, and lack of growth. Inositol has been shown to be an essential component for the growth and survival of human cell lines in tissue culture.[18]

Ascorbic acid (vitamin C)

Ascorbic acid (vitamin C) chemically is a sugar acid that readily undergoes oxidation to form dehydroascorbic acid. The structures of ascorbic acid and its oxidation are as follows:

Ascorbic acid   Dehydroascorbic acid
(reduced form)   (oxidized form)

Because of its property of undergoing oxidation, ascorbic acid is an effective reducing agent.

Good sources of ascorbic acid are fresh fruits and vegetables, including citrus fruits, green vegetables, tomatoes, and berries. Because of its ability to be oxidized, ascorbic acid is readily destroyed by oxidation through cooking, and as much as 50% of the ascorbic acid content of foods can be lost in this manner. Estimates of the daily requirement for ascorbic acid for the normal adult range from 45 to 80 mg (Table 23-1).

Physiologic and biochemical role. The metabolic role of ascorbic acid is probably related to the fact that ascorbic acid and dehydroascorbic acid form a readily reversible oxidation-reduction system, and it is thought that this vitamin plays a role in biologic oxidation and reductions in cellular respirations. Ascorbic acid is oxidized by cytochrome C in the presence of cytochrome C oxidase. Dehydroascorbic acid can be reduced by glutathione. Also, ascorbic acid may function in maintaining SH-activated enzyme systems in their reduced form.

A specific requirement for ascorbic acid occurs in tyrosine metabolism. This vitamin acts as a reducing agent in the parahydroxyphenylpyruvic acid oxidase reaction, which converts parahydroxyphenylpyruvic acid (formed by tyrosine) to homogentisic acid. The role of ascorbic acid in the foregoing reaction is nonspecific, however, since other reducing agents can replace the vitamin in the oxidation of parahydroxyphenylpyruvic acid.

Ascorbic acid appears to be necessary for the reduction of folic acid to tetrahydrofolic acid (THFA) in mammalian cells. THFA eventually functions in the transfer and utilization of one-carbon groups. Ascorbic acid also functions to catalyze the hydroxylation of proline to form the amino acid hydroxyproline. The subsequent distribution of the generated hydroxyproline occurs in collagen. Thus ascorbic acid plays a definite role in connective tissue metabolism in that it is required for the formation of collagen through the proline hydroxylation process.

The dramatic demonstration of the physiologic function of ascorbic acid is in the wound healing process. Scorbutic wounds (a deficiency of vitamin C) are characterized by a significant decrease in mature collagen fibrils associated with an accumulation of mucopolysaccharides or ground substance around a matrix of precollagenous fibers. Because of the absence of mature collagen, the tensile strength of the healing wound occurs, resulting in a normal healing process. The role of ascorbic acid in wound healing and collagen formation has been adequately reviewed.[19,20]

Clinical considerations. The manifestations of vitamin C deficiency occur because of the inability of the connective tissue to produce and maintain intercellular substances such as collagen, bone matrix, dentin, cartilage, and vascular endothelium. As a result of defective connective tissue formation, individuals with a vitamin C deficiency demonstrate alterations in bone formation tissue and in wound healing. The manifestations of defective connective tissue formation in vitamin C deficiency are listed in the outline below.

> Alterations in wound healing, manifested as
> > Lack of collagen
> > Poor healing process
> > Inadequate walling off of infections
> Alterations in the integrity of capillary walls, manifested as hemorrhages in
> > Skin
> > Mucous membranes
> > Muscles
> > Lungs
> > Joints
> > Gingivae (spongy, edematous, inflamed)
> Lack of formation of bone matrix, resulting in
> > Disorganization of epiphyseal line
> > Weakening of bones
> > Pathologic fractures
> > Resorption of alveolar bone with loosening and loss of teeth

Humans and other primates cannot synthesize vitamin C and must obtain it daily from their diet. Diets completely deficient in vitamin C are unusual, and there are few cases of serious vitamin C deficiency (scurvy). After a prolonged period of time without vitamin C (4 to 5 months), the following symptoms will occur in humans: weakness, anorexia, suppressed growth, anemia, lowered resistance to infection and fever, swollen and inflamed gums, loosened teeth, swollen wrist and ankle joints, petechial hemorrhages, fracture of ribs at costochondral junctions, and hemorrhaging due to capillary fragility in joints, muscle, and intestine.

It was suggested, as long ago as 1942, that vitamin C could be therapeutically beneficial in preventing the common cold.[21] Recently, Linus Pauling produced a number of reviews of previous data by other investigators.[22-25] He argued that these studies showed results which, if properly analyzed, indicated a substantial beneficial effect of vitamin C in preventing and treating the common cold. These studies suggested that daily ascorbic acid doses ranging from a few hundred milligrams up to several grams provided beneficial results in diminishing the incidence and severity of colds. Most recently, the clinical data relating to the efficacy of pharmacologic doses of ascorbic acid in relation to colds have been critically reviewed.[26] This review concluded that there is little evidence to suggest the effectiveness of ascorbic acid in preventing or treating the common cold and that the unrestricted use of ascorbic acid for these purposes should not be advocated on the basis of available evidence. Until the Pauling theory is subsequently verified or refuted by well-controlled experiments, it must be considered a hypothesis, at the very most.

Still another hypothesis has been set forth by Pauling that large quantities of vitamin C may suppress neoplastic cellular proliferation, and he suggests that the use of ascorbic acid be investigated in cancer management including prophylaxis, supportive therapy, and palliative treatment in advanced terminal cancer.[27]

Others have suggested that a prolonged marginal deficiency of vitamin C plays a contributory role in the initiation of periodontal disease.[28] This hypothesis probably stems from the fact that one of the manifestations of vitamin C deficiency is scorbutic gums (swollen, inflamed gingiva with loosening of the teeth). This hypothesis has not been substantiated by the findings of other investigators, however.[29,30] A deficiency of vitamin C may alter the local response to irritants and may lead to an increased severity of gingival disease (McBean and Speckmann[31]).

Ascorbic acid has been shown to interfere with the anticoagulation produced by heparin and dicumarol in animals.[32] Also, it has been reported that the vitamin caused a reduction in the desired prolongation of prothrombin time in a patient receiving warfarin.[33] Recently, it has been shown that vitamin C may inhibit the metabolism of drugs that undergo sulfate conjugation.[34]

Untoward effects have been reported with the use of vitamin C. A daily intake of 1 Gm of the vitamin may produce diarrhea. Also, acidification of the urine by the vitamin may cause precipitation of oxalate stones in the urinary tract.

Preparations. Ascorbic acid tablets, USP, contain 25, 50, 100, 250, 500, or 1000 mg of the vitamin, and solutions for oral use are also available. *Ascorbic acid injection*, USP, is available containing 50, 100, 250, or 500 mg/ml. Orange or lemon juice contain approximately 0.5 mg/ml of the vitamin.

FAT-SOLUBLE VITAMINS
Vitamin A

Vitamin A is an essential fat-soluble compound necessary for normal growth as well as maintaining the health and integrity of certain epithelial tissues. Vitamin A occurs in a variety of chemical forms in nature, and the term *vitamin A* is used to represent these various forms. Vitamin A_1 (retinol) is found exclusively in animal tissues and saltwater fishes. The structure of this compound is as shown below. Vitamin A_2 (3-dehydro-retinol) contains an additional double bond in the ring structure and is found in the tissues of freshwater fishes. A group of substances known as carotenes are present in plants and vitamin A may be derived from carotenes by the cleavage of these molecules. β-carotene is oxidatively cleaved in humans to form two molecules of a form of vitamin A known as vitamin A_1 aldehyde (retinal). The carotenes are found in various pigmented fruits and in vegetables including carrots, pumpkins, sweet potatoes, apricots, and peaches.

The recommended daily allowance for vitamin A is 4000 to 5000 IU (approximately 1.5 mg) for an adult (Table 23-1). Increased intake of the vitamin is required during pregnancy and lactation.

Vitamin A is essential for the maintenance of normal vision. Specifically, vitamin A is essential for the normal visual purple in the rod cells of the retina. Deficiency of the vitamin leads to impaired vision in dim light, called night blindness (nyctalopia). For a review of the actions of vitamin A on visual excitation see Wald.[35] Vitamin A is also essential for the maintenance of certain epithelial surfaces, such as the mucous membranes of the eyes and the mucosa of the respiratory, gastrointestinal, and genitourinary tracts. A deficiency of vitamin A results in keratinization of mucosa, and keratinization of the corneal mucosa leads to impairment of vision, a condition called xerophthalmia. Irritation and inflammation may occur on the corneal mucosa, leading to softening, deformation, and destruction of the cornea, a condition called keratomalacia. Keratinization may also occur in the oral cavity and mucosa. In the respiratory tract, ciliated columnar epithelium may be replaced by stratified squamous epithelium. The normal defense mechanism of cilia movement and mucus production is impaired, producing irritation and inflammation of these surfaces.

It has been suggested that vitamin A may play a significant role in the maintenance of the integrity and possibly the normal permeability of the cell membrane and the membranes of subcellular particles such as lysosomes and mitochondria.[36] Vitamin A deficiency decreases the activity of the osteoblasts and odontoblasts, thereby reducing the growth of bones and teeth. Excessive doses of the vitamin accelerate bone growth.

Since the human liver may store enough vitamin A to meet physiologic demands for as long as a year, a deficiency of the vitamin is

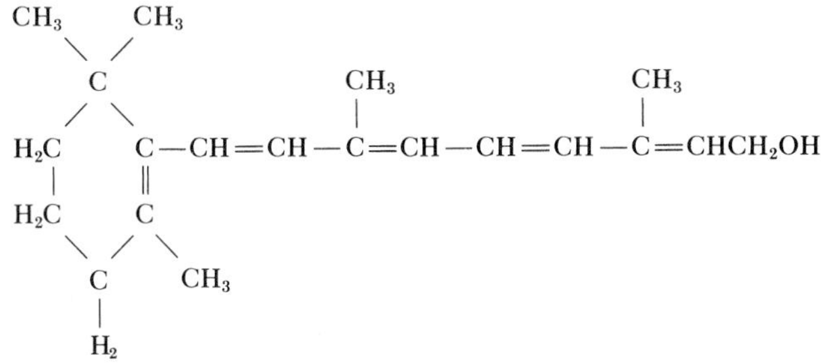

Vitamin A_1 (retinol)

usually rare. Deficiencies generally result from inadequate intake of the vitamin, malabsorption syndromes (especially disorders affecting fat absorption such as biliary tract disease), and severe liver disease.

Hypervitaminosis A is a toxic condition caused by excessive intake of the vitamin. Characteristics of the toxicity are itching skin, desquamation, coarse hair, painful subcutaneous swellings, gingivitis, hyperirritability, and limitation of motion. In infants, headache from increased intracranial pressure, gastrointestinal distress, jaundice, and hepatomegaly may occur. The margin of safety of vitamin A intake is large. Toxicity to the vitamin occurs in the adult only after the daily ingestion of several million units. Infants may show the effects of overdosage after a single dose of 350,000 units.

Preparations. Vitamin A, USP, is either fish-liver oil or a solution of natural or synthetic vitamin A. *Vitamin A capsules*, USP, contain 1.5 to 15 mg retinal (5000 to 50,000 units) per capsule. *Aquasol A* (water-miscible vitamin A) is a concentrate of vitamin A dispersed in water and encapsulated.

Vitamin D

The term *vitamin D* is used to refer to a group of closely related steroids produced by the action of ultraviolet light on certain provitamins. Vitamin D_3 (cholecalciferol) is produced in the skin of mammals from 7-dehydrocholesterol by the action of sunlight (irradiation). Vitamin D_2 (calciferol) is produced by the commercial irradiation of ergosterol. These reactions are as shown below. 7-Dehydrocholesterol occurs naturally in animal tissues and is synthesized from cholesterol in the skin and other peripheral tissues. Ergosterol occurs naturally in yeast and fungi. Vitamin D is generally used as the collective term for vitamins D_2 and D_3.

Vitamin D is required for normal mineralization of bone, and it is essential for the homeostatic regulation of plasma calcium concentration. Sources of vitamin D include food products of animal origin (eggs, cheese, milk, butter). The fish-liver oils are especially rich in vitamin D as well as vitamin A (cod-liver oil). Milk in the United States is fortified with vitamin D (as irradiated ergosterol), since the vitamin is intimately involved in calcium metabolism.

The recommended daily dietary allowance of vitamin D is 400 IU for a growing child or for a pregnant or lactating woman. The dietary allowance has not been established for the normal adult but is presumed to be of the same order of magnitude (Table 23-1). Some of the daily requirement for vitamin D is obviously satisfied by exposure of the individual to sunlight.

Vitamin D promotes normal mineraliza-

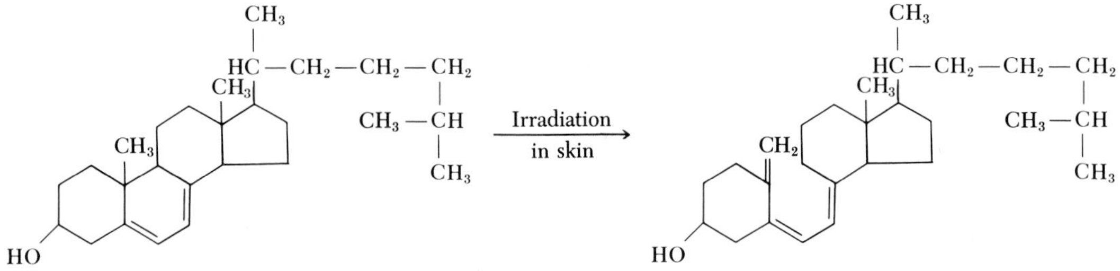

7-Dehydrocholesterol → (Irradiation in skin) → Vitamin D_3

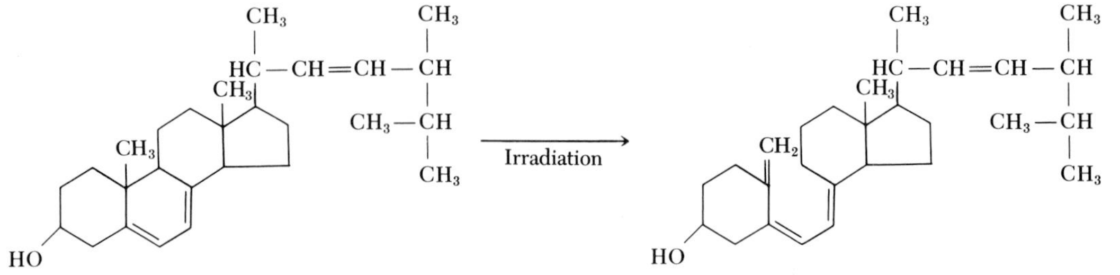

Ergosterol → (Irradiation) → Vitamin D_2 (calciferol)

tion of bone by providing an adequate supply of calcium to bone by means of its action to stimulate the intestinal absorption of this ion. Vitamin D_3 itself does not cause the active transport of calcium from the intestine. Experiments have shown that it is an active metabolite of vitamin D_3 found in the kidney which is responsible for the calcium transport across the intestine and for its other effects.[37] Once formed in the skin or taken in the diet, vitamin D_3 is carried to the liver where it is hydroxylated in the number 25 position to form 25-hydroxyvitamin D_3 (25-OH-D_3). This hydroxylation occurs in the liver microsomal fraction. The 25-OH-D_3 is then transported to the kidney and converted to the physiologically active 1,25-dihydroxyvitamin D_3 (1,25-$(OH)_2$-D_3 or 1,25-dihydroxy D_3). The active metabolite 1,25-dihydroxy D_3 may stimulate calcium transport through the intestine by inducing the formation of a calcium-binding protein in intestinal epithelial cells.[38]

The participation of vitamin D in the regulation of plasma calcium is by its action to promote mobilization of calcium from bone. The regulation of plasma calcium by this mechanism maintains those concentrations required for normal muscular and nervous function. Vitamin D, through its metabolite 1,25-dihydroxy D_3 also plays an integral part in the process of bone formation. It seems to be necessary for the initial calcification of bone matrix and probably exerts a prime action on the osteoblasts.

The actions of 1,25-dihydroxy D_3 are interrelated to parathyroid hormone (PTH). There is an increased formation of the D_3 hormone because of decreased plasma calcium—an effect mediated by way of PTH on the 1,25-dihydroxy D_3–forming mechanism in the kidney. The 1,25-dihydroxy D_3 together with PTH functions to mobilize calcium from previously formed bone. In addition, the 1,25-dihydroxy D_3 proceeds to the intestine where it functions directly to stimulate intestinal calcium absorption. These two phenomena result in the elevation of serum calcium to normal levels, which suppresses PTH secretion and hence 1,25-dihydroxy D_3 synthesis. Thus it has been suggested that 1,25-dihydroxy D_3 be regarded as a hormone derived from vitamin D_3 with the kidney as the endocrine organ and the intestine, bone, and possibly the kidney as target tissues. In-

creased formation of 1,25-dihydroxy D_3 is also mediated by decreased plasma phosphate (hypophosphatemia). The hormone also acts to stimulate the elevation of serum inorganic phosphate by enhancing the transport of the ion through the intestine. For a review of the mode of action of vitamin D, see DeLuca[39] or Haussler.[40]

In children, vitamin D deficiency results in *rickets*, whereas in the adult the disease state is *osteomalacia*. Rickets is characterized by a failure of mineralization of the osteoid matrix resulting in an excess of poorly mineralized osteoid tissue. The histologic characteristics of rickets include the failure of calcification of cartilage; overgrowth of cartilage; projection of masses of cartilage into the marrow cavity; disruption of osteochondral junctions; and weak, soft osteoid and cartilaginous tissues, which is easily bent, compressed, or fractured. The gross deformities of rickets include a squared appearance of the head due to excess osteoid, collapse of the ribs and protrusion of the sternum (pigeon breast syndrome), curvature of the spine, and bowing of the legs. Bone pain and muscle weakness may also be present.

In osteomalacia the basic changes are similar to those of rickets. There is inadequate mineralization resulting in an excess of osteoid matrix. Because of the weakness of the bones, there are deformities of weight-bearing bones as well as pathologic fractures. Adults with this condition also suffer from bone pain and muscle weakness. Causes of vitamin D deficiency are dietary insufficiency and malabsorption syndromes.

Like vitamin A, vitamin D may be ingested excessively, resulting in hypervitaminosis D. Signs and symptoms of vitamin D toxicity are associated with hypercalcemia. Initial symptoms include weakness, fatigue, headache, nausea, vomiting, and diarrhea. Prolonged hypercalcemia may result in the calcification of blood vessels, heart, lungs, and kidney. Daily quantities of vitamin D in the order of magnitude of 2000 IU/kg body weight can be toxic to adults and children.

Preparations. Vitamin D preparations are available as fish-liver oils with or without vitamin A, multivitamin preparations containing vitamin D, preparations containing vitamin D and calcium salts, and preparations of vitamin D alone.

Vitamin E

Compounds possessing vitamin E activity are known chemically as tocopherols. There are three such tocopherols designated as α-(alpha), β-(beta), and γ-(gamma) tocopherol. The structure of α-tocopherol is as follows:

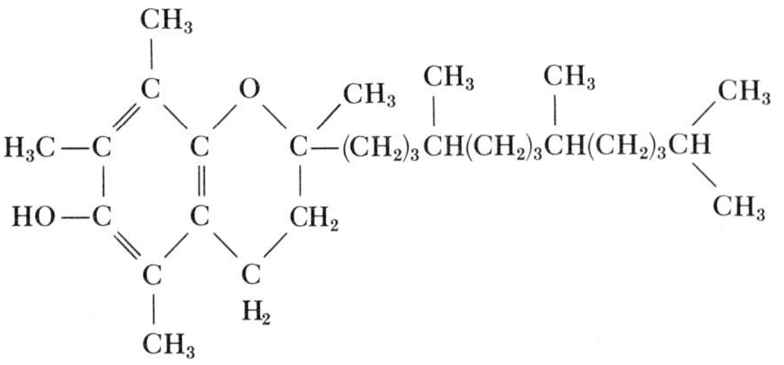

Vitamin E (α-tocopherol)

Vitamin E was originally isolated from wheatgerm oil and alpha-tocopherol is considered the most important vitamin E compound, since it elicits the greatest biologic activity in most bioassay systems. The metabolic role of vitamin E is not understood, although it appears that the vitamin functions as an antioxidant in mammalian tissues.

The best sources of vitamin E include vegetable oils such as soybean, corn, and cottonseed oils; other sources include fresh greens and vegetables. The daily requirement for vitamin E has been estimated to be 12 to 15 IU in adults (Table 23-1).

As an antioxidant, vitamin E probably prevents (1) the oxidation of essential cell constituents and (2) the formation of toxic oxidation products. Its physiologic role is best defined, however, from symptoms that have been observed in deficiency states. It has been reported that resistance of erythrocytes to hemolysis in the presence of hydrogen peroxide was related to vitamin E intake so that a shortened red blood cell survival time was alleviated by administration of the vitamin.[41] It has been suggested that degenerative changes of skeletal muscle cells occur in humans during vitamin E deficiency.[42] Also, a deficiency of the vitamin has been shown to result in muscular dystrophy in monkeys.[43] There has been no clinical evidence to show any beneficial effect of the vitamin in the treatment of this disease, however. Vitamin E deficiency in male rats results in reproductive failure and sterility (degeneration of the germinal epithelium within testicular tissue). In the female rat a deficiency leads to fetal death and resorption. In humans vitamin E has been used for the treatment of sterility and habitual abortion, but there is no conclusive evidence that the vitamin provides any beneficial effect in these conditions.

Vitamin E is generally thought to have a low toxicity. Levels of vitamin E greatly in excess of the normal dietary requirements have been administered to human subjects with no apparent adverse effects.

Preparations. Vitamin E, NF is a form of alpha-tocopherol that includes the isomers of alpha-tocopherol, alpha-tocopheryl acetate, or alpha-tocopheryl succinate. *Vitamin E capsules* (Aquasol E) contain 30 to 1000 IU of the vitamin.

Vitamin K

Vitamin K activity is elicited by at least two forms of the compound—vitamin K_1 (phylloquinone) and vitamin K_2 (the menaquinone series). The structures of these compounds are shown below.

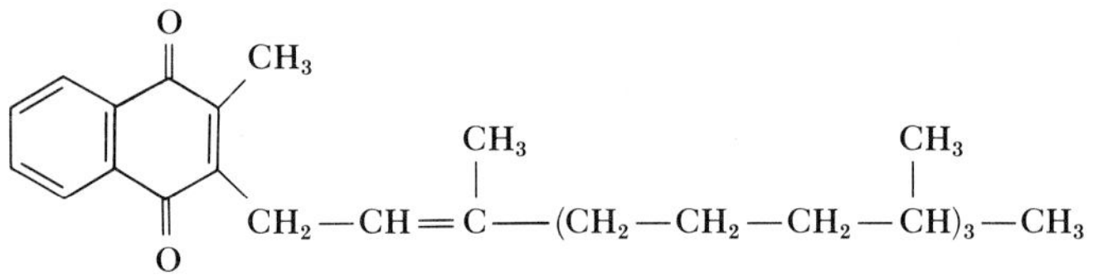

Vitamin K_1 (phylloquinone)

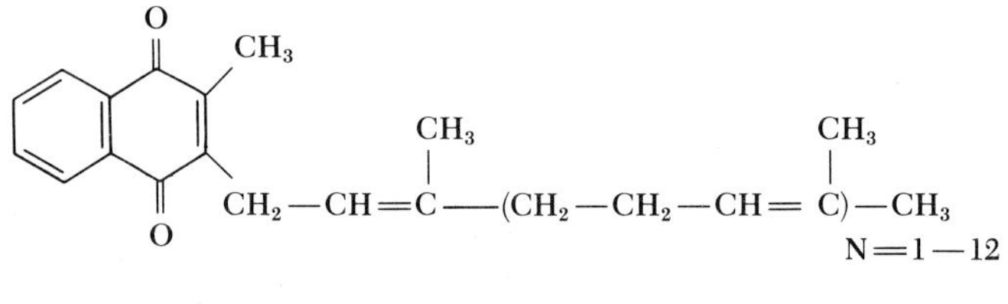

Vitamin K_2 (menaquinone series)

Vitamin K_1 occurs in green vegetables such as alfalfa, cabbage, and spinach as well as egg yolk, soybean oil, and liver. The menaquinones (vitamin K_2) are synthesized by grampositive bacteria, and microorganisms in the intestinal flora can provide some amounts of vitamin K to humans. Because of this source of supply, it is difficult to establish the requirement of this vitamin. Newborns do not have an established intestinal flora and are usually given a single dose of 1 mg vitamin K_1 at birth to prevent hemorrhagic disease.

Vitamin K is essential for the synthesis in the liver of prothrombin and for the bloodclotting factors VII, IX, and X. Prothrombin is the precursor of the active clotting agent thrombin, and the normal blood-clotting process does not occur without the presence of prothrombin and these clotting factors. Vitamin K deficiency is referred to as *hypoprothrombinemia*, and bleeding diathesis will result in the absence of the vitamin. Severe deficiency of vitamin K may result in hemorrhage due to the smallest trauma. Common sites of hemorrhage are operative wounds, skin (petechial bleeding), mucous membrane in the intestinal tract, and serosal surfaces.

The usual causes of vitamin K deficiency are malabsorption syndromes and inadequate intake. Other causes include hepatobiliary diseases where there is an obstruction to the bile flow, causing inadequate absorption of the fat-soluble vitamin, alterations in the normal bacterial flora that synthesize the vitamin such as after prolonged antibiotic use, and inadequate reserves in the newborn because of marginal levels in the mother.

A number of synthetic quinone derivatives possess vitamin K activity, with menadione (vitamin K_3) being the most active of these compounds.

The natural vitamins K_1 and K_2 are nontoxic in massive doses, and menadione is relatively nontoxic. Menadione has been implicated in producing hemolytic anemia in the newborn and hemolysis in those individuals suffering from an erythrocytic deficiency of glucose-6-phosphate dehydrogenase.[44]

Preparations. *Phytonadine*, USP (Mephyton, vitamin K_1), is available as 5 mg tablets and in ampules containing an emulsion of 2 or 10 mg/ml. Menadione, NF (vitamin K_3), is available in tablets containing 2 or 10 mg and as an injectable preparation containing 2, 10, or 25 mg/ml. *Menadione sodium bisulfite*, NF (Hykinone), is marketed in 5 mg tablets and in ampules containing 5 to 10 mg/ml.

REFERENCES

1. Nizel, A. E.: The science of nutrition and its application in clinical dentistry, ed. 2, Philadelphia, 1966, W. B. Saunders Co.
2. Umbreit, W. W.: Vitamin B_6 antagonists, Am. J. Clin. Nutr. 3:291-297, 1955.
3. Dreizen, S.: Oral indications of the deficiency states, Postgrad. Med. 49:97-102, 1971.
4. Rinehart, J. F., and Greenberg, L. D.: Vitamin B_6 deficiency in the rhesus monkey with particular reference to the occurrence of atherosclerosis, dental caries and hepatic cirrhosis, Am. J. Clin. Nutr. 4: 318, 1956.
5. Matsuda, T., and Toda, T.: Effects of vitamin B_6 on dental caries in rats, J. Dent. Res. 48:1460-1464, 1967.
6. Duvoisin, R. C., Yahr, M. D., and Cote, L. D.: Pyridoxine reversal of L-dopa effects in parkinsonism, Trans. Am. Neurol. Assoc. 94:81-84, 1969.
7. Cotzias, G. C.: Metabolic modification of some neurologic disorders, J.A.M.A. 210:1255-1262, 1969.
8. Ananth, J. V., Ban, T. A., and Lehmann, H. E.: Potentiation of therapeutic effects of nicotinic acid by pyridoxine in chronic schizophrenics, Can. Psychiatr. Assoc. J. 18:377-383, 1973.
9. Salkeld, R. M., Knorr, K., and Korner, W. F.: The effect of oral contraceptives on vitamin B_6 status, Clin. Chim. Acta 49:195-199, 1973.
10. Balogh, K., Petrucz, K., and Angyal, J.: Inhibition of bacterial growth in human saliva, J. Dent. Res. 39:886-891, 1960.
11. Stoohey, G. K.: Influence of thiamine on fluoride retention in the rat, J. Dent. Res. 53:139, 1974.
12. Food and Nutrition Board, National Research Council: Recommended dietary allowances, ed. 8, Publication no. 2216, Washington, D.C., 1974, National Academy of Sciences.
13. Hodges, R. E., Bean, W. B., Ohlson, M. A., and Bleiler, R.: Human pantothenic acid deficiency produced by omega-methyl pantothenic acid, J. Clin. Invest. 38:1421-1425, 1959.
14. Pratt, J. M.: Inorganic chemistry of vitamin B_{12}. New York, 1972, Academic Press, Inc.
15. FAO/WHO Expert Group: Requirements of ascorbic acid, vitamin D, vitamin B_{12}, folate and iron, World Health Organization Technical Report, Geneva, 1970, World Health Organization.
16. Herbert, V.: Nutritional requirements for vitamin B_{12} and folic acid, Am. J. Clin. Nutr. 21:243-252, 1968.
17. Herbert, V., and Tisman, G.: Effects of deficiencies of folic acid and vitamin B_{12} on central nervous system function and development, In Gaull, G., editor: Biology of brain dysfunction, vol. 1, New York, 1973, Plenum Press, Inc.
18. Eagle, H., Oyama, V. I., Levy, M., and Freeman, A. E.: *Myo*-inositol as an essential growth factor for normal and malignant human cells in tissue culture, J. Biol. Chem. 226:191-205, 1957.
19. Schwartz, P. L.: Ascorbic acid in wound healing—a review, J. Am. Diet. Assoc. 56:497-503, 1970.
20. Gould, B. S.: The role of certain vitamins in collagen formation, In Gould, B. S., editor: Treatise on collagen, vol. 2, New York, 1968, Academic Press, Inc.

21. Cowan, D. W., Diehl, H. S., and Baker, A. B.: Vitamins for the prevention of colds, J.A.M.A. **120:** 1268-1271, 1942.

22. Pauling, L.: Vitamin C and the common cold, San Francisco, 1970, W. H. Freeman & Co., Publishers.

23. Pauling, L.: Evolution and the need for ascorbic acid, Proc. Natl. Acad. Sci. U.S.A. **67:**1643-1648, 1970.

24. Pauling, L.: The significance of the evidence about ascorbic acid and the common cold, Proc. Natl. Acad. Sci. U.S.A. **68:**2678-2681, 1971.

25. Pauling, L.: Ascorbic acid and the common cold, Am. J. Clin. Nutr. **24:**1294-1299, 1971.

26. Dykes, M. H. M., and Meier, P.: Ascorbic acid and the common cold: evaluation of its efficacy and toxicity, J.A.M.A. **231:**1073-1079, 1975.

27. Cameron, E., and Pauling, L.: The orthomolecular treatment of cancer. I. The role of ascorbic acid in host resistance, Chem. Biol. Interact. **9:**273-283, 1974.

28. El-Ashry, G. M., Ringsdorf, W. M., and Cherashim, E.: Local and systemic influence in periodontal disease. II. Effect of prophylaxis and natural versus synthetic vitamin C upon gingivitis, J. Periodontol. **35:**250, 1964.

29. Glickman, L., and Dines, M. M.: Effect of increased ascorbic acid blood levels on the ascorbic level of treated and non-treated gingiva, J. Dent. Res. **42:**1152, 1963.

30. Shannon, I. L., and Gibson, W. A.: Intravenous ascorbic acid loading in subjects classified as to periodontal status, J. Dent. Res. **44:**355-361, 1965.

31. McBean, L., and Speckmann, E. W.: A review: the importance of nutrition in oral health, J.A.D.A. **89:** 109-114, 1974.

32. Hayes, K. C., and Hegsted, D. M.: Toxicity of the vitamins. In Committee on Food Protection, Food and Nutrition Board: Toxicants occurring naturally in foods, ed. 2, Washington, D.C., 1973, National Academy of Sciences.

33. Rosenthal, G.: Interaction of ascorbic acid and warfarin, J.A.M.A. **215:**1671, 1971.

34. Houston, J. B., and Levy, G.: Modification of drug biotransformation by vitamin C in man, Nature **225:** 78-79, 1975.

35. Wald, G.: The molecular basis of visual excitation, Nature **219:**800-807, 1968.

36. Wasserman, R. H., and Corradino, R. A.: Metabolic role of vitamins A and D, Ann. Rev. Biochem. **40:** 501-532, 1971.

37. Omdahl, J. L., and DeLuca, H. F.: Regulation of vitamin D metabolism and function, Physiol. Rev. **53:**327-372, 1973.

38. Taylor, A. N., and Wasserman, R. H.: Correlations between the vitamin D–induced calcium binding protein and intestinal absorption of calcium, Fed. Proc. **28:**1834-1838, 1969.

39. DeLuca, H. F.: Vitamin D: the vitamin and the hormone, Fed. Proc. **33:**2211-2219, 1974.

40. Haussler, M. R.: Vitamin D: mode of action and biomedical applications, Nutr. Rev. **32:**257-265, 1974.

41. Leonard, P. J., and Losowsky, M. S.: Relationship between plasma vitamin E level and peroxide hemolysis test in human subjects, Am. J. Clin. Nutr. **20:**795-798, 1967.

42. Mason, K. E.: Effects of nutritional deficiencies on muscle. In Bourne, G. H., editor: The structure and function of muscle, ed. 2, vol. 4, New York, 1973, Academic Press, Inc.

43. Dinning, J. S., and Day, P. L.: Vitamin E deficiency in the monkey, J. Exp. Med. **105:**395-402, 1957.

44. Zinkham, W. H., and Childs, B.: Effect of vitamin K and naphthalene metabolites on glutathione metabolism from normal newborns and patients with naphthalene hemolytic anemia, J. Dis. Child. **94:** 420-423, 1957.

PART THREE
Special topics

24

Emergency drugs

K. W. BESLEY

Emergency treatment is based on an accurate diagnosis of the problem and consists essentially of the maintenance of respiration and circulation. In dental emergencies the maintenance of these vital processes is generally accomplished by properly positioning the patient and delivering an adequate supply of oxygen (mechanical resuscitation). Drugs are usually only ancillary to these measures. It is impossible to maintain perspective on the subject of emergency drugs properly if it is divorced from diagnosis and the mechanical aspects of resuscitation. However, the intent of this chapter is a discussion of drugs and the emphasis is placed accordingly, with a review of the pharmacology, indication, and related physiology of several drugs that are useful in treating dental emergencies. The choice of drugs for a dental office emergency kit will depend on individual circumstances, experience, and personal preference.

The ultimate goal in any resuscitative effort is the maintenance of adequate tissue oxygenation. The practitioner must therefore assume that the essentials of airway management as well as support of respiration and circulation have been provided for prior to considering the use of drugs. The brain is unable to survive more than a few minutes under anaerobic conditions before irreversible changes take place. Although the heart and other organs are capable of metabolic adjustment in the form of anaerobic glycolysis, after a relatively short period of partial or complete lack of tissue perfusion and oxygenation, toxic products build up that may lead to an irreversible condition unless corrected. At this point mechanical means of ventilation and perfusion may not be enough, and chemical intervention becomes imperative. The time for drug support depends on the type of emergency. For example, in complete cardiopulmonary arrest no more than 5 to 10 minutes will be tolerated, even when mechanical ventilation and perfusion are provided. On the other hand, a convulsion or airway obstruction may require only mechanical support.

First in this chapter several drugs are listed that may be considered useful for dental office emergencies along with the indicated uses, dosages, and routes of administration. A discussion of the individual drugs then follows. A chart at the end of the chapter summarizes situations as to signs, symptoms, and treatment.

On the next page the list of emergency drugs with indications, adult dosages, and routes of administration is intended to act as a guide in setting up an emergency drug kit for most dental offices.

1. Epinephrine (Adrenalin)—1:1000
   Indications: anaphylaxis, cardiac arrest*
   Dose and route: 0.5 ml intravenously
2. Hydrocortisone sodium succinate (Solu-Cortef)—50 mg/ml
   Indications: cardiac arrest, anaphylaxis, acute adrenocortical insufficiency
   Dose and route: 2 ml intravenously, given slowly
3. Sodium bicarbonate—75 mg/ml
   Indication: cardiac arrest
   Dose and route: 10 ml per 5 minutes of cardiac arrest, intravenously

---

□ The opinions or assertions contained herein are the private ones of the writer and are not to be construed as official or as reflecting the views of the Navy Department or the naval service at large.

*The most controversial aspect of emergency drugs is the use of vasopressors and particularly epinephrine. A safe statement when dealing with dental office emergencies is to say that there are only two instances in which epinephrine is indicated—cardiac arrest and anaphylactic shock.

4. Diphenhydramine (Benadryl)—10 mg/ml
   Indications: acute allergic reaction,* extrapyramidal reaction to phenothiazine
   Dose and route: 5 ml intravenously
5. Aromatic spirits of ammonia—crush ampules
   Indications: syncope
   Dose and route: one ampule, by inhalation
6. Glyceryl trinitrate (nitroglycerin)—0.6 mg tablet
   Indication: angina pectoris
   Dose and route: one tablet sublingually
7. Morphine sulfate—15 mg/ml
   Indication: myocardial infarction
   Dose and route: 1 ml subcutaneously or intravenously
8. Phenylephrine hydrochloride (Neo-Synephrine Hydrochloride)—1:500
   Indications: toxic reaction to local anesthetic
   Dose and route: 1 to 2 ml intravenously
9. Dextrose in water—5%
   Indications: hypovolemia, intravenous route for drug administration
   Dose and route: 1000 ml intravenous drip
10. Anticonvulsant (individual choice)
    Indication: Severe or prolonged convulsion as in toxic reaction to local anesthetic†
    a. Diazepam (Valium)—5 mg/ml
       Dose and route: 1 to 8 ml intravenously (titrated)
    b. Pentobarbital sodium (Nembutal)—50 mg/ml
       Dose and route: 1 ml intravenously (careful titration)
11. Naloxone hydrochloride (Narcan)—0.4 mg/ml
    Indication: narcotic depression
    Dose and route: 1 ml intravenously or intramuscularly
12. Isoproterenol hydrochloride aerosol—0.25%
    Indication: bronchospasm
    Dose and route: one or two inhalations

DISCUSSION OF INDIVIDUAL DRUGS

Epinephrine. The inclusion of epinephrine in a dental office emergency kit is mandatory for the treatment of cardiac arrest and overwhelming anaphylaxis. However, it must be emphasized that these extreme conditions are the *only* situations that would require its use in the dental office emergency. There are a few clinicians who maintain the mistaken belief that epinephrine is the drug of choice in shock or shocklike states. There are three principal reasons for disputing this belief. First, in shock from almost any cause

*Response is delayed.
† Diazepam or barbiturates are not indicated in convulsion secondary to decreased cardiac output and cerebral anoxia. In this instance a neuromuscular blocking agent is the drug of choice.

there is decreased venous return to the heart because of peripheral venous pooling. Since the peripheral action of epinephrine is primarily on the arterial side, there is little gain in promoting peripheral vasoconstriction, which is already present because of the massive release of endogenous catecholamines (epinephrine and norepinephrine). At this point administration of epinephrine may further decrease venous return and tissue perfusion. Second, a possible deleterious effect is an increase in selective ischemia that takes place in certain viscera such as the kidney. Here, as in peripheral vessels, the blood supply is constricted in a compensatory effort to increase blood flow to the more vital brain and heart tissues. Perpetuation of this condition could be undesirable. Third, the possible precipitation of ventricular fibrillation in the ischemic and irritable myocardium is an important factor.[1] This could be especially disastrous in the dental office where defibrillation equipment is usually not available. In early treatment of shock states the patient will benefit more from measures aimed at correction of the primary cause such as hypovolemia rather than misdirected attempts at pharmacologic correction.

The primary reason for using epinephrine in the case of cardiac arrest and severe anaphylaxis is direct (beta) stimulation of the myocardium. An additional benefit in severe anaphylactic reactions is that epinephrine acts as a physiologic antagonist to the results of massive histamine release such as bronchiolar constriction, which leads to decreased oxygen exchange.

It must be emphasized that the beneficial effects of epinephrine are depressed in the presence of acidosis[2] that accompanies inadequate tissue perfusion. It is therefore mandatory that the administration of epinephrine must be preceded by appropriate mechanical resuscitative measures such as external cardiac massage and support of respiration. Intravenous fluid administration should accompany the use of any vasopressor drug.[3]

Sodium bicarbonate. Within a few minutes of cardiac arrest, metabolic acidosis reaches a critical level. Even when external cardiac massage is employed early, the build-up of lactic acid from hypoxic tissues requires compensatory measures. A safe rule of thumb is to administer 10 ml sodium bicarbonate intravenously for every 5 minutes of cardiac arrest. Critical acidosis may develop in any form of shock, but the process is seldom as rapid as in cardiac arrest unless the shock state is profound. The patient with severe chronic respiratory disease may develop acute acidosis from respiratory or circulatory failure. The usual manifestations are syncope, tachycardia, sweating, and tremors. In this case sodium bicarbonate is useful as adjunctive therapy. This is not to be confused with the acute asthmatic attack in which a drug such as isoproterenol is often employed to correct bronchiolar constriction. However, the dentist will normally be prepared for either of these eventualities by the patient's history.

Hydrocortisone sodium succinate. The concurrent use of hydrocortisone sodium succinate with other measures in the treatment of cardiac arrest, anaphylactic shock, and acute adrenocortical insufficiency is based on two general actions of the drug: hemodynamic and anti-inflammatory. The single 100 mg dose proposed here may result in potentiation of endogenous vasopressor drugs as well as protection against some of their toxic effects, and it may be given without fear of harmful side effects. This treatment is specific in acute adrenocortical insufficiency. The dentist is most likely to encounter this situation in patients receiving long-term steroid therapy or those who have been removed from such therapy within the past year. These patients may not respond normally to a stressful situation, since the effects of endogenous catecholamines will be minimized in the absence of sufficient steroid levels.

Although delayed, the anti-inflammatory action of corticosteroid drugs may be beneficial in the severe anaphylactic reaction. Several mechanisms have been proposed. First, the corticosteroids may inhibit the regranulation of mast cells once they have discharged their histamine. The actions of histamine are discussed in another chapter. Second, stabilization of cell and lysosomal membranes is a possible mechanism. In conditions such as cardiac arrest and anaphylactic shock, cell injury is partly caused by tissue ischemia and acidosis, which results in the release of the hydrolytic lysosomes and further cell damage. Some of this may be prevented by the corticosteroids.

Diphenhydramine (Benadryl). Diphenhydramine has been included in this discussion because it is indicated in the allergic reactions, often appearing as urticaria and pruritus after drug administration. Allergic reactions may be accompanied by some degree of respiratory distress. Since the action of antihistamines is competition with histamine for tissue receptor sites, a rapid reversal of allergic symptoms cannot be expected. However, eventual improvement in the sequelae of histamine release such as bronchiolar constriction, capillary dilation, and edema may be expected. This delayed action is of little value in a severe reaction and should not be relied on as primary therapy.

Diphenhydramine is often the drug of choice in the treatment of extrapyramidal reaction after the administration of phenothiazine drugs such as chlorpromazine (Thorazine), prochlorperazine (Compazine), promazine (Sparine), and trifluperazine (Stelazine). These drugs are sometimes used by the dentist for premedication or as antiemetics. Symptoms of extrapyramidal reactions from phenothiazine may include restlessness, spasms of neck or back muscles, rolling back of the eyes, trismus, difficulty in swallowing, and Parkinsonian type of movements. Not infrequently the patient is referred to the dentist for a spontaneous temporomandibular joint dislocation. Although it is seldom life threatening, the reaction can be a terrifying experience for the patient who is conscious but unable to control the abnormal muscular contractions. The intravenous administration of 2 to 5 ml diphenhydramine will reverse the majority of these symptoms in seconds or minutes. Although the response is usually rapid and dramatic, the fact should be pointed out that the reaction may recur in hours, days, or even several weeks. Therefore the patient should be so informed and observed even though phenothiazine therapy is discontinued. In the more severe reactions antiparkinsonian drugs may be required.

Aromatic spirits of ammonia. The signs, symptoms, and treatment of syncope are well known by every dentist. The typical beads of perspiration on the upper lip are seen fairly often and are automatically recognized as one of the signs of impending syncope. Also typical are the weak thready pulse, cold clammy skin, pallor, and dizzy feeling that may proceed to unconsciousness.

Loss of normal vasomotor tonus produces pooling of blood peripherally so that the normal blood volume becomes insufficient. Thus the practice of placing the patient in a supine position and elevating his feet is, in effect, giving a transfusion of whole blood by utilizing the forces of gravity. However, it should be emphasized that the object is to return blood to the heart for circulation to the brain; consequently, the head should not be more than about 10 degrees lower than the rest of the body. Extreme Trendelenburg position may result in an artificially increased pressure in the carotid sinus with a reflex decrease in blood pressure.

Inhaled ammonia irritates trigeminal nerve sensory endings, with a resulting reflex stimulation of medullary respiratory and vasomotor centers. The administration of oxygen will aid in combating tissue anoxia.

Syncope is usually psychogenic and represents only a transient problem in normal individuals. However, in the cardiac patient even a short period of tissue ischemia may be serious. The dentist must be aware that the signs and symptoms of syncope may represent a progressive or more serious condition.

Glyceryl trinitrate. The use of glyceryl trinitrate (nitroglycerin) for the relief of anginal pain is common, but its mechanism of action is not completely clear. It has been assumed for some time that dilation of the coronary arteries produces relief from the pain of myocardial ischemia. There are more potent coronary vasodilators that do not afford the same relief from anginal pain. However, the clinical effectiveness of glyceryl trinitrate has made it the most frequently used medication for relief of angina pectoris.

In patients who suffer from frequent anginal attacks, glyceryl trinitrate may be administered prior to the stress of dental treatment. When this prophylactic use is being considered, the practitioner should remember that some decrease in blood pressure may occur because of peripheral vasodilation. This becomes more important in patients taking drugs that tend to produce orthostatic hypotension. *Rauwolfia* drugs (reserpine), methyldopa (Aldomet), and hydralazine (Apresoline) are some of the more commonly used antihypertensive drugs that tend to produce orthostatic hypotension.

When glyceryl trinitrate is placed in an emergency kit, it should be marked with the date, since the effective shelf life is about 6 months.

Angina pectoris is characterized by a usually stress-related, sudden onset of crushing chest pain that may radiate to the left arm, shoulder, neck, or mandible. Shocklike symptoms may also be present. The usual treatment consists of a 0.6 mg tablet held under the tongue with the patient in a semiprone or sitting position. Relief will normally be obtained within 2 or 3 minutes. Removal of the stressful situation, calm reassurance, and the administration of a high flow of oxygen are important aspects of the treatment. Failure to respond to this treatment is a sign of myocardial infarction. Persistent pain may require the administration of morphine. A physician should be consulted as soon as possible when myocardial infarction is suspected.

Some of the commercially prepared drug kits contain amyl nitrite in crush ampules, which is a more potent coronary dilator but is more likely to produce nausea and vomiting. A disadvantage of placing amyl nitrite in the kit is that although the crush ampule is yellow, it may be mistaken for the white ampule of ammonia. The accidental use of a vasodilator in syncope could lead to a more serious condition, especially in the patient with some degree of cardiac insufficiency.

Morphine sulfate. Morphine sulfate is administered to the patient with acute myocardial infarction for the relief of pain and to allay apprehension. Also, the central depression produced reduces the amount of cardiac work through a reduction in the release of endogenous catecholamines.[4] The route of administration is usually subcutaneous, but intravenous injection is best if circulation is impaired.

Phenylephrine hydrochloride (Neo-Synephrine Hydrochloride). Phenylephrine hydrochloride is a vasopressor that acts directly on alpha-adrenergic tissue receptors. Stimulation of these receptors produces primarily an increase in vascular resistance in the peripheral, gastrointestinal, and renal arterioles. The heart is stimulated *indirectly* through an increase in venous return with a resulting increased arterial pressure and reflex slowing of the heart rate.[4] The reason for the selection of phenylephrine as the vasopressor of choice is its lack of direct myocardial stimulation. This is of importance in the dental office emergency where, in the face of an undiagnosed cardiac arrhythmia or irritable myocardium, the possibility of contributing to or producing ventricular fibrillation must be minimized. The use of phenylephrine hydrochloride in cases of severe or prolonged depression after the administration of a local anesthetic has the advantage of positive action when it is needed with little chance of deleterious effects. Other vasopressors that offer the same advantage are angiotensin amide (Hypertensin) and methoxamine hydroxide (Vasoxyl Hydroxide).

Many commercially available drug kits contain a vasopressor that acts on both alpha- and beta-adrenergic receptors. Here one of the actions is direct myocardial stimulation. This action is found in such drugs as norepinephrine, mephentermine (Wyamine), metaraminol (Aramine, Pressonex), and methamphetamine (Methedrine). It is my opinion that these drugs should not be used by the dentist in early treatment of dental office emergencies; their use should be relegated to a qualified physician.

5% dextrose in water. An intravenous route for drugs and fluid should be established in any serious dental office emergency. Most of the drugs used in an emergency situation are more effective if given intravenously. Fluid replacement is needed early in hypovolemia or peripheral vascular collapse. One of the ultimate results of shock in any form is a loss of intravascular fluid. Although the dentist is usually not directly responsible for the management of long-term fluid administration, he should at least get the ball rolling in any emergency. There are some instances where this is imperative. Such is the case when vasopressors are employed.[3] On the other hand, there are instances where the rate of fluid administration should be minimal until adequate monitoring such as central venous pressure is available. This is true, for example, in the patient with congestive heart failure and in children.

Although there are instances where solutions such as Ringer's lactate, physiologic saline, plasma expanders, or whole blood are more appropriate, the type of solution given initially in an emergency is not as important as establishing an intravenous route.

Anticonvulsants. The dentist has a choice of several drugs for use in the event of a serious convulsion occurring in the office, including diazepam (Valium), pentobarbital sodium (Nembutal), thiopental sodium (Pentothal Sodium), and succinylcholine (Anectine). The drug or drugs selected for an emergency kit will depend on the experience of the person dealing with the emergency.

It should be emphasized that in the majority of cases convulsive episodes are usually self-limiting and require only supportive care in the form of protection of the patient from physical harm and, in some cases, the administration of positive pressure oxygen. This is especially true of convulsion secondary to decreased cardiac output and cerebral hypoxia. In this instance, barbiturates are contraindicated and corrective measures should be directed toward tissue oxygenation. The most likely cause of a convulsive episode in the dental office is a toxic reaction to local anesthetic from overdose or idiosyncrasy. Here the problem is primarily one of central depression. Although the initial phase of the reaction may be manifested by stimulation in various forms, including convulsion, in dealing with lidocaine the stimulation is actually caused by depression of central inhibitory centers.[5] The eventual or, in some cases, initial response is respiratory and circulatory depression. It is logical therefore to be conservative in the use of anticonvulsant drugs, which may enhance this central depression. On the other hand, a convulsion may occasionally be severe enough to be life threatening in the form of respiratory embarrassment and require drug intervention. Each dentist must decide for himself, before the occasion arises, when to intervene chemically and what drug to use.

In recent years diazepam (Valium) has become popular as an anticonvulsant. It has the advantages of relative safety if the dose is carefully titrated and of versatility as to route of administration in that it can be given either intravenously or intramuscularly. Except in high doses and for children or elderly patients, diazepam has little potential for cardiovascular or respiratory depression. This is a definite advantage when it is compared with the barbiturates or neuromuscular blocking agents. In this respect slow intravenous administration is best to titrate dosage for the individual response. The range may

Table 24-1. Summary of dental office emergencies

Diagnosis	Signs and symptoms	Treatment
Syncope	1. Pulse weak and slow 2. Skin pale, cold, clammy 3. Dizziness or loss of consciousness	1. Supine position 2. 100% oxygen 3. Ammonia crush ampule

Toxic reaction to local anesthetic	1. Loss of central inhibitory centers
	  a. Apprehension, restlessness
	  b. Increase in blood pressure and respiratory rates, tachycardia
	  c. Convulsion
		1. Supine position
		2. Positive pressure oxygen
		3. Anticonvulsant of choice in *severe* case

	2. Signs of central depression
	  a. Decreased level of consciousness
	  b. Decreased blood pressure and respiratory rate, bradycardia
		1. Continue to support respiration as necessary
		2. IV infusion of 5% dextrose in water
		3. Phenylephrine, 1 ml IV if severe or prolonged

Cardiac arrest	1. Sudden collapse 2. Absence of carotid pulse 3. Dilated pupils 4. Cold, pale extremities or cyanosis	1. Sharp blow to precordium; repeat if necessary 2. External cardiac massage 3. Positive pressure oxygen 4. Epinephrine, 0.5 ml IV; repeat as needed 3 to 8 minutes 5. IV infusion of 5% dextrose in water 6. Sodium bicarbonate, 10 ml per 5 minutes of arrest 7. Hydrocortisone, 2 ml IV (slowly)
Allergic reaction 1. Mild	1. Urticaria 2. Pruritus	1. Diphenhydramine, 5 ml IV or IM 2. Epinephrine, 0.5 ml IV
2. Anaphylactic	3. Tightness in chest 4. Sudden collapse 5. Fall in blood pressure, tachycardia 6. Cardiac arrest	3. External cardiac massage and positive pressure oxygen as needed 4. IV infusion of 5% dextrose in water 5. Hydrocortisone, 2 ml IV (slowly)
Angina pectoris	1. Sudden, severe chest pain; may radiate to left arm, neck, or mandible 2. Extreme apprehension 3. Increased blood pressure, tachycardia	1. Sitting position 2. Oxygen 3. Nitroglycerin, 0.6 mg tablet sublingually 4. Reassurance
Myocardial infarction	1. Similar to angina but prolonged and no response to nitroglycerin 2. Arrhythmia	1. Sitting position 2. Oxygen 3. Morphine, 1 ml IM
Acute adrenal insufficiency	1. History of long-term steroid therapy 2. Weakness, syncope 3. Decreased blood pressure, tachycardia	1. Supine position 2. Oxygen 3. Hydrocortisone, 2 ml IV (slowly)
Extrapyramidal reaction (phenothiazines)	1. Restlessness 2. Eyes rolled back 3. Spasm of neck or back muscles (head extended) 4. Trismus 5. Difficulty in swallowing 6. Parkinsonian symptoms	1. Diphenhydramine, 5 ml IV
Respiratory depression (narcotics)	1. Shallow, slowed respirations 2. Tachycardia 3. Coma	1. Naloxone, 1 ml IV, IM, or SC
Bronchospasm	1. Dyspnea 2. Expiratory wheeze 3. Differentiate from obstruction or laryngospasm	1. Isoproterenol aerosol, 1 or 2 inhalations 2. 100% oxygen

be from 2 to 40 mg; if it is given intramuscularly, 5 to 10 mg increments would be appropriate.

Pentobarbital sodium (Nembutal) may also be administered intravenously or intramuscularly and is often included in the dental office emergency kit. It is a reasonable alternative to diazepam if the greater potential for respiratory and central depression is remembered. Careful titration of 50 mg increments will be the safest procedure.

Thiopental sodium (Pentothal Sodium) was an important anticonvulsant in dental emergency kits for many years because its ultrashort action presented less danger of prolonging or enhancing the central depression that may follow a convulsion. However, an extravascular injection of thiopental sodium, which is highly alkaline, may result in tissue necrosis and slough. Additionally, inadvertent intra-arterial injection may result in the loss of an extremity. For these reasons and because of the time-consuming inconvenience of having to mix a thiopental solution just prior to injection, we no longer consider this the drug of choice for dental emergency kits.

The neuromuscular blocking agents, such as succinylcholine (Anectine), are potent anticonvulsants, but their use requires special skill and equipment concerned with support of respiration in the paralyzed patient. They are therefore not recommended for use in the dental office. The actions of these drugs are discussed in another chapter.

Naloxone hydrochloride (Narcan). Naloxone is a pure narcotic antagonist with little pharmacologic activity of its own. For this reason it has largely replaced nalorphine (Nalline) as an emergency kit narcotic antagonist. Its use in the reversal of narcotic depression is extremely safe with one major precaution: the duration of action may be shorter than that of the narcotic being antagonized. It is therefore imperative that the patient be constantly observed for signs of returning respiratory depression.

An initial adult dose of 0.4 mg (1 ml) is usually given intravenously but may be given subcutaneously or intramuscularly. Onset of action is approximately 2 minutes when the intravenous route is used but will be slightly slower for the intramuscular or subcutaneous route. Basic resuscitation should continue until an adequate response is noted. It may be necessary to repeat the initial dose if spontaneous respiration does not occur within a reasonable time period. It should be emphasized that naloxone hydrochloride is effective in reversing respiratory depression due to opiate-derived drugs so that other causes must be considered when there is no response.

The mechanism of action is not firmly established, but it is likely that at least part of the effect is that of competitive antagonism whereby naloxone competes for receptor sites with the opioid.

Isoproterenol (Isuprel). Isoproterenol aerosol is indicated for the relief of acute bronchospasm associated with bronchial asthma or as an adjunct in the treatment of allergic reactions. The actions of isoproterenol are discussed in Chapter 13. Because of cardiac stimulation, isoproterenol should not be used in patients with known cardiac arrhythmias. Correct diagnosis is important to rule out dyspnea due to problems such as airway obstruction. In this case auscultation of the chest will give sufficient evidence of the expiratory wheeze of bronchospasm. If a patient with a sudden onset of respiratory difficulty has received a general anesthetic agent, the most likely cause is laryngospasm, and it should be treated accordingly. In any case 100% oxygen should be administered.

SUMMARY

Table 24-1 reviews some of the possible dental emergencies and suggested treatment.

REFERENCES

1. Goodman, L. S., and Gilman, A.: The pharmacological basis of therapeutics, ed. 4, New York, 1970, The Macmillan Co., p. 516.
2. Wood, W. B., Manley, E. S., Jr., and Woodbury, R. A.: Effects of CO_2-induced respiratory acidosis on depressor and pressor components of the dog's blood pressure response to epinephrine, J. Pharmacol. Exp. Ther. **139**:238-247, 1963.
3. Clauss, R. H., and Ray, J. E., III: Pharmacologic assistance to the failing circulation, Surg. Gynecol. Obstet. **126**:611-629, 1968.
4. DiPalma, J. R., editor: Drill's pharmacology in medicine, ed. 3, New York, 1965, McGraw-Hill Book Co., p. 260.
5. Monheim, L. M.: Local anesthesia and pain control in dental practice, St. Louis, 1969, The C. V. Mosby Co., p. 144.

25

Pharmacology of intravenous sedation

RICHARD L. WYNN

A variety of drugs can produce depression within the central nervous system, with the degree of depression ranging from mild sedation to death. Intravenous sedation is a useful technique in dentistry and utilizes those central nervous system depressant drugs which have the actions of sedation, antianxiety, or tranquilization. Sedative drugs consist of a variety of pharmacologic agents from several drug groups, including the barbiturates, the nonbarbiturate sedative-hypnotics, the narcotic analgesics, the psychosedatives, and the minor tranquilizers. The intent of this chapter on the pharmacology of intravenous sedation is to review the degrees of central nervous system depression that can be induced by drugs, to classify the central nervous system depressants according to the degree of depression they produce, and to discuss the pharmacology of each individual agent used in intravenous sedation techniques. Some of the information presented in this chapter has been discussed in Chapter 8, which examines the general use of these sedative drugs. Some repetition is necessary, however, to relate this information to the intravenous use of drugs for sedation. Although not a sedative, ketamine is also discussed with respect to its pharmacology, since it is a useful agent in intravenous techniques. Clinical considerations of intravenous agents are mentioned only briefly and only in the context of their pharmacologic effects. For more detailed discussion on clinical uses of these intravenous agents in dentistry and on intravenous techniques in general, the reader is referred to Chapter 26 and to several review articles.[1-6]

DEGREES AND MECHANISMS OF CENTRAL NERVOUS SYSTEM DEPRESSION

The depressant effects of drugs on the central nervous system are due to actions on the reticular activating system (RAS), the medulla, and the cerebral cortex. The so-called reticular core within the central nervous system is composed of an intertwining net of small neurons coursing through portions of the medulla and midbrain. Within this network exists the RAS, which is a complex group of neuronal pathways extending into the hypothalamus and thalamus. Normal activity within the RAS maintains a conscious alert state by projection of ascending neuronal activity through the thalamus and into the cerebral cortex. Depression of the neuronal activity within the RAS results in sedation and hypnosis. *Sedation* is defined as a state of drowsiness or mental clouding, and for the purposes of this discussion will be considered synonymous with tranquilization or antianxiety. During sedation, intermittent periods of hypnosis may occur in a patient from which he can be aroused. *Hypnosis* is a depression of the central nervous system resembling normal sleep. The patient can be aroused, and there is no analgesia present.

The medullary areas of the brain function to control autonomic reflexes of the circulation, heart, and lungs. These reflex areas are known as the vital centers, since damage to them is usually fatal. *Respiratory depression* results from the direct depression of respiratory control within the medulla. Both the respiratory drive and the mechanisms responsible for the rhythmic character of respiratory movements are depressed. Depression of excitatory pathways within the cerebral cortex in addition to the depression of the RAS result in loss of consciousness. *General anesthesia* is traditionally defined as a loss of consciousness from which a patient cannot be aroused and is accompanied by analgesia. With the advent of the so-called dissociative anesthetics, however, general anesthesia can also be defined as that state in which a patient is insensitive to pain, has a blockage of noxious reflexes, and exhibits generalized muscle relaxation, with or without the loss of consciousness.

CLASSIFICATION OF CENTRAL NERVOUS SYSTEM DEPRESSANTS

The central nervous system depressants can be classified according to the degree of depression produced by therapeutic doses (Fig. 15). The actions of *barbiturates* range from sedation to general anesthesia, depending on the specific barbiturate. For example, phenobarbital induces sedation and some hypnosis at therapeutic doses. Respiratory depression or general anesthesia is uncommon with this drug except in cases of overdosage. Other barbiturates such as thiopental or methohexital, however, induce hypnosis, respiratory depression, and general anesthesia at therapeutic doses. The actions of the *narcotic analgesics* differ slightly from those of the barbiturates in that their depressant effects range from sedation to respiratory depression with therapeutic doses. The *nonbarbiturate sedatives* most commonly induce sedation with little hypnosis at therapeutic doses. The nonbarbiturate hypnotics produce hypnosis at therapeutic doses rather than sedation. The *psychosedatives* and *minor tranquilizers* elicit sedative actions but have little hypnotic effects at therapeutic doses.

The nonbarbiturate sedatives include methyprylon (Noludar), chloral hydrate (Noctec), and ethchlorvynol (Placidyl). The nonbarbiturate hypnotics consist of methaqualone (Parest, Quaalude), glutethimide (Doriden), and ethinamate (Valmid). The nonbarbiturate sedatives and hypnotics are not available for intravenous administration and will not be included in this discussion.

Barbiturates

The barbiturates most useful in intravenous sedation include thiopental and methohexital. Thiopental is a sulfurated type of barbiturate and is considered to be the prototype of the intravenous anesthetics—those intravenous drugs inducing a true anesthesia. Methohexital is an oxybarbiturate, containing a methylated nitrogen atom on the ring structure. Both drugs are insoluble in water

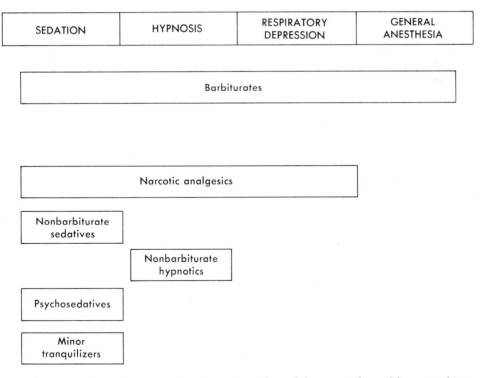

Fig. 15. Degree of central nervous system depression with usual therapeutic doses of depressant drugs.

and are supplied for clinical use as the water-soluble sodium salt. Included in each preparation is sodium carbonate, which makes the solutions strongly alkaline (pH 11). On injection the sodium carbonate is neutralized in the bloodstream, and the drugs revert back to their original chemical form from the sodium salts. Pentobarbital and secobarbital are also available for parenteral use and are effective as intravenous sedatives.

Barbiturates are general depressants to all tissues in the body, with the central nervous system being most sensitive to the depressant actions of these drugs. The barbiturates act on the RAS to depress the ascending neuronal conduction. Consciousness is not maintained, since there results a lack of ascending projection activity into the cerebral cortex. As a result, hypnosis ensues. With lower doses some projection activity apparently remains, resulting in sedation rather than hypnosis. Doses of the barbiturates above the hypnotic dose will cause a true anesthesia, which is due to the direct depression of excitatory pathways within the cerebral cortex in addition to the depression of the RAS.

Intravenous doses of thiopental, ranging from 2.0 to 3.5 mg/kg over a 15- to 30-second interval, will induce a general anesthesia. After induction supplemental doses may be given to maintain anesthesia, with the total dose not exceeding 1.0 Gm. Intravenous doses of methohexital ranging from 1.0 to 1.4 mg/kg will induce general anesthesia. The duration of action of the intravenous barbiturates at these doses is extremely short—approximately 10 to 15 minutes—and recovery may be accompanied by periods of restlessness.

Respiration must be carefully monitored when using these agents, since they are highly potent respiratory depressants. Respiratory effects of the barbiturates are a result of direct depressant actions on the medullary and pontine areas of respiratory control. Respiration is normally maintained by three physiologic influences: (1) a neurogenic control originating in the higher brain centers, which stimulates the medullary centers to drive respiration; (2) a chemical drive in which changes in blood pH and P_{CO_2} levels act on the medulla to control respiration; and (3) a hypoxic stimulus mediated by the chemoreceptors of the carotid and aortic

bodies. Hypnotic doses of a barbiturate depress the neurogenic control of respiration so that control is dominated by the chemical drive, with the hypoxic drive still functional. Anesthetic doses diminish both the chemical and hypoxic control. As intoxication doses increase, the chemical control is eventually inhibited with a shift in control of respiration to the hypoxic drive. At sufficiently high doses the hypoxic drive will also fail, and respiration will cease altogether. The margin between central nervous system depression and dangerous respiratory depression is sufficient to permit the barbiturates to be used as intravenous sedatives and anesthetics.

The effects of thiopental and methohexital on the cardiovascular system are mild and do not constitute a hazard in normal clinical practice. Myocardial contractility may be depressed by direct actions on the heart. Also, the medullary vasomotor center is depressed, resulting in a decreased heart rate. These drugs exert mixed effects on vascular resistance. Vascular resistance is usually decreased in the skin and increased in visceral tissues and in the central nervous system, resulting in an increase in total peripheral resistance. Studies with methohexital, however, have demonstrated that total peripheral resistance is most often decreased by this drug.[7]

Thiopental and methohexital rapidly penetrate all tissues because of their lipid solubility. This accounts for their rapid action, since they pass so rapidly into brain tissues. The rapid emergence from sleep after the intravenous administration of these two drugs is due to a redistribution from the brain to other tissues. The rate at which various tissues take up the drugs is related to blood flow. Thus the brain and other visceral organs exhibit maximum concentrations within 30 seconds after administration. Soon, however, skeletal muscle becomes saturated, whereas fat depots accumulate the drugs several hours after administration. As the muscle and fat take up the drugs, plasma levels fall and the drugs diffuse out of the brain. Consciousness is thus restored. Barbiturates may remain in the body fat for a period of days, which accounts for the cumulative effects of repeated doses of these drugs. Thiopental and methohexital are metabolized in the liver at a rate of 15% to 20% an hour.[8]

The metabolic products result from oxidation by liver microsomal enzymes. In general, the metabolic products thus formed retain no hypnotic activity and are eliminated by way of the kidney.

Complications associated with the use of intravenous barbiturates include laryngospasms and muscle twitching. Methohexital has a greater incidence of muscle movements and causes hiccough on frequent occasions. The use of any barbiturate is absolutely contraindicated in patients with a medical history of acute intermittent porphyria. In this disease the porphyrins, the components of hemoglobin, are produced in excess. Barbiturates ordinarily stimulate specific enzymes to increase the production of porphyrins. In the case of porphyria, barbiturates will cause exacerbation of the disease process itself and a fatal course is not uncommon. Most barbiturates are anticonvulsant in nature, and selected barbiturates are useful in the treatment of grand mal epilepsy.

Thiopental or methohexital should not be administered to patients who are taking other depressants or monoamine oxidase inhibitors, since serious drug interactions may occur. Monoamine oxidase inhibitors are used for antidepression effects in some neurotic patients. Patients taking these drugs have experienced severe barbiturate intoxication after therapeutic doses of barbiturates.

Narcotic analgesics

Narcotic analgesics useful in intravenous sedation techniques include morphine, meperidine (Demerol), alphaprodine (Nisentil), anileridine (Leritine), and fentanyl (Sublimaze).

Morphine. Morphine is a constituent of opium. A 3 to 15 mg intravenous dose of morphine produces euphoria, a sense of well-being. Drowsiness and mental clouding will occur with the drug and will last up to 2 hours. Respiration will be depressed in proportion to dose, with maximum depression occurring about 7 minutes after injection. No amnesia occurs with morphine, and there is little or no effect on the cardiovascular system when the drug is injected slowly. Although theoretically useful, the drug is rarely if ever used for intravenous sedation techniques in dentistry. Morphine can be used parenterally for severe pain. A dose of 10 to 15 mg subcutaneously will obtund severe pain of dental origin for about 6 hours.

The following are the central nervous systems effects after the administration of morphine. Analgesia occurs selectively by acting on the central nervous system at doses that do not induce sleep or affect other sensory pathways such as touch, hearing, or vision. Morphine induces hypnosis, which resembles normal sleep or that produced with low doses of barbiturates. Hypnotic effects of the drug are dose related and characterized by easy arousal. The probable mechanism is a depression of the reticular activating system. The medullary respiratory center is extremely sensitive to morphine. Death from overdoses of the drug is due to respiratory arrest. The mechanism of respiratory depression is a decrease in the sensitivity of the respiratory center to increases in P_{CO_2}. The vasomotor center may be depressed, resulting in a slowing of the heart and orthostatic hypotension.

Absorption of morphine is rapid after parenteral administration, and body distribution is favored in visceral tissues such as the lung, liver, kidney, and brain; it does not accumulate in fat tissues as the barbiturates do. Deactivation of the drug occurs through metabolism in the liver. Most of an administered dose is conjugated with glucuronic acid—a normal constituent of the body. A small amount of morphine is N-demethylated to normorphine. The drug is excreted by way of the kidney in the form of the glucuronic acid conjugate. Approximately 90% of an administered dose is excreted in 24 hours.

Morphine is contraindicated in patients suffering from biliary colic because of its ability to stimulate contractions within the bile duct. Patients suffering from severe asthma or chronic lung disease should not be given the drug because of its effect on respiration. The ability of morphine to cause constriction of the musculature of the bronchioles also contraindicates its use in the asthmatic patient. Morphine should be administered with caution in patients with conditions of hepatic insufficiency, since the liver is the site of deactivation of the drug.

Meperidine (Demerol). Meperidine is a synthetic narcotic analgesic and does not occur naturally like morphine. Although it is pharmacologically similar to morphine, it is much less potent, and 60 to 80 mg meperidine are equal in analgesic potency to 10 mg morphine. Like morphine it produces analgesia and sedation-hypnosis. Also, its medullary effects are similar to those of morphine. It causes respiratory depression and depresses the vasomotor reflexes to cause slowing of the heart and orthostatic hypotension. Meperidine is well absorbed by all routes of administration. Metabolism occurs in the liver with the formation of the glucuronic acid conjugates of two oxidative metabolites of the drug. The conjugates are subsequently excreted in the urine.

Meperidine is an excellent agent with which to produce conscious sedation in the ambulant dental patient. When administered intravenously in small incremental doses, meperidine produces a calmed, somewhat euphoric patient while providing some degree of analgesia. Adult intravenous doses range between 50 and 100 mg. In most cases little or no respiratory depression is seen, and at this dose dizziness is the most common complication. Postural hypotension may also occur if an erect posture is rapidly assumed. Meperidine should be administered with caution in patients medicated with the phenothiazine type of drugs, since enhancement of respiratory depression has been reported with these agents. Imipramine-like drugs are a group of antidepressant agents that are widely utilized in cases of endogenous depression and are represented by imipramine (Tofranil) and desipramine (Pertofrane). Both of these drugs have been shown to exert a dangerous supra-additive effect on meperidine-induced respiratory depression. Monoamine oxidase inhibitors have produced deep coma in the past and extreme hypotension resulting in a depression crisis when taken simultaneously with meperidine.[9,10]

Alphaprodine (Nisentil). Alphaprodine is a methylated derivative of meperidine. Pharmacologically, alphaprodine is similar to meperidine in all respects. The major differences between the two drugs are potency and duration of action. Alphaprodine is about twice as potent as meperidine. It exhibits greater sedative effects and respiratory depression at doses equal in analgesic potency to those of meperidine. Doses useful in intravenous sedation are 40 to 60 mg. Onset of action is 5 minutes with a duration of 45 minutes, compared with a duration of about 2

hours for meperidine. Care should be used when administering alphaprodine to children, since acute respiratory depression resulting in a death has occurred after a dose of approximately 20 mg was administered simultaneously with promethazine to a 28-month-old child.[11]

Anileridine (Leritine). Anileridine is chemically related to meperidine. It is approximately two and one half times as potent as meperidine, having an adult intravenous sedative dose of 25 mg. It is similar to meperidine in its pharmacologic effects and duration of action.

Fentanyl (Sublimaze). Fentanyl is also chemically related to meperidine. It is the most potent of the narcotics used in intravenous sedation, being about 500 times more potent than meperidine and 150 times more potent than morphine. Its intravenous dose ranges from 0.05 to 0.2 mg. The drug has an immediate onset of action and a duration of 30 minutes and is the shortest acting narcotic analgesic available for use in intravenous sedation. Profound respiratory depression is a feature of fentanyl, and muscle rigidity has been described after its use. The muscle rigidity results in occasional "stiff chest syndrome," which has caused a reduction of chest wall compliance to make lung inflation difficult. Fentanyl has not been found to cause clinically significant cardiovascular depression.

Psychosedatives (phenothiazines)

Phenothiazines with important sedative actions include chlorpromazine, promethazine, and propiomazine. Phenothiazines affect the reticular activating system and subcortical areas to cause drowsiness that is associated with easy arousal. They do not act on the cortex like barbiturates or narcotic analgesics, and they do not block ascending neuronal projections in the reticular activating system. Thus true hypnosis or general anesthesia is not produced by these drugs.

Phenothiazines are useful adjuncts for the control of fear and apprehension in many dental patients. Their contribution to intravenous sedation techniques is that they elicit psychomotor slowing and emotional quieting and allow the patient to be indifferent to environmental stimuli. These drugs elicit few side effects after the administration of single intravenous doses. Orthostatic hypotension is the most prevalent complication, and rare complications include respiratory depression and extrapyramidal reactions. Phenothiazines that are most useful in the production of conscious sedation include promethazine (Phenergan) and propiomazine (Largon) in intravenous doses of 25 to 50 mg and 10 to 20 mg, respectively. There is no overt effect on respiratory depression with low doses of the phenothiazines. Analgesia may or may not be demonstrated by the phenothiazines, depending on the compound. Chlorpromazine and other phenothiazines have consistent effects on the cardiovascular system, and they block the autonomic vasopressor tone of the peripheral vasculature. They cause direct relaxation of smooth muscle within the cardiovasculature to cause vasodilation. They also depress the contraction of the myocardium. The overall result of these three cardiovascular actions are hypotension and reflex tachycardia.

The phenothiazines are well absorbed by all routes of administration. They are also well distributed in tissues, and deactivation occurs through metabolism in the liver. The most common pathway of metabolic deactivation is the formation of glucuronic acid derivatives. Excretion occurs both in the urine and feces mostly as metabolites.

The use of phenothiazines is contraindicated in patients with myasthenia gravis because of their ability to cause relaxation of the skeletal musculature. Their use is also contraindicated in patients with epilepsy because of their ability to lower seizure thresholds within the central nervous system. Drug interactions between phenothiazines and central nervous system depressants are to be expected. These drugs will especially potentiate the respiratory depressant effects of meperidine, barbiturates, and morphine.

Minor tranquilizers (benzodiazepines)

Chlordiazepoxide (Librium) and diazepam (Valium) are the prototype drugs of a class of sedatives that differ chemically from other sedatives discussed so far. This class of sedatives is known as the benzodiazepines, which pharmacologically are classified as the minor tranquilizers.

Chlordiazepoxide as the prototype benzo-diazepine has a definite sedative action, and produces tranquilizing effects that are indistinguishable from sedation. Chlordiazepoxide exhibits anticonvulsant effects in animals. The drug has been advocated as a central-acting skeletal muscle relaxant, since it has been shown to abolish spastic rigidity in animals. Chlordiazepoxide, although available parenterally, has not been used as an intravenous sedative in dentistry.

Diazepam differs from chlordiazepoxide in several aspects. It is a more potent anticonvulsant and muscle relaxant, its potency being approximately two and one half times that of chlordiazepoxide; it has a shorter duration of action when taken orally; and it will produce amnesia in many individuals when administered intravenously. When injected intravenously, diazepam will elicit a calming effect in the dental patient. In most cases the patient will also experience euphoria. Perhaps the most unique action of diazepam, as mentioned earlier, lies in its amnesic properties. Approximately 50% of the patients experience retrograde amnesia in that they will not recall any of the events of the dental procedure. If amnesia is produced, its duration will be approximately 45 minutes. The intravenous dose useful for antianxiety and amnesic effects range from 2.5 to 15 mg. Diazepam has a complex metabolic fate, with the formation of the metabolic products probably occurring in the liver. Several metabolites appear in the urine and include the N-demethylated derivative, a hydroxylated compound, the N-demethylated hydroxylated compound (oxazepam), and the glucuronide conjugates.

Diazepam is an extremely safe drug with the doses used in intravenous sedation techniques. Perhaps the only complications are irritation at the injection site and postural hypotension. Diazepam has little if any effect on respiration or the cardiovascular system. The combination or concurrent use of diazepam with other drugs that the patient may be taking and that may produce additive or supra-additive effects should be avoided. These include barbiturates, phenothiazines, and the imipramine type of antidepressants such as imipramine (Tofranil) and amitriptyline (Elavil). Diazepam is suspected of having anticholinergic properties. Thus it is advised that the drug not be used in patients with glaucoma, since anticholinergic agents tend to enhance the glaucoma condition. In addition, diazepam should be used with caution in elderly patients, who are reportedly extremely sensitive to its effects.

Neuroleptanalgesia and dissociative drugs

Neuroleptanalgesia is defined as a state of central nervous system depression with tranquilization and intense analgesia produced without the use of barbiturates or volatile anesthetics. Dissociative analgesia is defined as a state where the patient is "dissociated" from his environment, resembling a state of catalepsy. In addition, amnesia and analgesia are present. If unconsciousness occurs in either case, the conditions are referred to as neuroleptanesthesia and dissociative anesthesia. Two drugs are required to produce the state of neuroleptanalgesia—a neuroleptic component and an analgesic component. *Neurolepsis* is a term applied to characterize a behavioral syndrome in animals and humans caused by these types of drugs. In experimental animals this syndrome consists of the loss of voluntary movement, cataleptic immobility, and inhibition of learned conditional behavior.

All the neuroleptic drugs useful in neuroleptanalgesia chemically consist of a four-carbon chain linked to an amino group and at least one aromatic group such as a phenyl group. Also, a keto group $(c=O)$ is required for high potency. Such a chemical structure is known as 4-phenylbutylamine or butyrophenone, the structure of which is as follows:

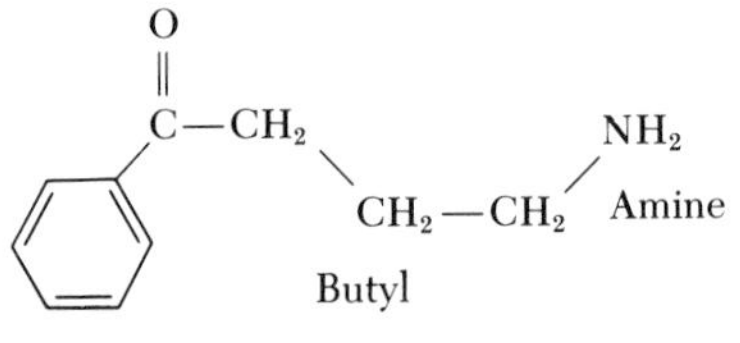

A butyrophenone derivative used in neuroleptanalgesia is haloperidol, an agent that exhibits much greater potency than butyrophenone itself. Another derivative is droperidol, which is approximately twice as potent a neuroleptic agent as haloperidol. Droperidol is the butyrophenone derivative most commonly used in neuroleptanalgesia at the present time. The structures of haloperidol and droperidol are as follows:

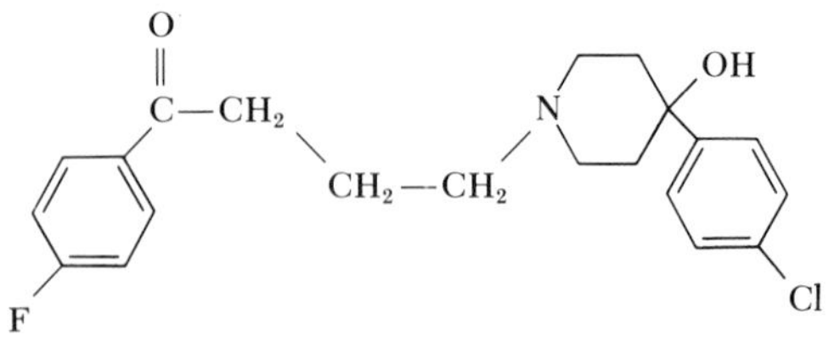

Haloperidol

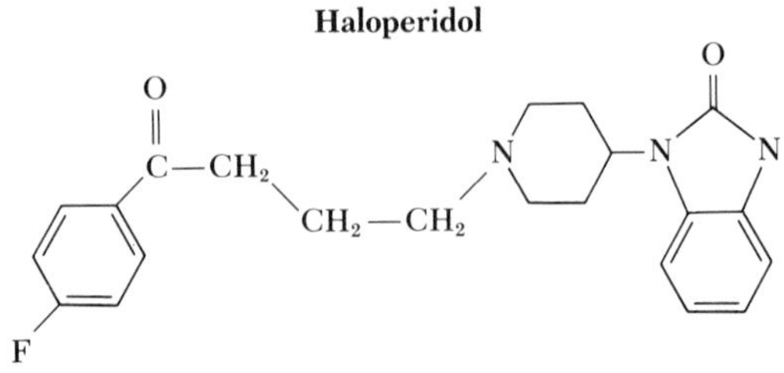

Droperidol

The analgesic component of the neuroleptanalgesic technique is fentanyl. The pharmacology and use of fentanyl in intravenous sedation was discussed earlier and in Chapter 26.

Droperidol is classified pharmacologically as a major tranquilizer. It has an inhibitory effect on voluntary behavior and a significant antipsychotic effect in humans. Effects on the basal ganglia result in extrapyramidal dyskinesias, which are similar to those extrapyramidal effects caused by the phenothiazines. Droperidol inhibits the chemoreceptor trigger zone in the medulla to prevent emesis. In the presence of droperidol, function is well maintained in the reticular activating system. Thus consciousness is maintained. The butyrophenones have little if any effect on the respiratory and circulatory (vasomotor) centers within the medulla. Droperidol is active with 5 minutes after injection, and its effects last between 6 and 12 hours.

Neuroleptanalgesia can be induced with a fixed 50:1 mixture of droperidol (2.5 mg/ml) and fentanyl (0.05 mg/ml) known as Innovar. Since droperidol has an extremely long duration of action (6 to 12 hours) compared with fentanyl (15 to 30 minutes), many clinicians believe it is unsafe to inject the two components as a fixed mixture. Thus the two agents are also available separately as Inapsine (droperidol, 2.5 mg/ml) and Sublimaze (fentanyl, 0.05 mg/ml). Clinical induction doses of Innovar result in a sedated but conscious patient with the following clinical symptoms. First, the patient appears resting, the eyes are closed and the face is expressionless. The patient will talk clearly and rationally when spoken to. Second, the patient will be in an immobilized state with an absence of any voluntary muscle movement. Third, profound analgesia will be present. Fourth, amnesia most likely will occur, although it will not always be complete.

Side effects resulting from the administration of Innovar are due to the actions of either the droperidol or fentanyl. Extrapyramidal effects of Parkinson's syndrome and dyskinesia are seen in a minority of patients. On rare occasions tetanus-like muscular contractions have been reported, which are caused by the droperidol. Other effects include muscular rigidity, hypotension, and respiratory depression, which are caused by the fentanyl.

Substances chemically related to hallucinogenic drugs such as lysergic acid diethylamide (LSD) have been proposed as anesthetics. The first of these, phencylidine, caused unfortunate psychological effects, including hallucinations. More recently a related drug, cyclohexylamine or ketamine (Ketalar) was synthesized and used clinically. Chemically, ketamine differs from all other drugs used in intravenous sedation and has a structure as follows:

Ketamine

Ketamine is used either intravenously or intramuscularly in doses of 1 to 2 mg/kg and 4 to 6 mg/kg, respectively. When so used, it causes dissociative anesthesia because during induction the patient feel dissociated from his environment, including even his own extremities. Analgesia and amnesia occur. Muscle relaxation is poor, but respiration is not affected. Overall, the patient appears awake, with the eyes open but detached from external stimuli. He does not respond to painful stimuli and does not become hypnotic.

The site of action of ketamine in the brain is considered to be in the thalamus and cortex. The mechanism within these areas is unknown, however. The midbrain reticular activating system is little affected. Also, there is no effect of the drug on medullary structures. Thus it has no sedative or hypnotic effects, since the reticular activating system is spared, and it has no effect on respiration, since the medulla is spared.

Ketamine elevates arterial blood pressure and pulse rates in patients. The pressor effect is probably due to an increase in cardiac output. Emergence phenomena are considered to be the most prevalent undesirable effect of ketamine. Vivid dreams are frequently noted by patients, some of which have been unpleasant, involving distortion of body image and temporal and spatial relationships. Diazepam and droperidol have been effective in preventing emergence phenomena.

Ketamine is not recommended for use in the adult patient or hypertensive patient. Muscular rigidity and heightened pharyngeal and laryngeal reflexes make oral procedures difficult. Actual operative time using ketamine is 30 to 50 minutes without supplemental doses, but the actual recovery times may be 2 to 3 hours.

REFERENCES

1. Foreman, P. A.: Pain control and patient management in dentistry—a review of current intravenous techniques, J.A.D.A. **80:**101-111, 1971.
2. Zauder, H. L., and Nichols, R. J.: Intravenous anesthesia, Clin. Anesth. **3:**317-358, 1969.
3. Trieger, N.: Intravenous sedation, Dent. Clin. North Am. **17:**249-261, 1973.
4. Dundee, J.: Comparative analysis of intravenous anesthetics, Anesthesiology **35:**137-148, 1971.
5. Kenney, W. M., and Rudo, F. G.: A review of intravenous sedation techniques in dentistry, J. Balto. Coll. Dent.-Surg. **29:**12-28, 1974.
6. Bennett, C. R.: Conscious-sedation in dental practice, St. Louis, 1974, The C. V. Mosby Co.
7. Bernhoff, A., Eklund, B., and Kaijser, L.: Cardiovascular effects of short-term anaesthesia with methohexitone and propanidid in normal subjects, Br. J. Anaesth. **44:**2-7, 1972.
8. Brand, L., Mark, L. C., Snell, M. M., Vrindten, P., and Dayton, P. G.: Physiologic disposition of methohexital in man, Anesthesiology **24:**331-335, 1963.
9. Shee, J. C.: Dangerous potentiation of pethidine by iproniazid and its treatment, Br. Med. J. **2:**507-509, 1960.
10. Vigran, I. M.: Potentiation of meperidine by pargyline, J.A.M.A. **187:**953-954, 1964.
11. Hine, C. H., and Pasi, A.: Fatality following use of alphaprodine, Clin. Toxicol. **5:**307-315, 1972.

26

Parenteral sedation and nitrous oxide analgesia

RONALD D. BAKER

Many experienced dental patients recognize the technologic progress made in their behalf, and consequently they have become more cooperative, appreciative, and less anxious patients. Most dental patients being treated in modern dental offices by aware, competent, and considerate dentists receive the benefits of comprehensive dental care in relative comfort with either oral or no sedation. There remain, however, a number of dental patients who, because of past experiences, hearsay, or their own psychological being, approach dental appointments with varied degrees of apprehension, dread, or reluctance. To manage these patients effectively, the dentist needs to consider more predictable methods of sedation. To this end, agents and techniques of parenteral sedation as well as nitrous oxide analgesia will be considered. It is not intended that this chapter will prepare the dentist to accomplish parenteral sedation or nitrous oxide analgesia. The objective here is only to familiarize the reader with considerations relative to these techniques that will provide a sound basis for supervised training in their administration.

PSYCHOLOGICAL ASPECTS OF PATIENT MANAGEMENT

At the outset the dentist's appreciation of the patient must be manifested to him by a careful consideration of his needs relative to the procedure or procedures to be accomplished. The psyche cannot be separated from the physical human being. Consequently, both aspects of the patient demand very close attention. Many successful practitioners credit the major portion of the high esteem in which their patients hold them simply to the rapport that they have developed

with each of them *personally.* Clearly, patient management requires the consideration of an individual with a sincere appreciation of his needs, desires, and fears. The dentist must have an empathy that is appreciated by the patient. With patient trust and confidence, in many instances one can achieve patient acceptance of unpleasant sensory situations that otherwise would cause severe, undesirable reactions.

The patient must be "examined" in his entirety, not just orally. The short discussion and observation period that this entails also serves as an ideal time to discuss what procedures the dentist plans and the conditions under which they will be accomplished. The patient needs to know what to expect, whether it be the type of preoperative sedation or steps in the procedure proper. The patient who is fully informed and thus properly prepared for the dentist's procedure will withstand it infinitely better than the one to whom it becomes a series of increasingly unpleasant surprises.

MEDICAL HISTORY

As the patient should be known to the dentist both orally and psychologically, so too should his medical status be completely appreciated. No practitioner should consider the administration of any type of medication, or indeed even routine dental care, without full comprehension of the medical status of his patient. It is repeatedly emphasized that the advances of medical science have succeeded in increasing the life-span of patients who previously would not have survived. Many of these patients with extensive medical problems do not consider themselves as unusual because they have grown accustomed to living with their malady. Others are hesitant to volunteer information regarding their condition. There are many well-designed formats to elicit the information required to assess the current status of a patient or determine if medical consultation may be indicated prior to dental therapy. It behooves each practitioner to choose the form that may best be actively integrated into his practice.

The dentist should ensure that the history form that is used not only delves into questions of general health but also provides space for listing medications that the patient is taking. This allows him to avoid drug interactions. Specific examples of drug interaction are noted when individual drugs are discussed later. This consideration is set forth for emphasis because this is an area that formerly was given little attention in discussions of drug prescription, and it is one that is becoming increasingly complex and important.

In summary, the dentist has the responsibility to ascertain the patient's medical status, including current or recent past medications, and to assess these factors in light of the physical and psychologic needs of the patient.

LIMITATIONS OF ORAL SEDATION

The routine use of drugs for premedication has generally been accomplished by oral administration. By utilizing the recommended dosage and thoroughly understanding the properties of the drugs used, oral premedication has proved to be exceedingly safe. This has resulted from the standardization of doses in tablets or capsules that provide a wide range of safety for the normal adult. There are, of course, people who will be oversedated by the administration of 100 mg secobarbital orally; however, the curve of safety relative to dosage with these drugs is so skewed toward providing safety that a goodly proportion of the population will have sedative effects of less than the desired degree. In effect, the safety of oral medications is achieved by using standardized dosages, with a resulting compromise in the consistency of sedation achieved. In the instances where adequate sedation is not attained, the dentist has not achieved the objective and has not properly prepared that patient for the procedure. To administer additional doses of oral medications to these patients

when it becomes apparent that more sedation is in fact required, will result in dosages beyond the standard. The premise of high degrees of safety is then lost. One must remember that once an oral medication is administered, the practitioner has lost all control of the effects of that dosage. Additionally, a protracted time period must be allowed to ensue before additional sedative effects are realized. Efficient office routine is thus disrupted.

There are certainly significant numbers of patients in daily practice who can be adequately premedicated with oral medication; however, the point to be realized is that standardized drug dosage yields widely variable results, not all of which can be considered as adequate sedation. In those patients in whom oral premedications have proved to be inadequate, in the severely anxious patient, in the obstructive child, and in the patient in pain, consideration should be given to the parenteral administration of premedicants.

INTRAMUSCULAR SEDATION

The intramuscular (IM) route of administration provides more certain absorption, a faster onset, and more predictable results than are obtained with oral sedation. The principal disadvantages of the IM over the oral route are more complicated delivery, less patient acceptance, and greater cost. As with oral premedication, there is an inability to remove the drug if overdosage or overreaction has occurred. In comparison with the intravenous route, IM administration has a slower onset. Like the oral route safe dosages still provide a range of sedative effects. The use of specific drugs in IM sedation are discussed later.

INTRAVENOUS SEDATION

The principal disadvantage of intravenous (IV) sedation is that the potent drugs being used make mandatory the avoidance of excessive dosages with resultant untoward depression of the cardiovascular, respiratory, or central nervous systems. It is a hazardous procedure unless the clinician is adequately trained. He must be equipped and competent not only to administer the drugs but also to treat and control adverse reactions and complications. For this reason IV sedation is discussed in some detail.

Intravenous practice, of recent interest in the United States, has long been accepted as routine in undergraduate teaching in Great Britain. Many practitioners regard IV sedation as involving more risks, being dangerous, or being in the realm of general anesthesia. It is, however, the most effective method of ensuring *predictable, adequate* premedication in *each* patient. By injection of the premedication drugs in small increments over an appropriate time span, with constant patient observation, each patient may be brought to that degree of sedation which ensures his comfort and provides the necessary degree of cooperation to enable the operator to accomplish the planned procedures. This is the principle of *titration* to achieve the desired effect. Since the clinician has continuous control over the amount of drug given, it is not necessary to administer more than is required for adequate sedation. Essentially, in the oral and IM routes the whole drug dosage is administered at one time, whereas in the IV administration small increments allow minute-to-minute control over the level of sedation. Individual patient variance is thus eliminated as a factor of dosage. As previously noted, certain training requirements and precautions are required of course, and a new set of potential complications evolve that the practitioner must be aware of and be prepared to avoid or treat.

Disadvantages of intravenous sedation

Initially, the introduction of intravenous sedation, as with any other newly introduced office technique, will require an increased expenditure of time. As facility increases and experience is gained, this disadvantage will be overcome, and indeed the time required for many procedures may be decreased because of the patient cooperation thus secured.

The technique requires the placement of a needle into a vein. Although many people dread this experience, it is usually met with more acceptance than intraoral injections. Although intravenous sedation requires the concomitant use of local anesthesia, the patient is put into such a relaxed, and at times amnesic, state that he does not find the intraoral injection objectionable. Many times the patient will not remember the intraoral injection or have hazy recollections of its administration.

The utilization of parenteral sedative techniques does require the maintenance of sufficient quantities of various drugs in the office. Secure storage facilities are required, and an increased risk of forced entry must be assumed.

Although the foregoing are considerations, the overwhelming restriction imposed by this technique is that the operator must have knowledge of the procedures and the agents used and also comprehend fully the implications, restrictions, and complications of its use. This is not the technique for the individual seeking an easy resolution to his sedation problems. Intravenous sedation must be approached in a totally committed manner. There exists a sufficient body of knowledge in texts and the literature in all phases of sedation to provide the didactic background that is required. The true student and dedicated, conscientious practitioner must realize that one chapter, one text, or one "short course" is inadequate preparation for introducing this technique into his practice. Additional requirements in the realm of emergency drugs, equipment, and their usage, and even the venipuncture technique are not added burdens but represent facets of practice that the dentist should already have prepared for in consideration of emergencies in his office.

If the disadvantages presented seem overwhelming, a point has been made. This technique is demanding in regard to competence and attention to detail; however, many of its facets should already be within the expected standard of practice. Additionally, the advantages of the use of intravenous sedation are such that its utilization should have consideration in the daily practice of a significant number of practitioners.

Complications of intravenous sedation

As with all new techniques, the operator must acquaint himself with a new set of complications. For the most part, complications are a result of lack of knowledge or inattention to detail.

Care must be taken at the time of drug infusion to prevent extravascular injection of the agent. This complication is the result of inattention and may be eliminated by developing good technique. The needle point must be carried a distance beyond vein entry to ensure intravascular drug administration.

Prior to and during the injection, aspiration will easily determine the adequacy of the venous system in use. If inadvertent extravascular administration occurs, it may be treated by the infiltration of up to 10 ml of a 1% solution of procaine hydrochloride in the area. This provides the following functions:

1. It dilutes the agent injected.
2. It causes vasodilation and hence speeds the absorption of the agent. Note that lidocaine will not afford this function.
3. Barbiturates are highly alkaline. The procaine hydrochloride will tend to neutralize the alkalinity of the barbiturates and prevent tissue slough.

The most serious mechanical error is intraarterial injection. This, like the extravascular injection, is an error of technique. It may be prevented by palpation of the contemplated injection site prior to tourniquet placement, knowledge of the anatomy of the upper extremity, and close observation of hydrostatic pressures affecting the syringe at the time intravascular puncture has been achieved. The patient may complain of a severe radiating pain progressing distally from the puncture site, which is a result of vasospasm of the violated artery. The vasospasm of the artery may cause blanching of the skin in its peripheral distribution. Thrombus formation may subsequently occur, and, when extensive, gangrene may follow with amputation sometimes being necessary. The treatment of intra-arterial injection may be divided into two phases:

1. *Immediate office treatment:* An attempt to maintain the needle in the artery should be made. If successful, 10 ml of 1% procaine hydrochloride is injected. This serves to dilute the agent (if one has been injected), relax the vasospasm, and ease the patient's pain.

2. *Consultation:* Depending on the results of the office therapy, consideration should be given to possible hospitalization and the performance of stellate ganglion (sympathetic interruption) blocks, or the administration of anticoagulants to the patient.

Perhaps the most common adverse sequela to intravenous utilization is the occurrence of thrombophlebitis. In these instances the vein will feel hard or ropelike along its path. This may be treated by resting the arm, elevating the arm, and applying hot soaks to the area. In some measure it may be prevented by dilution of intravenous agents, where this is possible.

Respiratory or circulatory depression, or both, from overdosage should not occur in the well-managed sedative regimen; however, the practitioner must be prepared to support respiration and circulation should overdepression occur.

The recovery room personnel as well as the person accompanying the patient must be impressed as to the patient's mental and physical limitations to avoid subsequent postoperative injuries. Written instructions and a discussion with the competent adult escort should ensure the safest transportation and care for the patient.

Precautions relating to intravenous sedation

Intravenous sedation must be accomplished by a strict aseptic technique. This involves a skin preparation usually accomplished with alcohol sponge wipedown. Today, a wide variety of prepackaged, sterile, disposable syringes, intravenous devices, and tubing is available, and their use is preferable for consistent maintenance of an aseptic routine.

The degree of patient monitoring necessary during drug administration and the operative procedure will vary directly with the degree of depression desired. With sedative techniques, pulse, respiration, and blood pressure monitoring should be adequate. There is an increasing variety of monitoring devices being made available to the profession. Depending on locale and practice, the acquisition of currently available devices may be advisable.

As with all procedures, a record should be maintained that indicates, at the least, presedation vital signs, time and dosages of drugs administered, and a statement of the patient's progress and condition when the procedure was concluded. Complete, accurate records are mandatory in this facet of dental practice.

Considerations in the performance of venipuncture

A detailed description of venipuncture technique is not within the purview of this text; however, a few significant points are vital enough to require emphasis.

Just as the dentist does not perform dental

procedures without knowledge of the anatomy involved, so too the dentist should not accomplish venipuncture without a knowledge of the structures in the area and their relationships. Although a detailed consideration of anatomy will not be presented, it is important that the arterial pathways of the upper extremity be partially defined. The arm is supplied by the brachial artery, which divides into the radial and ulnar arteries at or slightly distal to the cubital fossa. Although the venous pathways of the forearm are variable, three main vessels proceed toward the elbow: the median, basilic, and cephalic veins. The median vein, as its name implies, courses between the other two vessels on the medial surface of the forearm and ends in the area of the cubital fossa by sending branches to the basilic and cephalic veins. The median-basilic vein is usually more prominent and appears as the most likely suitable vein in this area. Just deep to the median-basilic vein, however, lies the brachial artery, with only a fascial layer intervening. In light of previous discussions on intra-arterial injections, it becomes apparent that this vein should be avoided despite its being a most attractive target.

The veins of the hand are located dorsally, a physiologic location to permit palmar action without impeding blood flow. When these veins are used for venipuncture, the patient may at times note some pain in the hand. This may be caused by the presence of arteriovenous shunts resulting in drug action initiating vasospasm of the arteries so affected.

In the distal forearm arterial pathways seldom border as closely on venous drainage routes. Veins in the dorsal hand as well as the distal forearm constitute the main area of interest in intravenous sedation techniques.

Contraindications to intravenous sedation

There are three overriding considerations that form absolute contraindications to the intravenous sedative technique. The first of these concerns the uninformed and incompletely trained operator, which has already been discussed. The second deals with the facilities available. Prior to entry into this field, the clinician's office must be equipped with a method of positive-pressure oxygen administration as well as a separate motor-driven suction apparatus. Additionally, the office suite must provide recovery space with both oxygen and suction availability. The office assistants must be trained as part of a team for the administration, intraoperative care, and recovery period observation. The third absolute contraindication consists of those systemic diseases and/or drug administration that compromise respiration or the cardiovascular system or that mandate the avoidance of specific drugs or procedures. The medical history and physical findings combined with the psychological nature of the patient determine the feasibility of these techniques.

PREMEDICANTS AND TECHNIQUES

A definition of the uses and delineation of the disadvantages of a few specific agents that I consider to be of most value for office sedation follow. In this way it is hoped that the reader will achieve a useful appreciation of these agents rather than have a broad overview of the subject, which serves little practical purpose.

Barbiturates

The barbiturates are excellent agents for the relief of apprehension. They do not have analgesic effects, unless the dosage is such that central nervous system depression renders the patient unconscious. Thus patients in pain who are given only barbiturates may lose cerebral control and become agitated or delirious. The barbiturates will depress the respiratory center, diminishing respiratory drive mechanisms, and hence cause a decreased respiratory minute volume. This becomes a consideration in the use of these drugs in patients with existing respiratory disease or compromise. Death from barbiturate overdosage is by way of profound respiratory depression. Concomitant use with many other drugs should be accomplished with a realization of possible interaction or synergism. The most commonly encountered of these would be the phenothiazines, alcohol, reserpine, and the antihistamines. Barbiturates increase the rate of coumadin metabolism and thus must be used with care in patients taking these drugs. Any barbiturate is contraindicated in patients with porphyria. These agents will pass the placenta barrier and also appear in the mother's milk. Elderly patients may not tolerate these drugs well and become confused.

As with all depressant drugs, ambulatory

patients must be accompanied by a responsible person when these drugs have been administered. The patient must be specifically warned about the length of time he must be cautious in his movements, driving a motor vehicle, cooking, signing legal papers, and so forth.

Intramuscular use. In the absence of pain these drugs may be utilized alone as premedicants. At least 30 minutes should intervene after injection before operative procedures are instituted. Vital signs should be monitored, and a well-equipped emergency kit and oxygen should be both available and familiar to the operator and his staff.

The dosage may be adjusted according to the procedure being contemplated, the degree of anxiety of the patient, and the patient's physical status. A muscular adult athlete may be expected to require a somewhat proportionally higher dosage than a slightly built individual, with all other factors being equal. The alcoholic will usually require an increased dose, unless liver disease is present. Clinical judgment will effect more exact and suitable individualized dosages as experience is gained with the technique. Intramuscular techniques will usually provide a more positive and predictable sedative level than do oral medications, but they too result in a range of sedative effects. The technique finds application where this range, more defined than with oral medication, is acceptable and desired by the operator and patient.

Pentobarbital (Nembutal) dosage: available in 50 mg/ml solution
  Normal adult—50 to 150 mg intramuscularly
  Children with normal height and weight relationships—1 to 2 mg/lb, up to 50 mg

Intravenous use. A convenient practice is to dilute 150 mg of pentobarbital (3 ml) with 7 ml sterile water for injection. This provides a 10 ml syringe, with each milliliter of solution containing 15 mg of the agent. An intravenous route is established, and 0.25 ml of the solution is first administered as a test dose. The patient is observed and the vital signs compared with preadministration values to detect significant untoward effects. If there are no such effects, an additional 3.75 to 4.75 ml of solution are administered, yielding a total injected dosage of 60 to 75 mg. This is accomplished over 30 to 45 seconds while the dentist converses with the patient. At this point an additional 60 sec-

onds are allowed to elapse to permit the assessment of the effects of the administered dosage. In *normal, healthy patients a 1-minute delay after injection of a quantity of these drugs may be expected to elicit nearly the full pharmacologic effect of that drug administration.** Additional increments of 15 mg (1 ml) are then injected until a relaxed, cooperative patient is secured without excessive depression or until cortical symptoms of dizziness or tiredness are achieved. Before each increment, a 45- to 60-second delay is mandatory to prevent excessive depression, that is, to assess at all times the current status of the patient. As the patient approaches the desired sedative levels, clearly observable signs occur, including slurred speech, the patient stating that the room is revolving, difficulty in focusing, talkativeness, a happy-drunk state; in other words the patient has become relaxed and no longer anxious. At any subsequent stage, additional increments may be added to maintain this level of sedation. One should appreciate that the dilution of the agent provides ease in administration of small additional fractions of the drug. Additionally, since the barbiturates are very alkaline in nature, this reduces the chemical insult to the vein, helping to prevent phlebitis. As in all intravenous administrations, care should be taken to avoid accidental intra-arterial injection.

During administration, pulse and blood pressure should be checked periodically, with clinically significant depression calling for cessation of further drug injections. During the dental procedure the degree of sedation, the patient's reactions, and his vital signs may be used to monitor the depression of systems.

If thought is given to the dosages required to achieve sedation and to those which are toxic, the difference, which represents the margin of error or conversely the degree of safety inherent with the drug, is wide enough so that pentobarbital may deserve consideration as the initial drug for the practitioner introducing intravenous technique into his practice. Goodman and Gilman state that although the lethal dose of barbiturates varies,

---

*Obviously, in sick or debilitated patients or those in shock this generalization is not true. The management of these patients must be individualized, preferably in a hospital setting.

"severe poisoning is likely to occur when more than ten times [10X!] the full hypnotic dose has been ingested at once."[1] Clearly, these drugs, if not abused, provide a wide range of safety not found with other premedicants.

The duration of sedative effects may extend for 2 to 4 hours. This technique is ideal to allay apprehension and provide sedation for procedures that may be time consuming and unpleasant for the patient. Adequate local anesthesia is a requirement in view of former discussions relative to barbiturates and pain. If the procedure is manifestly painful or will entail postoperative pain, consideration should be given to the utilization of subsequently described techniques.

Narcotics

Although morphine remains the standard on which other narcotics are judged, its uses in dentistry remain minimal. In contrast, meperidine (Demerol) has found wide clinical acceptance. Meperidine tends to produce sleepiness but produces euphoria to only a slight degree. Like the barbiturates meperidine will depress the respiratory center, with its effects lasting up to 4 hours. Meperidine has the potential to cause hypotension, although this primarily occurs in erect patients, with little such tendency in the recumbent position. This tendency toward postural hypotension forms one of the precautionary notes when releasing premedicated ambulatory patients.

Meperidine has an atropine-like effect, which may result in some degree of xerostomia. Like morphine the drug may cause the undesirable side effects of nausea, vomiting, and dizziness. It is primarily metabolized in the liver; hence, liver disease will result in retardation of its destruction. Meperidine passes the placental barrier.

Respiratory depression secondary to overdose can be antagonized by nalorphine, 5 to 10 mg intravenously, with repeated doses as necessary but not to exceed 40 mg. Recently naloxone (Narcan) has found increasing clinical use as the narcotic antagonist of choice. It does not have the opiate-like effects of nalorphine and levallorphan and hence exerts little, if any, pharmacologic effects beyond pure narcotic antagonism. Intravenous administration will usually bring reversal of narcotic-induced effects within 2 minutes. The duration of action is up to

2 hours, which may be *less than* the depressant effects of the narcotic. Continued observation until narcotic effects have ceased and repeated antagonist administrations are thus the rule for the treatment of narcotic-induced respiratory depression. The adult dose of naloxone is 0.4 mg (1 ml) intravenously, repeated as necessary in 2- to 3-minute intervals, up to 3 doses. Each dental office in which narcotics are administered should have a narcotic antagonist readily available.

It is vital to be absolutely certain that meperidine is not administered to any patient who has been recently or is now taking a monoamine oxidase inhibitor. The combination of meperidine and MAO inhibitor intake may result in delirium, convulsions, and possibly death. This drug has a moderate degree of safety, although not to the same degree as the barbiturates.

> Meperidine (Demerol) dosage: available in 50 mg/ml solution
> Normal adult—50 to 100 mg
> Children with normal height and weight relationships—0.5 mg/lb

Meperidine is seldom used alone as a premedicant drug, but rather it is used in combination with other agents. An intravenous technique that has received considerable recognition is the Jorgensen technique.[2] Many years ago Jorgensen combined the analgesic and sedative effects of meperidine with the sedative effects of pentobarbital. He also found that by administering the barbiturate first, the high incidence of nausea and vomiting with meperidine was eliminated. This produces a pleasant amnesic and analgesic state without the loss of consciousness. A significant advantage gained with the technique is that it tends to compress the time frame of reference for the patient so that a 2-hour appointment will seem like 30 minutes or less. The technique is as follows:

The patient should be made aware of the sequence of events at this appointment. He should be accompanied by a responsible person, one physically able to assist him, and should be aware of the physical and mental postoperative restrictions as noted previously. The supine position is preferable to avoid hypotensive episodes. Background distractions should be minimized, including instrument setup, talking between staff, and excessive movement in the room. A syringe of pentobarbital with the solution having a concentration of 10 mg/ml pentobarbital is prepared. An intravenous route is established, and a test dose of approximately 3 mg pentobarbital is administered to observe any untoward reaction. In the absence of a reaction, 10 mg (1 ml) of the agent is subsequently injected every 30 seconds until a light stage of sedation is achieved. With the observance of the first sign of cortical depression, such as noted earlier, a stage has been reached that Jorgensen considers to be the "baseline." The dose required to reach this stage will vary from 20 to 200 mg. With added experience in the technique, a variable additional increment may be added for more effective sedation. This augmentation will be in the range of 10% to 15% above baseline dosage. The syringe is removed and replaced with a fresh syringe. All traces of the barbiturate must have been cleared from whatever infusion system is utilized, since meperidine and the barbiturates together form an insoluble precipitate. The fresh syringe contains 25 mg meperidine and 0.32 mg scopolamine, which have been diluted to form 5 ml of solution. The dilute solution permits slow infusion to achieve constant dose control. As these medications are injected, the patient's pulse is monitored, and at the first sign of depression the injection is terminated. For the person who has taken over 100 mg pentobarbital to reach the baseline, the entire contents of the second syringe will probably be required. This dosage is not exceeded.

The sedation procedure is now complete and will last more than 2 hours. The scopolamine will produce amnesia and decrease the patient's memory of the procedure.

The technique is not without its disadvantages. Obviously, approximately 10 minutes will be required to achieve the sedative stage. The duration of action of the drugs employed results in a long time span of effect. These two aspects make the technique less desirable for short procedures.

Tranquilizing drugs

Diazepam (Valium) is one of a group of tranquilizing drugs that has found ready acceptance as a premedicant in dental practice. Additionally, it provides muscular relaxation and a degree of amnesia. The amnesia produced by the drug is not retrograde in type; that is, amnesia for events immediately prior to the injection is not usually expected.[3,4] Amnesia does follow the intravenous injection of diazepam closely. Driscoll and colleagues[5] studied the effects of intravenous diazepam sedation on multiple-extraction or impaction patients treated on an outpatient basis. The total titration dose of diazepam averaged 19.04 mg for patients with impaction and 18.4 mg for patients having extraction. These dosages did not result in significant changes in cardiopulmonary function. They were responsible for producing amnesia in 53.9% of patients for the intraoral injection as tested on the day of surgery and in 70.6% for the injection procedure as measured at the postoperative visit. Gregg and co-workers[6] also showed that amnesia was attained without significant alteration of the level of consciousness or depression of the cardiopulmonary systems. They showed that amnesia of controlled stimuli was a direct function of dose. In this regard it was shown that body weight was a significant variable in determining the levels of amnesia. Their study showed a peak effect of amnesia at a 10-minute interval from intravenous administration with a return to placebo level depending on dosage per body weight. The amnesia seen with diazepam thus may be clinically variable; however, depending on the noted variables, amnesia may be expected to persist for up to 45 minutes, with the latter portion of that time period having more cognitive breakthrough.

Diazepam is not analgesic so that adequate local anesthesia or combination with analgesics, where required, is indicated. Respiration is not depressed as with the barbiturates and narcotics. There is some evidence that respiratory function may be to a small degree more sensitive than the cardiovascular system, responding with slight respiratory depression.[7] If this characteristic is present, it is primarily due to a decrease in tidal volume. Respiratory depression with the doses of diazepam administered for outpatient dental procedures has not been a constant finding.[8] The cardiovascular system is not significantly affected,[9] although the relief of anxiety may result in some fall of blood pressure. The pulse rate may be unchanged, may decrease because of relief of anxiety, or as has been documented may increase in the first 10 minutes after administration and subsequently return to normal rates.[6,9] The patient may manifest lightheadedness, dizziness, and ataxia. Diazepam should be avoided in early pregnancy because its effects on the developing fetus are not yet fully realized. However, it is used in labor and delivery rooms with no significant cardiovascular or respiratory depression observable in neonates. Patients of advancing years may be somewhat more susceptible to the effects of this drug.

The metabolism of diazepam in the body is complex and has not been defined fully at this time. It is known that after intravenous injection of diazepam there is a moderately rapid decline in the plasma concentration. The degree of this decline is dose related and corresponds to the clinical period of sedative and amnesia effects. The plasma level will again show an increased concentration 6 to 8 hours after administration,[10] which is probably because of redistribution of the drug. It does form the basis of what must be strongly emphasized to the patient— that activities even for the protracted period of 8 to 10 hours must be limited. In the postoperative period relative loss of sedative effects or light stages of euphoria, as often are seen with this drug, makes these precautions and patient warnings even more important. Coupled with slow detoxification and excretion, extending for as long as 7 days, a hypnotically active metabolite called desmethyldiazepam increases in concentration for a 50-hour period after intravenous administration, and then it, too, is slowly metabolized over several days.[7] Patients with closely repeated dosages of diazepam may thus be expected to have higher than anticipated plasma levels. One must remember that this agent will potentiate many other sedative drugs such as the barbiturates, antihypertensives, and narcotics. Ingestion of alcohol should be avoided during periods of diazepam administration. The protracted metabolism of the drug should be considered when patients are counseled in this regard. The drug's duration of action is less than that of those previously considered, yielding approximately 1 hour of sedation. It is thus an excellent agent to consider where relatively short periods of sedation are required.

The intramuscular dosage of diazepam is as follows:

Normal adult—10 mg
Children (according to SAAD[11])
    Age 4 to 6 years—5 mg
    Age 7 to 10 years—7.5 mg
    Age 11 to 14 years—10 mg

The foregoing may be followed as a general rule, with the final determination being made on the basis of the weight or surface area of the child.

Intravenous technique. Diazepam is packaged in a 2 ml, amber-colored ampule with each milliliter of solution containing 5 mg diazepam; it is also available in a multiple-dose vial of 10 ml. It should be administered undiluted because it has some propensity to leave solution.

After mental and physical preparation of the patient, an intravenous route is established. Recent literature has suggested that small veins should be avoided. Past experience with the veins of the dorsum of the hand has evoked a "burning" response from the patient in the hand. It is recommended that the largest available suitable vein in the forearm or antecubital fossa be chosen for this injection. Additionally, the diazepam should be injected slowly to allow intravenous dilution of the drug, thus minimizing its irritating effects. Although the manufacturer does not recommend adding the drug to intravenous fluids, it is common practice to inject the agent slowly into a rapidly running intravenous infusion of 5% dextrose and water or Ringer's lactate solution. These precautions are to minimize the possibility of venous thrombosis or proximal phlebitis. As has been indicated earlier, this is the most commonly seen adverse sequelae to intravenous sedation.

Clinical experience with diazepam that has been administered properly has revealed a very low incidence of venous irritation. An initial dose of 2.5 mg (0.5 ml) is slowly administered, followed by a 60-second period of observation. During this time period the patient is observed for signs of an unusual response to the agent. Additional increments are injected at a rate not to exceed 5 mg (1 ml) per minute. During the slow injection phase the patient is observed for signs of adequate sedation, which are similar to those noted earlier for the intravenous use of barbiturates. Adequate sedative effects can also be expected when Verrill's sign has been achieved.[12] This is observed by having the patient look straight ahead. The upper eyelid will begin to droop, and when it covers one half of the iris (eye is at "half-mast"), no more drug is administered. Although some people will be effectively sedated with low dosages of diazepam, Verrill's sign is seldom achieved unless dosages in excess of 10 mg are given in the normal adult patient. Depending on the patient, his anxiety, the dentist's rapport with him, and the procedure itself, it will be found that 10 mg will provide adequate sedation in a great number of individuals, even though the aforementioned test point has not been reached. If one does proceed to "half-mast," no more than 20 mg should usually be administered to the routine dental outpatient. Even at 20 mg, however, there is a generous margin of safety with diazepam. Increments may be added during a procedure, within these guidelines, if they are required as the procedure progresses. The rapid decline of plasma levels coupled with delayed metabolism should induce caution as to the total dose administered during the course of one appointment. If a procedure has the potential for becoming protracted in time, perhaps another technique should be considered. With this agent the period of administration is sharply reduced from the Jorgensen technique. The efficient achievement of sedation combined with a short action makes the drug both practical and advantageous for short procedures.

The disadvantages of intravenous diazepam include a tendency for some patients to become talkative, especially when less drug is given than that required to achieve Verrill's sign. Additionally, there is a stringent requirement that patients who receive diazepam intravenously be accompanied by a responsible person and observe the noted restrictions in a lengthy postsedation period. This is especially true of diazepam because of its delayed metabolism and excretion and the commonly observed postoperative euphoria.

Combination of agents

Diazepam and meperidine. A slight modification of the intravenous diazepam administration and the Jorgenson technique affords advantages peculiar to both. In this technique for adults a 10 mg intravenous dose of diazepam is followed by 25 mg meperidine and 0.32 mg scopolamine. Added amnesia, relaxation, sedation, and analgesia are thus achieved. This combination offers advantages in the management of patients in pain at the inception of the procedure, for procedures that are in themselves painful, or in cases where considerable postoperative pain is anticipated. There have been reports

which show that a combination of diazepam and meperidine is responsible for significant alterations in blood gases. Respiratory depression can occur without clinical appreciation in the sedated patient. Dunsworth and associates,[13] while using diazepam and meperidine, showed an elevation in PCO_2 from 36.3 ± 3.6 preoperatively to 40.3 ± 5.7 at midsurgery and 39.2 ± 4.7 (mm Hg) in the 10 to 15-minute postoperative period. Dundee states that "A combination of diazepam and an opiate produced a greater degree of respiratory depression than would be expected from the individual drugs."[14] It has been theorized that the two drugs competed for the same detoxification enzyme. The need for the narcotic with the attendant possibility of respiratory depression must be carefully assessed as regards the patient's physical and mental condition and the proposed therapy. As with all drug therapy, the benefits to be gained should be greater than the attendant risks.

Innovar. Innovar is a combination of a narcotic, fentanyl (Sublimaze), and a tranquilizer, droperidol (Inapsine), in a 1:50 ratio. Each milliliter of Innovar contains 0.05 mg fentanyl and 2.5 mg droperidol. The combination produces an effect termed *neuroleptanalgesia*. This is a state of noticeable tranquilization and profound analgesia in which the patient, although conscious, is detached or mentally removed from his immediate surroundings. The patient will respond to commands, but when not so stimulated, he returns to a state of dissociation.

Fentanyl is a powerful narcotic with effects not unlike those of morphine. It differs significantly, however, in the following ways: The same analgesic effect is attained at approximately 1/100 the dose of morphine, its duration of action is significantly shorter, its effects on the cardiovascular system are more benign, it lacks emetic properties, and it does not cause histamine release. The latter action renders the agent suitable for use in asthmatic patients. Bradycardia, if produced by this agent, may be treated by the administration of atropine. Its main disadvantage relative to use in the routine dental outpatient is the great degree of respiratory depression it effects. Although this may be reversed with naloxone, respiration may have to be supported or controlled in the interim.

Droperidol is an active and highly potent tranquilizer with a significant antiemetic effect. Although it has minimal effect on the respiratory system, it can produce hypotension. It causes peripheral vascular dilation and reduction of the vasopressor effect of epinephrine. It will produce significant degrees of potentiation of other central nervous system depressants.

Innovar has found use in hospital anesthesia practice for diagnostic or surgical procedures where relief of pain and anxiety is required, for sedation with a low incidence of nausea or vomiting, or as an adjunctive agent in conjunction with local anesthesia. Skeletal muscle rigidity with thoracic ventilatory disruption may occur if the agent is administered too rapidly or in excessive amounts. This may be managed with muscle relaxants and controlled respirations. Patients who have received Innovar must be watched carefully. The respiratory depressant effect will last for a longer period of time than the perceived analgesic effect! Postoperative administration of depressant drugs must be limited and dosages reduced because of the profound potentiation mentioned earlier. Although Innovar has significant favorable qualities for use in a hospital environment, the possible adverse effects render it a drug to be used with extreme caution, if at all, by the general practitioner for outpatient premedication. The two agents combined in Innovar are now available separately, and their individual use might well be considered in conjunction with the preceding discussion.

Droperidol is available in 2 and 5 ml ampules with each milliliter having 2.5 mg of the drug. For preoperative sedation 1 to 2 ml may be administered; however, the possibility of hypotension with this agent should greatly minimize its use in the general dental practice. With its alpha-adrenergic blocking effects, hypotension that results from the administration of this agent should *not* be treated with epinephrine. Such use may result in a paradoxical further drop in blood pressure. With the other sedative agents that are available, specific indications should exist for the use of this agent over more routinely used drugs.

Fentanyl is available in 2 and 5 ml ampules, with each milliliter having 0.05 mg of the drug. Fentanyl has little hypnotic or sedative effect, but it is an excellent narcotic analgesic. It may be useful for controlling pain in the anxious patient, to supplement regional anesthesia during painful procedures, or in cases where postoperative pain may be expected.

As has been emphasized, the main disadvantage of this drug is its ability to cause severe respiratory depression. Apnea may be expected in doses in excess of 0.009 mg/kg.[15] Although this dosage would not be approached in supplementing sedation, with individual variation, it emphasizes the absolute need for a method of airway control with positive-pressure oxygen capability and narcotic antagonist availability. The duration of active analgesic effect is from 30 to 60 minutes when administered intravenously and from 1 to 2 hours when given intramuscularly. The onset of action is almost immediate with intravenous administration and within 10 minutes with intramuscular administration. As with the combination of these two agents, the respiratory depression will last longer than the analgesia obtained. Fentanyl should be used with caution in patients with respiratory disease as well as in those with liver and kidney disease.

The following dosages of fentanyl should be given*:

Normal adult—0.05 to 0.1 mg
1 to 2 ml given intramuscularly 30 to 60 minutes prior to procedure or *slowly* intravenously just prior to procedure
Child—0.02 to 0.03 mg per 20 to 25 pounds

NITROUS OXIDE ANALGESIA

The administration of nitrous oxide–oxygen inhalation analgesia in the dental office has undergone cyclic periods of enthusiasm and disfavor. Once again, this mode of sedation has become popular. The recent increase in its use is a result of continued use, with evangelistic recommendation by a few devotees, increased awareness of the patient, improvements in medical aspects of dental education, and a perfection of equipment.

One old misunderstanding that still exists is that many people equate nitrous oxide with general anesthesia. Although nitrous oxide is used as a part of general anesthetic procedures, the inhalation sedative technique does

---

*Dosage must be adjusted for the elderly, debilitated, or those receiving other depressant drugs.

not produce a state of general surgical anesthesia. The fact should be emphasized that when the anesthetic is properly administered, the patient remains conscious and protective reflexes remain operational. The nitrous oxide–oxygen sedative technique may be adapted to use in a wide range of dental office procedures offering increased patient cooperation and comfort. Local anesthesia may not be required with this technique for many procedures in operative dentistry.

The following discussion of nitrous oxide analgesia should only be considered a basic familiarization that will facilitate and reinforce adequate supervised training in the use of this technique.

Nitrous oxide–oxygen sedation defined

As a consequence of training requirements during World War I, Guedel amplified the definitions then existing as to the stages of anesthesia. Although these best relate to an agent of slow progression, such as ether, exploration of a portion of these definitions becomes significant with this technique. Stage I of general anesthesia was defined as that time period and sequence of physiologic events lasting from the beginning of the anesthetic procedure until such time as the patient lost consciousness. Stage II represented a period of delirium with uncoordinated movements. After this the level of surgical anesthesia was reached at stage III. Finally, the period from the cessation of respiration until cardiac failure was described as stage IV. Stage III was subdivided further into planes of surgical anesthesia. This chapter is restricted to dealing with a conscious patient so that attention is centered on stage I. This stage is of little interest in general anesthesia; however, it has become apparent that just as there are surgical levels within stage III, so too are there levels within stage I. Although these may be defined to some degree, an understanding of the physiologic effects in this stage is more important. Analgesia will be increased as the lower extent of the stage is approached and will reach 85% at the depths of this stage. Deeper into stage I, amnesia also progresses from minimal to nearly complete forgetfulness. The patient maintains his contact with the operator until near unconsciousness. However, while in the midplane area he will follow directions; with progression he may lose this response. Thus it can be seen that nearly complete amnesia and analgesia may take the patient close to that physiologic zone where he will pass into the excitement phase of stage II. Obviously, encroachment on this zone should be avoided. Progression of amnesia, analgesia, and relaxation may be achieved well into stage I, with only minimal decrease of protective reflexes. The important and significant consideration is that the area prior to and at the entrance into stage II be avoided.

Advantages

As has been implied, the nitrous oxide–oxygen technique has sufficient advantages to recommend its consideration in many dental care delivery systems. There is a rapid onset of sedative effects. Sensory changes are evident in less than 1 minute, and effective sedation is usually achieved in 3 or 4 minutes. This, of course, is in contrast to oral or intramuscular sedative techniques, in which a lengthy latent period is evident prior to sedation. Although intravenous sedative effects are quickly perceived, preparation and total administration time are greater than for nitrous oxide–oxygen sedation. Thus minimal preparation and a short time of onset are significant advantages of this technique. Additionally, of course, no intramuscular injection or venipuncture is required, which is appreciated by most people.

The technique allows for a very close control over the level of sedation achieved. In the conscious patient a change of the percentage of nitrous oxide administered results in rapid physiologic adjustment. Indeed, in patients with whom the technique is to be used for a series of procedures, the patient himself will learn to adjust his level to some degree by the amount of mouth breathing he does. This facility dispels fear of the procedure and provides ready acceptance, since the patient realizes that he has control over the technique and can quickly terminate its effects by total mouth breathing. In these instances where the technique is used in a series of procedures, it often becomes apparent that as the patient's approval of and confidence in the technique are achieved, decreased percentages of nitrous oxide are required for later treatments. This placebo effect further increases the overall safety of the technique.

Recovery is rapidly effected with full return to presedative psychomotor capacity. Thus the need for the patient to be accompanied may be eliminated.

The technique is highly effective in the management of the young patient. Children of 5 to 10 years of age may actually tolerate nasal masks used in this technique better than adults, since they relate the mask to space masks and other games. Thus a game may be played with the child, effecting a smooth sedative procedure. Many adults with claustrophobic tendencies may be able to be treated with this technique by means of good chairside rapport.

The nitrous oxide–oxygen technique will not only offer comfort to the patient and increase his acceptance of dental procedures but also will afford a more relaxed treatment administration; that is, the dentist should find himself with less tension and fatigue at the end of his office day.

Safety

As noted earlier, the following discussion is not intended to prepare the dentist to undertake nitrous oxide analgesia but to provide a basis for supervised training in this technique. Invariably, the complications that have occurred with the use of nitrous oxide–oxygen techniques have been the result of misuse or faulty installation of equipment. It remains the responsibility of the dentist to ensure that the installation or any subsequent alteration or repair of equipment is accomplished in such a manner as to provide proper administration of the gases. Obviously, an installation that crossed oxygen and nitrous oxide lines could be disastrous if 100% of nitrous oxide were given under the assumption that it were oxygen!

All cylinders are now colored in a standard manner. Nitrous oxide cylinders are blue and oxygen cylinders are green. One may remember this easily by considering oxygen as the "good green gas." As systems may be of a central nature, wall mounted, or mobile, cylinders of varying sizes are available. The cylinders are additionally "pin coded" as an added measure of safety. This "pin index safety system," by providing matching pins in the apparatus' yoke and holes in the cylinders, prevents inadvertent mixing of cylinders and lines.

Combination with other sedative regimens will increase the potential danger of entering into a general anesthetic state. The dentist should appreciate the limits of each technique and select the appropriate technique for the patient in consideration of the procedures to be accomplished. If the dentist combines inhalation sedation with other modes of sedation, he *must* be trained in and prepared for the eventuality that general anesthesia might be produced.

Contraindications

Since the nasal passages are utilized as passages for gaseous exchange, upper respiratory obstruction or coryza is an absolute contraindication for this technique. Other respiratory diseases must also be carefully evaluated, if present, since this technique requires a normally functioning respiratory system for safe administration.

Since patients experience euphoria or altered sensorium with nitrous oxide analgesia, emotional instability in a patient is an absolute contraindication to its use. It should be noted that this is not a unique consideration to nitrous oxide sedation but should be a consideration in other sedative techniques as well.

Systemic disease that renders a patient at risk for a particular procedure requires similar consideration relative to the analgesic technique. Use of nitrous oxide–oxygen in pregnant patients in the first trimester should also be avoided.

Pharmacology

Nitrous oxide is an inorganic, colorless, nonirritating gas that exhibits a faint sweet smell. It is 1.5 times heavier than air. Nitrous oxide is carried in solution in the plasma, being fifteen times more soluble than nitrogen. It undergoes no chemical change in the body and is eliminated unaltered mostly through the lungs, with small amounts through the skin, sweat, and urine.

The main physiologic effects of nitrous oxide are exerted on the central nervous system, hence the effects of analgesia and amnesia. Although there is sensory depression, auditory perception is not affected to the same degree. As a result, a tranquil, quiet environment is a requirement for nitrous oxide–oxygen analgesic procedures. The circulatory system is not significantly affected except that a peripheral vasodilation may occur. This property may facilitate venipuncture should an intravenous route be desired. The respiratory system is not affected significantly. Nitrous oxide does not stimulate secretions as some other inhalation agents do.

The degree of uptake in the lungs is in part a measure of the alveolar tension of that particular gas. Nitrous oxide quickly establishes an equilibrium between alveolar concentration and plasma concentration. Thus changes in the applied concentration of the agent result in rapid physiologic effectiveness. This, too, is the reason why a continuous flow of the agent should result in a more even level of sedation. This quick physiologic response based on the physical properties of the agent forms a part of the safety margin of the technique as well as being responsible for the rapid recovery. It does, however, provide a precautionary consideration at that time when the administration of nitrous oxide ceases.

During the administration of nitrous oxide, an equilibrium has been established between alveolar nitrous oxide and that dissolved in the blood. When nitrous oxide administration ceases, there will be relatively small amounts of nitrogen in the alveoli and the bloodstream as a result of displacement by the nitrous oxide. If at the end of a procedure the patient is permitted to breathe room air, nitrogen will begin to reenter the bloodstream. However, as was noted earlier, the nitrous oxide is more soluble in the blood than is nitrogen. Since the room air contains no nitrous oxide, the nitrous oxide will flood out of the bloodstream to establish a new equilibrium. Since the same quantity of blood will release more nitrous oxide into the alveoli than it can dissolve nitrogen, there will be a net increase in alveolar gas volume. This essentially causes a decreased concentration of oxygen. Thus the patient might be hypoxic even with the administration of over 20% oxygen. This process is known as diffusion hypoxia. By permitting the patient to breathe 100% oxygen for 4 to 5 minutes at the end of the sedative procedure, the nitrous oxide may be washed out of the bloodstream without hypoxia occurring.

Physical properties of the gases

It is important to realize that nitrous oxide, when compressed for medical utilization, forms a liquid which is in equilibrium with overlying gas. This equilibrium will remain, with nearly constant gauge pressure being noted, until most of the liquid has been transformed into gas and utilized. At this point the gauge pressure will drop rapidly, and replacement of the cylinder is imminent. On the other hand, oxygen under pressure remains a gas in a compressed state. The gauge pressure falls more evenly, and gauge pressures more accurately reflect the amount of oxygen remaining.

Equipment

Numerous analgesia machines are currently available. With the decision to include nitrous oxide–oxygen analgesia in one's practice, a survey of the existing machines on the market is in order. A few generalizations can be made relative to the equipment in current use.

This brief discussion of the properties of nitrous oxide should have made the informed reader aware that this technique can be best managed by the utilization of moderate to high *continuous* flow of gases. Intermittent or demand flow machine usage may result in a bouncing-ball sedative course and has no overriding advantage to recommend this use.

Modern machines are equipped with flowmeters, whereby minute delivered volumes of oxygen and nitrous oxide can be determined. Most machines now in production have built-in safety systems that will prevent the delivery of nitrous oxide unless a suitable concentration of oxygen is also being delivered. This may vary with machines but should not be less than 20%. Some manufacturers build in alarm systems that also signal the loss of adequate oxygen pressures. Most machines are so built that even with normal oxygen pressures oxygen flows of less than 20% are not possible. The modern machines also offer direct instant oxygen flooding or flushing of the system as a facilitating means of applying oxygen in an emergency.

Although face masks have no place in dental analgesic regimens, they should be available for the application of positive pressure during emergency situations.

Nasal masks and cannulas are available for use with this technique. The cannula presents distinct disadvantages in that its diameter allows air dilution during inhalation, which may significantly alter applied concentrations of the agents. For example, if a 40% nitrous oxide–60% oxygen mixture is set on the flowmeters, the patient would receive a nitrous oxide concentration much less than this if a nasal cannula were used. Essentially, the concentrations set on the machine are invalid if a nasal cannula is used with this technique. If the effects are diluted by room air intermingling to the point where adequate sedation is not achieved, the dentist may abandon the technique. In these cases the technique is wrongfully rejected, since the actual cause of failure remains undetected. At the very least, utilization of the cannula makes the relation between flowmeter readings and sedative levels empirical.

The rebreathing or reservoir bag functions to permit a constant source of gases for the patient to breathe. It may also be used in conjunction with the face mask for positive-pressure oxygen administration.

Procedure

Prior to the beginning of the sedative procedures, the operator should assure himself that the equipment is functioning properly. The procedure and sequence of events and sensations within the appointment should be explained to the patient. In keeping with the discussions of hearing perception, background noise should be kept to an absolute minimum. Practitioners must remember that not only is the patient conscious but an altered sensorium may cause a misunderstanding of remarks passed between staff members. Additionally, fanciful dreams occurring during the procedure may, on recovery, be interpreted as having actually occurred. Consequently, a female staff member must be in attendance when female patients are being treated. Aberrant sensations may lead to unfounded accusations unless this requirement is strictly adhered to.

The patient should neither come to the appointment in a fasting state nor should he have ingested a large meal in the past 3 hours. The incidence of nausea and vomiting is low with nitrous oxide–oxygen analgesia.

At the onset it should be appreciated that there is an individual variance of reaction to similar percentages and gas flows. Initially, a high flow of 8 to 10 L/min is used to begin the analgesic sequence. Commencing with 100% oxygen allows a gradual introduction of nitrous oxide as well as a washing out of

nitrogen in the lungs, permitting a more efficient sedative induction. The nasal mask is adapted comfortably to the patient's face, and the patency and adequacy of gas flow are determined. The patient may have to be cautioned to maintain normal nasal breathing. Nitrous oxide can then be introduced at a level of 25%. The dentist should remember that at least 25% oxygen should be maintained during administration, and liter flow of oxygen should not be below 2 L/min. The concentration of nitrous oxide can be adjusted in increments of approximately 5% to achieve the proper level of sedation. The level of sedation may be evaluated as follows:

1. Perhaps the best indicator of the sedation level of the patient is his response to questions. The patient may exhibit a slurred speech or a slow response. He may often relate that he experiences a feeling of well-being or of euphoria. He may remember the questioning but simply at that time does not have the mental drive remaining to respond quickly.

2. The patient will be relaxed and cooperative. There will be almost no response to local anesthetic injections. The patient may remember the injection, but it is an unremarkable memory. If a series of injections are accomplished, he may remember them as a decreased number or even as one event. Inappropriate movement may be indicative of a patient too deep in stage I.

3. The patient will maintain with ease an open-mouth position in the desired planes, whereas increased depth is associated with a tendency to close his mouth.

4. The eyes may be closed but opened easily by the operator. The pupils are normal in the desired planes of sedation but may become large in the plane approaching anesthesia. At that level the eyeballs may be eccentric or rolling.

5. In relative analgesia planes, respiration will be normal. The respiratory rate will decrease and become irregular as general anesthesia is approached.

6. The pulse rate and blood pressure are not suitable aids to determine the level of depression. While the patient is in the proper plane of analgesia there should be little change in pulse or blood pressure. Pain in this plane as well as an increasing depth may be the cause of increased pulse rate or blood pressure rise.

As nitrous oxide levels are varied or as the time of sedative induction increases, the patient will report subjective symptoms of the relative analgesia. The first symptoms related may be tingling sensations in the fingers, toes, lips, or tip of the tongue. These may become apparent at levels of 20% nitrous oxide. With increased concentrations the patient will state that he felt a warm wave of relaxation pass over him. He develops an attitude of euphoria, sometimes together with a feeling of detachment. Progression will also cause increased degrees of drowsiness. Above 50% nitrous oxide the patient may have exaggerated dreams, requiring the precautions mentioned earlier.

In almost all instances adequate relative analgesia can be achieved at applied concentrations of nitrous oxide of 50% or less. Even at 50% care must be taken, since more susceptible individuals may pass into early general anesthesia at this level.

Essentially then, by starting at 25% applied nitrous oxide and progressing, as required, in increments of approximately 5% increased concentrations, a relative analgesia state should be safely achieved in almost all patients prior to a 50% administration. As the procedure continues, the rate of flow of the gases may be decreased, although at least 2 L/min oxygen should always be administered. At the end of the procedure, 5 to 8 L/min oxygen is administered for 4 or 5 minutes to avoid diffusion anoxia.

It is interesting and valuable for the dentist to question patients as to their subjective reactions under sedation. In addition to the features already mentioned, the patient will often indicate that the frame of time the procedure occupied in his consciousness has been dramatically decreased. The operating time may appear to be one third or one half as long as it was in reality. By relating the subjective symptoms to the sedative course, the operator will gain added insight into the regimen of inhalation analgesia.

CONCLUSION

There are many varied, yet correct methods to achieve adequate preoperative sedation. The end result, however, is successful only if the patient has suffered no ill effects and an optimal environment for treatment has been provided. Comprehension, by reading texts and the literature, by participation in education courses, and by attendance at professional meetings form the basis for intelligent, successful, and ethical application of any sedative technique. I hope that this chapter will be an additional aid in the preparation of the practitioner to control pain and anxiety in his practice.

REFERENCES

1. Goodman, L. S., and Gilman, A.: The pharmacological basis of therapeutics, ed. 4, New York, 1970, The Macmillan Co., p. 116.
2. Jorgensen, N. B., and Hayden, J., Jr.: Premedication, local and general anesthesia in dentistry, Philadelphia, 1967, Lea & Febiger, pp. 30-32.
3. Clarke, P. R., Eccersley, P. S., Frisby, J. P., et al.: The amnesic effect of diazepam (Valium), Br. J. Anaesth. **42:**690, 1971.
4. Pandit, S. K., Dundee, J. W., and Keilty, S. R.: Amnesic studies with intravenous premedication, Anaesthesia **26:**421, 1971.
5. Driscoll, E. J., Smilack, E. H., Lightbody, P. M., et al.: Sedation with intravenous diazepam, J. Oral Surg. **30:**332, 1972.
6. Gregg, J. M., Ryan, D. E., Levin, K. H., et al.: The amnesic actions of diazepam, J. Oral Surg. **32:**651, 1974.
7. Dundee, J. W., and Wyant, G. M.: Intravenous anaesthesia, London, 1974, Churchill Livingstone, pp. 252, 257.
8. Schechter, H. O., and Cosentino, B. J.: Combinations of psychotherapeutic drugs and local anesthesia for dental procedures, J. Oral Surg. **28:**280, 1970.
9. Dundee, J. W., and Wyant, G. M.: Intravenous anaesthesia, London, 1974, Churchill Livingstone, pp. 255-257.
10. Baird, E. S., and Hailey, D. H.: Delayed recovery from a sedative, Br. J. Anaesth. **44:**803, 1972.
11. Drummond-Jackson, S. L., editor: Intravenous anaesthesia, ed. 5, London, 1971, The Society for the Advancement of Anaesthesia in Dentistry, p. 244.
12. O'Neil, R., Verrill, P. J., and Aellig, W. H.: Intravenous diazepam in minor oral surgery, Br. Dent. J. **128:**15, 1970.
13. Dunsworth, A. R., Thornton, W. E., Byrd, D. L., et al.: Evaluation of cardiovascular and pulmonary changes during meperidine-diazepam anesthesia, J. Oral Surg. **33:**18, 1975.
14. Dundee, J. W., and Wyant, G. M.: Intravenous anaesthesia, London, 1974, Churchill Livingstone, p. 258.
15. Dundee, J. W., and Wyant, G. M.: Intravenous anaesthesia, London, 1974, Churchill Livingstone, p. 212.

BIBLIOGRAPHY

Allen, G. D.: Dental anesthesia and analgesia, Baltimore, 1972, The Williams & Wilkins Co.
Langa, H.: Relative analgesia in dental practice: inhalation analgesia with nitrous oxide, Philadelphia, 1968, W. B. Saunders Co.
McCarthy, F. M.: Emergencies in dental practice: Prevention and treatment, ed. 2, Philadelphia, 1972, W. B. Saunders Co.

27

Pharmacologic considerations in patients with systemic disease

WILLIAM K. BOTTOMLEY

The level of medical expertise continues to progress at an amazing rate. Sophisticated diagnostic procedures and therapeutic modalities allow successful treatment of disease processes that, in some instances, would have been hopeless only a few years ago. As a result the dental profession is confronted with a population surviving a multitude of systemic diseases largely because of the drug regimens prescribed for them.

Admittedly, the physician is held accountable for the management of the patient's primary diagnosis, but once the dentist has any pharmacologic or, in a broad sense, psychogenic input with this patient, he shares the responsibility for maintaining the health status of the patient. It logically follows that a prudent course of action for the dentist in planning treatment for a patient with a systemic disease should include a consultation with the physician to arrive at a safe, successful pharmacotherapeutic approach in achieving total health care.

For purposes of organization in the following discussion, systemic disease is treated as disease of organ systems. The contents of this chapter necessitate the acceptance of a few basic premises. No discussion of therapeutics can be all-encompassing. The very nature of dosage regulation to allow for individual response to drugs dictates the use of generalizations. I have strived to make the following discourse function at all times as a practical and expedient reference.

In general, the drug regimen for a systemic disease can be predicted by allowing vari-

ances for individual response, dose-effectiveness of a drug, and degrees of severity of systemic debilitation. Representative examples of drugs most likely to be encountered in each systemic disease are discussed in respect to their effect on the oral cavity and dental treatment. When a drug interaction affects dosage requirements and one of the interacting drugs is withdrawn, dosage adjustments may be necessary. Therefore any possible interaction of these drugs with those which the dentist might employ are given priority attention.

When a drug the dentist might institute is said to be contraindicated, because of either interaction with drugs being employed for a systemic condition or because of potential deleterious side effects in a specific disease condition, it is implied that the drug would be given in prolonged or repeated doses.

Successful pharmacotherapeutic patient management is, of course, predicated on the dentist's having taken a competent medical-drug history.

In consonance with pharmacotherapeutic influences on the dental management of a patient with systemic disease, it is equally important to consider the effects of systemic diseases on dental procedures as well as the effect of dental treatment on systemic health problems. The Council on Dental Education of the American Dental Association, recognizing a need for more knowledge in this phase of patient management, has recommended that dental school curricula reflect a greater emphasis on the physical evaluation of patients. A section at the end of this chapter addresses disease states of special interest in dental practice. The salient features and prominent influences of these

□ The opinions or assertions contained herein are the private ones of the writer and are not to be construed as official or as reflecting the views of the Navy Department or the naval service at large.

systemic conditions on dental treatment are briefly discussed.

CARDIOVASCULAR SYSTEM
Antianginals

Nitroglycerin (Angibid, Nitro-Bid, Nitroglyn, Nitrong, Nitrospan)
Erythrityl tetranitrate (Cardilate)
Pentaerythritol tetranitrate (Antora, Duotrate, Neo-Corovas, Pentryate, Peritrate, Steps, Tetrasule, Vaso-80 Unicelles; *with other components:* Cartrax, Corovas, Miltrate, Papavatral, Pentritol)
Isosorbide dinitrate (Isordil, Sorbitrate)
Propranolol hydrochloride (Inderal)
SIGNIFICANCE:

Used in management of angina pectoris.
Ask the patient to bring his medication to treat himself prior to stressful dental procedures. The dentist should maintain a minimal supply of sublingual nitroglycerin tablets for emergency use.
Adverse effects include a sudden fall in blood pressure and orthostatic hypotension. Halitosis is a side effect of isosorbide dinitrate.

Cardiotonics

Digitalis (Digitora, Pil-Digis)
Digitoxin (Crystodigin, Digitaline Nativelle, Myodigin, Purodigin)
Digoxin (Davoxin, Lanoxin)
SIGNIFICANCE:

Used in the treatment of congestive heart failure and atrial fibrillation.
Barbiturates are contraindicated, since they may decrease the effects of these drugs.
Quinidine polygalacturonate (Cardioquin)
SIGNIFICANCE:

Used for prevention of cardiac arrhythmias.
An intravenous injection of epinephrine can precipitate a fibrillation in patients taking this drug.
Propranolol hydrochloride (Inderal)
SIGNIFICANCE:

Used in the management of cardiac arrhythmias.
Side effects include orthostatic hypotension and hypoglycemia.
Procainamide hydrochloride (Pronestyl)
SIGNIFICANCE:

Used in the management of ventricular arrhythmias.

The neuromuscular blocking action of streptomycin, neomycin, kanamycin, and surgical muscle relaxants may be potentiated.
An intravenous injection of lidocaine (Xylocaine) may add to the neurologic effects of this drug, producing ventricular tachycardia and severe hypotension.

Hypotensives

Reserpine (Butaserpine, Rau-Sed, Serpasil; *with other components:* Diupres, Diutensen-R, Eskaserp, Exna-R, Hydromox R, Hydropres, Metatensin, Naquival, Regroton, Renese-R, Salutensin, Solfo-Serpine, Unitensen-R)
Deserpidine (Harmonyl; *with methylclothiazide:* Enduronyl)
Methyldopa (Aldomet)
Guanethidine sulfate (Ismelin)
Hydralazine hydrochloride, (Apresoline)
Propranolol hydrochloride (Inderal)
SIGNIFICANCE:

Used in the treatment of hypertension.
Barbiturates may potentiate the hypotensive action.
Aspirin may contribute to the ulcerogenic effect of these drugs.
Side effects include dryness of the mouth, sore tongue, and orthostatic hypotension.

Diuretics

Spironolactone (Aldactone; *with hydrochlorothiazide:* Aldactazide)
Ethacrynic acid (Edecrin)
Acetazolamide (Diamox)
Furosemide (Lasix)
Chlorothiazide (Diuril; *with methyldopa:* Aldoclor)
Hydrochlorothiazide (Esidrix; *with other components:* Aldoril, Butizide, Dyazide, Esimil, Hydropres, Oretic, Ser-Ap-Es)
SIGNIFICANCE:

Used in the management of fluid retention and hypertension.
Aspirin may interfere with the diuretic action.
Side effects include dry mouth and increased thirst. This should alert the dentist to a possible electrolyte imbalance.
Acetazolamide may produce facial paresthesia.
Symptoms of gout may occur. This could

be manifested as a temporomandibular joint syndrome.

The possibility of orthostatic hypotension is enhanced.

Be alert for oral manifestations of diabetes mellitus from a possible diabetogenic effect of the diuretics.

SPECIFIC CONSIDERATIONS

The American Heart Association recommendations for the prevention of infective endocarditis in patients with congenital heart defects or a history of rheumatic fever are presented in Appendix C. The same regimen is recommended for outpatients with *heart prostheses.*

Patients with heart and other organ transplants

Ordinarily the dental management of these patients is intimately coordinated with the attending physician. However, if an emergency arises, the drug regimen for subacute bacterial endocarditis (SBE) prophylaxis may be instituted until the physician can be contacted.

The use of aspirin is contraindicated because of its ulcerogenic potential.

Patients with coronary bypasses

The current consensus is that the fact of a patient having had a bypass procedure does not dictate the necessity of prophylactic antibiotic coverage for dental treatment.

RESPIRATORY SYSTEM
Antituberculous preparations

Isoniazid (Nydrazid, Triniad, Uniad; *with other components:* Niadox, Pasna Tri-Pack Granules)

SIGNIFICANCE:

Used in the treatment of active tuberculosis.

Epinephrine may enhance its neurovascular side effects.

p-Aminosalicylic acid (PAS-C, Rezipas)

SIGNIFICANCE:

Potentiates the action of isoniazid.

Vitamin C increases the possibility of crystalluria.

Aspirin is contraindicated if aminosalicylic acid toxicity is suspected because of its additive effect.

Cardinal signs of toxicity are nausea and vomiting.

Streptomycin
Rifampin (Rifadin, Rimactane)

SIGNIFICANCE:

Used in combination therapy for tuberculosis.

Streptomycin may enhance the neuromuscular blockade action of surgical skeletal muscle relaxants.

Adverse effects of rifampin include leukopenia and jaundice.

Bronchial dilators

Ephedrine hydrochloride (*with other components:* Amesec, Bron-Sed, Calcidrine, Co-Xan, Dainite, Duovent, KIE, Lufyllin-EPG, Mudrane, Quadrinal, Quelidrine, Tedral, Verequad)

Pseudoephedrine hydrochloride (Actifed, Bronchobid Duracap, Deconamine, Dimacol, Disophrol, Emprazil, Fedahist, Isoclor, Rondec, Sudafed)

SIGNIFICANCE:

Used in the treatment of bronchial asthma.

Asthmatics may be allergic to aspirin.

Side effects include dry mouth.

Antihistamines

The three commonly used antihistamines listed represent only a small part of the large number of these drugs that are currently marketed.

Chlorpheniramine maleate (Teldrin; *with other components:* Allerest, Aristomin, Chlor-Trimeton Maleate, Colrex, Coricidin, Coriforte, Corilin, Co-Tylenol, Deconamine, Dehist, Demazin, Desa-Hist, Dextro-Tussin, Dor-C, Drinus, Duadacin, Extendryl, Fedahist, Histabid, Histaspan, Hycomine Compound, Isoclor, Napril, Narine, Narspan, Neotep, Nilcol, Nolamine, Novahistine, Oralen, Oraminic, Ornade, Pediacof, Quelidrine, Ryna-Tussadine, Sinodec, Sinovan, Sinulin, Tusquelin, Tussend, Tuss-Ornade, Tussi-Organidin, Wesmatic)

Pyrrobutamine phosphate (*with other components:* Co-Pyronil)

Brompheniramine maleate (Dimetane; *with other components:* Dimetapp, Drixoral)

SIGNIFICANCE:

Used for the symptomatic relief of allergenic states.

Barbiturates may cause additive depressant effects.

Side effects include dry mouth. If antihistamines are dispensed by the dentist, the patient should be cautioned that he may experience drowsiness; the drugs are potentiated by ethyl alcohol; and antihistimines potentiate the effects of tricyclic antidepressants (see discussion on Neuromuscular system).

SPECIFIC CONSIDERATIONS

Barbiturates, narcotics, and other central nervous system depressants should be used with caution in patients with emphysema to avoid respiratory embarrassment.

BONES AND JOINTS
Antiarthritics

Phenylbutazone (Butazolidin; *with other components:* Sterazolidin)
Indomethacin (Indocin)
Ibuprofen (Motrin)
Oxyphenbutazone (Tandearil)
SIGNIFICANCE:
Used for the relief of pain and the reduction of inflammation in rheumatoid arthritis.
Aspirin in concomitant administration may precipitate symptoms of gout, especially with phenylbutazone.
Toxic effects may manifest as fever, sore throat, and lesions in the mouth (symptoms of blood dyscrasia).

GASTROINTESTINAL SYSTEM
Antispasmodics and anticholinergics

Propantheline bromide (Pro-Banthine; *with phenobarbital:* Probital)
Belladonna (Prydon; *with other components:* B & O Supprettes, Barbidonna, Bar-Don, Belbarb, Belladenal, Bucladin, Butibel, Chardonna, Decholin-BB, Denol, Donnatal, Gourmase PB, Kinesed, Phen-O-Bel, Sidonna, Trac)
SIGNIFICANCE:
Used in the treatment of peptic ulcer.
Aspirin should be avoided because of its ulcerogenic contribution.
Side effects include dry mouth.

Connective tissue medication

Salicylazosulfapyridine (Azulfidine)
SIGNIFICANCE:
Used in the treatment of regional enteritis (Crohn's disease).
The dentist should be alert for oral extension of the intestinal lesions.

Antacids

The following active ingredients are components of various brand-name preparations, which are listed in parentheses:
Aluminum hydroxide
Magnesium hydroxide
Calcium carbonate
Dihydroxyaluminum sodium carbonate
Magnesium trisilicate (Aludrox, Amphojel, Camalox, Creamalin, Delcid, Ducon, Gaviscon, Gelusil, Maalox, Mylanta, Riopan, Rolaids, Titralac, Tricreamalate, Trisogel, Tums)
SIGNIFICANCE:
Used in the prevention and treatment of peptic ulcers.
They interfere with the absorption of tetracyclines.
Aspirin should be avoided in these patients because of its ulcerogenic potential.

UROGENITAL SYSTEM
Ion-exchange resin

Sodium polystyrene sulfonate (Kayexalate)
SIGNIFICANCE:
Used in the treatment of hyperkalemia attributable to grossly impaired kidney function.
Potassium salts, such as K penicillins, should be avoided.

SPECIFIC CONSIDERATIONS

Vitamin C in large doses causes acidification of the urine, which could cause the precipitation of urate, oxalate, or cystine stones in the urinary tract. The dosage of potentially nephrotoxic antibiotics (tetracyclines, kanamycin, neomycin, cephaloridine) should be adjusted in patients with reduced renal function to prevent additional renal damage and damage to other organs. The blood concentration of the antibiotics can be reduced by increasing the interval between doses or by decreasing the individual doses.

EXAMPLE: tetracycline in reduced doses
1.00 Gm/24 hr if BUN is 50 mg/100 ml
0.75 Gm/24 hr if BUN is 75 mg/100 ml
0.50 Gm/24 hr if BUN is 100 mg/ml

ENDOCRINE SYSTEM
Estrogens

Norethynodrel and mestranol (Enovid)
Norethindrone and mestranol (Norinyl, Ortho-Novum)

Norethindrone acetate and ethynyl estradiol (Norlestrin)
SIGNIFICANCE:
 Used for contraception and occasionally in the treatment of acne.
 Patients may demonstrate oral manifestations of pregnancy gingivitis.
 Oral contraceptives can interfere with the absorption of folate, resulting in anemia.
Conjugated estrogens (Estratab, Femogen, Formatrix, Premarin, Trexinest)
SIGNIFICANCE:
 Used in the treatment of hypermenorrhea, endometriosis, and osteoporosis.
 These patients may display dry, atrophic, sensitive oral tissue.

Thyroid

Sodium levothyroxine (Letter, Levoid, Synthroid; *with other components:* Euthroid, S-P-T, Thyrolar)
Sodium liothyronine (Cytomel)
Thyroid globulin (Proloid)
SIGNIFICANCE:
 Used as replacement therapy for diminished or absent thyroid function.
 Barbiturates are preferred drugs for sedation.

Antithyroid

Isothiouracil sodium (Itrumil)
Methimazole (Tapazole)
SIGNIFICANCE:
 Used in the treatment of hyperthyroidism.
 Epinephrine injected intravascularly can precipitate a thyroid crisis.
 Barbiturate preoperative sedation is recommended to relieve anxiety and stress.
 Side effects include sore throat and loss of taste.

Corticoids

Dexamethasone (Decadron, Gammacorten, Hexadrol)
Prednisone (Delta-Dome, Deltasone; *with other components:* Arthralgen with Prednisone, Deltasmyl, Sterazolidin)
Meprednisone (Betapar)
Prednisolone (Ataraxoid, Delta-Cortef)
Triamcinolone (Aristocort, Kenacort; *with other components:* Aristomin)
Cortisone acetate (Cortone Acetate)
SIGNIFICANCE:
 Used in the treatment of inflammatory conditions, as immunosuppressive agents and in antineoplastic therapy.

 Adjust dosage before stressful dental procedures (consult the patient's physician).
 Antibiotics should be instituted prophylactically before any dental procedure that predisposes to infection or that can induce a bacteremia.
 Aspirin is contraindicated because of the ulcerogenic contribution.
 Oral manifestations of diabetes mellitus may be observed with prolonged corticoid therapy. (Diabetes mellitus is discussed under Metabolic system.)
 Hypertension and mood swings are frequent side effects of protracted corticoid therapy.

THE BLOOD AND BLOOD-FORMING SYSTEMS
Anticoagulants

Sodium warfarin (Coumadin, Panwarfin)
Bishydroxycoumarin (Dicumarol)
SIGNIFICANCE:
 These are oral anticoagulants used by outpatients for the treatment of venous thrombosis and embolism.
 Vitamin K (Synkayvite) is the antidote.
COMMON DRUGS THAT INCREASE THE ACTION OF ORAL ANTICOAGULANTS:
 Acetaminophen (Nebs, Neopap, Temlo, Tempra, Tenlap, Tylenol; *with other components:* Arthralgen, Bancaps, Codalan, Coldene, Colrex, Dialog, Duacin, Esgic, Excedrin, Gaysal, Midrin, Ornex, Panitol, Parafon Forte, Percogesic, Prolaire-B, Scotgesic, Sinubid, Sinulin, Sinutab-II, Supac, T-Caps, Trind, Tussagesic, Vanquish)
 Aspirin (Ecotrin, Empirin, Measurin; *with other components:* Alka-Seltzer, Anacin, A.S.A. Compound, Aspergum, Bufferin, Colban, Cope 1, Coricidin, Darvon Compound, Defensin, Dristan, Excedrin, Fizrin, 4-Way Cold Tablets, Midol, P-A-C, Sal-Fayne, Stanback, Trigesic)
 Choline salicylate (Arthropan)
 Salicylamide (*with other components:* Sal-Eze, Zarumin)
 Cephaloridine (Loridine)
 Diazepam (Valium)
 Kanamycin (Kantrex)
 Narcotic analgesics
 Tetracyclines
COMMON DRUGS THAT DECREASE THE ACTION OF ORAL ANTICOAGULANTS:
 Barbiturates (Amytal, Phenobarbital, Seconal)

Chlordiazepoxide (Librium)
Ethchlorvynol (Placidyl)
Glutethimide (Doriden)
Meprobamate (Equanil, Kesso-Bamate, Meprospan, Miltown; *with other components:* Bamadex, Deprol, Pathibamate)

Heparin sodium

SIGNIFICANCE:

This is an intramuscularly or subcutaneously administered anticoagulant.

Protamine sulfate, given intravenously is the antidote.

Since an increasing number of drugs are found to display varying interactions with different anticoagulants, it would be prudent for the physician to do frequent prothrombin times after the addition or withdrawal of *any* other drugs that are taken repeatedly by patients receiving anticoagulants.

Immunosuppressants

Azathioprine (Imuran)
Cyclophosphamide (Cytoxan)
Corticosteroids (see Endocrine system)

SIGNIFICANCE:

Used to suppress antibody formation and subsequent rejection in transplant patients.

Consultation with the patient's physician should precede any dental treatment.

Antibiotic coverage prophylactically is recommended for all dental treatment.

Oral candidiasis should be anticipated.

Antineoplastic agents

Busulfan (Myleran)
Mercaptopurine (Purinethol)
Cyclophosphamide (Cytoxan)
5-Fluorouracil (Efudex)
Chlorambucil (Leukeran)
Methotrexate
Cytarabine (Cytosar)
Corticosteroids (see Endocrine system)

SIGNIFICANCE:

Used primarily in the treatment of leukemias, lymphomas, and carcinoma.

Consultation with the patient's physician should precede any dental treatment.

Oral lesions may occur as a manifestation of the disease process or as a sequela of the drug therapy.

Oral candidiasis is a common sequela.

These patients may have an increased bleeding tendency.

Antibiotic coverage prophylactically is in-

dicated because of the increased susceptibility to infection.

METABOLIC SYSTEM

Antidiabetic agents

Insulin
Chlorpropamide (Diabinese)
Tolbutamide (Orinase)
Acetohexamide (Dymelor)
Tolazamide (Tolinase)
Phenformin hydrochloride (DBI)

SIGNIFICANCE:

Used in the treatment of diabetes mellitus. The sulfonylureas (acetohexamide, chlorpropamide, tolbutamide) and tolazamide stimulate endogenous insulin production.

Sulfonylureas may prolong the effects of barbiturates.

Aspirin enhances the response to sulfonylureas and may precipitate a hypoglycemic coma.

Sulfonamides may potentiate the effects of the sulfonylureas.

Epinephrine increases insulin requirements and inhibits pancreatic insulin release.

Corticosteroids increase insulin requirements.

Infection increases insulin requirements. Therefore all precautions to prevent infection should be exercised.

Antigout agents

Allopurinol (Zyloprim)
Probenecid (Benemid)
Sulfinpyrazone (Anturane)
Colchicine (*with other components:* Colbenemid, Salpacine)

SIGNIFICANCE:

Allopurinol interferes with the formation of uric acid.

Probenecid and sulfinpyrazone promote the urinary excretion of uric acid (uricosurics).

Colchicine relieves the pain of acute attacks of gout.

Aspirin interferes with the action of probenecid and sulfinpyrazone.

When probenecid is administered along with a penicillin or a cephalosporin, it increases the serum concentration of the antibiotic. This action is useful in the treatment of endocarditis and osteomyelitis.

Probenecid prolongs the action of the

sulfonylureas (see Antidiabetic agents).
Sulfinpyrazone potentiates the action of
the sulfonylureas and insulin.

NEUROMUSCULAR SYSTEM
Tranquilizers (ataractics)
Phenothiazines
> *Prochlorperazine maleate* (Compazine;
> *with other components:* Combid, Eska-
> trol)
> *Thioridazine hydrochloride* (Mellaril)
> *Trifluoperazine hydrochloride* (Stelazine)
> *Chlorpromazine hydrochloride* (Thorazine)
> *Propiomazine hydrochloride* (*with other*
> *components:* Largon)

SIGNIFICANCE:
Used in the management of anxiety and
tension.
They potentiate other depressants.
Possible side effects include orthostatic
hypotension, oral manifestations of a
blood dyscrasia, and uncontrolled movement of the muscles of the face, tongue,
and jaw (extrapyramidal reactions).

Other tranquilizers
> *Diazepam* (Valium)
> *Chlordiazepoxide hydrochloride* (Librium)
> *Hydroxyzine hydrochloride* (Atarax, Vista-
> ril; *with other components:* Ataraxoid,
> Cartrax, Enarax, Marax)
> *Flurazepam hydrochloride* (Dalmane)
> *Meprobamate* (Equanil, Meprospan,
> Meprotabs; *with other components:*
> Deprol, Milpath)

SIGNIFICANCE:
Used in the management of tension, anxiety, and insomnia.
These drugs are potentiated by barbiturates, meperidine hydrochloride, MAO
inhibitors, and other antidepressants.
Side effects include dryness of mouth.
Diazepam is contraindicated in patients
with acute narrow angle glaucoma.
The use of diazepam during pregnancy is
contraindicated.

Antidepressants
Monoamine oxidase inhibitors (MAOI)
> *Isocarboxazid* (Marplan)
> *Nialamide* (Niamid)
> *Pargyline hydrochloride* (Eutonyl)
> *Phenelzine sulfate* (Nardil)
> *Tranylcypromine sulfate* (Parnate)

SIGNIFICANCE:
Used in the treatment of depression.

An intravascular injection of epinephrine could precipitate a hypertensive
crisis.
These drugs potentiate the effects of sedatives, hypnotics, and analgesics, especially increasing the central nervous
system depressant effect of barbiturates,
meperidine hydrochloride, and morphine.

Tricyclic antidepressants
> *Amitriptyline hydrochloride* (Elavil; *with*
> *other components:* Etrafon, Triavil)
> *Desipramine hydrochloride* (Norpramin,
> Pertofrane)
> *Imipramine hydrochloride* (Tofranil)
> *Nortriptyline hydrochloride* (Aventyl Hy-
> drochloride)
> *Protriptyline hydrochloride* (Vivactil)
> *Doxepin hydrochloride* (Sinequan)

SIGNIFICANCE:
Used in the treatment of depression.
An intravascular injection of epinephrine
can precipitate an exaggerated hypertensive reaction.
Vitamin C and barbiturates can decrease
the effects of these drugs.
Meperidine hydrochloride and antihistamines enhance the action of these drugs.

Anticonvulsants
Phenytoin, formerly termed diphenylhy-
dantoin sodium (Dilantin)
SIGNIFICANCE:
Used in the control of seizures, in the
treatment of cardiac arrhythmias, and in
the treatment of neuralgias.
Stress and phenobarbital can decrease the
effect of this drug.
Librium enhances the effect of Dilantin.
Folic acid depresses its action.
Side effects include gingival hyperplasia
and oral manifestations of a blood dys-
crasia, especially anemia.
Primidone (Mysoline)
SIGNIFICANCE:
Used to control seizures.
Side effects include gingival pain.
Clonazepam (Clonopin)
SIGNIFICANCE:
Used to control seizures.
Side effects include reduced salivation.

Parasympathomimetics
Pyridostigmine bromide (Mestinon)
Neostigmine bromide (Prostigmin)

SIGNIFICANCE:

Used in the symptomatic control of myasthenia gravis.

Promotes increased salivation.

Skeletal muscle relaxants—general

Carisoprodol (Rela, Soma)

Chlorzoxazone (*with acetaminophen:* Parafon Forte)

Orphenadrine (Disipal, Norflex; *with other components:* Estomul, Norgesic)

Methocarbamol (Robaxin)

SIGNIFICANCE:

Used in the treatment of muscle spasms, pain, and stiffness.

Other central nervous system depressants may enhance the effect of these drugs.

Robaxin should be used with caution in myasthenic patients receiving pyridostigmine bromide (Mestinon).

Orphenadrine may interact with Darvon, resulting in mental confusion, anxiety, and tremors.

Skeletal muscle relaxants—surgical

Succinylcholine chloride (Anectine, Sucostrin)

SIGNIFICANCE:

Used to produce muscle relaxation during operative procedures.

Kanamycin, neomycin, and streptomycin may enhance the effects of these drugs.

Sedatives. See Chapter 6.

Analgesics. See Chapters 9 and 10.

DISEASE STATES OF SPECIAL INTEREST

Asthma. Infection, allergies, and hypersensitivities are the primary causes of asthmatic attacks. The psychophysiologic stress of dental treatment may also provoke an attack. An asthmatic may have multiple allergies that have not been identified. Therefore the dentist should be judicious with the introduction of any medication to this patient, especially aspirin-containing drugs. A frequent side effect of antihistamines used to treat this condition is the reduction of salivary flow, which in turn adversely affects caries rate, periodontal status, tissue sensitivity, and the retention of complete dentures.

Emphysema. The reduced oxygenation of the blood resulting from pulmonary emphysema stimulates a compensatory erythrocytosis. Surgery on these patients should be preceded by an evaluation of the coagulation status. In severe emphysema a daily regimen of tetracycline is often prescribed as a prophylactic measure against a bacterial infection of the lungs. Tetracyclines tend to impair prothrombin utilization, thereby further promoting a potential bleeding diathesis.

Hypertension. In cases where the numerical values of 90 mm Hg for diastolic pressure and 140 mm Hg for systolic pressure are exceeded on a consistent basis, the patient is considered to be hypertensive. In general, the higher the blood pressure is above the limits of normal the greater will be the potential of a cardiovascular accident. Elective dental treatment should be delayed until medical control of the blood pressure is demonstrated. Sedation with 5 mg diazepam (Valium) given 1 hour before the dental appointment may be indicated in cases where anxiety is a complicating factor.

Congestive heart failure. The clinical signs of distended neck veins and cyanosis are indications of the degree of severity of congestive heart failure. Conservative measures of short appointments, an upright sitting position, and sedation for anxiety are indicated with this disease state. Oxygen support should be immediately available.

Angina. Chest pain is recognized and interpreted by the patient on the basis of previous experience. Angina is usually provoked by exhaustion, anxiety, or pain. Therefore the precautions of brief, early-morning dental appointments, appropriate sedation, and adequate local anesthesia should be taken. Sublingual nitroglycerin tablets should be available for immediate administration if needed.

Myocardial infarction. Elective dental treatment should be delayed for at least 3 months after a myocardial infarction. These patients may be extremely anxious and intolerant of any pain. The same precautions should be applied in patients with this condition as in patients with angina. Anticoagulant therapy might be an additional complicating factor. If the clinical signs and symptoms of shortness of breath (SOB), intermittent chest pain, flushed face, and obvious obesity are present, a consultation with the patient's physician is indicated.

Anticoagulation. Therapy with anticoagulants always presents the threat of excessive bleeding with any procedure that may initiate some bleeding. However, at the controlled therapeutic level routine dental procedures, including single extractions and subgingival curettage may be accomplished without complications. Medications that either enhance the action of the anticoagulant or otherwise contribute an additional anticoagulant effect, for example, aspirin, should be avoided.

Rheumatic heart disease, congenital heart disease, and heart murmurs. With a history of any of these conditions, the primary dental concern is the increased susceptibility toward infective endocarditis. The cardiac status of the patient should be evaluated by the attending physician and a copy of the written consultation placed in the dental record. For any intervening dental treatment that will cause bleeding, the administration of antibiotics prophylactically is a judicious precaution. (See Appendix C.)

Pacemaker. There is a lack of consensus about the management of this condition. Precautions most usually implemented are avoiding the use of any electronic equipment, including vitalometers and the Cavitron, and using the prophylactic antibiotic regimen recommended for subacute bacterial endocarditis.

Prosthetic heart valves. There are two primary concerns regarding dental treatment for patients with heart valve prostheses, bacteremia, and excessive bleeding. Outpatients should be covered with the prophylactic antibiotic regimen recommended for subacute bacterial endocarditis. A current prothrombin time should be requested, since these patients are taking anticoagulants.

Hepatic failure. Clinical signs and symptoms that reflect the extent of hepatic failure are weakness, fatigability, jaundice, ascites, and ankle edema. The primary concern to the dentist is the impaired coagulation status due to the development of a thrombocytopenia and a hypoprothrombinemia. The bleeding and prothrombin times should be evaluated before surgical treatment is initiated.

Hepatitis. The clinical signs and symptoms of jaundice, fever, malaise, and nausea indicate an acute viral hepatitis. Elective dental procedures should be delayed until the liver function tests have returned to normal. When it becomes necessary to treat a high-risk patient, the dentist should wear a face mask, glasses, and disposable gloves. The instruments should be washed with a 1% solution of sodium hypochlorite and then autoclaved.

Malabsorption syndrome. Oral signs and symptoms of glossitis, cheilosis, and anemia should suggest malnutrition, which may be secondary to malabsorption. Laboratory tests for the levels of iron, vitamin B_{12}, and folates should be conducted before treatment is initiated. Treatment on an empirical basis may mask serious underlying physiologic defects.

Renal failure. During a period of acute renal failure, only emergency dental treatment should be entertained because of the multiple systemic complications and the high risk of an infection that may be difficult to control. Chronic or irreversible end-stage renal failure is treated by hemodialysis.

Dialysis. Complications influencing the dental management of a patient being treated by intermittent hemodialysis include an increased susceptibility to infection, a bleeding tendency due to inadequate platelet factor III activity, the possibility of hypertension, a predisposition toward osteodystrophy complicated by secondary hyperparathyroidism, and a high rate of nonicteric viral hepatitis. Antibiotic coverage and close monitoring of the bleeding time are basic recommendations. Dental treatment is best accomplished in the morning of the day after dialysis.

Renal transplantation. The patient's host resistance to infection is depressed by immunosuppressive drug therapy. Aseptic necrosis of bone and impaired stress response are major sequelae of the steroid therapy employed. The periodontal status of these patients should be closely monitored because of the greater susceptibility to infection and the diabetogenic effect of the steroids. Treatment of the dialysis and renal transplant patient should be closely coordinated with the attending physician.

Seizure disorder. Anxiety generated by dental treatment or pain during the treatment allowed by inadequate anesthesia may precipitate a seizure in patients taking anticonvulsant medication. A history of a recent seizure indicates poor therapeutic control. For best results the patient's appointment should be in the morning, when he is rested and shortly after he has taken his medication.

Stroke. All efforts should be directed toward keeping the patient calm, comfortable, and free of pain. Any event that effects a sudden, exaggerated rise in blood pressure has the potential of precipitating a cardiovascular accident. The patient should have a morning appointment when he is rested, premedication for anxiety should be given where indicated, and the operation should be performed with good anesthesia.

Anemia. A deficiency of hemoglobin may be manifested orally by a loss of papillae on the tongue, a glossitis, and a generally pale color of all the mucous membranes. Constitutional symptoms of headache and fever may also be present. The patient should be referred to a physician for the diagnosis and treatment of the etiology of the anemia.

Leukemia. The malignant proliferation of immature white cells decreases the host resistance to infection and tends to crowd out the cells in the marrow that produce the red blood cells and platelets. Oral signs and symptoms include swollen gingivae, unprovoked bleeding, and secondary infection. Dental treatment should consist of conservative, supportive care directed toward improving oral comfort and preventing oral infections. It is imperative to maintain good oral hygiene.

Thrombocytopenia. A deficiency in platelets may be manifested orally as ecchymotic areas and gingival bleeding. Referral for immediate diagnosis and therapy is essential. Any dental therapy that initiates bleeding could result in a life-threatening situation.

Hyperpituitarism. Acromegaly is the result of hyperfunction of eosinophil cells of the anterior pituitary after closure of the epiphyses. There is a general increase in size of the orofacial structures, which may lead to a provisional diagnosis of the condition. There is a high incidence of diabetes mellitus in acromegalics, which may be manifested as a poor response to oral healing and exacerbated periodontal disease.

Hypopituitarism. A deficiency of hormones produced by the anterior pituitary gland can affect the size, shape, and eruption rate of the teeth in children. These may be subtle changes but may constitute the first clinical evidence of hypopituitarism. In adults the hormonal deficiency affects the dependent glands and results in general constitutional symptoms.

Addison's disease. The diagnosis of adrenal insufficiency is based on the signs and symptoms of weakness, weight loss, low blood pressure, nausea, and vomiting. Pigmentation of the mucous membranes and a glossitis from malnutrition are oral signs of this condition. Elective dental treatment should be delayed until replacement steroid therapy is regulated.

Cushing's disease (syndrome). An excessive amount of adrenal cortical hormones, whether endogenous or exogenous, may result in hypertension, hirsutism, edema, thinning of the skin, elevated blood glucose level, and osteoporosis. Oral infections and periodontal disease may be more difficult to control. Candidiasis is more prevalent. Sedation and good pain control are prime considerations for dental treatment, since there is no steroid reserve to respond to stress.

Pheochromocytoma. Oral candidiasis and headaches may be early dental complaints to indicate hypersecretion of epinephrine and norepinephrine due to an adenoma of the adrenal medulla. Supporting evidence of hypertension, sweating, and tremors should prompt medical consultation.

Diabetes (mellitus). The primary dental concerns with the diabetic are a reduced host response to infection and a tendency toward candidiasis. In the adult who displays an unexplained exacerbation of periodontal disease and decreased salivary flow, undiagnosed or uncontrolled diabetes should be ruled out.

A patient with diagnosed diabetes who goes into a coma of clinically unrecognizable origin should be given a small amount of sugar (glucose) as a precautionary measure until medical attention is available.

Hyperparathyroidism. Dental radiographic findings of loss of the lamina dura and distortion of the normal trabecular pattern of the bone, producing a ground-glass appearance, are frequent indications of hyperparathyroidism. Immediate medical treatment should be instituted.

Hypoparathyroidism. Hypoparathyroidism may be manifested as recurrent oral candidiasis, circumoral paresthesia, and spasm of the facial muscles. The patient should be referred for medical treatment.

Hyperthyroidism. Only emergency dental

treatment is indicated for patients with uncontrolled hyperthyroidism. Adequate sedation and pain control are necessary to prevent a hyperthyroid crisis. The classic clinical features are restlessness, sweating, tremors, and protruding eyes.

Hypothyroidism. An insidious hyposecretion of the thyroid may develop in adults, resulting in edema, increased weight, brittle hair, drowsiness, and an intolerance to cold. These features may appear in patients who are being given inadequate thyroid supplement. There are no contraindications for dental treatment, and the patient should be referred for medical correction of the condition.

Scleroderma. Tissues affected by scleroderma will display an extremely diminished response to injury or infection because of the compromised blood supply to the area. Radiographic findings of widened periodontal ligament spaces may be an early indication of diffuse scleroderma. Periodontal disease is particularly difficult to manage. Where facial masking is progressive, extraction of posterior teeth is recommended while there is mechanical accessibility.

Myasthenia gravis. Dental treatment may need to be modified because of the easy fatigability of the patient's head and neck muscles. The parasympathomimetic effects of the pharmacotherapy may increase salivary flow. If the border of a prosthesis encroaches on the parotid papilla, salivary drainage can be impeded because of impaired muscle action.

Ulcers (duodenal/gastric). Antacid medications and milk reduce the efficacy of tetracyclines. Oral signs of anemia may indicate a chronic blood loss or an iron deficiency due to inadequate acid in the stomach, as a result of the antacid medication, to convert ingested iron to the ferrous state for absorption.

Postradiation therapy. The primary adverse sequelae after radiation therapy are an inordinate risk of local infection due to the compromised vascular supply to the area irradiated and xerostomia due to inactivation of the salivary glands. Dental procedures that may result in bleeding require extended prophylactic antibiotic coverage. A 0.5% solution of sodium carboxymethyl cellulose will relieve the xerostomia. Candidiasis is a frequent occurrence in this condition.

Glaucoma. The use of antisialagogues is contraindicated because they tend to increase the pressure in the anterior chamber of the eye.

Arthritis (rheumatoid and degenerative). The objective of pharmacotherapeutics in arthritic conditions is to relieve pain and reduce inflammation. Most of these medications have the potential of depressing marrow activity. Oral ulcerations and gingival hemorrhage may be the first clinical signs of this adverse side effect. Immediate medical referral is imperative when a toxic response to medication is suspected.

BIBLIOGRAPHY

American Medical Association Council on Drugs: AMA drug evaluations, ed. 2, Acton, Mass., 1973, Publishing Sciences Group, Inc.

Clin-Alert, Louisville, Ky., Science Editors, Inc.

American Dental Association Council on Dental Therapeutics: Accepted dental therapeutics, ed. 36, Chicago, 1975, American Dental Association.

Hansten, P. D.: Drug interactions, Philadelphia, 1971, Lea & Febiger.

The medical letter on drugs and therapeutics, New Rochelle, N.Y., The Medical Letter, Inc.

Penna, R. P.: A screening procedure for drug interactions, J. Am. Pharm. Assoc. 10:66-67, 1970.

Physician's desk reference, ed. 25, Oradel, N.J., 1976, Medical Economics, Inc.

28

Pharmacologic management of certain common oral disease entities

SAM V. HOLROYD
WILLIAM K. BOTTOMLEY

To present treatment in its proper context, the introductory paragraph or paragraphs on each condition briefly review the occurrence, etiology, and principal signs and symptoms of the disease. No attempt is made to present complete diagnostic criteria. Sample prescriptions are included to facilitate the treatment procedure. (All doses are for adults unless otherwise indicated.)

ACUTE NECROTIZING ULCERATIVE GINGIVITIS

Acute necrotizing ulcerative gingivitis (ANUG) has been called *Vincent's infection, trench mouth,* and numerous other names. Although ANUG is less prevalent than it was in years past, it remains a disease of importance in dental practice. The etiology of ANUG appears to have both bacteriologic (spirochetes and fusiform bacilli) and predisposing (local irritants, physical and mental stress, debilitation) components. Basic to diagnosis is the typical pseudomembranous ulcer that begins at the tips of the interdental papillae. This painful spreading ulcer is usually associated with a distinctive odor and increased salivation. Systemic signs and symptoms are not necessarily present, but cervical lymphadenopathy, an elevated temperature, general malaise, nausea, and headache may be experienced.

The principal treatment of ANUG is *not* pharmacologic and includes the removal of irritants, the establishment of good oral hygiene, and a regimen of adequate rest and nutrition. However, certain drug categories should be discussed in regard to the treatment of ANUG.

Mouthwashes. Mouthwashes facilitate oral hygiene by their flushing action. For this reason they are useful during the treatment of ANUG. Hydrogen peroxide in a 1% to 1.5% solution or a physiologic saline solution may be used. The evidence is unconvincing that the oxygen-releasing agents are any more effective than saline rinses in home care of ANUG. The local effects of a dilute solution of an obtundent mouthwash, such as Cepacol, may be useful in some cases.

R Hydrogen peroxide, 3%
Disp: 8 oz
Sig: Dilute to half strength with warm water and rinse mouth every 2 hours.

Analgesics and antipyretics. In severe cases of ANUG the mouth is very painful and the temperature is sometimes elevated. An antipyretic analgesic should be prescribed in these cases, and aspirin or acetaminophen (Tylenol) is usually adequate. Instructions to the patient to take two 5-grain aspirin or acetaminophen tablets every 4 hours if needed for pain is generally adequate. However, sometimes a prescription may be necessary even for these very commonly used drugs.

R Aspirin, 5 gr
Disp: 100 tablets
Sig: Take 2 tablets every 4 hours as needed for pain.

R Acetaminophen, 5 gr
Disp: 100 tablets
Sig: Take 2 tablets every 4 hours as needed for pain.

Food supplements. The oral tissues may be so painful in some cases of ANUG that eating becomes difficult. Certain commercially prepared food supplements (Meritene,

□ The opinions or assertions contained herein are the private ones of the writers and are not to be construed as official or as reflecting the views of the Navy Department or the naval service at large.

Nutrament, Provimalt, Sustagen) may be used as meal substitutes if an adequate soft diet cannot be obtained or if the patient prefers the supplements. These food supplements provide required vitamins and minerals as well as the necessary carbohydrate, fat, and protein. There is no convincing evidence that the vitamin preparations are helpful in ANUG, but it is probably well to prescribe them in those cases where an inadequate vitamin intake has preceded the onset of the condition. In these cases any of a large number of multiple vitamin preparations should suffice.

R Meritene
Disp: 1 lb can
Sig: Take three servings daily. Prepare as indicated on can.

Antibiotics. There is no question that many antibiotics will improve the clinical course of ANUG. However, because of the rapid and dramatic recovery of patients with the condition after local treatment, antibiotics are infrequently required and their routine use is to be condemned. One should consider administering them only in severe cases where the patient's resistance to infection is low or there is evidence of significant systemic involvement. When antibiotics must be given, penicillin, erythromycin, and the tetracyclines are effective. Although clinical reports are lacking, lincomycin and clindamycin will also probably be effective. Patients with rheumatic or congenital heart disease should, of course, be premedicated with penicillin in accordance with the recommendations of the American Heart Association before debridement.

R Penicillin V tablets, 250 mg
Disp: 40 tablets
Sig: Take 1 tablet at bedtime and 1 hour before each meal.*

Topical caustics. Caustic drugs should not be used on the lesions of acute necrotizing ulcerating gingivitis.

PRIMARY HERPETIC GINGIVOSTOMATITIS

Primary herpetic gingivostomatitis (primary herpes) is a common disease that is caused by the herpes simplex virus. It is principally a disease of infants and children and is frequently associated with pneumonia, meningitis, and upper respiratory infections. Primary herpes is seldom seen in adolescents or adults. The painful lesions may appear throughout the gingival, labial, buccal, palatal, glossal, and pharyngeal mucosa. They appear as depressed yellow-white ulcers circumscribed by an area of erythema. Systemic signs and symptoms that are generally associated with these lesions include high temperature, headache, refusal to take food, lymphadenopathy, and general malaise. The systemic reaction is usually less severe in adults than in children. In infants and young children primary herpes can be dangerous because of the problems of dehydration, acidosis, contact spread to the hands and eyes, and visceral dissemination.

Therapeutic agents generally have little or no effect on the course of primary herpes, and treatment is essentially supportive. Drugs in the following groups are used.

Analgesics and antipyretics. Although the course of the primary herpes infection may be subclinical, many children experience a high temperature, which may reach 105° F but usually recedes shortly after the lesions appear. In view of the temperature and extremely painful nature of the lesions, an antipyretic analgesic such as aspirin or acetaminophen is indicated. One should note that in the use of aspirin and acetaminophen to control high temperature in children, careful attention must be given to dosage. This is particularly true in primary herpes because the patient may be dehydrated. Fluid intake is often minimal in this disease because of the painful oral condition, and absorption of fluids may be hindered by a disturbance of gastrointestinal function. Sponging with tepid water frequently controls high temperatures effectively and thus allows minimal dosage with antipyretics. Dehydration and acidosis that may be associated with high temperatures in children can be dangerous and should receive prompt inpatient attention.

See earlier statement on analgesics and antipyretics.

Mouthwashes and topical obtundents. Mouthwashes, particularly those with local obtundent activity, may partially relieve the painful local symptoms of primary herpetic

---

*Dosage for treatment of ANUG when an antibiotic is indicated—not for subacute bacterial endocarditis prophylaxis.

gingivostomatitis and thereby encourage the adequate intake of food and liquid. Viscous lidocaine, dyclonine hydrochloride in 0.5% aqueous solution, diphenhydramine (Benadryl), Kaopectate, gentian violet, methylene blue, and combinations of these medications have been used topically to provide temporary symptomatic relief. We recommend the local anesthetics. The application of sodium carboxymethyl cellulose paste (Orabase Emollient) to the lesions may also reduce the discomfort.

> ℞ Benadryl powder, 0.5% with dyclonine, 0.5% in physiologic saline
> Disp: 8 oz
> Sig: Rinse with 1 teaspoonful every 2 hours.

> ℞ Benadryl elixir, 12.5 mg/5 ml
> Disp: 4 oz
> Sig: Rinse with 1 teaspoonful for 2 minutes before each meal.

> ℞ Benadryl elixir, 12.5 mg/5 ml with Kaopectate, 50% mixture by volume
> Disp: 8 oz
> Sig: Rinse with 1 teaspoonful every 2 hours.

> ℞ Xylocaine viscous, 2%
> Disp: 450 ml
> Sig: Rinse with 1 tablespoonful every 4 hours.

Food supplements. In situations where a nutritious soft diet cannot be consistently obtained, the food supplements previously mentioned should be employed. If the soft diet is preferred, supplementation with a daily multiple vitamin and mineral preparation may be helpful, particularly in infants and children. Specific curative effects of individual vitamins are not established.

See earlier statement on food supplements.

Topical caustics. The results of the application of caustics such as silver nitrate, phenol, and trichloroacetic acid are not impressive, and their use is generally discouraged.

Corticosteroids. Since the etiologic agent in primary herpes is viral, the use of the adrenocorticosteroids may result in a serious and possibly fatal spread of the infection. Consequently, these drugs are *contraindicated* in primary herpes.

Antibiotics. Because of the viral nature of primary herpes, antibiotics are not considered helpful unless a secondary bacterial infection is present. However, some clinicians routinely start antibiotics in the severely affected infant or child.

See earlier statement on antibiotics.

RECURRENT HERPES LABIALIS

The lesions of recurrent herpes labialis, which are relatively common, are caused by the herpes simplex virus. The painful lesions occur at the vermilion border of the lip, where they may appear initially as an area of erythema followed by vesicle formation. Rupture of the vesicle leaves an encrusted ulceration. The lesions are usually single, last about 1 week, and heal without scarring. Elevated temperature and other signs and symptoms of systemic involvement associated with primary herpes are not usually seen with herpes labialis.

In treatment the practitioner is essentially concerned with the painful and unesthetic lip lesion. Many substances have been placed on these lesions to accelerate healing, but although numerous favorable reports have appeared, confirming studies have not been reported. The application of a lubricating agent seems to lessen the pain. Adrenocorticosteroid applications to cutaneous herpes simplex infections have been associated with serious disseminated infection with the herpes simplex virus.[1] Consequently, as in the case of primary herpes, the use of corticosteroids is contraindicated in herpes labialis.

Antiviral agents. The topical application of 0.5% idoxuridine (Stoxil) ophthalmic ointment is not effective on lip lesions, probably because of the poor penetrability of the active ingredient. An antiviral agent recently approved for the treatment of herpes simplex (type I) is 9-B-D-arabinofuranosyladenine (Vira-A). Early tests indicate a 10% ointment is effective against the herpes labialis form.

Photochemical inactivation. Viruses can be inactivated by treatment with certain heterotricyclic dyes, for example 0.1% proflavine, and subsequent exposure to ordinary fluorescent light. Because of the possibility that this treatment might mutagenize cells into cancer cells, it is not recommended.

Vitamins. Water-soluble bioflavonoid–ascorbic acid complex, an essential constituent for normal capillary permeability and fragility, is valuable in reducing the signs and symptoms associated with recurrent herpes simplex (type I) virus infections. As with all agents used, the therapy is more effective when instituted in the early prodromal stage of the disease process.

> ℞ Citrus bioflavonoids and ascorbic acid capsules, 200 mg

Disp: 20 capsules

Sig: Take 1 capsule three times per 24 hours for 3 days.

RECURRENT APHTHOUS STOMATITIS

Recurrent aphthous stomatitis is a relatively common condition that is seen most frequently after 20 years of age. Investigative evidence indicated that a transitional L form of an alpha streptococcus was the etiologic agent; however, vaccinations against this organism proved ineffective.[2-5] Recent studies have disclosed an association between recurrent aphthae and deficiencies of vitamin B_{12}, folic acid, and iron.[6] Hematologic screening should precede the initiation of vitamin therapy. The painful lesions of aphthous stomatitis are similar in appearance to those of primary herpes, but the associated systemic signs and symptoms are absent or much less severe. In some cases a low-grade fever, cervical lymphadenopathy, leukocytosis, and debilitation may occur.[7]

Symptomatic control by previously mentioned drugs is indicated: aspirin for pain and fever; obtundent mouthwashes for discomfort, particularly to allow the maintenance of an adequate diet; and food supplements where nutrition cannot be maintained otherwise.

Topical adrenal steroids have been beneficial in some cases.[5,8,9] However, in view of the problem of adrenocortical atrophy during steroid medication, the use of these drugs in recurrent aphthous stomatitis should be limited to short-term topical application in severe cases. A convenient form of steroid for intraoral application is 0.1% triamcinolone acetonide in a sodium carboxymethyl cellulose emollient paste (Kenalog in Orabase), which is to be applied two or three times daily. Since the use of steroids is contraindicated in fungal or viral lesions of the oral cavity, the practitioner must be certain of his diagnosis of an aphthous lesion. Relief from discomfort will be obtained in some cases if the emollient paste alone is applied to the lesions after meals and at bedtime.

Since recurrent aphthous stomatitis is believed to be caused by a streptococcus, tetracycline medication has been employed. Graykowski and co-workers[5] found the following antibiotic regimen to be helpful in about 70% of the cases studied: Each dose of 5 ml (1 teaspoonful) of a 250 mg/5 ml tetracycline suspension is held in the mouth for 2 minutes and then swallowed four times per 24 hours for 5 to 7 days. The patient should be instructed not to eat for 1 hour after medication. The dose given is for an adult. Unfortunately, the numerous tetracycline syrups do not seem to be effective. Apparently, it is necessary to prescribe the tetracycline powder for reconstitution to a suspension. This is only available in a 1.5 Gm bottle, which is reconstituted with distilled water to 30 ml (250 mg/5 ml). A 6-day regimen for an adult would require four bottles (120 ml).

The literature does not reflect any consistency in regard to the use of silver nitrate, smallpox and poliomyelitis vaccinations, antihistamines, gamma globulin, and vitamins in the treatment of recurrent aphthous stomatitis.

Ŗ Kenalog in Orabase, 0.1%

Disp: 5 Gm tube

Sig: Apply to lesion after each meal and at bedtime.

Ŗ Achromycin V oral suspension (Lederle), 1.5 Gm

Disp: Four 1.5 Gm bottles (Do not premix.)

Sig: Rinse with 1 teaspoonful for 2 minutes after each meal and at bedtime and swallow. (To prevent deterioration, mix one bottle at a time with water when it is to be used. Fill bottle to the top with tap water. Shake well before using.)

CANDIDIASIS (MONILIASIS)

Candidiasis is infection by the fungus (yeast) *Candida albicans*. Other species of *Candida* are infrequently pathogenic in humans. The infection of mucous membrane by *C. albicans* (thrush) is fairly common. The most frequent sites are the oral and vaginal mucosa; skin is less frequently involved. Visceral involvement is even less common and is generally associated with a strong predisposing component. The principal visceral involvement is aspiration pneumonia. Less frequently, hematogenous spread may involve the kidney, brain, meninges, heart, thyroid, pancreas, liver, and adrenals.[10]

Oral candidiasis. C. albicans is a normal inhabitant of the oral cavity. A disease state is manifested when the fungus is capable of unusually accelerated growth. Predisposing factors that increase the susceptibility to candidal overgrowth include (1) suppression of normal oral flora by antibacterial therapy (this is particularly important in the use of long-term and/or broad-spectrum antibiotics), (2) debilitation (may be caused by age or disease), (3) diabetes, (4) therapy with adrenal steroids, (5) antineoplastic therapy, (6) malnutrition, (7) pregnancy (increased incidence of vaginal candidiasis), and (8) infancy.

The diagnosis of oral candidiasis is based on the presence of the characteristic lesions plus a history of predisposition. Diagnosis can be confirmed by a microscopic study of smears taken from the lesions. The characteristic oral lesions of acute candidiasis are white, milk curd–like patches that adhere to the mucosa. Removal of the lesions leave red areas or bleeding points.

Oral candidiasis in chronic form may be manifested as an angular cheilitis, a denture stomatitis, or hyperplastic candidiasis.[11] No systemic signs or symptoms are caused by oral candidiasis.

The treatment of oral candidiasis consists of the topical application of the antifungal drug nystatin (Mycostatin). When the aqueous suspension (100,000 U/ml) is used, the usual adult dosage is 2 ml four times per 24 hours. Zegarelli[12] has recommended a dose of up to 3 ml after each meal and prior to bedtime. The suspension should be swished in the mouth for 2 minutes before swallowing. Nystatin suspension is supplied in 60 ml bottles with a dropper calibrated at 1 ml. Cohen[11] has recommended the use of nystatin tablets. A tablet (500,000 units) is dissolved in the mouth four times per 24 hours. Nystatin vaginal tablets (100,000 units) may be used as lozenges. This modality supplies continuous therapy to the affected area, decreasing the duration of the clinical signs and symptoms. Regardless of whether the suspension or tablet is used, treatment should continue for at least 14 days and not be discontinued until two successive smears are negative[13] or at least until 48 hours after the signs of infection have disappeared. Treatment may require 4 to 6 weeks or longer to eliminate this rather tenacious infection. This is particularly true of chronic hyperplastic candidiasis.

℞ Nystatin oral suspension, 100,000 U/ml
Disp: 60 ml
Sig: Take 2 ml four times per 24 hours. Hold in mouth for 2 minutes and swallow.

℞ Nystatin oral tablets, 500,000 U/tablet
Disp: 30 tablets
Sig: Let tablet dissolve in mouth, four times per 24 hours.

℞ Nystatin vaginal tablets, 100,000 U/tablet
Disp: 30 tablets
Sig: Let tablet dissolve in mouth, three times per 24 hours.

ANGULAR CHEILITIS/CHEILOSIS

Angular cheilitis (inflammation of the angles of the mouth) may be characterized by simple redness or may exhibit fissures, erosion, ulcers, and crusting. The area may be painless, may burn, or may be otherwise painful. Angular cheilitis may be caused by reduced vertical dimension with consequent accentuation of the commissural skin folds and drooling. It may also be caused by infection, allergic reactions, trauma, and nutritional deficiencies. In angular cheilitis from a nutritional deficiency (principally a lack of riboflavin), the lesion takes on a more "macerated" appearance and is generally given the more specific name, *angular cheilosis.*

The cause of angular cheilitis is usually multiple. Consequently, treatment must encompass all etiologic factors. Lesions from nutritional deficiency result principally from lack of riboflavin but are generally associated with multiple deficiencies. These lesions should be resolved by the establishment of adequate dietary intake. Temporary use of meal supplements or multiple vitamin preparations, particularly those heavy in the B-complex vitamins should be helpful. Allergy-induced angular cheilitis is rare and should be resolved by determining and eliminating the allergenic agent. Lesions induced by trauma, such as stretching and pulling during prolonged dental procedures, should heal without treatment after the traumatogenic component is removed. However, the traumatic angular lesion may become secondarily infected before complete healing obtains. Angular cheilitis caused by a reduced vertical dimension should be resolved by reestablishing an acceptable interocclusal distance. However, the cheilitis is frequently caused by both a loss of vertical dimension and infection.

Most cases of angular cheilitis that require pharmacologic management are caused by infection. The presence of infection by *C. albicans* or bacteria should be suspected in all cases of angular stomatitis that do not respond quickly to the removal of other etiologic components. Severe cases of angular cheilitis or any case that does not respond to other indicated procedures should be cultured to determine the presence of *C. albicans* or bacteria as etiologic agents. If *C. albicans* is a causative factor, the indicated treatment is the local application of nystatin ointment (100,000 U/Gm) two to six times per 24 hours until at least 48 hours after the lesion has disappeared. Nystatin ointment is available in 30 Gm tubes. If the infecting agent is bacterial rather than fungal, the lesion is likely to be resolved by keeping the area clean and by eliminating other etiologic factors. In cases where pharmacologic intervention is required to eliminate bacterial involvement, a bacitracin-neomycin preparation (Bacimycin Ointment: bacitracin 500 units, neomycin 23.5 mg/Gm) may be applied three or four times per 24 hours. This ointment is available in 15 Gm tubes. An alternative agent is 3% chlortetracycline ointment, applied three or four times per 24 hours. The 3% chlortetracycline preparation is available in 15 and 30 Gm tubes. Some infections may be due to a mixture of fungal and bacterial organisms. A preparation of nystatin-neomycin-triamcinolone acetonide (Mycolog) is effective in providing quick clinical improvement and symptomatic relief in mixed infections. Mycolog is available as an ointment in 15 and 20 Gm tubes.

Ŗ Allbee with C capsules
Disp: 100 capsules
Sig: Take 1 capsule with each meal.

Ŗ Nystatin ointment, 100,000 U/Gm
Disp: 30 Gm
Sig: Apply to affected area after each meal and at bedtime.

Ŗ Bacimycin ointment
Disp: 15 Gm
Sig: Apply to affected area after each meal and at bedtime.

Ŗ Chlortetracycline, 3% ointment
Disp: 15 Gm
Sig: Apply to affected area after each meal and at bedtime.

Ŗ Mycolog ointment
Disp: 15 Gm
Sig: Apply to affected area after each meal and at bedtime.

LICHEN PLANUS

Lichen planus is a relatively common skin disease that frequently involves mucous membranes. It is a disease of adults, with no sex predisposition. The etiology is unknown, but it is invariably precipitated by stress. Clinically, it has variable forms with the most characteristic being a white network on an erythematous base. The hyperkeratotic form is asymptomatic. The symptoms of oral erosive lichen planus vary in intensity from a slight sensitivity to acidic liquids and spicy foods to extreme discomfort with any contact of the affected area.

Treatment is directed toward improving the host response and the general nutritional state. Regimens of niacinamide plus vitamins B and C at twenty times the prophylactic dose for 4 weeks have been reported to be beneficial. The topical application of anti-inflammatory agents improves the clinical symptoms. Ointments of 0.1% betamethasone valerate (Valisone) and 0.05% flurandrenolone (Cordran) are frequently employed. When these ointments are covered with Kenalog in Orabase, it prolongs their duration of action. Rinsing with an elixir of dexamethasone (Decadron) is a common treatment. In severe cases systemic steroids combined with antibiotics may be necessary to control the disease process.

Ŗ Valisone ointment, 0.1%
Disp: 15 Gm tube
Sig: Apply to affected area after each meal and at bedtime.

Ŗ Cordran ointment, 0.05%
Disp: 15 Gm tube
Sig: Apply to affected area after each meal and at bedtime.

Ŗ Kenalog in Orabase, 0.1%
Disp: 5 Gm tube
Sig: Coat the lesion after each meal and at bedtime.

Ŗ Decadron elixir, 0.5 mg/5 ml
Disp: 100 ml
Sig: Rinse with 1 teaspoonful for 1 minute after each meal and at bedtime. Do not swallow.

BURNING TONGUE SYNDROME AND SYMPTOMATIC GEOGRAPHIC TONGUE

Either local irritants or systemic deficiencies or a combination of the two may result in sensitivity of the tongue. The ultimate treatment is based on the diagnosis, which in some instances requires a thorough medical evaluation to rule out nutritional deficiencies, malabsorption syndrome, endocrine disturbances, blood dyscrasias, secretory impairment, and allergic states.

Symptomatic relief may be achieved by

rinsing with elixir of diphenhydramine hydrochloride (Benadryl). It coats the tissue temporarily, has mild topical anesthetic qualities, and if swallowed provides some sedation.

R Benadryl elixir, 12.5 mg/5 ml
Disp: 8 oz
Sig: Rinse with 1 teaspoonful for 2 minutes before each meal and swallow.

PERICORONITIS

Pericoronitis is the inflammation of tissues around the crown of a tooth. Although the term could be applied to any tooth, it generally refers to a common and painful inflammatory reaction around partially erupted lower third molars. In these teeth a flap of gingiva (operculum) covers part of the occlusal surface. The presence of food debris and bacteria between the operculum and tooth generates an inflammatory response. The swelling that results enlarges the operculum and frequently results in the development of periodontal pockets on one or more tooth surfaces. The edema thus enlarges the pocket area in which bacteria can grow and more debris can become entrapped.

Patients usually experience intermittent occurrences of mild inflammation and slight swelling of the soft tissues prior to more serious involvement. The component of infection that may be minimal initially can progress quickly to present a serious cellulitis.

When treatment is instituted early, only gentle debridement of the cul-de-sac areas by curet or saline irrigation may be required. The patient is usually instructed to continue warm saline rinses for a day or so. The problem will recur in most cases periodically until tooth eruption and/or degeneration or excision of the operculum has eliminated the debris-collecting area. If the full mouth treatment plan includes removal of the tooth involved, early extraction to avoid further episodes is desirable.

In the more severe cases of pericoronitis, debridement is still the primary treatment. However, other considerations must be made. Swelling may reach the point that the opposing maxillary third molar may traumatize the mandibular soft tissues. If the lower molar is ultimately to be removed, extraction of the opposing maxillary third molar is often helpful in alleviating the acute episode. Swelling may also interfere with opening and chewing. In these cases one must force fluids and ensure adequate nutritional intake. If this cannot be accomplished by the use of a soft diet, the nutritional supplements previously discussed should be employed to ensure adequate nutrition. Pain, induced by swelling and infection, will frequently require analgesics. Aspirin will be adequate in most cases, but more potent drugs will be required in some.

Infection will be resolved in most healthy patients by local and supportive treatment. However, the practitioner must be aware that infection associated with pericoronitis may abscess locally or may spread rapidly into alveolar bone and through fascial spaces. The following are rare but serious results: retropharyngeal, peritonsillar, masseter, and temporal space abscesses; laryngeal edema; Ludwig's angina, cavernous sinus thrombosis; and acute meningitis.[14] Consequently, indications that infection associated with pericoronitis are spreading in spite of local treatment, especially in elderly, debilitated, or otherwise unhealthy patients, should be treated vigorously with antibiotics. The selection of an antibiotic for cases of pericoronitis is based on the same principles discussed in Chapter 20.

R Penicillin V tablets 250 mg
Disp: 40 tablets
Sig: Take 2 tablets at once followed by 1 tablet 1 hour before each meal and at bedtime.

ALVEOLAR OSTEITIS ("DRY SOCKET")

Alveolar osteitis occurs after 2% to 3% of all extractions.[15-17] It occurs predominately in lower molar areas, where the incidence may be much higher. The occurrence after the removal of impacted lower third molars has been reported to be as high as 25%.[18] The incidence of alveolar osteitis is increased by trauma, lack of aseptic techniques, and the presence of thick, relatively avascular bone.

Alveolar osteitis is caused by the loss or necrosis of the blood clot, resulting in unprotected bone within the extraction socket. The exposed bone is extremely painful, becomes to some degree necrotic, and is generally secondarily infected. The loss or necrosis of the original clot may result from its being rinsed out by the patient or may result from infection of, or inadequate blood supply to, the clot.

In addition to the absence of a clot or the presence of an ill-formed clot, the signs and symptoms include constant pain localized to or radiating from the site of a recent extraction and an associated foul odor. Swelling, elevated temperature, and lymphadenopathy indicate the presence of infection.

The treatment of alveolar osteitis consists essentially of (1) debriding the socket, usually with warm saline; (2) maintaining an antiseptic-analgesic pack in the socket until the osseous walls become covered by granulation tissue; (3) control of pain; (4) control of infection if present; and (5) supportive therapy, such as ensuring adequate rest, nutrition, and fluid intake.

Dressing. The socket dressing usually consists of a strip of gauze that contains obtundent and antiseptic agents. This dressing keeps debris out of the socket and provides analgesic and antiseptic effects. The dressings are placed after the socket has been carefully debrided. They are generally changed daily but may have to be changed two or three times a day to provide adequate pain relief. Although plain eugenol has been used effectively, several pastes and a wide variety of ingredients have been recommended for incorporation into the gauze. None of the more commonly recommended mixtures has any great advantage over the others. Some examples are (1) a paste containing equal parts of thymol iodide powder and benzocaine crystals dissolved in eugenol,[19] (2) equal parts guaiacol and eugenol, (3) guaiacol (3 Gm), benzocaine (3 Gm), Peruvian balsam (9 Gm).[20]

Food supplements. The severe and often prolonged pain of alveolar osteitis may alter the patient's food intake to the point where dietary inadequacies develop that could conceivably delay recovery. Patient instruction in soft diets and/or the use of the food supplements previously mentioned should ensure adequate dietary intake.

See earlier statement on food supplements.

Analgesics. Both local (dressing) and systemic analgesics will be required in almost all cases of alveolar osteitis. Although aspirin may be adequate in some cases, more potent analgesics such as codeine will be frequently required.

R Codeine tablets, ½ gr
Disp: 12 tablets
Sig: Take 1 tablet with 2 aspirin tablets every 4 hours as needed for pain.

Antibiotics. Antibiotics that may be necessary when infection is associated with alveolar osteitis should be selected and prescribed as for other oral infections. One must be aware that what begins as an osteitis may progress to osteomyelitis. Consequently, the practitioner must recognize the presence of overt infection and institute early treatment. Thoma[21] has also pointed up the importance of a differential diagnosis between alveolar osteitis and osteomyelitis.

There is some indication that sulfonamide and tetracycline cones placed in extraction sites may reduce the incidence of alveolar osteitis. In a recent, controlled double-blind study, Hall and co-workers[22] found a statistically significant reduction in the incidence of "dry sockets," from 19% (control third-molar extractions) to 7% (tetracycline-treated extraction sites). In this study a 50 mg tetracycline hydrochloride tablet was dissolved in 1 ml tap water and absorbed in a gelatin sponge (Gelfoam), which was placed in the experimental extraction sites.

The favorable results reported from the local application of sulfonamides and tetracyclines in reducing the occurrence of alveolar osteitis do not justify their routine use. Aseptic technique, proper suturing when indicated, and minimal trauma in healthy patients should decrease the occurrence of alveolar osteitis. In cases where negative factors are present in third-molar extractions, such as broken aseptic technique, considerable trauma, and an unhealthy patient, the use of local tetracycline prophylaxis such as that reported by Hall and co-workers[22] may be justified.

XEROSTOMIA

The condition of reduced salivary flow may result from a disease process, the treatment of disease, drug therapy, and the generalized decrease in secretions associated with aging. Sjögren's syndrome, salivary gland aplasia, and Mikulicz's disease are classic disease conditions that depress salivary gland activity. Radiation therapy in excess of 800 rads induces irreparable changes in the structure of the salivary glands, adversely affecting the amount and composition of the saliva. Antihistamines, tranquilizers, diuretics, and atropine-like drugs tend to decrease salivary production. Xerostomia is a frequent symptom in women after 40 years of age. Often it is associated with the hormonal and glandular changes observed with menopause. The etiology of the salivary discrepancy must be identified before effective, long-term therapy can be instituted.

The immediate symptoms can be relieved by the application of sodium carboxymethyl cellulose. It is a nonirritating agent that moistens and lubricates the oral tissues and may be used for prolonged periods without adverse effects.

R Sodium carboxymethyl cellulose, 0.5% aqueous solution
Disp: 8 oz
Sig: Use as a rinse as frequently as needed to relieve symptoms of dry mouth.

POSTIRRADIATION CARIES

The lack of proper oral plaque control and the qualitative and quantitative changes in saliva after radiation therapy to the dental region can produce an extremely accelerated rate of dental caries. This is characteristically manifested by generalized cervical decay within the first year after therapy. Recommended prophylactic and therapeutic measures include the institution of a meticulous oral hygiene program and the self-application of 1% sodium fluoride gel per 24 hours in a flexible bite guard. This regimen should be continued indefinitely.

R Fluoride gel, 1% sodium fluoride
Disp: 2 oz.
Sig: Place 5 to 10 drops in bite guard and apply for 5 min/24 hr.

ROOT SENSITIVITY

Hypersensitivity of exposed root surfaces is a common dental complaint. Pain in an area of exposed root may be precipitated by mechanically touching the area, by heat or cold, or by sweet or sour foods.

Root hypersensitivity may be caused by occlusal trauma or may result from the irritation of organic matter in exposed dentinal tubules.[14] Hypersensitive root surfaces not caused by occlusal trauma generally result from (1) exposure of roots by periodontal surgery, (2) extensive root planing, and/or (3) accumulation of tooth accumulated materials (TAM) on exposed roots. In cases where occlusal trauma is the cause, occlusal adjustment is the treatment. The treatment of root sensitivities of other etiology can be highly frustrating. Basic to all treatment is ensuring that the root surface be kept free of TAM. This serves two purposes: (1) irritants

are removed and (2) direct contact by desensitizing agents is possible.

A wide variety of both simple and complex agents, including high concentrations of poppycock, have been painted, burnished, electroplated, tapped, poured, pushed, and brushed on sensitive roots. The consistency of results has not been terribly impressive. Treatments can be divided into those provided in the dental office and those instituted at home by the patient.

Agents applied by the dentist

No attempt is made to discuss the myriad of agents that have been used by the dentist to reduce root sensitivity. The following agents should be adequate for effective practice.

Glycerin. One of the most simple treatments for root hypersensitivity has been to burnish glycerin into the cleaned and dried sensitive area with a ball burnisher or orangewood stick. The results are not highly predictable, and the mechanism of action is unknown. It is likely that any favorable effects result from the burnishing action rather than from any direct effect of the glycerin.

Sodium fluoride. Various mixtures of sodium fluoride have been applied to hypersensitive root areas. Although results have been neither consistent nor highly impressive, success has been obtained in some cases. There is no evidence that the more exotic mixtures of sodium fluoride are any more effective than straight 2% topical solution applied by cotton swab or placed in pumice for rubber cup application to clean, dry root surfaces.

Stannous fluoride. A number of stannous fluoride mixtures have also been applied to hypersensitive root areas. There is no evidence that the more exotic mixtures of stannous fluoride are any more effective than straight 10% topical solution applied by cotton swab or placed in pumice for rubber cup application to clean, dry root surfaces. The application of a 9% stannous fluoride paste should be equally effective or ineffective.

Adrenal steroids. Bowers and Elliott[23] evaluated the effectiveness of a prednisolone preparation against root hypersensitivity. This preparation had been used earlier to prevent sensitivity in cavity preparations.[24,25] They found that one or two applications of the following solution "appeared effective in the treatment of sensitivity due to incisal (occlusal) fractures, extensive occlusal adjustment or odontoplasty, periodontal surgery and post scaling and root planing procedures."[23]

Components	Percentages by weight
Parachlorophenol	25
Metacresyl acetate (Cresatin)	25
Gum camphor	49
Prednisolone	1

The solution was applied with a cotton pellet to clean, dry sensitive areas. This prednisolone solution deteriorates rapidly and is not likely to be effective after 90 days. Sensitivity resulting from gingival recession was reduced but not as dramatically as in other cases. Although no side effects of the prednisolone solution were observed in this study, an effort should be made to limit systemic absorption by restricting the solution to tooth surfaces as much as possible.

Prichard[26] and others have used an ophthalmic solution of prednisolone (Metimyd) successfully. This 0.5% prednisolone solution is applied to clean, dry tooth surfaces. Each milliliter of this ophthalmic solution contains 5 mg prednisolone acetate, 100 mg sodium sulfacetamide, and preservatives. It is available in 5 ml bottles. The antibacterial action of sulfacetamide would have no purpose when this solution is used for desensitization. Although no studies are available, it might be equally effective and more rational to eliminate the unnecessary but active ingredient sulfacetamide by using an ophthalmic solution that contains 0.5% prednisolone as the only active ingredient. Such a solution is available (Optival) in 5 ml bottles.

The dentist should become familiar with the pharmacology and precautions related to adrenal steroids prior to their use. In view of the broad pharmacologic effects of systemically absorbed adrenal steroids, these drugs should not be used for root hypersensitivity unless contact with soft tissues can be minimized. This is not likely to be possible in cases of generalized hypersensitivity.

Agents applied by the patient

Home brushing of hypersensitive areas with concentrated sodium chloride solutions and 0.5% stannous fluoride have been recommended. The results are poorly documented. In cases where there is generalized tooth sensitivity, the self-application of 1%

sodium fluoride gel for 5 min/24 hr in a flexible bite guard has been beneficial.

Desensitizing toothpastes deserve some discussion. Many practitioners believe that optimal effects occur when office treatment is followed by the use of a desensitizing toothpaste. The degree of usefulness of these pastes is rather vague.

Hazen and co-workers[27] conducted a double-blind clinical comparison of four dentifrices: (1) 0.76% sodium monofluorophosphate with insoluble sodium metaphosphate as the abrasive (pH 5.5); (2) a control having the ingredients of (1) minus the sodium monofluorophosphate; (3) a commercial dentifrice containing 1.4% formalin (pH 8.5); and (4) a commercial dentifrice containing 0.4% stannous fluoride with insoluble sodium metaphosphate as the abrasive (pH 4.8 to 5.2). Patients with chronic root sensitivity were randomly provided with one of the preceding dentifrices and instructed to brush in the usual manner at least twice daily. The patients were examined for root sensitivity after approximately 2 and 4 weeks. All dentifrices reduced tooth hypersensitivity after 4 weeks of use; however, only dentifrice (1) showed a statistically significant improvement over the control dentifrice.

Until further double-blind comparisons of desensitizing dentifrices are available, it is not possible to assess the practical superiority, if any, of special desensitizing dentifrices over regular dentifrices. Unquestionably, improved tooth cleaning is effective against root hypersensitivity regardless of the type of dentifrice used.

REFERENCES

1. Burket, L. W.: Oral medicine, ed. 5, Philadelphia, 1965, J. B. Lippincott Co., p. 109.
2. Barile, M. F., Graykowski, E. A., Driscoll, E. J., and Riggs, D. B.: L Form of bacteria isolated from recurrent aphthous stomatitis lesions, Oral Surg. 16:1395-1402, 1963.
3. Graykowski, E. A., Barile, M. F., and Stanley, H. R.: Periadenitis aphthae: clinical and histopathologic aspects of lesions in a patient and of lesions produced in rabbit skin, J.A.D.A. 69:118-126, 1964.
4. Stanley, H. R., Graykowski, E. A., and Barile, M. F.: The occurrence of microorganisms in microscopic sections of aphthous and nonaphthous lesions and other oral tissues, Oral Surg. 18:335-341, 1964.
5. Graykowski, E. A., Barile, M. F., Lee, W. B., and and Stanley, H. R., Jr.: Recurrent aphthous stoma-

titis: clinical, therapeutic, histopathologic, and hypersensitivity aspects, J.A.M.A. **196:**637-644, 1966.

6. Wray, D., Ferguson, M. M., Mason, D. K., et al.: Recurrent aphthae: treatment with vitamin B$_{12}$, folic acid, and iron, Br. Med. J. **2:**490-493, 1975.

7. Ship, I. I., Merritt, A. D., and Stanley, H. R.: Recurrent aphthous ulcers, Am. J. Med. **32:**32-43, 1962.

8. Burket, L. W.: Oral medicine, ed. 5, Philadelphia, 1965, J. B. Lippincott Co., p. 117.

9. Browne, R. M., Fox, E. C., and Anderson, R. J.: Topical triamcinoline acetonide in recurrent aphthous stomatitis, Lancet **1:**565-567, 1968.

10. Braude, A. I.: Moniliasis (candidiasis) in Harrison's principles of internal medicine, ed. 6, New York, 1970, McGraw-Hill Book Co.

11. Cohen, L.: A synopsis of medicine in dentistry, Philadelphia, 1972, Lea & Febiger.

12. Zegarelli, E. V.: Therapeutic management of certain acute and chronic soft tissue diseases of the mouth, Dent. Clin. North Am. **14:**733-741, Oct., 1970.

13. Candida infections, Med. Lett. Drugs Ther. **12:**29, 1970.

14. Grant, D. A., Stern, I. B., and Everett, F. G.: Orban's periodontics, ed. 3, St. Louis, 1968, The C. V. Mosby Co.

15. Adkisson, S. R., and Harris, P. F.: Statistical study of alveolar osteitis, U.S. Armed Forces Med. J. **7:**1749, 1956.

16. Lehner, T.: Analysis of 100 cases of dry socket, Dent. Pract. **8:**275, 1958.

17. Hansen, E. H.: Alveolitis sicca dolorosa (dry socket): frequency of occurrence and treatment with trypsin, J. Oral Surg. **18:**409, 1960.

18. Quinley, J. F., Roger, R. Q., and Gores, R. J.: Dry socket after mandibular odontectomy and use of soluble tetracycline hydrochloride, Oral Surg. **13:**38, 1960.

19. Kruger, G. O.: Textbook of oral surgery, ed. 3, St. Louis, 1968, The C. V. Mosby Co.

20. American Dental Association Council on Drugs: Accepted dental therapeutics 1971/72, Chicago, 1971, American Dental Association.

21. Thoma, K. H.: Oral surgery, ed. 5, St. Louis, 1969, The C. V. Mosby Co.

22. Hall, H. D., Bildman, B. S., and Hand, C. D.: Prevention of dry socket with local application of tetracycline, J. Oral Surg. **29:**35-37, 1971.

23. Bowers, G. M., and Elliott, J. R.: Topical use of prednisolone in periodontics, J. Periodontol. **35:**486, 1964.

24. Fry, A. E., Watkins, R. E., and Phatok, N. M.: Topical use of corticosteroids for the relief of pain sensitivity of dentin and pulp, Oral Surg. **13:**594, 1960.

25. Masteller, J. H.: Prednisolone for postoperative thermal sensitivity, J. Prosth. Dent. **12:**1176, 1962.

26. Prichard, J. F.: Advanced periodontal disease, Philadelphia, 1965, W. B. Saunders Co.

27. Hazen, S. P., Volpe, A. R., and King, W. J.: Comparative desensitizing effect of dentifrices containing sodium monofluorophosphate, stannous fluoride and formalin, Periodontics **6:**230-232, 1968.

28. Research News, vol. 26, no. 1, University of Michigan, July, 1975.

29

Drug interactions

RICHARD L. WYNN

Drug interactions usually result in undesired drug effects. This phenomenon is defined as the action of an administered drug on the effectiveness or toxicity of another drug administered earlier, simultaneously, or later. It is a problem of growing concern to the health professions and is directly related to increased incidence of multiple drug therapy. One study has shown that hospitalized patients received an average of fourteen different medications during confinement.[1] Another study has observed that the incidence of drug interactions ranged from 4% to 5% when two drugs were used to 45% when more than two drugs were used.[2]

Dental professionals have more than just an academic interest in this drug problem. Much of the population receiving dental treatment is receiving concurrent drug therapy in the form of prescribed medication or as over-the-counter self-medication. Every dentist should be aware that medication prescribed by him may interact with other drugs to produce undesired effects in his patient. Taking a complete medical history and familiarity with the pharmacologic actions, therapeutic uses, and side effects of individual drugs are both usually sufficient for the dentist to predict the consequences of drug therapy. Often, however, unexpected drug interactions may occur to the surprise of the prescriber. Therefore a review of the current status of drug interactions in dentistry is necessary. It is the intent of this chapter to serve as a guide in preventing drug interactions. Important interactions that have occurred or could possibly occur through the use of dental drugs are also reviewed.

MECHANISMS

Interactions between two or more drugs result in antagonism or enhancement of pharmacologic effects. Antagonism occurs when one drug decreases the effect of another. Enhancement occurs when one drug increases the effect of another. In some cases enhancement and even antagonism result in a hazardous situation to the patient.

Drug enhancement or antagonism results when drug effects are additive or subtractive or when one drug influences one or more of the following aspects of the other: intestinal absorption, plasma protein binding, tissue protein binding, biotransformation, renal excretion, action at receptor sites, and alteration of normal body constituents. The following examples illustrate these mechanisms of drug interactions.

Intestinal absorption. Certain compounds such as antacids and ferrous sulfate contain divalent metal ions such as calcium, magnesium, and ferrous iron or trivalent ions such as aluminum, which will impair the absorption of tetracyclines because of the formation of a metal-tetracycline complex.

Plasma protein binding. In most cases that fraction of any drug bound to plasma protein is biologically inactive. It is the unbound or "free" drug fraction that produces pharmacologic or toxic effects. Many weakly acidic drugs can compete for the same binding sites on plasma proteins. Hence, one acidic drug may be displaced by another, thereby increasing the concentration of its free fraction. This effect tends to increase the pharmacologic effectiveness and in some cases the toxicity of the displaced drug. The highly bound oral anticoagulant bishydroxycoumarin has induced hypoglycemia by displacing tolbutamide from plasma protein.[3]

Tissue protein binding. Drugs may also be displaced from tissue protein by other drugs that have a greater binding affinity for the same binding sites. When the antimalarial agent pamaquine was administered to patients previously medicated with quina-crine, the pamaquine was displaced from tissue sites and resulted in increased plasma concentrations.[4]

Biotransformation. The stimulation and inhibition of the metabolism of one drug by another are well-known mechanisms of drug interactions.[5] Phenobarbital stimulates the metabolism of zoxazolamine, hexobarbital, and bishydroxycoumarin by inducing the formation of microsomal enzymes respon-sible for their metabolism. This results in a decrease in activity of these compounds. Cholinesterase inhibitors enhance the actions of acetylcholine and some of its congeners by preventing the enzymatic hydrolysis of these agents. The enzyme monoamine oxi-dase (MAO) metabolizes drugs such as me-peridine, chloral hydrate, some minor tran-quilizers, sympathomimetic amines, barbitu-rates, and amphetamines. The inhibition of MAO by MAO inhibitors (MAOIs) could consequently enhance the actions of these drugs.

Renal excretion. Probenecid inhibits the renal tubular secretion of penicillin, thus increasing plasma levels of the latter. Al-though some therapeutic advantage has been taken of this, higher penicillin levels are more directly obtained by increasing the dosage.

Action at receptor sites. Atropine inhib-its the activity of acetylcholine and its con-geners by competing at muscarinic receptor sites.

Body constituents. Alterations in body constituents by some drugs will affect the pharmacologic actions of others. Hypo-kalemia (lowered serum potassium levels) caused by thiazide diuretics will promote arrhythmias in the presence of digitalis.

DENTAL DRUG INTERACTIONS

The following discussion of dental drug interactions includes those which are po-tentially most significant to the patient and which can be caused by drugs routinely pre-scribed in dentistry. For purposes of ac-curacy, differentiation is made between clini-cal reports and those interactions only ob-served in animal studies.

Addicting analgesics

In general, the central nervous system depression produced by morphine and meperidine is enhanced by alcohol, seda-tives, hypnotics, antihistamines, and other central nervous system depressants. Serious reactions have occurred clinically through the use of meperidine. The simultaneous administration of this drug with monoamine oxidase inhibitors has led to a deep coma and extreme hypotension, resulting in a de-pressor crisis.[6,7] This effect is believed to be partially caused by an inhibition of meperi-dine degradation.[8]

Both the respiratory depression and the analgesia produced by narcotic analgesics can be enhanced by various drugs. For exam-ple, the phenothiazine derivatives including propiomazine, chlorpromazine, and prom-azine have dangerously exaggerated and pro-longed the respiratory depression of meperi-dine.[9-11] The inherent hypotensive action of these phenothiazines is an additional com-plication to the sedative action of morphine and meperidine. Imipramine-like antide-pressants exert a supra-additive effect on morphine- and meperidine-induced respira-tory depression.[12] Phenothiazines are also able to reduce the dose of morphine required to produce a given level of analgesia.[13] Con-comitant administration of meperidine with diazepam, amphetamines, or neostigmine results in an enhancement of its analgesic effect.[13-15] The analgesic potency of codeine is enhanced by the simultaneous administra-tion of aspirin, an effect that is clinically beneficial.[16]

Animal studies have indicated some po-tential clinical interactions involving the nar-cotic agents. In rats the anticholinergic ac-tion of scopolamine potentiates the sedative action of morphine.[17] The combined action of atropine and morphine has been investi-gated in mice, and it was shown that the anti-cholinergic effects of atropine were enhanced by this narcotic.[18] The ganglionic blocker mecamylamine has potentiated the analgesia produced by morphine in rats.[19] Reserpine, however, caused a decrease in the analgesic effect of meperidine as shown by the in-crease in the analgesia ED50 for meperidine in reserpinized rats.[20] Preliminary reports indicate that the antibacterial furazolidone enhances meperidine depression in humans[21] and that the beta-blocking agent propranolol potentiated the central nervous system de-pression induced by morphine.[22] Addicting analgesics may enhance the response to oral anticoagulants.[23,24] Clinical significance of this effect has not been established, however, and it is unlikely that short-term administration of these drugs will have appreciable effects on oral anticoagulant response.

Nonaddicting analgesics

Bleeding episodes have occurred after the administration of salicylates to patients receiving anticoagulant therapy with the coumarin derivatives.[25] This reaction was probably caused by a decrease in blood prothrombin levels and subsequent increase in prothrombin time caused by the salicylates. Salicylates are also able to displace the coumarin type of anticoagulants from protein binding sites in plasma. This action results in increased peak plasma concentrations of the free (unbound) anticoagulant with a resultant decreased plasma half-life of the drug.[26] Acetaminophen, like salicylates, will also potentiate anticoagulant drugs by increasing the normal physiologic prothrombin times.[27]

Several other clinical interactions involving salicylates have been reported. The uricosuric action of both aspirin and probenecid was inhibited when the two drugs were administered simultaneously.[28] This action may result in an undesirable situation in patients suffering from gout. The nonsteroidal antiinflammatory agent phenylbutazone has been observed to inhibit the uricosuric activity of aspirin.[29] Aspirin has reportedly caused hypoglycemic coma in diabetic patients receiving sulfonylurea hypoglycemic agents.[30] Plasma protein displacement of the sulfonylureas by aspirin or other salicylates appears to be the mechanism of this effect.[31] It has also been reported that administration of salicylates during a tapering of corticosteroid dosage in 4 patients resulted in an increased plasma level of unbound salicylates with concomitant salicylate intoxication in one of the patients.[32] When acetanilid was administered to patients receiving chlorpromazine therapy, there occurred an increase in the nonmetabolized chlorpromazine serum levels, an action that resulted in a potentiation of the effects of the drug.[33]

Other actions of salicylates, although not observed clinically, may be of importance. Aspirin, indomethacin, and phenylbutazone, when administered together, may cause enhanced irritation to the gastrointestinal tract. Any combination of these drugs may also cause enhancement of their ulcerogenic effects. Animal studies have indicated that acetazolamide, a specific inhibitor of carbonic anhydrase, enhances the oral absorption of salicylates to provide increased blood levels of these analgesics.[34] Apparently, acetazolamide lowers the gut pH, which favors absorption of the salicylates. In vitro studies indicate that salicylates may displace phenytoin, an antiepileptic agent, from plasma protein binding sites to result in a potentiation in the actions of the latter.[35] There is no clinical supporting evidence for this effect, however.[36] It has been noted that salicylates can cause as much as 50% decrease in sodium and chloride ion excretion in humans—an action that may antagonize thiazide diuretics.[37] Manufacturers' information concerning propoxyphene has indicated that this analgesic may potentiate the toxic effect of the skeletal muscle relaxant orphenadrine. Symptoms of this interaction are reported to be mental confusion, anxiety, and tremors. It is interesting to note that these symptoms are those which occur during a hypoglycemic episode and that both propoxyphene and orphenadrine have been reported to induce hypoglycemic activity when given alone.[38,39]

Anti-infectives

Various anti-infective drugs are able to enhance the effect of simultaneously administered coumarin anticoagulants in humans. A mechanism suggested for this effect is the interference of vitamin K synthesis in microorganisms of the gastrointestinal tract by anti-infective drugs.[40] Specifically, penicillin G has been reported to increase the prothrombin time response to oral anticoagulants.[24] Other agents likely to cause problems of this nature are tetracyclines and sulfonamides. The intestinal absorption of some anti-infectives in humans can be impaired by various agents. For example, antacids and milk that contain divalent and trivalent metal ions prevent absorption of tetracyclines.[41] According to one report, over 5% of the patients receiving tetracyclines also received such antacids.[42] The simultaneous administration of 40 mg ferrous sulfate with tetracycline resulted in a 50% to 90% lower serum level of this antibiotic.[43] Also, the concomitant administration of sodium bicarbonate reduces the absorption of oral tetracycline in humans. One suggested mechanism for this effect is the insolubility of the drug at higher pH in the stomach resulting from the bicarbonate.[44] Another report has suggested that the tetracycline capsule itself is responsible for the decrease in absorption because the capsule does not dissolve in neutral or basic solutions.[45] Lincomycin failed to clear up a severe dental infection because the absorption of the drug was inhibited by cyclamates that were inadvertently ingested with the drug.[46]

Tetracyclines and erythromycin effectively antagonize the antimicrobial activity of simultaneously administered penicillin, and the simultaneous administration of either of these two agents with penicillin to treat infection is contraindicated.[47-49] The mechanism of this effect probably results from the fact that penicillin is most effective against bacteria during the stage of rapid multiplication, and tetracyclines reduce this rapid rate of bacterial multiplication. There is some evidence to indicate an antagonism between lincomycin and erythromycin,[50] although a mechanism of action and clinical significance have yet to be established. Lincomycin and erythromycin have similar antimicrobial activity, and indications for their simultaneous use in dentistry should be rare, if at all. The possibility of antagonism is further reason to avoid any use of the two drugs together.

Some important clinical interactions have been observed with penicillins and cephalosporins. Probenecid produces increased plasma levels of unbound penicillin.[51] This action occurs by two mechanisms: the inhibition of the renal tubular secretion of penicillin and the displacement of penicillin from plasma protein binding sites. Also, salicylates, sulfonamides, and para-aminobenzoic acid have been shown in humans to displace penicillin from protein binding sites in the serum.[52] Both of these interactions of penicillin cause an enhancement of its antimicrobial activity in vivo. Probenecid and phenylbutazone interact with cephalosporins by competing for renal tubular secretion. This results in a decrease in the renal secretion of cephalosporins and an increase in the serum levels—most likely causing an increase in its antimicrobial action in the tissues.[53]

Sulfonamides can displace certain sulfonylurea hypoglycemics from plasma protein, particularly tolbutamide, thereby increasing the plasma levels of free drug. This action has resulted in a hypoglycemia coma.[54] Sulfonamides can also cause an increase in anticoagulant response caused by displacement of coumarin-like anticoagulants from plasma protein binding sites. Sulfamethoxypyridazine competes specifically with warfarin for the same binding sites on human serum albumin.[40] Animal studies have indicated that sulfonamides can be displaced from plasma albumin binding sites by agents having greater binding affinity, that is, phenylbutazone and salicylic acid. Clinically, this action has resulted in increased activity of the sulfonamides.[55] It has been demonstrated in vitro that sulfonamide drugs can displace penicillins from plasma protein binding sites.[56] This action may be responsible for the apparent synergism reported for the two drugs.

Sedatives, hypnotics, and tranquilizers

As a general rule, any combination of alcohol, barbiturates, antihistamines, and other central nervous system depressants should be considered with caution, since enhancement of sedation by one another will result. Severe barbiturate intoxication occurred in a patient treated with a MAOI.[57] Phenobarbital has decreased the effectiveness of coumarin anticoagulants and phenytoin in humans by stimulating the formation of hepatic microsomal enzymes necessary for the metabolism and subsequent elimination of these agents.[58] Phenobarbital reportedly has the capability of reducing the plasma concentration and enhancing the renal elimination of the tricyclic antidepressants desipramine and nortriptyline[59] and the analgesic aminopyrine.[60] These effects are also caused by stimulation of metabolic enzymes responsible for the metabolism and elimination of these agents. Phenobarbital also interacts with griseofulvin to reduce the blood levels of this antifungal agent in humans. This effect is reportedly the result of an increased metabolism of griseofulvin.[61] More recently, it has been reported that the intestinal absorption of griseofulvin was inhibited when phenobarbital was administered simultaneously in humans.[62] Codeine has been shown to stimulate the onset and duration of sleep induced by secobarbital in humans—an interaction that results in synergism.[63] Caffeine is able to counteract the hypnotic effect of pentobarbital when administered concomitantly. The effects induced by 250 mg caffeine plus 100 mg pentobarbital were indistinguishable from placebo.[64]

An interaction of potential clinical significance has been reported concerning the potentiation of the hypnotic effects of pentobarbital by quinine in animals. Apparently, quinine acts to inhibit the metabolism and subsequent elimination of pentobarbital from the body.[65] Magnesium and aluminum hydroxides retard gastrointestinal absorption of sodium pentobarbital in rats.[66] This effect resulted in a lowering of blood levels of the barbiturate, which caused a prevention or delay in the onset of sleep. Long-term administration of diazepam has reduced sleep time and serum levels of pentobarbital in rats and humans—an effect attributed to the stimulation of enzymes responsible for the deactivation of the latter.[67]

Chlordiazepoxide has been shown to potentiate the side effects of amitriptyline, which resulted in a condition resembling brain damage.[68] The administration of chlordiazepoxide with antacids reduces the rate of its absorption. Specifically, magnesium and aluminum hydroxide mixture prolonged the mean chloridazepoxide absorption halftime from the gastrointestinal tract from 11 to 24 minutes and delayed achievement of peak blood concentration by 0.5 to 3.0 hours.[69] Patients receiving diazepam and phenytoin (an antiepileptic agent) or chlordiazepoxide and phenytoin may have higher blood levels of the antiepileptic than patients receiving phenytoin therapy without either of the other two drugs.[70] Also, a case of phenytoin toxicity has been reported in which a diazepam derivative, nitrazepam, might have contributed to the high phenytoin plasma levels.[71] Chloral hydrate and glutethimide promote the metabolism of coumarins in humans, thus decreasing their effectiveness.[72]

Miscellaneous agents

Atropine exerts an additive effect when administered simultaneously with various agents. It was shown to potentiate the phenothiazine sedation in humans by an additive central nervous system depressant effect, and it elicited an additive anticholinergic effect with isoniazid.[21,73] Nasal bleeding, acute dryness of the mouth, fissures of the tongue, and cracked lips occurred when diphenhydramine in combination with methaqualone was administered to a patient previously medicated with the antipsychotic agent thioridazine.[74] It was also reported that diphenhydramine in combination with the anticholinergic drugs trihexyphenidyl and imipramine caused a loss of dentition in a patient as a result of prolonged xerostomia.[75] Pyridoxine (vitamin B_6) reportedly reduces the clinical benefits of the antiparkinsonian agent levodopa.[76] Patients taking B-complex vitamins simultaneously with levodopa should be sure that vitamin B_6 is not present. Two cases have been reported in which ascorbic acid (vitamin C) impaired

Table 29-1. Clinically significant dental drug interactions occurring with analgesics

Dental drug	Interacting drug	Resultant effect
Salicylates	Coumarin anticoagulants	Enhanced anticoagulation; possible bleeding episodes
Aspirin	Probenecid; phenylbutazone	Decreased uricosuria
	Sulfonylurea hypoglycemics	Enhanced hypoglycemia
Acetaminophen	Coumarin anticoagulants	Enhanced anticoagulation
Meperidine	Monoamine oxidase inhibitors (MAOIs)	Hypotension and coma
	Phenothiazines; imipramine antidepressants; furazolidone	Enhanced respiratory depression
	Diazepam; amphetamines; neostigmine	Enhanced analgesia
Morphine	Imipramine antidepressants; propranolol	Enhanced respiratory and CNS depression
	Phenothiazines	Enhanced analgesia
Codeine	Aspirin	Enhanced analgesia

the response to warfarin, an oral anticoagulant.[77,78] A subsequent study in several patients revealed no evidence of this interaction, however,[79] and more evidence is needed to determine the clinical significance of this interaction. Finally, replacement of folic acid in folate-deficient patients receiving phenytoin may increase the metabolism of the latter with a resultant decrease in serum phenytoin levels.[80]

PREVENTION

Available to the dentist are extensive compilations of drug interaction information that can be used in preventing possible interactions that could occur through drug prescribing.[81–86] These compilations include descriptions of interactions observed both clinically and in laboratory animals. A classification and description of those interactions of clinical importance to dentistry, however, may be a more efficient approach toward prevention. Drug interactions that may occur in dental practice are summarized in Tables 29-1 to 29-4. The interactions listed are those which have been reported to occur clinically by drugs used in dental practice. For simplicity and ease of reference the interactions are described according to the resultant effects only. The reader is referred to the text for information concerning the mechanisms of these interactions. Drugs

Table 29-2. Clinically significant dental drug interactions occurring with anti-infectives

Dental drug	Interacting drug	Resulting effect
Penicillin	Coumarin anticoagulants	Enhanced anticoagulation
	Probenecid; salicylates; sulfonamides	Enhanced antimicrobial action
	Tetracyclines; erythromycin	Decreased antimicrobial action
Erythromycin	Lincomycin	Decreased antimicrobial action
Tetracyclines	Coumarin anticoagulants	Enhanced anticoagulation
	Antacids; milk; ferrous sulfate; sodium bicarbonate	Decreased oral absorption
Sulfonamides	Coumarin anticoagulants	Enhanced anticoagulation
	Tolbutamide	Increased hypoglycemia
	Salicylates; phenylbutazone	Increased antimicrobial action
Cephalosporins	Probenecid; phenylbutazone	Enhanced antimicrobial action

Table 29-3. Clinically significant dental drug interactions occurring with sedatives-hypnotics

Dental drug	Interacting drug	Resulting effect
Barbiturates	Monoamine oxidase inhibitors (MAOIs)	Severe CNS depression
Phenobarbital	Coumarin anticoagulants	Decreased anticoagulation
	Phenytoin	Decreased effectiveness of phenytoin
	Aminopyrine; tricyclic antidepressants	Enhanced metabolism and renal excretion of these agents
	Griseofulvin	Oral absorption of griseofulvin inhibited
Pentobarbital	Caffeine	Hypnotic effect inhibited
Secobarbital	Codeine	Enhanced hypnotic activity
Benzodiazepines (Librium, Valium)	Phenytoin	Enhanced phenytoin toxicity
Chlordiazepoxide (Librium)	Antacids	Decreased oral absorption
Chloral hydrate	Coumarin anticoagulants	Decreased anticoagulation

Table 29-4. Clinically significant dental drug interactions occurring with miscellaneous drugs

Dental drug	Interacting drug	Resulting effect
Atropine	Phenothiazines	Enhanced sedation
Diphenhydramine	Phenothiazines; anticholinergics (trihexyphenidyl, imipramine)	Acute dryness of mouth
Pyridoxine (vitamin B$_6$)	Levodopa	Inhibits antiparkinson action of levodopa
Ascorbic acid (vitamin C)	Coumarin anticoagulants	Decreased anticoagulation
Folic acid	Phenytoin	Decreased effectiveness of phenytoin

Table 29-5. Drugs used in dental practice having implications in drug interactions

Product	Generic ingredients that have been implicated in drug interactions
Achromycin-V	tetracycline HCl
APC Demerol	aspirin, meperidine HCl
ASA with Codeine Compound	aspirin, codeine phosphate
Ascodeen	aspirin, codeine phosphate
Bancaps-C	acetaminophen, butabarbital sodium, codeine phosphate
Benadryl HCl	diphenhydramine HCl
Compocillin VK	phenoxymethylpenicillin potassium
Darcil	phenethicillin potassium
Darvon	propoxyphene HCl
Darvon with ASA	aspirin, propoxyphene HCl
Darvon Compound	aspirin, propoxyphene HCl
Darvon Compound-65	aspirin, propoxyphene HCl
Darvo-Tran	aspirin, propoxyphene HCl
Declomycin	demethylchlortetracycline HCl
Demerol HCl	meperidine HCl
Demerol APAP	acetaminophen, meperidine HCl
Empirin Compound with Codeine	aspirin, codeine phosphate
Equagesic	aspirin
Fiorinal with Codeine	isobutylallylbarbituric acid, aspirin, codeine phosphate
Librium	chlordiazepoxide
Maxipen	phenethicillin potassium
Medadent	aspirin
Mepergan	meperidine HCl, promethazine
Mysteclin-F	tetracycline phosphate complex
Nembutal Sodium	pentobarbital sodium
Noctec	chloral hydrate
Pentids	potassium penicillin G
Pen-Vee K	phenoxymethylpenicillin potassium
Phenaphen	aspirin
Phenaphen with Codeine	aspirin, codeine phosphate
Phenergan HCl	promethazine HCl
Rondomycin	methacycline HCl
Seconal Sodium	secobarbital sodium
Sumycin	tetracycline phosphate
Terramycin HCl	oxytetracycline HCl
Tetracyn HCl	tetracycline HCl
Tetrex HCl	tetracycline phosphate complex
Tylenol with Codeine	acetaminophen, codeine phosphate
Valium	diazepam
Vibramycin Hyclate	doxycycline hyclate
V-Cillin-K	phenoxymethylpenicillin potassium
Zactirin Compound	aspirin

normally prescribed in dental practice that can involve themselves in interactions are listed in Table 29-5. The generic ingredients that have been implicated in drug interactions are indicated for each trade name drug. Specific interactions of clinical significance for these generic components are described in the text and listed in Tables 29-1 to 29-4.

Practitioners are encouraged to maintain up-to-date drug interaction information such as that discussed in this chapter. The dentist's responsibility to his patients must include predicting possible adverse situations from potential interactions between prescribed drugs and medication the patient has previously taken. The dentist should also not neglect to look for possible adverse situations already present from previous multiple-drug therapy.

In conclusion, it should be noted that a known potential for interaction between two drugs is not an absolute contraindication to their concomitant use. As has been previously noted, some interactions serve therapeutic purposes. Additionally, one must recognize that drug interactions are dose related. One aspirin tablet is unlikely to cause severe hemorrhagic episodes in a patient taking a coumarin anticoagulant. However, the intended use of a course of aspirin in a patient taking these anticoagulants is best discussed with the physician maintaining the anticoagulant dosage. Similarly, the usual dosages of aspirin are unlikely to upset the blood glucose balance of a patient taking hypoglycemics. However, both the dentist and the patient must be aware of this potentiality, and intended high or prolonged doses of aspirin in the patient with poorly controlled diabetes should be discussed with the patient's physician.

When is a potential interaction an absolute contraindication to the use of a specific drug? If not absolutely contraindicated, what doses can be safely used? Answers to these questions can be determined only by (1) knowing the potentialities of the interaction, (2) being aware of the patient's overall health and medical status, and (3) an ability and willingness to discuss intended therapy with the other practitioner (physician or dentist) who has instituted earlier therapy.

REFERENCES

1. Cluff, L. E., Thornton, G. F., and Seidle, L. G.: Studies on the epidemiology of adverse drug reactions, J.A.M.A. **188**:976-983. 1964.
2. Stuart, D. M.: Drug metabolism, Pharm. Index, Sept.-Oct., 1968.
3. Kristensen, M., and Hansen, J. M.: Potentiation of the tolbutamide effect by Dicumarol, Diabetes **16**:211, 1967.
4. Zubrod, C. G., Kennedy, T. J., and Shannon, J. A.: Studies on the chemotherapy of the human malarias. VIII. The physiological disposition of pamaquine, J. Clin. Invest. **27**:114-120, 1948.
5. Burns, J. J., and Conney, A. H.: Enzyme stimulation and inhibition in the metabolism of drugs, Proc. R. Soc. Med. **58**:955-960, 1965.
6. Shee, J. C.: Dangerous potentiation of pethidine by iproniazid and its treatment, Br. Med. J. **2**:507-509, 1960.
7. Vigran, I. M.: Potentiation of meperidine by pargyline, J.A.M.A. **187**:953-954, 1964.
8. Eade, N. R., and Renton, K. W.: The effect of phenelzine and tranylcypromine on the degradation of meperidine, J. Pharmacol. Exp. Ther. **173**:31-36, 1970.
9. Hoffman, J. C., and Smith, J. C.: The respiratory effects of meperidine and propiomazine in man, Anesthesiology **32**(4):325-331, 1970.
10. Lambertsen, C. T., Wendel, H., and Longenhagen, J. B.: The separate and combined respiratory effects of chlorpromazine and meperidine in normal men controlled at 46 mm Hg alveolar P_{CO_2}, J. Pharmacol. Exp. Ther. **131**:381-393, 1961.
11. Morton, W. R., and Turnbull, W.: Promazine and meperidine (Sparidol-50), an efficient combination for preoperative medication, Can. Med. Assoc. J. **90**:1257-1259, 1964.
12. Goodman, L. S., and Gilman, A.: The pharmacological basis of therapeutics, ed. 4, New York, 1970, The Macmillan Co., pp. 250-251.
13. Goodman, L. S., and Gilman, A.: The pharmacologic basis of therapeutics, ed. 4, New York, 1970, The Macmillan Co., p. 258.
14. Niswander, K. R.: Effect of diazepam on meperidine required of patients during labor, Obstet. Gynecol. **34**:62-67, 1969.
15. Christensen, E. M., and Gross, E. G.: Analgesic effects in human subjects of morphine, meperidine and methadone, J.A.M.A. **137**:594-597, 1948.
16. Houde, R. W., Wallenstein, S. L., and Beaver, W. T.: Clinical measurement of pain. In deStevens, G., editor: Analgetics, New York, 1965, Academic Press, Inc., pp. 75-122.
17. Herz, A.: The effect of central inhibiting and stimulating actions of morphine by anticholinergic, nicotinolytic and antihistaminics in the rat, Arch. Exp. Pathol. Pharmakol. **241**:253-263, 1961.
18. Eerola, R.: The combined action of morphine and atropine: an experimental study with mice, Ann. Med. Exp. Biol. Fenn. **40**:83-90, 1962.
19. Gupta, G. P., and Dhawan, B. N.: Potentiation of morphine analgesia by mecamylamine, Arch. Int. Pharmacodyn. Ther. **134**:54-60, 1961.
20. Sethy, V. H., Pradham, R. J., Mandrekar, S. S., and Sheth, V. K.: Role of brain amines in the analgesic action of meperidine hydrochloride, Psychopharmacologia **17**:320-326, 1970.
21. Hartshorn, E. A.: In Franke, D. E., editor: Handbook of drug interactions, Cincinnati, 1970, D. E. Franke.
22. Dunphy, T. W.: The pharmacist's role in the prevention of adverse drug interactions, Am. J. Hosp. Pharm. **26**:366-377, 1969.

23. Weiner, M.: Effect of centrally active drugs on the action of coumarin anticoagulants, Nature **212:** 1599-1600, 1966.

24. Anticoagulant therapy—a selected bibliography, 1968, Endo Laboratories, p. 49.

25. Roos, J., and van Joost, H. E.: The cause of bleeding during anticoagulant treatment, Acta Med. Scand. **178:**129-131, 1965.

26. Sandler, A. I.: Interactions of oral coumarin anticoagulants. In Franke, D. E., editor: Handbook of drug interactions, Cincinnati, 1970, D. E. Franke, pp. 72-74.

27. Antlitz, A. M., Mead, J. A., and Tolentino, M. A.: Potentiation of oral anticoagulant therapy by acetaminophen, Curr. Ther. Res. **10:**501-508, 1968.

28. Krakoff, I. H.: Clinical pharmacology of drugs which influence uric acid production and excretion, Clin. Pharmacol. Ther. **8:**124-138, 1967.

29. Hussar, D. A.: Therapeutic incompatibilities: drug interactions, Hosp. Pharm. 3(8):14-24, 1968.

30. Peaston, M. J. T., and Finnegan, P.: A case of combined poisoning with chlorpropamide, aspirin and paracetamol, Br. J. Clin. Pract. **22:**30-31, 1968.

31. Wishinsky, H.: Protein interactions of sulfonylurea compounds, Diabetes 2(supp.):18-25, 1962.

32. Klinenburg, J. R., and Miller, F.: Effect of corticosteroids on blood salicylate concentrations, J.A.M.A. **194:**601-604, 1965.

33. Huang, C. L., and Hirano, K.: The effect of antipyretic analgesics on the metabolism of chlorpromazine in man, Biochem. Pharmacol. **16:**2023-2026, 1967.

34. Schnell, R. C., and Miya, T. S.: Increased ileal absorption of salicylic acid induced by carbonic anhydrase inhibition, Biochem. Pharmacol. **19:**303-305, 1970.

35. Lunde, P. K. M.: Plasma protein binding of diphenylhydantoin in man: interaction with other drugs and the effect of temperature and plasma dilution, Clin. Pharmacol. Ther. **11:**846, 1970.

36. Toakley, J. G.: "Dilantin" overdosage, Med. J. Aust. **2:**639-640, 1968.

37. McDougal, M. R.: Interaction of drugs with aspirin, J. Am. Pharm. Assoc. **10:**83-85, 1970.

38. Widerholt, I. C.: Recurrent episodes of hypoglycemia induced by propoxyphene, Neurology **17:** 703-706, 1967.

39. Buckle, R. M., and Guillebaud, J.: Hypoglycaemic coma occurring during treatment with chlorpromazine and orphenadrine, Br. Med. J. **4:**599-600, 1967.

40. Hussar, D. A.: Oral anticoagulants—their interactions, J. Am. Pharm. Assoc. **10:**78-82, 1970.

41. Kunin, C. M., and Finland, M.: Clinical pharmacology of the tetracycline antibiotics, Clin. Pharmacol. Ther. **2:**51-69, 1961.

42. Risk of drug interaction may exist in 1 of 13 prescriptions, J.A.M.A. **220:**1287, 1972.

43. Neuvonen, P. J., Gothoni, G., Hackman, R., and Bjorkstein, K.: Interference of iron with the absorption of tetracyclines in man, Br. Med. J. **4:**532-534, 1970.

44. Barr, W. H., Adir, J., and Garrettson, L.: Decrease of tetracycline absorption in man by sodium bicarbonate, Clin. Pharmacol. Ther. **12:**779-784, 1971.

45. Elliott, G. R., and Armstrong, M. F.: Sodium bicarbonate and oral tetracycline, Clin. Pharmacol. Therap. **13:**459, 1972.

46. Francis, L., and Kutscher, A. H.: Why teach pharmacology to dental students—multidisciplinary commentary, J. Dent. Educ. **34:**51-58, 1970.

47. Lepper, M. H., and Dowling, H. F.: Treatment of pneumococcic meningitis with penicillin compared with penicillin plus aureomycin: studies including observations on an apparent antagonism between penicillin and aureomycin, Arch. Intern. Med. **88:**489-494, 1951.

48. Jawetz, E.: The use of combinations of antimicrobial drugs, Ann. Rev. Pharmacol. **8:**151, 1968.

49. Ritschel W. A.: Therapeutic incompatibilities between penicillin and other antibiotics administered intravenously, Drug Intelligence 3:355, 1969.

50. A second look at lincomycin (Lincocin), Med. Letter **11:**107, 1969.

51. Gibaldi, M., and Schwartz, M. A.: Apparent effect of probenecid on the distribution of penicillins in man, Clin. Pharmacol. Ther. **9:**345-349, 1968.

52. Kunin, C. M.: Clinical pharmacology of the new penicillins. II. Effect of drugs which interfere with binding to serum proteins, Clin. Pharmacol. Ther. **7:**180-188, 1966.

53. Kabins, S. A.: Interactions among antibiotics and other drugs, J.A.M.A. **219:**206-212, 1972.

54. Christensen, L. K., Hasen, J. M., and Kristensen, M.: Sulphaphenazole-induced hypoglycemic attacks in tolbutamide-treated diabetics, Lancet **2:**1298-1301, 1963.

55. Anton, A. H.: A drug induced change in the distribution and renal excretion of sulfonamides, J. Pharmacol. Exp. Ther. **129:**282-288, 1960.

56. Kunin, C. M.: Enhancement of antimicrobial activity of penicillins and other antibiotics in human serum by competitive serum binding inhibitors, Proc. Soc. Exp. Biol. Med. **117:**69-72, 1964.

57. Domino, E. F., Sullivan, T. S., and Luby, E. D.: Barbiturate intoxication in a patient treated with MAO inhibitor, Am. J. Psychiatry **118:**941-943, 1962.

58. Cucinell, S. A., Conney, A. H., Sansur, M., and Burns, J. J.: Drug interaction in man. I. Lowering effect of phenobarbital on plasma levels of bishydroxycoumarin (Dicumarol) and diphenylhydantoin (Dilantin), Clin. Pharmacol. Ther. **6:**420-429, 1965.

59. Hammer, W., and Sjoqvist, F.: Plasma levels of monomethylated tricyclic antidepressants during treatment with imipramine-like compounds, Life Sci. **6:**1895-1902, 1967.

60. Kampffmeyer, H. G.: Failure to detect increased elimination rate of phenacetin in man after treatment with phenobarbital, Klin. Wochenschr. **42:** 1237, 1238, 1969.

61. Bushfield, D., Child, K. J., and Atkinson, R. M.: An effect of phenobarbitone on blood levels of griseofulvin in man, Lancet **2:**1042-1043, 1963.

62. Riegelman, S., Rowland, M., and Epstein, W. L.: Griseofulvin-phenobarbital interaction in man, J.A.M.A. **213:**426-431, 1970.

63. Bellville, J. W., Forrest, W. H., Shroff, P., and Brown, B. W.: The hypnotic effects of codeine and secobarbital and their interaction in man, Clin. Pharmacol. Ther. **12:**607-612, 1971.

64. Forrest, W. H., Bellville, J. W., and Brown, B. W.: The interaction of caffeine with pentobarbital as a nighttime hypnotic, Anesthesiology **36:**37-41, 1972.

65. Boulos, B. M., Short, C. R., and Davis, L. E.:

Quinine and quinidine inhibition of pentobarbital metabolism, Biochem. Pharmacol. **9:**723-732, 1970.

66. Hurwitz, A., and Sheehan, M. B.: The effects of antacids on the absorption of orally administered pentobarbital in the rat, J. Pharmacol. Exp. Ther. **179:**124-131, 1972.
67. Heubel, F.: Interferenz von diazepam und pentobarbital an der ratte und am menschen, Arch. Exp. Pathol. Pharmakol. **264:**246-247, 1969.
68. Kane, F. J., and Taylor, T. W.: A toxic reaction to combine Elavil-Librium therapy, Am. J. Psychiatry **119:**1179-1180, 1963.
69. Greenblatt, D. J., Shader, R. I., Harmatz, J. S., Franke, K., and Koch-Weser, J.: Influence of magnesium and aluminum hydroxide mixture on chlordiazepoxide absorption, Clin. Pharmacol. Ther. **19:**234-239, 1976.
70. Vajda, F. J. E.: Interaction between phenytoin and the benzodiazepines, Br. Med. J. **1:**346, 1971.
71. Treasure, T., and Toseland, P. A.: Hyperglycaemia due to phenytoin toxicity, Arch, Dis. Child. **46:**563, 1971.
72. Cucinell, S. A., Odessky, L., Weiss, M., and Dayton, P. G.: The effect of chloral hydrate on bishydroxycoumarin metabolism, J.A.M.A. **197:**366-368, 1966.
73. Gershon, C., Neubauer, H., and Sundland, D. M.: Interaction between some anticholinergic agents and phenothiazines: potentiation of phenothiazine sedation and its antagonisms, Clin. Pharmacol. Ther. **6:**749-754, 1965.

74. Kessell, A., Williams, A. G., Young, J. D. C., and Jensen, G. R.: Side effects of a new hypnotic: drug potentiation, Med. J. Aust. **2:**1194-1195, 1967.
75. Winer, J. A., and Bahn, S.: Loss of teeth with antipressant drug therapy, Arch. Gen. Psychiatry **16:** 239-240, 1967.
76. Cotzias, G. C.: Metabolic modification of some neurologic disorders, J.A.M.A. **210:**1255-1262, 1969.
77. Rosenthal, G.: Interaction of ascorbic acid and warfarin, J.A.M.A. **215:**1671, 1971.
78. Smith, E. C.: Interaction of ascorbic acid and warfarin, J.A.M.A. **221:**1166, 1972.
79. Hume, R.: Interaction of ascorbic acid and warfarin, J.A.M.A. **219:**1479, 1972.
80. Baylis, E. M.: Influence of folic acid on bloodphenytoin levels, Lancet **1:**62, 1971.
81. Hansten, P. D.: Drug interactions, ed. 2, Philadelphia, 1973, Lea & Febiger.
82. Evaluation of drug interactions, ed. 2, Washington, D.C., 1976, American Pharmaceutical Association.
83. Swidler, G.: Handbook of drug interactions, New York, 1971, John Wiley & Sons, Inc.
84. Garb, S.: Clinical guide to undesirable drug interactions and interferences, New York, 1971, Springer Publishing Co., Inc.
85. Cohon, M. S.: Therapeutic drug interactions, Madison, Wis., 1970, The University of Wisconsin Medical Center.
86. Carson, J. A.: Drug interaction manual, Danville, Ill., 1970, Danville Pharmaceutical Publishing Co.

30

Drug abuse

BARBARA F. ROTH-SCHECHTER

The following chapter is directed toward familiarizing the reader with a discussion of the presently most widely abused psychoactive drugs (drugs capable of changing behavior or inducing psychosis-like reactions or both). The concept of using drugs to produce profound effects on mood, thought, and feeling is as old as civilization itself; only the kind of substances used for that purpose seems to change. Because of the vastly increased number of drugs made available to the clinician in recent history, the number and kind of misused substances expanded by an equal extent. The agents used for their psychoactive properties can be conveniently subdivided into those which are otherwise of therapeutic value (narcotics, sedatives, alcohol, sympathomimetic central nervous system stimulants) and those which are of no known therapeutic value (the psychedelics of various chemical groups). This chapter will deal with the various aspects of their abuse only; for their pharmacologic properties and therapeutic usefulness the reader is referred to their respective chapters. The legal aspects covering dispensing are presented in Chapter 4.

DEFINITIONS AND GENERAL ASPECTS

If abuse is defined as misuse of any drug in a way unacceptable to present medical understanding and/or social customs,[1] any discussion on drug abuse in its broadest sense would have to include a presentation of a vast spectrum of drugs, for example, agents like laxatives, vitamins, and antibiotics, to name just a few widely misused groups of drugs. This chapter, however, will discuss only the abuse of drugs that produce changes in mood and behavior, drugs misused for their psychoactive properties.

In this frame of reference *psychological dependence* is defined as a state of mind in which the individual believes he is unable to maintain optimal performance without having taken his drug and therefore knows no limits in his means of securing it. Psychological dependence varies in severity from mild desire to compulsive obsession (compulsive drug use) with the attainment of the drug. With prolonged self-administration the individual probably will (but does not have to) develop tolerance to and physical dependence on the drug. *Tolerance* to a psychoactive drug is characterized by the necessity to increase the dosage continually to achieve the desired effect, or otherwise the effect obtained with the same dose is continually diminishing. In this discussion of abuse of psychoactive drugs the type of tolerance referred to is central tolerance, that is, consisting of a definite, decreased responsiveness of brain tissue to constantly increasing amounts of drug. Tolerance of metabolic origin, that is, tolerance attributable to an accelerated rate of metabolism of the drug, is excluded in this discussion. Suffice it to say that development of metabolic tolerance is an insignificant factor contributing to the tolerance observed in humans to most of the psychoactive drugs.

Physical dependence refers to the altered physiologic state resulting from constantly rising drug concentrations. The presence of physical dependence is established by the occurrence of a *withdrawal syndrome*, a combination of many drug-specific symptoms that occur on acute discontinuance of drug administration. At present, it is generally agreed that physical dependence and withdrawal syndrome are caused by drug-induced changes at the cellular level. Most widely investigated have been those occurring in the central nervous system. Established alterations include changes in neurotransmitter levels, various enzyme levels and/or activities, permeability and excitability characteristics, and many more. Of course, any definite cause-effect relationship remains to be established.

Addiction is a term that has been almost as much misused as the drugs it attempts to characterize. Any use of this term has to be preceded by its definition. The present discussion will concern the specific symptomatology introduced earlier.

Drugs that produce tolerance and physical dependence can be grouped according to their ability to substitute for each other (Table 30-1). For example, different narcotics can be administered to maintain a desired effect, and no withdrawal syndrome will be experienced; however, a barbiturate cannot be substituted for a narcotic. Therefore narcotics and barbiturates do not belong to the same group of dependence-producing drugs. This phenomenon of substitution and withdrawal suppression between different drugs is called *cross-tolerance* or *cross-dependence*, and it is observed between the members of the same group but not between groups (Table 30-1). Cross-tolerance may be partial or complete and appears to be determined more by the pharmacologic action of the drug rather than by its chemistry.

Although most characteristics of drug abuse are determined by the individual drug involved, two more generalizations can be made: The time required to produce physical dependence is shortest when a rapidly metabolized drug is involved and is longest when a slowly metabolized drug of the same group is compared. Equally, the time course of withdrawal reactions can be related to a large extent to the half-life of the drug. Those with the longest half-life may not produce any symptoms for several days after withdrawal, those with the shortest half-life will produce acute reactions within hours after withdrawal.

NARCOTIC ANALGESICS

Heroin, methadone, and morphine are presently the most popular but not the only members of narcotic analgesics that are being abused. The narcotics sold illegally on the street may be adulterated with quinine, lidocaine, mannitol, or almost anything else imaginable. The present discussion can only focus on the pharmacology of the nonadulterated narcotics, primarily the aforementioned drugs. When relevant, other agents are mentioned. In addition to being analgesics, the opium alkaloids produce a state in humans described as complete satiation of all drives. Morphine and its derivatives elevate the mood, causing euphoria in many patients; they relieve fear and apprehension and produce a feeling of peace and tranquility. They also suppress hunger, reduce sexual desires, and diminish an individual's response to provocation. However, routine function and productive work of an individual are not incompatible with regular use of these drugs. Thus, in the presence of morphinelike drugs, the abuser is a satisfied, complacent, and highly cooperative individual. It seems worth while emphasizing here that this is in stark contrast to the alcohol abuser, who, in the presence of *his* drug is generally quarrelsome, dissatisfied, highly uncooperative, and of reduced productivity to society. In addition to its drive-reducing properties, when morphine is administered intravenously, it will produce a comfortable warm flushing of the skin, likened by abusers to sexual orgasm. Undoubtedly, initial abuse will be reinforced by these "positive" experiences described so far. With the development of physical

Table 30-1. Drugs that produce tolerance and dependence

Group	Tolerance	Physical dependence	Psychological dependence
Narcotic analgesics	++++	+++	++++
Sedative hypnotics, alcohol, and minor tranquilizers	++	++++	++
CNS stimulants except cocaine	++++	±(?)	++++
Cocaine	0	0	++++
Hallucinogens, LSD, marihuana	++	0	+

dependence (see later), however, the driving motivation to obtain the drug gradually becomes more and more "negative." The fear of having to experience the withdrawal syndrome and its suffering begins to override any other motivation. Only then does the addict resort to criminal activities and violence, these then being secondary effects of opioid dependence and not psychopharmacologic actions of the drugs.

Pattern of abuse. Heroin and other narcotic analgesics are administered by the abuser mostly by the parenteral route. The signs and symptoms of an acute overdose are the same for almost all members of this group. They consist of fixed pinpoint pupils, cyanosis and/or depressed respiration, hypotension and shock, slow or absent reflexes, and drowsiness or coma. The rate at which physical dependence and tolerance develop depends on the frequency of administration. Tolerance does not develop to *all* pharmacologic effects of narcotics. It primarily develops to the euphorigenic, analgesic, sedative, and respiratory depressant actions. Tolerance rarely develops to miotic and constipatory actions.

It is equally significant that with the development of tolerance the lethal dose is greatly increased. Thus, as long as intake is maintained, excessively large doses can eventually be tolerated without any respiratory or cardiovascular complications. Cross-tolerance with all other narcotic analgesics is a common finding and is apparently independent of the chemical configuration of the narcotic. There is no cross-tolerance between the narcotics and the sedative hypnotics or with alcohol. Symptomatology and time course of the withdrawal syndrome are determined by the specific drug abused, the dose and rate of drug administration, the duration of abuse, and of course, the general physiologic state of the individual. Discontinuation of drug administration will result in the withdrawal syndrome beginning at the time of the abuser's next scheduled dose, or it can be precipitated within minutes by the administration of a narcotic antagonist.

In the case of morphine or heroin the first signs of withdrawal are yawning, lacrimation, rhinorrhea, and perspiration, followed by a restless, tiring sleep. With further abstinence anorexia, tremors, irritability, weakness, and excessive gastrointestinal activity are experienced. Heart rate is rapid, blood pressure is elevated, and chills alternate with excessive sweating. The presence of gooseflesh and widely dilated pupils is considered one objective sign of narcotic withdrawal. Peak intensity is usually reached between 48 and 72 hours after the last dose of heroin or morphine. All of these physiologic symptoms are increasingly accompanied by varying degrees of desperation and fear. The individual undergoing withdrawal is usually fully aware of the fact that at any point in this ordeal the administration of a dose of narcotic would completely block all withdrawal symptoms and alleviate his misery. Without any treatment observable symptoms disappear around the eighth day after the last dose.

Management of acute overdose and withdrawal. If hypopnea due to a narcotic overdose (coma, pinpoint pupils) is suspected, narcotic antagonists should be used immediately. This is safe, since apnea due to barbiturates or other drugs will not be made worse by treatment with naloxone (Narcan), the drug of choice. If respirations do not increase within minutes, opiate overdose is unlikely. If no narcotic antagonist is available, manual or mechanical artificial respiration with the use of oxygen and airway is necessary. Drugs to raise the blood pressure and plasma expanders are used for the treatment of shock; other signs and symptoms have to be treated individually and supportively.

The immediate withdrawal reaction from a street narcotic is only moderately distressing to the patient because of poor drug quality. Most patients can be made comfortable with the administration of methadone, 20 mg orally. For the relief of tension a phenothiazine or a benzodiazepine is sufficient.

The underlying principles in long-term withdrawal and rehabilitation reactions to opiates are (1) substitution of a physiologically equivalent drug and (2) gradual weaning from the substitute. Pharmacologically, this treatment is based on (1) the existence of cross-tolerance between morphinelike drugs and (2) the inverse relationship between duration of drug action and intensity of withdrawal symptomatology outlined earlier.

Medically, methadone detoxification and methadone maintenance are presently advocated by many as treatments of choice. In either case, methadone is administered orally and as such does not produce the usual narcotic euphoria. It will produce a definite tolerance to all other opiate-like drugs, and it wholly or partly, depending on dose, will block the effects of heroin. If detoxification and abstinence are the ultimate goals, methadone is administered throughout the initial psychotherapeutic phase. Because of the long half-life of methadone, in psychologically prepared individuals, it can then be slowly withdrawn without the occurrence of profound withdrawal symptoms.

Methadone maintenance is advocated as the most successful long-term treatment for many heroin abusers.[2] Methadone maintenance can be considered an open-ended therapeutic regimen, where the patient is "maintained" with no narcotic hunger, no need to increase the dose, and no fear of withdrawal symptoms until some unspecified time. The overall objective of this approach is to return the individual as a useful member of society. Aside from impotence and constipation, there are no other presently known side effects from using oral methadone for as long as several years.

The most recent drug advocated for the same purpose is alpha-acetylmethadol, a congener of methadone.[3] It has the same set of effects as methadone, differing only in that acetylmethadol is effective for a 2- to 3-day period in contrast to the 24-hour relief afforded by methadone.

Another approach to the long-term management of narcotic abuse is long-term blockade of the narcotic receptor. This is achieved by maintaining the patient on a specific narcotic antagonist (naloxone, cyclazocine) after the completion of withdrawal. Although these drugs do not reduce narcotic craving, they do prevent the positive reinforcement from "shooting" the narcotic because of the blockade. However, cyclazocine has some agonist actions and thus poses an abuse potential of its own. A discussion of advantages and disadvantages of methadone maintenance and the use of narcotic antagonists is beyond the scope of this chapter. Both approaches are presently under active clinical investigation, and their impact and success of conquering opiate abuse remain to be established.

SEDATIVE HYPNOTICS AND ALCOHOL

Previously, this group of abused psychoactive drugs included only the barbiturates and alcohol. But the introduction of many new sedatives and antianxiety agents in the past 20 years has extended the range considerably. It now additionally includes drugs like glutethimide, meprobamate, chlordiazepoxide, diazepam, and methaqualone. Still, barbiturates are the most widely misused among the sedative drugs. In this context of their abuse, drugs in the category of central nervous system depressants can be discussed together.

At least four different types of barbiturate-like drug abusers can be identified. However, they do not constitute clear-cut entities but overlap to some extent. In the first group are those individuals abusing the drug for its sedative effect to deal with their various states of emotional distress. The second group of abusers seek the drug for its paradoxical action of excitation, which seems to constitute a release phenomenon in which the drug impairs certain psychological inhibitory mechanisms. A similar paradoxical stimulation is observed in many individuals after tolerance has been developed. Such individuals often use a combination of amphetamines plus barbiturates to obtain more elevation of mood than either drug can produce alone. The mechanism of this superadditive effect is not yet understood. The third group of individuals misuse barbiturates to counteract abuse effects of various stimulant drugs to obtain a cyclical pattern of stimulation-sedation. In the fourth category a sedative hypnotic is abused, together with other types of drugs, such as alcohol or opiates or both. The purpose of such combination may be an attempt to counteract withdrawal effects from the first drug, or it can be to obtain effects that surpass those of either drug alone.

Initial symptomatology obtained with any of the drugs of this category resembles the well-known symptomatology of alcohol intoxication. The symptoms of the paradoxical reaction can range from mild elation to excessive stimulation; symptoms from abuse of sedative hypnotics in combination with other drugs are unpredictable. With varying onset, determined by the drug abused, the symptoms consist of general sluggishness, difficulty in thinking, comprehension, and attention, slowness in speech, faulty sensory judgment, and sometimes quarrelsomeness and moroseness.

Under prolonged misuse of these drugs, again, either depressive or stimulative actions may be the overriding manifestation. Several psychological changes occur in either situation: Emotional instability, hostile and paranoid ideations, and suicidal tendencies are common.

Pattern of abuse. In the majority of cases central nervous system (CNS)–depressant drugs are administered by the oral route, yet parenteral administration is not uncommon, either. An acute overdose of any one of the CNS depressants produces essentially the same syndrome, with major complications arising from the depression of respiratory and cardiovascular functions: An overdose can lead to coma with depressed respiration and hypotension. The pupils may be unchanged or small, and lateral nystagmus is present. Confusion, slurred speech, and ataxia are always present. In comparison with the narcotic analgesics, barbiturates and sedative hypnotics have a slower onset of tolerance and physical dependence. Furthermore, tolerance to the sedative effects is not accompanied by a comparable increase in the lethal dose of these drugs. There is complete cross-tolerance between all members of this general CNS–depressant type, including alcohol.

The withdrawal syndrome is equally similar for all these drugs, but only its time course depends to a great extent on the half-life of disappearance of the drug in question. The benzodiazepines and the long-acting barbiturates may not produce symptoms for as long as 48 hours after withdrawal, and the reaction may be attenuated over time, with seizures not appearing until a week or more after discontinuation of the drug. The first signs of the withdrawal syndrome from CNS depressants are insomnia, weakness, and a tremulous restlessness. Often a high temperature and a large degree of agitation occur. Delirium and convulsions may be culminating in cardiovascular collapse and loss of the temperature-regulating mechanism. Meprobamate and short-acting barbiturates, on the other hand, produce acute reactions similar to those from alcohol.

Alcohol-withdrawal syndrome is clearly a CNS–depressant withdrawal syndrome, but it does have additional features worth pointing out. It begins within a few hours after the last drink and consists of the same initial symptoms as those from general CNS depressants: nausea, vomiting, weakness, anxiety, and perspiration. Extensive tremors are then accompanied by alcohol-specific hallucinations. These develop into the well-known delirium tremens. Hyperthermia and cardiovascular complications are more common than in barbiturate withdrawal, whereas seizures and convulsions are less common and less severe. Without treatment, recovery from alcohol withdrawal is within 7 days; that from other CNS depressants varies depending on the drug involved.

Management of acute overdose and withdrawal. The most important consideration after an acute overdose of a CNS depressant is support of the cardiovascular and respiratory functions. An airway must be established and maintained. Early gastric lavage after intubation and dialysis can assist in removal of the drug. Analeptic drugs and stimulants may be harmful and are not to be given.

In contrast to withdrawal from narcotics, withdrawal from CNS depressants can be life threatening, and the patient should be hospitalized. Abrupt withdrawal of any CNS depressant, including alcohol, is not considered safe medically. The two major principles of treatment are (1) replacement of the abused drug with a pharmacologically or physiologically equivalent drug in the acute situation and (2) gradual withdrawal of the equivalent drug for prolonged withdrawal. Drugs like pentobarbital, paraldehyde, and chloral hydrate have been standard agents for substitution during acute withdrawal of CNS depressants, but sedatives without respiratory depressant action have been found to be safer.[4] Chlordiazepoxide or diazepam is considered by many to be the drug of choice. Chlorpromazine and hydroxyzine by comparison have been found considerably less efficacious, and they also pose the danger of lowering seizure threshold, thus aggravating the tendency of withdrawal seizures. Gradual withdrawal of the substitute drug together with psychotherapy can then be accomplished over a matter of weeks.

At the time of its discovery, disulfiram was hailed as the panacea in the postwithdrawal treatment of chronic alcoholism. Given by itself, disulfiram is a relatively nontoxic substance in humans. However, it significantly alters the metabolism and thus the effects of subsequently administered ethyl alcohol. Biochemically, this results in the accumulation of acetaldehyde, and consequently the resulting clinical syndrome is referred to as acetaldehyde syndrome. It consists of pulsating headache, dyspnea, nausea, and vomiting, followed by hypotension, weakness, and vertigo. The reaction starts a few minutes after the intake of alcohol and lasts between 30 minutes and several hours. It must be appreciated that disulfiram thus is not a cure of chronic alcoholism but merely afford the volunteer a crutch to stop drinking by acting as a deterrent.

SYMPATHOMIMETIC CENTRAL NERVOUS SYSTEM STIMULANTS

The sympathomimetic CNS stimulants are abused for their ability to produce at least initially, a euphoric elevation of mood and a sense of increased energy and alertness. Although they do not seem to improve physical performance per se, these drugs may improve competitive performances by decreasing fatigue and boredom. Almost all CNS stimulants are also appetite suppressants and have an entire spectrum of sympathomimetic effects. (See Chapter 10.)

The most widely abused members of this class are amphetamine, dextroamphetamine, diethylpropion, methylphenidate, and cocaine. The pharmacology of cocaine is presented in Chapter 14. Although cocaine produces CNS stimulatory effects much like the amphetamines, there are significant differences in some characteristics of their abuse (Table 30-1). The discussion of abused CNS stimulants focuses on the amphetamines, and deviations from that pattern are pointed out when necessary. CNS stimulants are administered by the oral as well as intravenous route. Some abusers develop a mild form of psychic dependence in which, although believing that the drugs are essential to maintain their daily routine, the abusers do not increase the dosage much beyond usual therapeutic limits. The more prevalent pattern of abuse is the one in which the person self-administers the drug with increasing frequency and in increasing amounts.

Symptoms and signs of an acute overdose of CNS stimulants consist of the following: The pupils are dilated and reactive, blood pressure and pulse are elevated, and cardiac arrhythmias may occur. The patient has a dry mouth, is sweating, and has a slight-to-moderate temperature. Fine tremors may be present, and most often the patient exhibits a hyperactive stereotyped behavior.

Tolerance develops to the central sympathomimetic effects, no tolerance seems to develop to the tendency to induce a toxic psychosis at higher doses. Modest levels of prolonged abuse of stimulants do not produce any withdrawal reaction of consequence—in most cases only general fatigue and prolonged sleep. Withdrawal from some of the monumental doses used (as much as 10 Gm methamphetamine taken intravenously daily) will precipitate a withdrawal syndrome consisting of muscular achiness, a ravenous appetite with abdominal pain, which is followed by a long period of sleep. On awakening a profound psychological depression, sometimes suicidal, sets in. During that period definite electroencephalographic abnormalities have been observed.

The effects of cocaine are similar to those observed after the intravenous administration of amphetamines. However, its action is brief, which may be the reason for the absence of tolerance to and withdrawal reactions from this drug. (See Table 30-1.)

Management of acute overdose and withdrawal. Treatment of an acute overdose of a CNS stimulant includes a phenothiazine for the CNS symptoms and a short-acting receptor blocking agent if hypertension is severe. Abrupt withdrawal without any medication is not life threatening, but individuals can be made more comfortable with sedatives or tranquilizers for a few days. If severe depression occurs, a tricyclic antidepressant is indicated. One should also keep in mind that prolonged abuse of CNS stimulants is accompanied by prolonged appetite suppression, and thus nutritional deficiencies are likely to have occurred. Part of the long-term management of withdrawal is correction of the nutritional disturbances.

The most serious sociologic problem with stimulant abuse, especially in a young population of abusers, is the induction of mental abnormalities. Although it was formerly believed that many of the reactions observed during use of or withdrawal from stimulants were exaggerations of preexisting psychopathology, experimental evidence suggest that amphetamine psychosis can be quickly induced in previously unaffected volunteer subjects.[5]

There are several other therapeutically useful drugs that are misused for their psychoactive properties that do not fall into any of the pharmacologic categories discussed earlier. Of these, the anticholinergics (scopolamine, phencyclidine) deserve special mention, since their misuse is still fairly common. The principal signs of acute intoxication with anticholinergics are dry mouth, blurred vision, dilated pupils, rapid pulse, fever, and delirium. The treatment of choice is an intramuscular injection of physostigmine. Tolerance and dependence to these drugs have not been reported.

PSYCHEDELICS (HALLUCINOGENS)

Although the drugs discussed below are usually grouped in a separate category, their central actions are not really substantially different from many other centrally active stimulant drugs. It seems that their separate coverage is perpetuated because of two factors: (1) They are capable of inducing states of altered perception and (2) they do not have any general therapeutic usefulness of medical acceptance. The drugs to be discussed in this limited presentation are some of the indolealkylamines, such as lysergic acid diethylamide (LSD), psilocybin, psilocin, dimethyltryptamine (DMT), some of the phenylethylamines such as mescaline, and some of the cannabinols such as marihuana. Clearly, this selection represents only a fraction of those substances released on the illicit drug market. Furthermore, it must be appreciated that it is common for hallucinogens to be mislabeled and/or adulterated.

In general, psychedelics will affect perceptions in such a way that all sensory input is perceived with heightened awareness. Sounds are perceived to be brighter and clearer; colors seem stronger and more brilliant. Flat objects seem to stand out in three dimensions. Taste, smell, hearing, sight, and touch seem to be more acute. One sensory impression may be translated or merged into another; for example, music may appear as a color, and colors may seem to have a taste. Judgment of reality and surroundings is often greatly impaired; most pronounced is the user's loss of his sense of time. Furthermore, these agents have clearly been shown to exacerbate latent personality disorders and

psychoses. Lastly, none of the drugs in this category induces definite physical dependence, yet prolonged use of them is believed to be associated with a deterioration of the personality.

Pattern of abuse. Qualitative and quantitative differences between the three types of psychedelics to be discussed warrant separate coverage, but certain general statements about their abuse pattern can be made.

Psychedelic-induced dependence is psychological, not physical. Tolerance develops within days and disappears as rapidly. These two characteristics combined favor periodic rather than continuous abuse of psychedelic drugs.

Indolealkylamines. Lysergic acid diethylamide (LSD) is by far the most potent indolealkylamine psychedelic, and it is therefore discussed as the representative example. LSD is abused for its "mind-expanding" abilities. This is a misnomer, since it only refers to the hallucinogenic activity of the drug. There are so many descriptions of "good trips," "bad trips," and "flashbacks" available referring to the perceptual changes that occur after the ingestion of LSD that it is believed to be unnecessary to repeat them here. LSD has additional sympathomimetic effects, manifesting themselves in a rise in blood pressure, tachycardia, hyperreflexia, nausea, piloerection, and increased body temperature.

A high degree of tolerance develops rapidly to the behavioral effects of LSD. This is not accompanied by physical dependence on the drug, and thus no withdrawal syndrome appears during any drug-free period. There is almost complete cross-tolerance between LSD, STP, psilocybin, psilocin, and mescaline, but none between amphetamines and LSD or marihuana.

Symptoms of an acute overdose include widely dilated pupils, flushed face, elevated blood pressure, and the experience of visual and temporal distortions, hallucinations, and derealization. Acute adverse reactions occurring during the use of LSD include panic reactions, paranoia, and accidental death from misperceptions. Prolonged use can cause long-lasting mental disturbances, varying from depressions to schizophrenic manifestations. In neither the acute nor the chronic situation does the user lose consciousness, and he is highly suggestible throughout his experiences. These two facts constitute the psychiatric basis for treatment on an individual basis, providing reassurance and in general just "talking him down." Some drugs, particularly chlorpromazine, have been used to handle either situation, but their use requires simultaneous psychiatric consultation. Any patient who had adverse reactions with the use of LSD should be cautioned about taking marihuana or antihistamines, which are known to trigger flashbacks or acute recurrence of a psychedelic-like state.

Phenylethylamines. Mescaline is the prototype of the phenylethylamines subgroup of psychedelics. As mentioned earlier, mescaline exhibits cross-tolerance with LSD, and it does not differ significantly in its effects from LSD, although its duration is longer.

Cannabinols. Marihuana has become an all-inclusive term for the many ingredients obtained from flowering tops of *Cannabis sativa*. The more concentrated resin is known as hashish, but all marketed "marihuana" presumably has as the active ingredient tetrahydrocannabinol. Although applicable to effects obtained with any drug, the following statement is particularly true for marihuana: The subjective effects experienced with it vary considerably with the preparation used, the dose, the set, and the setting. With sufficiently high doses and in the right setting, essentially all behavioral effects of LSD can be obtained with marihuana, yet in a different setting no behavioral changes may be experienced. Usually the cannabinols produce fewer and milder sympathomimetic actions and more sedative symptoms. Tolerance of considerable proportion can be de-veloped within days, and cannabinols are the only psychedelics that produce some minor effect on withdrawal (restlessness, insomnia, anorexia), possibly indicating a small degree of physical dependence. Of particular interest to the dentist is the fact that prolonged, high-level abuse of marihuana may manifest itself in xerostomia.

Since there is no physical dependence and thus no withdrawal syndrome to speak of with the psychedelics, pharmacologic treatment has to concern itself only with the adverse reactions of these drugs. Excessive behavioral effects have to be treated symptomatically. Panic reactions and "bad trips" in general should be handled on a highly individual basis by psychiatrically experienced professionals. The use of phenothiazines as successful adjuvants in managing the acute psychotic reaction is widely accepted.

REFERENCES

1. Jaffe, J. H.: Drug addiction and drug abuse. In Goodman, L. S., and Gilman, A. Z., editors: The pharmacological basis of therapeutics, ed. 4, New York, 1970, The Macmillan Co.
2. Dole, V. P., Nyswander, M. E., and Kreek, M. J.: Narcotic blockade, Arch. Intern. Med. **118**:304-309, 1966.
3. Jaffe, J. H., and Senay, E. C.: Methadone and *l*-methadyl acetate: use in management of narcotics addicts, J.A.M.A. **216**:1303-1305, 1971.
4. Kaim, S. C., Klett, C. J., and Rothfeld, B.: Treatment of the acute alcohol withdrawal state: a comparison of four drugs, Am. J. Psychiatry **125**:1640-1646, 1969.
5. Griffith, J. D., Cavanaugh, J. H., Held, J., and Oates, J. A.: Experimental psychosis induced by the administration of *d*-amphetamine. In Costa, E., and Garrattini, S., editor: International Symposium on Amphetamines and Related Compounds, New York, 1970, Raven Press, pp. 897-904.

Appendices

Dosages of drugs prescribed in dental practice[1-3]

Dosages of drugs prescribed in dental practice

Drugs	Children's dose*	Adult dose	Commonly used preparations
Analgesics			
Aspirin			
Oral	65 mg/kg/24 hr (maximum dose 3.6 Gm) divided into 4-6 doses or 60 mg (1 grain)/ year of age/dose, 5 times/24 hr (maintain hydration) (maximum dose 600 mg)	600 mg q.4h.	75 and 300 mg tablets
Acetaminophen (Nebs, Tempra, Tylenol)			
Oral	Under 1 year: 60 mg q.6-8h. 1-3 years: 60-120 mg q.6-8h. 3-6 years: 120 mg q.6-8h. Over 6 years: 240 mg q.6-8h.	300-600 mg q.4h.	300 mg tablets 60 mg/0.6 ml drops (15 ml bottle with dropper) 120 mg/5 ml syrup
Propoxyphene HCl (Darvon)			
Oral	Not recommended	32-65 mg q.6-8h.	See Chapter 9
Codeine phosphate Codeine sulfate			
Oral	As a single sedative or analgesic dose 0.8-1.5 mg/kg	15-60 mg q.4-6h.	15, 30, 60 mg tablets
SC	0.8 mg/kg	30 mg q.4-6h.	15, 30, 60 mg/ml solutions
Meperidine HCl (Demerol)			
Oral, IM, or SC	For pain: 0.5-0.8 mg/lb q.4-6h. For preoperative use: 1-2 years: 13 mg 3-4 years: 18 mg 5-6 years: 25 mg 7-8 years: 37 mg 9-12 years: 50 mg 13 years: 75 mg	50-100 mg q.4-6h.	50 and 100 mg tablets 50 mg/5 ml oral elixir 50 and 100 mg/ml IM, SC solutions
Morphine sulfate			
SC	0.12-0.2 mg/kg q.4h. (Not over 10 mg) (Infants ½ dose)	10-15 mg	10, 15, 30 mg/ml solutions

Continued.

*Children's dosages must be individualized. Consequently, these dosages are estimates that frequently require adjustment based on clinical observation.

Dosages of drugs prescribed in dental practice—cont'd

Drugs	Children's dose	Adult dose	Commonly used preparations
Pentazocine (Talwin) Oral	Not recommended	50-100 mg q.3-4h. (Not over 600 mg/24 hr)	50 mg tablets
IM, SC, IV	Not recommended	30 mg q.3-4h. (Not over 360 mg/24 hr)	30 mg/ml solution

Antibiotics

Drugs	Children's dose	Adult dose	Commonly used preparations
Penicillin G (Pentids, Pfizerpen, Sugarcillin) Oral	Children under 12 years (adult dose for over 12 years) 25,000-90,000 U (15-56 mg)/ kg/24 hr in 3-6 divided doses 1 hour before or 2 hours after meals	125-250 mg q.6h.	125, 250, 500 mg tablets 125, 250 mg/ml syrups
IM	20,000-50,000 U/kg/24 hr in 4-6 doses	200,000-600,000 units q.4h.	200,000-1,000,000 U/ml solution
Phenoxymethylpenicillin, Penicillin V (Compocillin, Pen-Vee, V-Cillin) Oral	Children under 12 years (adult dose for over 12 years) 25,000 to 90,000 U (15-56 mg)/ kg/24 hr in 3-6 divided doses 1 hour before or 2 hours after meals	125-250 mg q.6h.	125, 250, 300 mg tablets 125 and 250 mg/ml solutions
Phenoxyethylpenicillin, phenethicillin (Darcil, Maxipen, Syncillin) Oral	Children under 12 years (adult dose for over 12 years) 25,000-90,000 U (15-56 mg)/ kg/24 hr in 3-6 divided doses 1 hour before or 2 hours after meals	125-250 mg q.6h.	125 and 250 mg tablets 125 mg/5 ml solution
Procaine penicillin G (Duracillin, Wycillin) IM	100,000-300,000 U/dose, 1-2 doses/24 hr	600,000 U/24 hr	600,000 U/ml solution
Benzathine penicillin G (Bicillin, Permapen) IM	600,000-1,200,000 units monthly	1,200,000 U/month	300,000 U/ml solution

Dosages of drugs prescribed in dental practice—cont'd

Drugs	Children's dose	Adult dose	Commonly used preparations
Ampicillin (Omnipen, Penbritin, Polycillin) Oral	50-200 mg/kg/24 hr in 4 doses	250 mg q.6h.	250 and 500 mg capsules 125 and 250 mg/5 ml suspension
Cloxacillin (Tegopen) Oral	50 mg/kg/24 hr divided into 4 doses	500 mg-1 Gm q.4-6h.	125-250 mg capsules 125 mg/5 ml solution
Methicillin (Dimocillin, Staphcillin) IM or IV	25 mg/kg q.6h.	1 Gm q.4-6h. (IM)	1, 4, 6 Gm vials
Nafcillin (Unipen) Oral	25-50 mg/kg/24 hr divided into 4 doses	250 mg-1 Gm q.4-6h.	250 mg capsules 250 mg/5 ml solution
IM	25 mg/kg/24 hr divided into 2 doses	500 mg q.4-6h.	500 mg vials
Tetracycline, chlortetracycline, and oxytetracycline (Achromycin, Aureomycin, Terramycin) Oral	20-40 mg/kg/24 hr divided into 4 doses	250 mg q.6h.	125 and 250 mg tablets 125 mg/5 ml solution
Methacycline (Rondomycin) Demethylchlortetracycline (Declomycin) Oral	6-12 mg/kg/24 hr divided into 2 or 4 doses	600 mg/24 hr in 2 or 4 divided doses	150 and 300 mg tablets and capsules 75 mg/5 ml solution
Doxycycline (Vibramycin) Oral	Children under 100 lb: 2 mg/lb weight divided into 2 doses on first day; 1 mg/lb/24 hr thereafter	100 mg q.12h. first day, 100 mg/24 hr thereafter	50 and 100 mg capsules 25 mg/5 ml solution
Erythromycin (E-Mycin, Erythrocin, Ilotycin) Oral	See Chapter 20	250 mg q.6h.	125 and 250 mg tablets 125 mg chewable tablets 100 mg/ml drops 125 and 250 mg/5 ml solution

Continued.

Dosages of drugs prescribed in dental practice—cont'd

Drugs	Children's dose	Adult dose	Commonly used preparations
Lincomycin (Lincocin) Oral	30-60 mg/kg/24 hr divided into 3 doses (not used in infants under 1 month of age)	500 mg q.6h.	250 and 500 mg capsules 250 mg/5 ml solution
Clindamycin (Cleocin) Oral	8-16 mg/kg/24 hr (4-8 mg/lb/24 hr) divided into 3-4 equal doses (not used in infants under 1 month of age)	150-300 mg q.6h.	75 and 150 mg capsules
Nystatin (Mycostatin) Topical	See Chapter 20	See Chapter 20	See Chapter 20
Sedative hypnotics Chloral hydrate Orally as single-dose hypnotic or sedative Rectally as single-dose sedative	12.5-50 mg/kg (not over 1 Gm) (see pp. 59-60) 4-20 mg/kg (not over 1 Gm)	0.5-2 Gm	250 and 500 mg capsules 500 mg/5 ml solution 500 mg suppository
Pentobarbital sodium (Nembutal) Orally as single sedative dose	2-5 mg/kg	100 mg	50 and 100 mg capsules 20 mg/5 ml solution 50 mg/ml parenteral solution
Secobarbital sodium (Seconal) Orally as single-sedative dose	2-6 mg/kg	100 mg	50 and 100 mg capsules 50 mg/ml parenteral solution
Phenobarbital Orally as single sedative dose	0.5-2 mg/kg	16-32 mg	16, 32, and 64 mg tablets 20 mg/5 ml solution
Antihistamines Dimenhydrinate (Dramamine) Oral	5 mg/kg/24 hr divided into 3-4 equal doses	50 mg q.6h.	50 mg tablets 12.5 mg/4 ml solution 100 mg suppositories
Diphenhydramine (Benadryl) Oral	5 mg/kg/24 hr divided into 3-4 equal doses	50 mg q.6h.	25 and 50 mg capsules 12.5 mg/5 ml solution
Antisialagogue Propantheline (Pro-Banthine) Orally as single-dose antisialogogue	0.3 mg/kg (maximum 7.5 mg)	15 mg	7.5 and 15 mg tablets

REFERENCES

[1]Silver, I. K., Kempe, D. H., and Bruyn, H. B.: Handbook of pediatrics, ed. 7, Los Altos, Calif., 1967, Lange Medical Publications.

[2]Physician's desk reference, ed. 27, Oradell, N.J., 1973, Medical Economics, Inc.

[3]American Medical Association Council on Drugs: AMA drug evaluations—1971, Chicago, 1971, American Medical Association.

Management of dental problems in patients with cardiovascular disease

Advances in medical science and other factors have resulted in an increasing number of people who are living into the advanced years. The latest figures released by the Office of National Vital Statistics reveal the life expectancy of the American citizen in 1960 to be 69.7 years and for 1961 the preliminary estimates reveal an expectancy of 70.2 years.

As life expectancy increases, certain disease processes become prominent. Approximately 60 per cent of individuals over 60 years of age have some chronic disease. Cardiovascular problems are an important segment of this group. It is estimated that there are over ten million people in the United States with some form of cardiovascular disease, and the various forms of cardiovascular problems are responsible for 54 per cent of all deaths in this age group.

Patients with cardiovascular diseases are of particular interest to the dentist since they have a decreased ability to recover from

□ This appendix consists of a report of a working conference jointly sponsored by the American Dental Association and the American Heart Association, and held in April, 1963, to discuss the "Medical-Dental Management of Patients with Cardiovascular Disease." This report and subsequent additions, all of which are reproduced verbatim, represent the recommendations of this conference. The text was approved by the Committee on Medical Education of the American Heart Association, Incorporated, and the Council on Dental Therapeutics of the American Dental Association.

The report, entitled "Management of Dental Problems in Patients With Cardiovascular Disease," was printed in the *Journal of the American Dental Association*, vol. 68, pp. 333-342, March, 1964. Copyright 1964 by the American Dental Association. The health questionnaire was revised subsequent to original publication and appears in revised form (copyright 1967 and 1964, respectively). All material in this appendix is used by permission.

stress. Therefore, the dentist is often required to alter his treatment so that it will have no ill effect on the patient's over-all condition.

However, dental treatment should not be denied a patient because of a cardiovascular problem. With only a few exceptions, dental treatment, when properly performed, is safe. Maintenance of the oral cavity in a state of health is possible for these patients and should be the goal of the dental profession. Generally speaking, a fully ambulatory patient without cardiac symptoms, who can come to the office, is suitable for outpatient care.

Management of dental problems in patients with cardiovascular disease requires close cooperation between the physician and dentist. The physician must be aware of the dentist's problem, and, in turn, the dentist should know the medical problem and the limitations it imposes. There is need for mutual understanding, respect, and cooperation between the physician and dentist if the best interest of the patient is to be served. When dental treatment is necessary, the dentist should discuss the problem with the patient's physician and proceed only after there has been agreement on the course of action. The physician should know what type of dental treatment is involved and the drugs and medicaments to be used so he can intelligently evaluate the problem and give sound advice.

Should a medical history be taken by the dentist?

An adequate medical history should always be taken for the protection of the patient since most cardiovascular diseases can be detected in this manner. The history should contain the name of the patient's physician and reveal pertinent information regarding any previous illness, bleeding tendencies, unusual symptoms or allergies, and drugs or medicaments the patient is taking. Specific questions regarding cardiovascular disease should be included. When a history of cardiovascular disease is obtained, or if any bleeding problem or medicaments the patient is taking suggest cardiovascular disease, the dentist should consult the patient's physician before proceeding with dental treatment.

A sample questionnaire that is extremely useful to the dentist is included.

Periodic re-evaluation of this medical history is of great importance and must be kept current. This can be accomplished chiefly by obtaining the following information from the patient on succeeding visits:

1. Has there been any change in the patient's health since the last history was recorded?

2. Is the patient receiving any new drugs (medication)?

What preventive dental procedures are indicated when it is discovered that the patient has cardiovascular disease?

Because of the progressive nature of many cardiovascular diseases and the decreased ability of patients to tolerate stress, preventive dental procedures should be instituted early in the course of such conditions. When a diagnosis of cardiovascular disease is first made, the physician should refer the patient to a dentist for complete oral and dental evaluation, and any required treatment should be completed at this time. Periodic re-examination and performance of any treatment necessary to maintain the oral cavity in a state of health is essential.

What drugs commonly taken by patients with cardiovascular disease require special precautions?

To avoid reactions, special precautions must be taken by the dentist when he is treating a patient who is taking one of the following drugs:

1. Diuretics and antihypertensive drugs. These drugs may predispose to orthostatic hypotension and patients may faint when changed from a relatively prone position to a sitting or standing position.

2. Nitroglycerine. A patient who takes nitroglycerine for angina pectoris should al-ways have a supply of fresh tablets immediately available when he visits the dentist. If an angina attack occurs during dental treatment, all procedures must be interrupted, and nitroglycerine should be taken according to previous instructions from the patient's physician.

3. Rauwolfia compounds, guanethidine or ganglionic blocking agents. These drugs potentiate the response to vasoconstricting drugs. Therefore, the injection of local anesthetics containing vasoconstrictors should be carefully administered *in order to avoid intravascular injection* since any resulting blood pressure changes may be extremely hazardous. The frequency of syncope is also increased in patients taking these drugs.

Should saliva-inhibiting drugs be administered to a patient with cardiovascular disease?

Saliva-inhibiting drugs such as atropine and methantheline should not be administered to a patient with cardiovascular disease until his physician has been consulted since the dosage of either drug, commonly used in dental practice, often produces tachycardia.

Is it good practice to premedicate the cardiovascular patient to prevent apprehension?

In cardiac patients with coronary, hypertensive, or syphilitic heart disease, or with congestive heart failure from any cause, preanesthetic sedation with short-acting barbiturates is advised. Apprehension may thus be decreased and blood pressure rises minimized or prevented in the waiting room period, as well as in the dental chair. Because of their short-acting period and wide use, pentobarbital in a dosage of 50 to 100 mg., or secobarbital in a dosage of 50 to 100 mg., are satisfactory for most adults, *although dosage must be on an individual basis and the drug carefully administered.*

Since occasional patients react unfavorably, or even paradoxically, to these drugs, patients should be carefully questioned as to whether they have taken the drug previously. The medication should be given in the waiting room at least 45 minutes before the surgical procedure. Tranquilizing (ataractic) drugs may, on occasion, be used instead. All individuals who take barbiturates should have someone accompany them to the dentist's office as a precautionary measure.

CAUTION: Dangerous hypotensive episodes or orthostatic hypotension may occur when sedatives are given to patients being treated for cardiovascular disease with certain drugs such as ganglionic blocking agents or hydralazine (Apresoline), guanethidine (Ismelin), methyldopa (Aldomet), phenothiazines and Rauwolfia drugs. These agents also prolong the action of analgesics, sedatives and tranquilizers. Therefore, special caution must be exercised when administering sedatives to patients taking these drugs.

Is it necessary to administer prophylactic antibiotic therapy to prevent bacteremia and bacterial endocarditis?

Bacteremia is frequently associated with extraction of teeth, other oral surgical procedures, and manipulation of periodontal tissue. The frequency and severity of bacteremia in dental procedures are related to the degree of trauma.

Prophylactic therapy against subacute bacterial endocarditis is indicated for all patients with rheumatic fever scarred valves or congenital heart defects. Unfortunately there is, at the present time, no known antibiotic dosage regimen which is completely effective in preventing bacteremia and bacterial endocarditis following traumatic dental procedures. The majority of such patients, however, can be protected from endocarditis by the administration of appropriate antimicrobial agents. The drug of choice is penicillin. Treatment schedules, originally outlined by a special committee of the American Heart Association and reviewed in 1960, are recommended and are found in [Appendix C].*

What type of anesthetic should be given for dental procedures when the patient has cardiovascular disease?

Local anesthesia, properly administered, is generally the anesthesia of choice. It is particularly important to provide complete and total local anesthesia and to eliminate apprehension to minimize the discharge of endogenous epinephrine. The following procedures should be followed in the administration of local anesthetics:

1. Use adequate premedication.

---

*Appendix C now contains 1977 revised treatment schedules.

2. If a patient is known to react to a specific local anesthetic, another anesthetic of different chemical structure should be used.

3. Reduce pain at the injection site.

4. Use the smallest quantity of the lowest concentration anesthetic compatible with the problem at hand.

5. Use minimal concentrations of vasoconstrictors.

6. Inject slowly with minimal pressure.

7. Multiple injections should be spaced in time.

8. Following injection, keep patient under close observation. If unusual reactions develop, promptly instigate any indicated resuscitative and/or supportive measures.

Why is it important to avoid intravascular injection?

The intravascular injection of local anesthetics is a real danger to anyone, and particularly to those patients with cardiovascular disease. Without special precautions, the concentration of local anesthetics and/or added vasoconstrictors may be inadvertently *built up*, and death or serious cardiovascular complications may result. Intra-arterial injections provoke distant anesthesia and blanching of the immediate area, while intravenous injection may cause central nervous system stimulation or depression and produce hypertensive crises or dangerous degrees of myocardial ischemia. Intravenous injection is probably the cause of most reactions to local anesthesia in dentistry. The instruments sometimes used by dentists do not allow for preliminary aspiration. However, *aspirating cartridge syringes, now on the market*, provide increased safety for the patient with fewer anesthetic failures, as well as fewer anesthetic "reactions."

Intravascular injection can be avoided, provided that the following precautions are observed:

1. Use a needle no smaller than 25-gauge. Smaller needles often prevent aspiration.

2. Prevent intravascular injection by aspirating before injection.

3. If the position of the needle is changed during injection, reaspirate before continuing the injection.

4. If blood is aspirated, the cartridge should be discarded and another cartridge used.

When are general anesthetics indicated on patients with cardiovascular disease?

General anesthesia or general analgesia is hazardous in patients with cardiovascular disease, particularly those with ischemic heart disease, e.g., angina pectoris, myocardial infarction or coronary insufficiency. However, for the extremely apprehensive patient or for complicated surgical procedures, general anesthesia may be indicated. These patients are ideally treated in a hospital environment or one with comparable facilities.

Is it safe to use a vasoconstrictor in the local anesthetic for the cardiovascular patient?

A vasoconstrictor agent is generally indicated as a component of a local anesthetic preparation because it ensures more profound anesthesia and limits the rate of absorption of the local anesthetic agent. The concentrations of vasoconstrictors normally used in dental local anesthetic solutions are not contraindicated in patients with cardiovascular disease when administered carefully *and with preliminary aspiration.* The following concentrations can be used: epinephrine, 1:50,000-1:250,000; levarterenol, 1:30,000; levonordefrin, 1:20,000; and phenylephrine, 1:2,500.

The special precautions in administering local anesthetics listed above should be meticulously followed.

When gingival retraction or hemostasis is required for dental procedures on patients with cardiovascular disease, should agents containing vasoconstrictors be used?

The use of vasoconstrictors for gingival retraction or hemostasis is potentially dangerous and should be avoided.

How may the dentist determine the extent of the dental procedures that may be accomplished at one time?

All dental procedures are not of the same magnitude and since patients with cardiovascular disease have varying capacities to withstand stressful situations no hard and fast rule can be set forth as to the amount of dental work that should be done at any one time. The following, however, can be used as a guide in determining the extent of the procedure:

1. The number of teeth to be extracted or the extent of any dental procedures to be completed at one time should be determined by the amount of trauma involved and the patient's ability to withstand the trauma. This ordinarily calls for discussion of the problem with the patient's physician.

2. Patients who have chest pain, marked periodic pallor or exhibit breathlessness, alteration in consciousness, faintness, and/or have a very labile or rapid pulse should not be subjected to extensive or traumatic procedures without prior medical consultation, since these symptoms may indicate serious heart disease.

3. Dental procedures should be avoided for a period of at least three months after the patient has had a coronary heart attack. However, in cases of a dental emergency prior to the lapse of three months, minimal dental procedures should be handled in consultation with the patient's physician.

4. Serious heart disease is unlikely in those people who can do strenuous exercise (such as rapid stair climbing) without discomfort and such patients can tolerate dental procedures well.

If a patient is taking an anticoagulant drug, should the drug be withdrawn if a surgical procedure is necessary?

The use of anticoagulants is increasing, and many physicians believe that patients with coronary artery disease should be kept on this therapy permanently. Some types of actual or threatened strokes are also considered indications for the long-term use of anticoagulant drugs.

The reported results of either continuing or stopping anticoagulant therapy for dental extraction are somewhat conflicting. The sudden withdrawal of anticoagulant drugs, especially if any vitamin K preparations are administered, may cause thrombosis or embolism. Conversely, if anticoagulant drugs are continued at full doses, profound bleeding may occur.

Therefore, when periodontal surgery, extractions or other dental surgical procedures are planned, the physician, in consultation with the dentist, should *gradually* reduce the dosage of oral anticoagulants to maintain the prothrombin times at approximately 1½ times the control level. Dental surgical procedures may then be carried out without undue bleeding, if the operative site is sufficiently limited to permit the effective use of local procedures for hemostasis, including use of an absorbable hemostatic agent, sutures, and prolonged pressure applied to a gauze dressing placed over the wound.

No modification in dosage is required for injection of local anesthetics but prolonged pressure over the injection area may be desirable to prevent hemorrhage.

How can a cardiac emergency be recognized? If a cardiac emergency occurs, how should it be treated?

A cardiac emergency may occur in a dental office in a patient with known cardiac disease or it may be the patient's first manifestation of cardiac disease. Such emergencies should be suspected when the patient experiences chest pain, persistent breathlessness or prolonged fainting and unconsciousness. When confronted with any of these problems, the following therapy should be carried out:

1. Be calm: It is of the UTMOST IMPORTANCE that the dentist remain calm and reassure the patient.
2. Chest pain
   a. Place patient in sitting position.
   b. Administer oxygen.
   c. Have the patient place a fresh tablet of nitroglycerine under his tongue (if patient is using the drug).
   d. Call physician.
   e. Do not administer epinephrine.
3. Persistent breathlessness
   a. Place patient in sitting position.
   b. Administer oxygen.
   c. Call physician.
4. Fainting
   a. Place patient in recumbent position with legs raised.
   b. Have patient inhale aromatic spirits of ammonia.
   c. Administer oxygen.
5. Unconsciousness
   a. Place patient in recumbent position with legs raised.
   b. Make sure airway is patent and administer oxygen.
   c. If patient is not breathing, give artificial respiration.
   d. If the pulse cannot be detected after 30 seconds or if an audible heart beat with ear on chest cannot be detected after 30 seconds, institute external closed chest cardiac resuscitation and other required resuscitative procedures. (Information about closed chest cardiac resuscitation is available from your local heart association.)

HEALTH QUESTIONNAIRE

Name _____ Sex _____ Age _____

Address _____

Telephone _____ Height _____ Weight _____

Date _____ Occupation _____ Marital status _____

Directions

If your answer is YES to the question, put a circle around "YES."
If your answer is NO to the question, put a circle around "NO."
Answer all questions and fill in blank spaces when indicated.
Answers to the following questions are for our records only and will be considered confidential.

1. Are you in good health	YES NO
a. Has there been any change in your general health within the past year	YES NO
2. My last physical examination was on _____	
3. Are you now under the care of a physician	YES NO
a. If so, what is the condition being treated _____	
4. The name and address of my physician is _____	

5. Have you had any serious illness or operation .... YES NO
   a. If so, what was the illness or operation _____
6. Have you been hospitalized or had a serious illness within the past five (5) years .... YES NO
   a. If so, what was the problem _____

7. Do you have or have you had any of the following diseases or problems:

a. Rheumatic fever or rheumatic heart disease	YES NO
b. Congenital heart lesions	YES NO
c. Cardiovascular disease (heart trouble, heart attack, coronary insufficiency, coronary occlusion, high blood pressure, arteriosclerosis, stroke)	YES NO
(1) Do you have pain in chest upon exertion	YES NO
(2) Are you ever short of breath after mild exercise	YES NO
(3) Do your ankles swell	YES NO
(4) Do you get short of breath when you lie down, or do you require extra pillows when you sleep	YES NO
d. Allergy	YES NO
e. Asthma or hay fever	YES NO
f. Hives or a skin rash	YES NO
g. Fainting spells or seizures	YES NO
h. Diabetes	YES NO
(1) Do you have to urinate (pass water) more than six times a day	YES NO
(2) Are you thirsty much of the time	YES NO
(3) Does your mouth frequently become dry	YES NO
i. Hepatitis, jaundice or liver disease	YES NO
j. Arthritis	YES NO
k. Inflammatory rheumatism (painful swollen joints)	YES NO
l. Stomach ulcers	YES NO
m. Kidney trouble	YES NO
n. Tuberculosis	YES NO
o. Do you have a persistent cough or cough up blood	YES NO
p. Low blood pressure	YES NO
q. Venereal disease	YES NO
r. Other _____	

8. Have you had abnormal bleeding associated with previous extractions, surgery, or trauma: .... YES NO
   a. Do you bruise easily .... YES NO
   b. Have you ever required a blood transfusion .... YES NO

Continued.

If so, explain the circumstances _____

_____

9. Do you have any blood disorder such as anemia	YES	NO
10. Have you had surgery or x-ray treatment for a tumor, growth, or other condition of your mouth or lips	YES	NO
11. Are you taking any drug or medicine	YES	NO

If so, what _____

12. Are you taking any of the following:

a. Antibiotics or sulfa drugs	YES	NO
b. Anticoagulants (blood thinners)	YES	NO
c. Medicine for high blood pressure	YES	NO
d. Cortisone (steroids)	YES	NO
e. Tranquilizers	YES	NO
f. Aspirin	YES	NO
g. Insulin, tolbutamide (Orinase), or similar drug	YES	NO
h. Digitalis or drugs for heart trouble	YES	NO
i. Nitroglycerin	YES	NO
j. Other _____		

13. Are you allergic or have you reacted adversely to:

a. Local anesthetics	YES	NO
b. Penicillin or other antibiotics	YES	NO
c. Sulfa drugs	YES	NO
d. Barbiturates, sedatives, or sleeping pills	YES	NO
e. Aspirin	YES	NO
f. Iodine	YES	NO
g. Other _____		

14. Have you had any serious trouble associated with any previous dental treatment	YES	NO

If so, explain _____

_____

15. Do you have any disease, condition, or problem not listed above that you think I should know about	YES	NO

If so, please explain _____

16. Are you employed in any situation which exposes you regularly to x-rays or other ionizing radiation	YES	NO

Women

17. Are you pregnant	YES	NO
18. Do you have any problems associated with your menstrual period	YES	NO

Remarks:

_____   _____
SIGNATURE OF PATIENT   SIGNATURE OF DENTIST

Prevention of bacterial endocarditis

A STATEMENT PREPARED BY THE COMMITTEE ON PREVENTION OF RHEUMATIC FEVER AND BACTERIAL ENDOCARDITIS OF THE AMERICAN HEART ASSOCIATION

Edward L. Kaplan, M.D., Chairman; Bascom F. Anthony, M.D., Alan Bisno, M.D., David Durack, M.B., D.Phil., Harold Houser, M.D., H. Dean Millard, D.D.S., Jay Sanford, M.D., Stanford T. Shulman, M.D., Max Stillerman, M.D., Angelo Taranta, M.D., Nanette Wenger, M.D.

Bacterial endocarditis remains one of the most serious complications of cardiac disease. The morbidity and mortality remain significant despite advances in antimicrobial therapy and cardiovascular surgery. This infection occurs most often in patients with structural abnormalities of the heart or great vessels. Effective measures for prevention of this infection by physicians and dentists are highly desirable.

Dental treatment, or surgical procedures or instrumentation involving the upper respiratory tract, genitourinary tract, or lower gastrointestinal tract, may be associated with transitory bacteremia. Bacteria in the bloodstream may lodge on damaged or abnormal valves such as are found in rheumatic or congenital heart disease or on endocardium near congenital anatomic defects, causing bacterial endocarditis or endarteritis. However, it is not possible to predict specific patients with structural heart disease in whom this infection will occur, nor the specific causal event.

Prophylaxis is recommended in those situations most likely to be associated with bacteremia since bacterial endocarditis cannot occur without a preceding bacteremia. Certain patients (e.g., those with prosthetic heart valves) appear to be at higher risk to develop endocarditis than are others (e.g., those with mitral valve prolapse syndrome). Likewise, certain dental (e.g., extractions) and surgical (e.g., genitourinary tract surgery) procedures appear to be much more likely to initiate significant bacteremia than are others. These factors, although difficult

to quantitate, have been considered in developing these recommendations.

Since there have been no controlled clinical trials, adequate data for comparing various methods for prevention of endocarditis in man are not available. However, an experimental animal model permitting consistent induction of bacterial endocarditis with microorganisms which often cause the infection in man has allowed experimental evaluation of both prophylaxis and treatment. Data from these studies, although derived from animal rather than clinical investigations, represent the only direct information on the efficacy of prophylaxis that is presently available. This information has influenced formulation of the current recommendations. The significant morbidity and mortality associated with infective endocarditis and the paucity of conclusive clinical studies emphasize the need for continuing research into the epidemiology, pathogenesis, prevention, and therapy of infective endocarditis.

When selecting antibiotics for bacterial endocarditis prophylaxis one should consider both the variety of bacteria that is likely to enter the bloodstream from any given site and those organisms most likely to cause this infection. Certain species of microorganisms cause the majority of cases of infective endocarditis, and their antimicrobial sensitivity patterns have been defined. The present recommendations are based on a review of available information about the organisms responsible for endocarditis including their in vivo and in vitro sensitivity to specific antibiotics and the pharmacokinetics of these drugs.

□ From Circulation **56**:139A, July, 1977.

In general, *parenteral administration* of antibiotics provides more predictable blood levels and is preferred when practical, especially for patients thought to be at high risk. Optimal prophylaxis requires close cooperation between physicians, and between physicians and dentists.

Dental procedures and upper respiratory tract surgical procedures

Patients at risk to develop infective endocarditis should maintain the highest level of oral health to reduce potential sources of bacterial seeding. Even in the absence of dental procedures, poor dental hygiene or other dental disease such as periodontal or periapical infections may induce bacteremia. Patients without natural teeth are not free from the risk of bacterial endocarditis. Ulcers caused by ill-fitting dentures should be promptly cared for since they may be a source of bacteremia.

Antibiotic prophylaxis is recommended with _all_ dental procedures (including routine professional cleaning) that are likely to cause gingival bleeding. Chemoprophylaxis for dental procedures in children should be managed in a similar manner to the way in which it is handled in adults. Although not a procedure, one exception to this is the spontaneous shedding of deciduous teeth; there are no data to suggest a significant risk of bacteremia accompanying this common event.

Devices which utilize water under pressure to clean between teeth and dental flossing may improve dental hygiene, but they also have been shown to cause bacteremia. However, bacterial endocarditis associated with the use of these devices has not been reported. Present data are insufficient to make firm recommendations with regard to their use in patients susceptible to endocarditis. However, caution is advised in their use by patients with cardiac defects, especially when oral hygiene is poor.

Several studies suggest that *local gingival degerming* immediately preceding a dental procedure provides some degree of protection against bacteremia. However, use of this technique is controversial, since gingival sulcus irrigation itself could theoretically induce bacteremia. If local degerming is employed, it should be used only as an adjunct to antibiotic prophylaxis.

Since alpha hemolytic streptococci (e.g., viridans streptococci) are the organisms most commonly implicated in bacterial endocarditis following dental procedures, antibiotic prophylaxis should be specifically directed toward them. Certain procedures on the upper respiratory tract (e.g., tonsillectomy or adenoidectomy, bronchoscopy—especially with a rigid bronchoscope—and surgical procedures involving respiratory mucosa) also may cause bacteremia. Since bacteria entering the bloodstream after these procedures usually have similar antibiotic sensitivities to those recovered following dental procedures, the same regimens are recommended.

The table on p. 353 contains suggested regimens for chemoprophylaxis for dental procedures or surgical procedures and instrumentation of the upper respiratory tract. The order of listing does not imply superiority of one regimen over another although parenteral administration is favored when practical. The committee also favors the combined use of penicillin and streptomycin or the use of vancomycin in the penicillin allergic patient (regimen B) in those patients felt to be at high risk (e.g., prosthetic valves).

For dental procedures and surgery of the upper respiratory tract
Regimen A—Penicillin

1. *Parenteral-oral combined:*
   Adults: Aqueous crystalline penicillin G (1,000,000 units intramuscularly) _mixed with_ *Procaine Penicillin G* (600,000 units intramuscularly). Give 30 minutes to 1 hour prior to procedure and then give penicillin V (formerly called phenoxymethyl penicillin) 500 mg orally every 6 hours for 8 doses.†
   Children: * *Aqueous crystalline penicillin G* (30,000 units/kg intramuscularly) _mixed with_ *Procaine Penicillin G* (600,000 units intramuscularly). Timing of doses for children is the same as for adults. For children less than 60 lbs. the dose of penicillin V is 250 mg orally every 6 hours for 8 doses.†
2. *Oral:* ‡
   Adults: Penicillin V (2.0 gm orally 30 minutes to 1 hour prior to the procedure and then 500 mg orally every 6 hours for 8 doses.)†
   Children: * *Penicillin V* (2.0 gm orally 30 minutes to 1 hour prior to procedure and then 500 mg orally every 6 hours for 8 doses.† For children less than 60 lbs. use 1.0 gm orally 30 minutes to 1 hour prior to the pro-

Prophylaxis for dental procedures and surgical procedures of the upper respiratory tract

	Most congenital heart disease;[3] rheumatic or other acquired valvular heart disease; idiopathic hypertrophic subaortic stenosis; mitral valve[4] prolapse syndrome with mitral insufficiency	Prosthetic heart valves[5]
All dental procedures that are likely to result in gingival bleeding[1,2]	Regimen A or B	Regimen B
Surgery or instrumentation of the respiratory tract[6]	Regimen A or B	Regimen B

[1]Does not include shedding of deciduous teeth.

[2]Does not include simple adjustment of orthodontic appliances.

[3]E.g., ventricular septal defect, tetralogy of Fallot, aortic stenosis, pulmonic stenosis, complex cyanotic heart disease, patent ductus arteriosus or systemic to pulmonary artery shunts. Does *not* include uncomplicated secundum atrial septal defect.

[4]Although cases of infective endocarditis in patients with mitral valve prolapse syndrome have been documented, the incidence appears to be relatively low and the necessity for prophylaxis in all of these patients has not yet been established.

[5]Some patients with a prosthetic heart valve in whom a high level of oral health is being maintained may be offered oral antibiotic prophylaxis for routine dental procedures except the following: parenteral antibiotics are recommended for patients with prosthetic valves who require extensive dental procedures, especially extractions, or oral or gingival surgical procedures.

[6]E.g., tonsillectomy, adenoidectomy, bronchoscopy, and use surgical procedures of the upper respiratory tract involving disruption of the respiratory mucosa. (See text).

cedure and then 250 mg orally every 6 hours for 8 doses.)†

For patients allergic to penicillin:

Use *either* Vancomycin (see Regimen B)

or use

Adults: Erythromycin (1.0 gm orally 1½-2 hours prior to the procedure and then 500 mg orally every 6 hours for 8 doses.)†

Children: Erythromycin (20 mg/kg orally 1½-2 hours prior to the procedure and then 10 mg/kg every 6 hours for 8 doses.)†

Regimen B—Penicillin plus streptomycin

Adults: Aqueous crystalline penicillin G (1,000,000 units intramuscularly)
mixed with
Procaine penicillin G (600,000 units intramuscularly)
plus
Streptomycin (1 gm intramuscularly).
Give 30 minutes to 1 hour prior to the procedure; then penicillin V 500 mg orally every 6 hours for 8 doses.†

*Children:** Aqueous crystalline penicillin G* (30,000 units/kg intramuscularly)
mixed with
Procaine penicillin G (600,000 units intramuscularly)
plus
Streptomycin (20 mg/kg intramuscularly).
Timing of doses for children is the same as for adults. For children less than 60 lbs the recommended oral dose of penicillin V is 250 mg every 6 hours for 8 doses.†

For patients allergic to penicillin:

Adults: Vancomycin (1 gm intravenously over 30 minutes to 1 hour). Start initial vancomycin infusion ½ to 1 hour prior to procedure; then *erythromycin* 500 mg orally every 6 hours for 8 doses.†

*Children:** Vancomycin* (20 mg/kg intravenously over 30 minutes to 1 hour).** Timing of doses for children is the same as for adults. *Erythromycin* dose is 10 mg/kg every 6 hours for 8 doses.†

Footnotes to regimens:

†In unusual circumstances or in the case of delayed healing, it may be prudent to provide additional doses of antibiotics even though available data suggest that bacteremia rarely persists longer than 15 minutes after the procedure. The physician or dentist may also choose to use the parenteral route of administration for all of the doses in selected situations.

*Doses for children should not exceed recommendations for adults for a single dose or for a 24-hour period.

**For vancomycin the total dose for children should not exceed 44 mg/kg/24 hours.

‡For those *patients receiving continuous oral penicillin for secondary prevention of rheumatic fever,* alpha hemolytic streptococci which are relatively resistant to penicillin are occasionally found in the oral cavity. While it is likely that the doses of penicillin recommended in Regimen A are sufficient to control these organisms, the physician or dentist may choose one of the suggestions in Regimen B or may choose oral erythromycin.

Cardiac surgery

Patients undergoing cardiac surgery utilizing extracorporeal circulation—especially those requiring placement of prosthetic heart valves or needing prosthetic intravascular or intracardiac materials—are at risk to develop infective endocarditis in the perioperative and postoperative periods. Because the morbidity and mortality of infective endocarditis in such patients are high, maximal preventive efforts are indicated, including the use of prophylactic antibiotics.

Early postoperative infective endocarditis following these surgical procedures is most often due to *Staphylococcus aureus* (coagulase positive) or *Staphylococcus epidermidis* (coagulase negative). Streptococci, gram negative bacteria, and fungi are less frequently responsible. No single antibiotic regimen is effective against all these organisms. Furthermore, the prolonged use of broad spectrum antibiotics may itself predispose to superinfection with unusual or highly resistant microorganisms. Therefore, antibiotic prophylaxis at the time of open heart surgery should be directed primarily against staphylococci and should be of short duration. The choice of antibiotic should be influenced by each individual hospital's antibiotic sensitivity data, but *penicillinase resistant penicillins* or *cephalosporin antibiotics* are most often selected. Antibiotic prophylaxis should be started shortly before the operative procedure and usually is continued for no more than three to five days postoperatively to reduce the likelihood of emergence of resistant microorganisms. The physician or surgeon should consider the effects of cardiopulmonary bypass on serum antibiotic levels and time the doses accordingly.

Careful preoperative dental evaluation is recommended so that any required dental treatment can be carried out *several weeks prior* to cardiac surgery whenever possible. Such measures may decrease the incidence of late postoperative endocarditis (occurring later than 6-8 weeks following surgery) which is often due to the same organisms which are responsible for causing infective endocarditis in the unoperated patient.

Status following cardiac surgery

Following cardiovascular surgery the same precautions should be observed that have been outlined for the unoperated patient undergoing dental, gastrointestinal, genitourinary, and other procedures. As far as is known, the risk of endocarditis probably continues indefinitely; it appears particularly significant in patients with prosthetic heart valves. Exceptions are patients with an uncomplicated secundum atrial septal defect repaired by direct suture without a prosthetic patch, and patients who have had ligation and division of a patent ductus arteriosus; these patients do not appear to be at increased risk of developing endocarditis. For these two defects, prophylaxis for prevention of infective endocarditis is not necessary following a healing period of six months after surgery. Although prophylactic antibiotics are often given intraoperatively, there is no evidence to suggest that patients who have undergone coronary artery operations are at risk to develop endocarditis in the months and years following surgery unless there is another cardiac defect present; prophylactic antibiotics to protect against endocarditis are not needed in these postoperative patients.

Other indications for antibiotic prophylaxis to prevent endocarditis

In susceptible patients chemoprophylaxis to prevent endocarditis is also indicated for surgical procedures on *any infected or contaminated tissues,* including incision and drainage of abscesses. Antibiotic prophylaxis for the indicated dental and surgical procedures should also be given to those patients who have had a documented previous episode of infective endocarditis, even in the absence of clinically detectable heart disease.

Indwelling vascular catheters, especially those which reside in one of the cardiac chambers, present a continual danger. Particular care should be given to maintaining the sterility of these catheters and to avoiding unnecessarily prolonged use.

Indwelling transvenous cardiac pacemakers appear to present a low risk of endocarditis; however dentists and physicians may choose to employ prophylactic antibiotics to cover dental and surgical procedures in these patients. The same recommendations apply to renal dialysis patients with implanted arteriovenous shunt appliances. Although no firm recommendation can be made on the basis of current information, antibiotic prophylaxis for prevention bacteremia provoked by dental and surgical procedures also deserves consideration in patients with ventriculoatrial shunts placed to relieve hydrocephalus since there are documented cases of infective endocarditis in these patients.

Prophylactic antibiotics are *not* required in diagnostic cardiac catheterization and angiography since, with standard techniques, the occurrence of endocarditis following these procedures has proven to be extremely uncommon.

It is important to recognize that antibiotic doses used to prevent recurrences of acute rheumatic fever ("secondary" rheumatic fever prophylaxis) are *inadequate* for the prevention of bacterial endocarditis (see reference). Special attention should be paid to these patients and appropriate antibiotics should be prescribed *in addition* to the antibiotic they are receiving for prevention of group A beta hemolytic streptococcal infections (the addition of an aminoglycoside to appropriate doses of penicillin, or the use of erythromycin or vancomycin).

Warning

The committee recognizes that it is not possible to make recommendations for all possible clinical situations. Practitioners should exercise their clinical judgment in determining the duration and choice of antibiotic(s) when special circumstances apply.

Furthermore, since endocarditis may occur despite antibiotic prophylaxis, physicians and dentists should maintain a high index of suspicion in the interpretation of any unusual clinical events following the above procedures. Early diagnosis is important to reduce complications, sequelae, and mortality.

SELECTED REFERENCES

1. American Heart Association Committee on Prevention of Rheumatic Fever: Prevention of Rheumatic Fever, Circulation **55**:1, 1977.
2. Durack, D. T. and Petersdorf, R. G.: Chemotherapy of experimental streptococcal endocarditis. I. Comparison of commonly recommended prophylactic regimens, J. Clin. Invest. **52**:592, 1973.
3. Durack, D. T., Starkebaum, M. S., and Petersdorf, R. G.: Chemotherapy of experimental streptococcal endocarditis. VI. Prevention of enterococcal endocarditis, J. Lab. Clin. Med. (in press), 1977.
4. Editorial: Prophylaxis of bacterial endocarditis, Faith, Hope, and Charitable Interpretations, Lancet **1**:519, 1976.
5. Everett, E. D., and Hirschman, J. V.: Transient bacteremia and endocarditis prophylaxis. A review, Medicine **56**:61, 1977.
6. Finland, M.: Current problem in infective endocarditis, Mod. Con. Cardiovasc. Dis. **41**:53, 1972.
7. Parker, M. T., and Ball, L. C.: Streptococci and aerococci associated with systemic infection in man, J. Med. Microbiol. **9**:275, 1976.
8. Pelletier, I. L., Jr., Durack, D. T., and Petersdorf, R. G.: Chemotherapy of experimental streptococcal endocarditis. IV. Further observations on prophylaxis, J. Clin. Invest. **56**:319, 1975.
9. Sande, M. A., Levison, M. E., Lukas, D. S., and Kaye, D.: Bacteremia associated with cardiac catheterization, N. Eng. J. Med. **281**:1104, 1969.
10. Sande, M. A., Johnson, W. D., Hook, E. W., and Kaye, D.: Sustained bacteremia in patients with prosthetic cardiac valves, N. Eng. J. Med. **286**:1067, 1972.
11. Scopp, I. W., and Orvieto, L. D.: Gingival degerming by povidone-iodine irrigation. Bacteremia reduction in extraction procedures, J. Am. Dent. Assoc. **83**:1294, 1971.
12. Sipes, J. N., Thompson, R. I., and Hook, E. W.: Prophylaxis of infective endocarditis: A reevaluation, Ann. Rev. Med. **28**:371, 1977.
13. Sullivan, N. M., Sutter, V. L., Mims, M. M., Marsh, V. H., and Finegold, S. M.: Clinical aspects of bacteremia after manipulation of the genitourinary tract, J. Infect. Dis. **127**:49, 1973.

BOOKS

1. Infective Endocarditis—An American Heart Association Symposium, edited by E. L. Kaplan and A. V. Taranta. American Heart Association Monograph Series No. 52. American Heart Association, Dallas, Texas, 1977.
2. Infective Endocarditis, edited by Donald Kaye, University Park Press, Baltimore, Maryland, 1976.
3. Subacute Bacterial Endocarditis, by Andrew Kerr, Jr., Charles C Thomas, Publisher, Springfield, Illinois, 1955.

Board review questions

The purpose of these board review questions is to review key points in each chapter as a means of (1) emphasizing important points, (2) checking comprehension of what has been read, and (3) providing a review for board examination. It is suggested that you read or study each chapter and then (1) mark the answers to each question and (2) check answers in the text. For the most part, answers are in sequence within the text.

CHAPTER 1: INTRODUCTION

1. The term *drug* may be defined as any (a) chemical substance, (b) compound that affects biologic systems, (c) substance that is effective in the treatment of disease, (d) organic chemical.

2. The dentist should be prepared to obtain the maximum advantage from available drugs while inducing minimal disadvantages. He should also know how medically prescribed drugs have altered the functions of his patients. Assume that a patient tells you that he is taking a medically prescribed drug and he only knows its proprietary name. In which of the following reference sources would you be able to locate information most conveniently about the indications and adverse potentialities of this drug? (a) *The United States Pharmacopeia*, (b) *The National Formulary*, (c) *Accepted Dental Therapeutics*, (d) *Physicians' Desk Reference*.

3. The "official" name of a drug, that is, the one used in the USP or NF is the _____ name. (a) chemical, (b) trade, (c) generic, (d) proprietary.

4. A *multiple-entity drug* is one that (a) is effective against more than one disease state, (b) affects more than one organ system, (c) contains more than one ingredient, (d) contains more than one active ingredient.

5. An advantage to using trade names is that they (a) simplify drug identification, (b) allow the least expensive product to be dispensed, (c) are more familiar to the pharmacist and consequently are less likely to be dispensed incorrectly, (d) are convenient time-savers when one writes a prescription for a multiple-entity preparation, (e) eliminate the need for learning a large number of generic names.

6. One should learn generic names because they (a) are usually shorter and easier to remember than trade names, (b) eliminate the need for learning a large number of trade names, (c) identify the manufacturer, (d) identify the chemical nature of the drug.

7. The federal control of narcotics and drugs considered to have a potential for abuse is administered by the (a) Food and Drug Administration, (b) Federal Trade Commission, (c) Department of Health, Education, and Welfare, (d) Department of Justice, (e) Internal Revenue Service.

CHAPTER 2: GENERAL PRINCIPLES OF DRUG ACTION

1-3. The log dose–effect curve is a plot of dose against effect. Questions 1 to 3 refer to the following figure.

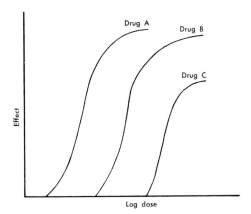

1. What is the potency relationship between drug A and drug B? (a) A is more potent, (b) B is more potent, (c) they are of equal potency, (d) a conclusion cannot be drawn.
2. What is the potency relationship between drug B and drug C? (a) B is more potent, (b) C is more potent, (c) they are of equal potency, (d) a conclusion cannot be drawn.
3. What is the efficacy relationship between drug A and drug C? (a) A is more efficacious, (b) C is more efficacious, (c) they are of equal efficacy, (d) a conclusion cannot be drawn.

4. The ED50 of a drug is (a) the effective dose of a drug in 50% of the subjects tested, (b) one half the effective or therapeutic dose, (c) the dose that gives 50% of the maximum effect.

5. Enteral routes of administration are (a) oral and rectal, (b) oral and topical, (c) topical and inhalation, (d) rectal and topical.

6. The more predictable drug response is obtained by _____ administration. (a) oral, (b) SC, (c) IM, (d) IV.

7. The topical application of drugs to mucous membranes (a) precludes the development of systemic blood levels, (b) only allows slow absorption, (c) allows faster absorption than that obtained from skin, (d) produces only local effects.

8. Which of the following drug characteristics will *increase* the tendency of a drug to cross cell membranes? (a) nonionized and high lipid solubility, (b) nonionized and low lipid solubility, (c) ionized and high lipid solubility, (d) ionized and low lipid solubility.

9. If you inject a drug with a pH of 6.5 and a pKa of 8.1 into a tissue with a pH of 7.4, to what extent would you expect this drug to be ionized in the tissues? (a) over 50%, (b) 50%, (c) under 50%.

10. Other factors being equal, would a weakly acidic drug with a pKa of 3.4 be absorbed more readily in the stomach or in the intestine? Why? (a) stomach—because it will be more highly ionized there, (b) stomach—because it will be less highly ionized there, (c) intestine—because it will be more highly ionized there, (d) intestine—because it will be less highly ionized there.

11. A drug that is bound to plasma protein is usually inactive pharmacologically. What happens to a drug that is so bound? (a) Most protein-bound drug is metabolized before it can be released to the active form. (b) As unbound drug is distributed to the tissues, bound drug dissociates itself from protein to reestablish an equilibrium between bound and unbound fractions. (c) After most unbound drug is released from the vascular system to the tissues, the bound fraction dissociates slowly and provides a longer duration of action. (d) Protein-bound drug remains bound until

NOTES

it passes through capillary cell walls, at which time the protein moiety is removed and the active drug form enters the tissues.

12. Drug A characteristically becomes 50% bound to plasma protein. A patient receives a maximal dose of drug A followed by an average dose of drug B. Drug B has a greater affinity for the same protein sites that bind drug A. How will the administration of drug B alter the effects of drug A? (a) Therapeutic and adverse effects of drug A will be intensified. (b) Only the therapeutic effects of drug A will be intensified. (c) Therapeutic and adverse effects of drug A will be reduced in intensity. (d) There will be no change in the intensity of either therapeutic or adverse effects.

13. The tissue distribution of drugs depends on both tissue affinities (guanethidine for heart and skeletal muscle, thiopental for fat) and differential passage across specialized cell membranes (blood-brain barrier, placenta). Most drugs are thought to pass the placenta by (a) active transport, (b) simple diffusion in accordance with their degree of lipid solubility, (c) simple diffusion in accordance with their degree of water solubility, (d) passage through membrane pores.

14. Tissue redistribution is particularly important in regard to (a) tetracyclines, (b) guanethidine, (c) quinine, (d) thiopental.

15. Agonists are drugs that (a) block tissue receptor sites, (b) activate tissue receptor sites, (c) reverse the effect of other drugs on tissue receptor sites.

16. To be therapeutically useful the selective effect of drugs on cellular components must be _____.

17. Most drugs are metabolized to products that are more easily excreted because they are _____ than the original compound. (a) less polar and more lipid soluble, (b) less polar and less lipid soluble, (c) more polar and more lipid soluble, (d) more polar and less lipid soluble.

18. Can you give an example of an inactive compound that is metabolized to an active agent?

19. Can you give an example of an active drug that is converted to another active drug before being inactivated?

20. The fact that pentobarbital can decrease the anticoagulant effect of coumarin is an example of enzyme (a) destruction, (b) binding, (c) induction, (d) inhibition.

21. What is an example of a drug that is excreted by active secretion in renal tubules? (a) phenobarbital, (b) penicillin, (c) procaine, (d) alcohol.

22. If a child's dose is calculated, the most accurate determination will be based on his (a) age, (b) weight, (c) body surface area.

CHAPTER 3: ADVERSE DRUG REACTIONS

Drug actions that are clinically desirable are termed *therapeutic effects.* Undesirable actions are termed *adverse effects.* The clinician's objective is to obtain maximal therapeutic effects while experiencing minimal adverse effects. Adverse drug effects occur frequently. Consequently, the clinician must be as concerned with a drug's adverse potentialities as with its therapeutic applicability. This chapter has only discussed definitions and general principles; adverse reactions to specific drugs are discussed in other appropriate chapters.

1. Reactions that cannot be explained by known mechanisms are termed (a) side effects, (b) idiosyncrasy, (c) allergic reactions, (d) teratogenic effects.

2. Which of the following can occur at therapeutic dosage levels in healthy patients? (a) idiosyncratic responses, (b) allergic reactions, (c) teratogenic effects, (d) all except *b,* (e) all of the above can occur.

3. The LD50 of a drug is (a) the dose (mg/kg) that kills 50% of the treated animals, (b) one half the dose that kills all of the treated animals, (c) 50% of the lethal dose in humans, (d) 50% of the lethal dose in an experimental animal.

4. The therapeutic index can be expressed (a) in mg/kg, (b) as $\dfrac{LD50}{ED50}$, (c) as $\dfrac{ED50}{LD50}$, (d) as *a* and *b*, (e) as *a* and *c*.

CHAPTER 4: PRESCRIPTION WRITING

1. How many milligrams of aspirin are contained in a 5-grain tablet? (a) 200, (b) 300, (c) 400, (d) 600.

2. The "average" man is considered to weigh about 70 kilograms. Approximately how many pounds does he weigh? (a) 145, (b) 155, (c) 165, (d) 170.

3. How would you abbreviate instructions if you wanted a patient to take 1 tablet every 6 hours? (a) 1 tab. t.i.d., (b) 1 tab. q.h.4, (c) 1 tab. q.4.h., (d) 1 tab. q.i.d.

4. If you want a patient to start taking a drug as soon as the prescription is filled, you might use the following abbreviation: (a) stat., (b) s.o.s., (c) p.c., (d) a.c.

5. A liquid preparation of K penicillin V contains 125 mg/5 ml. If you want the patient to take 250 mg each dose you would prescribe _____ per dose. (a) 1 teaspoon, (b) 2 teaspoons, (c) 1 tablespoon, (d) 2 tablespoons.

6-11. The following drugs and doses are frequently prescribed in dental practice. Write the "bodies" of prescriptions for each of the following in the space provided and check against the text.

6. An adult has a periapical abscess. You have provided local and supportive treatment. You determine that antibiotic therapy is also indicated and wish to prescribe potassium penicillin G for 5 days. (Dose: 250 mg at bedtime and 1 hour before meals.)
Ŗ:

7. You wish to prescribe a liquid preparation of penicillin V (125 mg/5 ml) for a child for 10 days. (Dose: 125 mg every 6 hours.)
Ŗ:

8. You wish to prescribe an antibiotic for an adult. The bactericidal potency of penicillin is not required and you decide to prescribe tetracycline HCl tablets for 5 days. (Dose: 250 mg every 6 hours.)
Ŗ:

9. You are prescribing 100 mg secobarbital sodium to be taken 1 hour before an appointment for preoperative sedation.
Ŗ:

10. You are prescribing 30 mg codeine sulfate to be taken with two aspirin tablets every 4 hours. You wish coverage for 24 hours.
Ŗ:

11. You are prescribing penicillin V as prophylaxis against subacute bacterial endocarditis for an adult with a history of rheumatic heart disease.
Ŗ:

12. Which of the following laws required that certain drugs be sold by prescription only? (a) The Food, Drug and Cosmetic Act of 1938, (b) The Durham-Humphrey Law of 1952, (c) The Kefauver-Harris Bill of 1962, (d) The Drug Abuse Control Amendments of 1965.

13. Which of the following laws prohibited the refilling of a prescription unless directions to the contrary are indicated on the prescription? (a) The Food, Drug, and Cosmetic Act of 1938, (b) The Durham-Humphrey Law of 1952, (c) The Kefauver-Harris Bill of 1962, (d) The Drug Abuse Control Amendments of 1965.

14. Which of the following laws required that a manufacturer demonstrate a drug's *effectiveness* as well as safety before it could be marketed? (a) The Food, Drug and Cosmetic Act of 1938, (b) The Durham-Humphrey Law of 1952, (c) The Kefauver-Harris Bill of 1962, (d) The Drug Abuse Control Amendments of 1965.

15. As established by The Controlled Substance Act of 1970, which drugs can be prescribed only by practitioners who are registered with the DEA? (a) Schedule I drugs, (b) Schedule II drugs, (c) Schedule III drugs, (d) Schedule IV drugs, (e) Schedule V drugs.

16. Which "schedule" of drugs has the *lowest* potential for abuse? (a) Schedule I drugs, (b) Schedule II drugs, (c) Schedule III drugs, (d) Schedule IV drugs, (e) Schedule V drugs.

CHAPTER 5: GENERAL ANESTHETICS

1-3. Regarding the early history of general anesthesia, match the anesthetic agent in column B with the man responsible for its early development. Each agent will be used once.

Column A	Column B
1. Horace Wells	(a) Nitrous oxide
2. W. T. G. Morton	(b) Ethyl ether
3. J. Y. Simpson	(c) Chloroform

4. According to the Meyer-Overton theory, general anesthetics (a) inhibit oxidative enzymes that are involved in glucose metabolism in neural tissue, (b) depress the transmission of nerve impulses by forming microcrystals in cerebral tissues, (c) have a potency that is roughly proportional to their oil-water solubility.

5. What stage of general anesthesia is characterized by excitement? (a) Stage I, (b) Stage II, (c) Stage III, Plane 1, (d) Stage III, Plane 3, (e) Stage IV.

6-14. Select the characteristic that is *not* descriptive of the drug indicated.
   6. Nitrous oxide. (a) nonflammable gas, (b) high patient acceptability, (c) potent anesthetic, (d) produces analgesia at 65% concentration.
   7. Cyclopropane. (a) highly explosive, (b) frequently produces cardiac arrhythmias, (c) potent anesthetic, (d) stormy induction.
   8. Ethylene. (a) explosive, (b) potent anesthetic, (c) disagreeable odor and taste, (d) poor patient acceptability.
   9. Diethyl ether. (a) irritating to mucous membranes, (b) slow induction and slow recovery, (c) explosive, (d) produces nausea and vomiting, (e) poor muscle relaxation.
   10. Vinyl ether. (a) more potent than diethyl ether, (b) rapid and smooth induction, (c) more dangerous than diethyl ether, (d) best for long procedures.
   11. Halothane. (a) not explosive, (b) highly potent, (c) irritating to mucous membranes, (d) produces incomplete muscle relaxation, (e) tends to produce hypotension, (f) sensitizes heart to epinephrine.
   12. Chloroform. (a) flammable liquid, (b) potent anesthetic, (c) induction rapid, (d) produces liver damage.
   13. Ethyl chloride. (a) nonflammable liquid, (b) principal use is anesthesia by topical refrigeration, (c) inhalation produces cardiac arrhythmias, (d) hepatotoxic.

14. Trichloroethylene. (a) nonflammable liquid, (b) causes cardiac arrhythmias, (c) may become habituating, (d) produces good muscle relaxation for long procedures.

15. Which of the following is *not* true of thiopental anesthesia? (a) smooth induction, (b) rapid induction, (c) moderate muscle relaxation, (d) progressive respiratory depression.

16. Anesthesia by intravenous barbiturates is contraindicated in patients with (a) asthma, (b) porphyria, (c) hyperactive cough reflexes, (d) hyperactive laryngeal reflexes, (e) all of the above conditions.

17. What is the principal difference between thiopental and the newer IV barbiturates—thiamylal and methohexital? The latter (a) are slightly more potent, (b) have different contraindications, (c) causes less muscle relaxation, (d) have less effect on the cardiovascular system.

18. Which of the following is or are true of ketamine anesthesia? (a) rapid induction, (b) profound analgesia with light sleep, (c) stimulation of the cardiovascular system, (d) moderate muscle relaxation, (e) depressed laryngeal reflexes, (f) frequently induced undesirable mental effects, (g) all except *c* and *d* are true, (h) all except *d* and *e* are true, (i) all are true, (j) none is true.

CHAPTER 6: SEDATIVE-HYPNOTIC DRUGS

1. An important problem in using barbiturates is that (a) their adverse potentialities are not well known, (b) they are habit forming and addictive, (c) they are inconvenient to administer, (d) all of the above are true, (e) none of the above is true.

2. Why are the barbiturates converted to their sodium salts? (a) so that parenteral solutions can be prepared, (b) to make them less toxic, (c) to increase their stability.

3. What is a common property of methohexital, thiamylal, and thiopental? (a) all contain sulfur, (b) all are used for general anesthesia, (c) both *a* and *b*, (d) neither *a* nor *b*.

4. Which of the following barbiturates would be most likely to show a prolonged effect in a patient with renal impairment? (a) phenobarbital and secobarbital, (b) pentobarbital and amobarbital, (c) thiopental and thiamylal, (d) phenobarbital and barbital.

5. A sedative dose of a barbiturate should be expected to produce (a) respiratory depression, (b) minor analgesia, (c) decreased BMR, (d) all of the above effects, (e) none of the above effects.

6. You have a patient who is a barbiturate addict. If he continues to receive barbiturates required by his addiction, you would expect him to (a) become progressively depressed in time and to develop little tolerance to barbiturates, (b) become progressively depressed in time and to develop significant tolerance, (c) retain relative normality of function, but require increasing doses because of the rapid and extensive development of tolerance, (d) retain relative normality of function without need for increasing doses.

7. If a patient is taking dicumarol and a barbiturate, the withdrawal of the latter would _____ the effect of this coumadin anticoagulant. (a) increase, (b) decrease, (c) have no effect on.

8. In comparing the nonbarbiturate sedatives with the barbiturates, one may say that the former are (a) more potent and better known, (b) more potent, although not as well known, (c) less potent but better known, (d) less potent and not as well known.

9. Which of the following drugs is (are) so highly irritating to mucosa that it (they) should not be administered to patients with ulcers or gastro-

enteritis? (a) bromides, (b) chloral hydrate, (c) paraldehyde, (d) ethinamate, (e) *a* and *b*, (f) *b* and *c*, (g) *c* and *d*.

10. Why would you question the use of paraldehyde in a patient with bronchopulmonary disease? (a) A significant amount is eliminated by the respiratory route. (b) It causes bronchiolar constriction. (c) Oral doses irritate the larynx. (d) It directly and extensively depresses respiration.

11. Teratogenic studies are insufficient to recommend which of the following for use in pregnant women? (a) ethinamate, (b) ethchlorvynol, (c) glutethimide, (d) none is recommended.

CHAPTER 7: PSYCHOTHERAPEUTIC DRUGS
CHAPTER 8: MINOR TRANQUILIZERS AND CENTRALLY ACTING MUSCLE RELAXANTS

1. The most widely used antipsychotic drugs are the (a) *Rauwolfia* alkaloids, (b) phenothiazines, (c) butyrophenones, (d) thioxanthines.

2. The prolonged duration of action of phenothiazines results from the fact that (a) a large part of the dose enters the enterohepatic circulation and is slowly released into general circulation, (b) they are not metabolized to any significant extent by the liver and must be eliminated by the kidney, (c) their metabolic conjugates are pharmacologically active and slowly excreted, (d) their metabolic conjugates are pharmacologically active and are retained in body fat.

3. Which of the following is one most likely to see during the long-term use of phenothiazines? (a) tolerance to antipsychotic effects, (b) euphoria, (c) "neuroleptic syndrome," (d) loss of intellectual function, (e) all of the above.

4. Tolerance to the sedative effect of phenothiazines (a) develops in 1 to 2 days, (b) develops in 1 to 2 weeks, (c) develops in 2 to 4 months, (d) does not develop.

5. The time necessary to develop the full antipsychotic effect to phenothiazines is (a) 1 to 2 days, (b) 1 to 2 weeks, (c) 2 to 4 months, (d) 4 to 6 months.

6. The antiemetic effect of phenothiazines results from depression of (a) the vomiting center, (b) the chemotherapeutic trigger zone, (c) both *a* and *b*, (d) neither *a* nor *b*.

7. Chlorpromazine is not useful in controlling nausea and vomiting associated with (a) uremia, (b) gastroenteritis, (c) carcinomatosis, (d) drug therapy, (e) motion sickness.

8. The sympatholytic effect of phenothiazines accounts for the tendency of these drugs to cause (a) orthostatic hypotension with compensatory tachycardia, (b) hypertension with compensatory bradycardia, (c) increased salivation, (d) xerostomia.

9. Toxic or side effects of phenothiazines include (a) extrapyramidal stimulation, (b) antimuscarinic effects: xerostomia, urinary retention, and inhibition of sweating, (c) both *a* and *b*, (d) neither *a* nor *b*.

10. Haloperidol is sometimes a desirable alternative to chlorpromazine as an antipsychotic drug in patients with coronary or cerebrovascular disease because it produces (a) less hypotension, (b) less hypertension, (c) more sedation, (d) bradycardia.

11. When compared with phenothiazines, the thioxanthines can be described as (a) more potent and less toxic, (b) more potent and more toxic, (c) less potent and less toxic, (d) less potent and more toxic.

12. Which of the following are produced by meprobamate? (a) central tolerance and physical dependence, (b) sedation and muscle relaxation, (c) anticonvulsive effects, (d) all of the above.

13. Which of the following are produced by chlordiazepoxide? (a) central tolerance and physical dependence, (b) sedation and muscle relaxation, (c) anticonvulsive effects, (d) all of the above.

14. Diazepam (Valium) and chlordiazepoxide (Librium) have become extensively used drugs in recent years. Their pharmacologic effects are similar. What are the principal differences between these agents? (a) Only chlordiazepoxide produces muscle relaxation. (b) Diazepam is shorter acting, has a higher margin of safety, and when used IV produces amnesia. (c) Only diazepam has anticonvulsant properties. (d) All the above are known differences.

15. Overdose with CNS depressants is always a problem. Which of the following has a greater potential for fatal overdose? (a) pentobarbital, (b) meprobamate, (c) chlordiazepoxide, (d) diazepam.

16. Hydroxyzine (Atarax, Vistaril) has sedative, antihistaminic, antispasmodic, and antiemetic actions. It has been used as a CNS depressant and to treat or prevent nausea and vomiting. Why is it not used against nausea occurring during pregnancy? (a) It is not effective against nausea occurring during pregnancy. (b) Fetal abnormalities have been caused by hydroxyzine in experimental animals. (c) Fetal anoxia is more likely to occur after the use of this particular minor tranquilizer. (d) It frequently causes methemoglobinemia.

17. In a normal individual the tricyclic antidepressants have effects similar to the phenothiazines. However, the depressed patient responds with an elevation of mood and (a) increased mental and physical activity without euphoria, (b) increased mental and decreased physical activity, (c) reduced preoccupation with suicide, (d) euphoria, (e) both *a* and *c*, (f) both *b* and *d*.

18. You are least likely to see which of the following adverse effects associated with the use of the tricyclic antidepressants? (a) fine tremors and blurred vision, (b) dry mouth and constipation, (c) orthostatic hypotension and tachycardia, (d) psychological and physical dependence.

19. Why do the effects of monoamine oxidase inhibitors (MAOIs) last for several days or even weeks after their use is discontinued? (a) Their inhibition of MAO is irreversible and new enzyme must be synthesized. (b) They conjugate with protein and consequently are very slowly excreted by the kidneys. (c) They are not metabolized by the liver and renal excretion is slow. (d) Their metabolic products are active and have a strong affinity for lipids.

20. Which of the following statement(s) relative to MAOIs is (are) false? (a) Their antidepressant action is described as euphoric stimulation and occurs in normal as well as depressed patients. (b) High doses of MAOIs may cause excessive CNS stimulation resulting in manic reactions and hallucinations. (c) They antagonize the effect of sympathomimetic amines. (d) All of the above are false.

21. The mechanism of action that makes lithium effective in controlling the manic phase of manic depression is (a) unknown, (b) related to enzyme inhibition, (c) caused by depletion of CNS catecholamines, (d) a result of both *b* and *c*.

CHAPTER 9: NONNARCOTIC ANALGESICS

1. Which of the following does *not* have antipyretic effects? (a) salicylates, (b) mefenamic acid, (c) aniline derivatives, (d) propoxyphene.

2. In addition to their analgesic effects, some salicylates are used therapeutically as (a) keratolytic agents, (b) counterirritants, (c) flavoring in cooking, (d) all of the above.

3. What effects of aspirin result from both peripheral and hypothalamic actions? (a) analgesic, (b) antipyretic, (c) anti-inflammatory, (d) all of the above.

4. High doses of aspirin (a) stimulate metabolism, (b) increase the tendency of blood platelets to adhere to endothelium, (c) do both of the above, (d) do neither of the above.

5. Buffering cannot be relied on to reduce gastrointestinal upset after the use of aspirin. The reason for this is probably because of aspirin's (a) overwhelming acidity, (b) systemic effect, (c) direct, nonacidic effects, (d) chelating tendencies.

6. Allergic reactions to aspirin are not rare. They may be characterized by (a) asthmatic symptoms, (b) angioneurotic edema, (c) anaphylactic shock, (d) only *a* and *b*, (e) all of the above.

7. The treatment of a severe toxic reaction to aspirin requires (a) immediate hospitalization and the use of IV fluids to correct acidosis and electrolyte imbalance, (b) IV cortisone and vasopressors, (c) gastric lavage, parenteral sedatives, forced fluids, and rest, (d) IV glucose and support of respiration.

8. An arthritic patient has been taking 20 grains/24 hr of aspirin for 3 months. You might expect to see (a) hyperprothrombinemia and electrolyte imbalance, (b) hypoprothrombinemia and inhibited platelet function, (c) acidosis and prolonged prothrombin time, (d) decreased prothrombin time and inhibited platelet function.

9. An oral dose of aspirin would normally be expected to produce a peak blood level in about (a) 15 minutes, (b) 30 minutes, (c) 1 hour, (d) 2 hours.

10. The renal excretion of aspirin would be increased by (a) acidification of the urine, (b) alkalinization of the urine, (c) diuresis, (d) *a* and *c*, (e) *b* and *c*.

11. What is a significant clinical distinction of phenylbutazone when compared with salicylates or other pyrazolones? (a) greater analgesic potency, (b) greater antipyretic potency, (c) greater anti-inflammatory potency, (d) less toxicity.

12. Mefenamic acid should be administered with particular caution in (a) diabetics, (b) hypertensives, (c) asthmatics, (d) psychotics.

13. The principal pharmacologic difference among the aniline derivatives is their (a) toxicity, (b) analgesic potency, (c) antipyretic potency, (d) *a* and *b*.

14. You would not expect cross-allergy to exist between acetaminophen and (a) aspirin, (b) phenacetin, (c) acetanilid, (d) any of the above drugs.

15. Overdoses with acetaminophen have been associated with (a) anaphylactic shock and serum sickness, (b) agranulocytosis and aplastic anemia, (c) hepatic necrosis and renal failure, (d) all of the above.

16-24. Match the drug in column A with the statement in column B. Each item in both columns will be used only once.

Column A	Column B
16. Aspirin	(a) Methemoglobinemia
17. Aminopyrine	(b) Xerostomia
18. Phenylbutazone	(c) Agranulocytosis
19. Mefenamic acid	(d) Weak acid
20. Acetanilid	(e) Slow onset
21. Phenacetin	(f) The *P* in APC
22. Acetaminophen	(g) Popular aspirin substitute
23. Propoxyphene	
24. Ethoheptazine	

CHAPTER 10: NARCOTICS

1. The principal differences between the narcotic analgesics are their (a) potencies and variety of adverse potentialities, (b) potencies, rates of onset, and durations, (c) chemical structures, (d) overall pharmacologic effects.

2. The narcotic analgesics tend to produce (a) addiction, (b) respiratory depression, (c) sedation, (d) emesis, (e) constipation, (f) only *a* and *b*, (g) only *c* and *d*, (h) all of the above.

3. All opium alkaloids (a) are obtained from the unripe seed capsules of *Papaver somniferum*, (b) are addicting, (c) are analgesics, (d) depress smooth muscle, (e) are characterized by all of the above.

4. Tolerance does *not* develop to which of the following effects of morphine? (a) analgesia, (b) sedation, (c) euphoria, (d) respiratory depression, (e) miosis.

5. Respiratory depression is an important clinical consideration relative to the use of morphine. Quantitatively, this effect generally parallels (a) analgesic potency, (b) molecular weight, (c) euphoric depth, (d) all of the above, (e) none of the above.

6. Morphine causes nausea and vomiting by (a) direct gastrointestinal effects, (b) stimulation of the emetic trigger zone, (c) stimulation of the vomiting center, (d) all of the above mechanisms.

7. Morphine and codeine produce constipation by (a) affecting specific medullary centers, (b) increasing water absorption from the gastrointestinal tract, (c) reducing gastrointestinal secretions and motility, (d) increasing the tone of the gastrointestinal musculature.

8. Which of the following series of effects can be caused by morphine? (a) urinary retention, depression of the vasomotor center, and dilation of the biliary duct, (b) bronchiolar constriction, miosis, convulsions, and urinary retention, (c) urinary retention, increased intracranial pressure, and depression of the vagus, (d) increased intracranial pressure, diuresis, and stimulation of the vagus.

9. The morphine addict may appear completely normal except for (a) sedation and dilated pupils, (b) minor disorientation and lacrimation, (c) constipation and miosis, (d) anorexia and irritability.

10. The diagnostic triad of morphine overdose consists of (a) "pinpoint" pupils, tremor, and vomiting, (b) tremor, perspiration, and chills, (c) dilated pupils, coma, and tremors, (d) coma, depressed respiration, and "pinpoint" pupils.

11. Codeine can be considered a weak morphine. However, it equals morphine as an antitussive and may have greater _____ effects. (a) constipating, (b) emetic, (c) euphoric, (d) excitatory.

12. Which of the following effects are most likely to be seen after a therapeutic dose of codeine? (a) emesis and constipation, (b) minor respiratory depression and nausea, (c) constipation and miosis, (d) euphoria and constipation, (e) all of the above.

13. Unless a patient has developed a tolerance to narcotics, maximal analgesic potency is usually obtained with _____ mg codeine. (a) 30, (b) 60, (c) 90, (d) 120.

14-18. Match the drug with the most relative characteristic given. Each characteristic will be used once.

Drug	*Characteristics*
14. Dihydrocodeinone	a. Principal current use is as an antitussive
15. Dihydromorphinone	b. More potent and more addicting than codeine; ingredient in Percodan
16. Oxymorphone	
17. Oxycodone	c. Cannot be legally manufactured or imported into the United States
18. Heroin	
	d. Rapid onset, rapid duration; analgesic potency about five times that of morphine
	e. Analgesic potency and tendency to produce undesirable effects eight to ten times greater than that of morphine

19. Which of the following effects are *not* likely to be associated with the use of meperidine? (a) sedation, (b) constipation, (c) addiction, (d) nausea, (e) relaxation of gastrointestinal musculature, (f) none of the above is associated with the use of meperidine.

20. Meperidine is most likely to be valuable in dental practice in cases where (a) the pain cannot be controlled by morphine, (b) the patient is allergic to morphine, (c) the patient has developed tolerance to morphine, (d) rapid analgesia and sedation are desirable.

21. Alphaprodine, anileridine, and piminodine are most similar to (a) meperidine, (b) morphine, (c) codeine, (d) methadone.

22. What characteristic of methadone has made it useful as a narcotic substitute for addicts? (a) It does not cause addiction. (b) Users do not suffer from mental depression. (c) Withdrawal from methadone appears to be accomplished more easily than from morphine. (d) Methadone cannot be used orally. (e) All of the above.

23. Pentazocine appears to be a more potent analgesic than codeine, but less potent than morphine. In addition to analgesia, it also (a) produces sedation, (b) reduces an elevated temperature, (c) has anti-inflammatory properties, (d) does both *a* and *b*, (e) does both *b* and *c*.

24. The fact that pentazocine is classified as a Schedule III drug means that it is (a) not considered to be addicting, (b) considered to be less addicting than Schedule II drugs, (c) considered to be more addicting than morphine, (d) considered to be more addicting than codeine.

25. Propoxyphene produces analgesia and (a) antipyresis, (b) weak anti-inflammatory effects, (c) sedation, (d) no other therapeutic effects.

26. Overdose by which of the following can be antagonized by nalorphine? (a) aspirin, (b) acetaminophen, (c) mefenamic acid, (d) propoxyphene, (e) all of the above, (f) none of the above.

27. When used alone, the analgesic potency of ethoheptazine is probably (a) inferior to that of aspirin, (b) slightly but consistently superior to a placebo, (c) more potent than mefenamic acid, (d) more potent than acetaminophen.

28. Which of the following has an antipyretic effect? (a) propoxyphene, (b) acetaminophen, (c) ethoheptazine, (d) all of the above.

29. In which of the following cases would nalorphine or levallorphan increase or initiate respiratory depression? (a) when used alone, (b) when used in a patient depressed by morphine, (c) when used in a patient depressed by a barbiturate, (d) in both *a* and *b*, (e) in both *b* and *c*, (f) in both *a* and *c*.

30. Levallorphan is a newer narcotic antagonist than nalorphine. What is its principal difference from nalorphine? (a) greater potency, (b) greater safety, (c) broader pharmacologic effects, (d) all of the above, (e) none of the above.

31. Papaverine is a benzylisoquinoline opiate that has had limited use as an (a) analgesic, (b) cough suppressant, (c) sedative, (d) peripheral vaso-dilator.

CHAPTER 11: CENTRAL NERVOUS SYSTEM STIMULANTS

1. The principal site of action of strychnine is the (a) cerebral cortex, (b) mid-brain, (c) brain stem, (d) hindbrain, (e) spinal cord.

2. Strychnine causes excessive motor impulses that lead to heightened re-flexes, stiffness of facial and cervical muscles, and possible convulsions by (a) stimulating excitatory neurons, (b) depressing inhibitory neurons, (c) both *a* and *b*, (d) neither *a* nor *b*.

3. The major site of action of picrotoxin in reversing respiratory depression caused by barbiturates is the (a) cerebral cortex, (b) midbrain, (c) medulla, (d) spinal cord.

4. The primary use(s) of pentylenetetrazol is (are) to (a) reverse respiratory depression caused by barbiturates, (b) assist in the diagnosis of epilepsy, (c) evaluate the effectiveness of anticonvulsants against petit mal epilepsy, (d) do both *a* and *b*, (e) do both *b* and *c*, (f) do all of the above.

5. Why is the effectiveness of amphetamines as anorexigenic agents limited? (a) They are not potent anorexigenic drugs. (b) Significant tolerance to the anorexigenic effect develops within 3 to 4 weeks. (c) Their effectiveness is limited because of both *a* and *b*. (d) Their effectiveness is not limited because of either *a* or *b*.

6. Which of the following signs and symptoms would you expect to see in a patient taking amphetamines? (a) increased heart rate and hypertension, (b) restlessness and irritability, (c) insomnia, (d) both *a* and *b*, (e) both *b* and *c*, (f) all of the above.

7. The xanthines allay drowsiness and fatigue and at certain doses increase the force of contraction of the heart, increase heart rate and cardiac output, and stimulate respiration. They act to a greater extent on the _____ than any of the other CNS stimulants discussed. (a) cerebral cortex, (b) mid-brain, (c) medulla, (d) spinal cord.

8. In addition to action as CNS stimulants, the xanthines also have _____ properties. (a) diuretic, (b) antidiuretic, (c) histaminic, (d) antihistaminic, (e) diuretic and antihistaminic, (f) histaminic and antidiuretic.

CHAPTER 12: ANTICONVULSANT DRUGS

1. Anticonvulsants control the symptoms but do not treat the cause of the disease. Theories to explain the mechanism of action of anticonvulsants state that these drugs may prevent epileptic seizures by (a) increasing the activity of inhibitory neurons, (b) impeding the spread of discharges throughout the cortex, (c) weakening the discharge of ectopic foci, (d) any one or all of the above mechanisms.

2. When an epileptic is treated with phenobarbital, which of the following are likely to develop in time? (a) tolerance to the sedative effects, (b) tolerance to the anticonvulsant effects, (c) physical dependence, (d) only *b* and *c*, (e) none of the above, (f) all of the above.

3. Phenytoin produces gingival hyperplasia in 20% to 30% of patients. Al-though infrequent, phenytoin, also has caused (a) adverse hepatic and hematologic effects, (b) ataxia and hirsutism, (c) elevated blood cholesterol and phosphatase levels, (d) both *a* and *b*, (e) both *b* and *c*, (f) both *a* and *c*, (g) all of the above, (h) none of the above.

4. Why would mephenytoin *not* be selected over phenytoin as the drug of choice for prophylaxis against grand mal seizures? Mephenytoin is (a) not effective against grand mal seizures, (b) less potent than phenytoin, (c) more toxic than phenytoin, (d) both *b* and *c*.

5. Although ethosuximide is considerably less toxic than trimethadione, it has caused (a) insomnia, diarrhea, and fatigue, (b) dermatitis, headache, and liver damage, (c) blood dyscrasias, (d) all of the above except c, (e) all of the above.

6. Relative to structure-activity relationship, primidone is a useful anticonvulsant because it is (a) chemically related to trimethadione, (b) oxidized to phenobarbital in humans, (c) oxidized to trimethadione in humans, (d) oxidized to phenytoin in humans.

7. Phenacemide is a potent and highly toxic anticonvulsant that is used when other drugs have failed in cases of _____ seizures. (a) grand mal, (b) petit mal, (c) psychomotor, (d) all of the above.

8-18. Indicate whether the drug listed is used principally against (a) grand mal, (b) petit mal, (c) psychomotor, (d) grand mal and psychomotor, (e) grand mal, petit mal, and psychomotor.
   8. Phenobarbital
   9. Metharbital
   10. Phenytoin
   11. Mephenytoin
   12. Ethotoin
   13. Trimethadione
   14. Paramethadione
   15. Ethosuximide
   16. Methsuximide
   17. Primidone
   18. Phenacemide

CHAPTER 13: AUTONOMIC DRUGS

1-6. Indicate which division of the autonomic nervous system would be stimulated to cause the effect listed.
   1. Secretion of thin, watery saliva
   2. Secretion of thick, viscid saliva
   3. Bradycardia
   4. Constriction of pupil
   5. Decrease in peristalsis
   6. Increase in gastrointestinal secretions

7. Acetylcholine is the specific neurotransmitter at (a) all parasympathetic synapses, (b) sympathetic preganglionic synapses, (c) neuromuscular junctions, (d) at a and b, (e) at a, b, and c.

8. Acetylcholine is the neurotransmitter at sympathetic postganglionic synapses that affects (a) salivary glands, (b) sweat glands, (c) the adrenal medulla, (d) the adrenal cortex, (e) all of the above.

9. Why has the attempt to use choline esters to promote salivation been unsuccessful? (a) They affect too many other body systems. (b) They cause xerostomia. (c) They are too expensive. (d) Their effect on salivation is too weak.

10. What is the mechanism of the parasympathomimetic effects of physostigmine, neostigmine, and malathion? (a) They stimulate parasympathetic receptors directly. (b) They cause the release of acetylcholine. (c) They inhibit the enzyme that metabolizes acetylcholine. (d) They simulate anticholinesterase.

11. Most anticholinergic drugs act by (a) destroying acetylcholine, (b) complexing with the active sites on the acetylcholine molecule, (c) activating the sympathetic division of the autonomic nervous system, (d) blocking cholinergic receptors.

12. Atropine and scopolamine have similar pharmacologic effects. Which of the following actions does only scopolamine have? (a) reduction of salivation, (b) prevention of cardiac slowing during general anesthesia, (c) CNS depression, (d) mydriasis, (e) cycloplegia.

13. If you prescribe atropine to reduce salivary flow you should advise the patient that the following side effects may be experienced: (a) dryness and burning of the throat, (b) vasodilation of skin capillaries with flushing, (c) blurred vision, (d) all of the above.

14. Anticholinergic drugs should be used with considerable caution in patients with cardiovascular disease and are contraindicated in patients with (a) glaucoma, (b) prostate hypertrophy, (c) intestinal obstruction, (d) any of the above.

15. What is the effect of stimulating alpha-adrenergic receptors?

16. What is the effect of stimulating beta-adrenergic receptors?

17. How can epinephrine cause both vasodilation of capillaries in striated muscle and vasoconstriction in skin capillaries?

18. Both small and large doses of epinephrine cause an increase in (a) the strength of contraction, (b) heart rate, (c) cardiac output, (d) oxygen utilization, (e) all of the above, (f) all except *b*, (g) all except *d*.

19. Norepinephrine does not normally cause (a) vasoconstriction in the skin, (b) increased systolic blood pressure, (c) decreased diastolic blood pressure, (d) bradycardia.

20. Why would norepinephrine be a poor substitute for epinephrine in a severe allergic response? (a) It does not relax bronchial smooth muscle. (b) It does not increase both systolic and diastolic blood pressure. (c) It dilates pulmonary arterioles. (d) It would be a poor substitute for all of the above reasons.

21. Norepinephrine will produce significant tissue necrosis used as the vasoconstrictor in a local anesthetic solution or if injected subcutaneously. This damage results from (a) severe local vasoconstriction, (b) direct irritation to the tissues, (c) damage caused by the high pH of norepinephrine solutions, (d) thrombosis of local blood vessels.

22. Since isoproterenol (Isuprel) stimulates only beta receptors, it has all the following effects except one. Which one of these actions does it *not* have? (a) increases heart rate, (b) increases strength of cardiac contraction, (c) increases systolic and diastolic pressure, (d) decreases bronchial spasm.

23. The amphetamines are (a) indirect adrenergic stimulants and CNS stimulants, (b) indirect adrenergic stimulants and CNS depressants, (c) direct adrenergic stimulants and CNS stimulants, (d) direct adrenergic stimulants and CNS depressants.

CHAPTER 14: LOCAL ANESTHETICS

1. The synthesis of procaine by _____ in 1905 initiated a new era in local anesthesia. (a) Niemann, (b) Koller, (c) Halstead, (d) Einhorn.

2. The heading "Trends in Local Anesthesia in Dentistry" in this chapter indicates a movement toward (a) more potent and more toxic local anesthetics, (b) less potent and more toxic local anesthetics, (c) more potent and less toxic local anesthetics, (d) less potent and less toxic local anesthetics.

3. Local anesthetics are converted to salts for clinical use because the latter are (a) less toxic but more potent, (b) more stable and have a greater water solubility, (c) more stable and have a greater fat solubility, (d) more potent and cause less local tissue damage.

4. What is the most potent and most toxic local anesthetic in current use? (a) lidocaine, (b) mepivacaine, (c) proparacaine, (d) dibucaine.

5. Local anesthetics inhibit the propagation of nerve impulses (a) along nerve fibers, (b) at sensory endings, (c) at myoneural junctions, (d) at synapses, (e) at *a* and *b* only, (f) at all the above sites.

6. Some local anesthetics are used as cardiac antiarrhythmic agents. This is possible because they (a) depress the excitability of heart muscle, (b) reduce conduction rate, (c) increase conduction rate, (d) do both *a* and *b*, (e) do both *a* and *c*.

7. The rate at which a local anesthetic leaves the injection site and enters systemic circulation is increased by the application of (a) cold and the absence of a vasoconstrictor in the solution, (b) cold and the presence of a vasoconstrictor, (c) heat and the absence of a vasoconstrictor, (d) heat and the presence of a vasoconstrictor.

8. Severe liver disease would *least* affect the metabolism of which of the following agents? (a) procaine, (b) lidocaine, (c) mepivacaine, (d) prilocaine.

9. The presence of infection in an injection area may reduce the effectiveness of a local anesthetic because (a) the low pH of the area may inhibit the liberation of the salt from the free base form, (b) the low pH of the area may inhibit the liberation of free base, (c) the high pH of the area may inhibit the liberation of the salt from the free base form, (d) the high pH of the area may inhibit the liberation of free base.

10. Certain antihistamines, such as tripelennamine and diphenhydramine, have significant local anesthetic actions. The anesthesia produced by these drugs may be characterized as (a) potent and long acting, (b) potent and short acting, (c) weak and long acting, (d) weak and short acting.

11. Vasoconstrictors, which may be included in local anesthetic solutions, function to (a) prolong and increase the depth of anesthesia, (b) reduce the toxic effects of the drug, (c) increase the toxic effects of the drug, (d) provide both *a* and *b*, (e) provide both *a* and *c*.

12. A working conference of the American Dental Association and American Heart Association has said that the concentration of vasoconstrictors normally used in dental local anesthetics are not contraindicated in patients with cardiovascular disease when administered carefully and with preliminary aspiration. The N.Y. Heart Association has also stated that vasoconstrictors are *not* contraindicated in patients with cardiovascular disease but, as a guideline, recommended the following as a maximum dose of epinephrine for any one session: (a) 0.1 mg (10 ml of a 1:100,000 solution), (b) 0.2 mg (20 ml of a 1:100,000 solution), (c) 0.3 mg (30 ml of a 1:100,000 solution), (d) 0.4 mg (40 ml of a 1:100,000 solution).

13-17. According to Monheim, how many milliliters of the following 2% local anesthetic solutions represent the *maximum* recommended dose for a healthy adult?
13. procaine (a) 10, (b) 20, (c) 30, (d) 40
14. lidocaine (a) 5, (b) 10, (c) 15, (d) 20
15. mepivacaine (a) 5, (b) 10, (c) 15, (d) 20
16. prilocaine (a) 5, (b) 10, (c) 15, (d) 20
17. tetracaine (a) 1, (b) 1.5, (c) 2, (d) 2.5

18. The most frequent cause of a high blood level of local anesthetic after a dental injection is (a) the injection of an excessive volume, (b) the injection of an excessive concentration, (c) intravascular injection, (d) inadequate hepatic function, (e) inadequate renal function.

19. You have established that a patient had an allergic reaction to procaine 6 months ago. Which of the following would be contraindicated? (a) a topical spray containing tetracaine, (b) a topical spray containing lidocaine, (c) mepivacaine by injection, (d) prilocaine by injection, (e) all of the above, (f) none of the above.

20. Which of the following is *not* true of procaine? (a) rapid onset, (b) short duration, (c) potency one half that of lidocaine, (d) one of the safest local anesthetics, (e) effective topically.

21. Which of the following is *not* true of lidocaine? (a) rapid onset, (b) short

duration, (c) spreads well through tissues, (d) effective topically, (e) neither *a* nor *b* is true of lidocaine, (f) neither *b* nor *c* is true of lidocaine.

22. Compared to lidocaine, mepivacaine can is said to be (a) profoundly more potent, (b) significantly less toxic, (c) faster acting, (d) longer acting, (e) equivocal.

23. Which of the following is *least* effective topically? (a) lidocaine, (b) mepivacaine, (c) tetracaine, (d) cocaine, (e) benzocaine, (f) dyclonine.

24. Compared to lidocaine, prilocaine is (a) less potent, (b) less toxic, (c) longer acting, (d) all of the above, (e) none of the above.

25. A unique toxicity of prilocaine is that in some patients it causes (a) methemoglobinemia, (b) disorientation, (c) brain rot, (d) pregnancy, (e) all of the above.

26. Pyrrocaine is most similar therapeutically and chemically to (a) lidocaine, (b) prilocaine, (c) procaine, (d) tetracaine, (e) propoxycaine.

27. Which of the following is *not* true of tetracaine? (a) slow onset, (b) long duration, (c) low potency, (d) high toxicity, (e) rapidly absorbed topically, (f) effective topically.

28. Compared to tetracaine, propoxycaine has (a) greater potency, (b) greater toxicity, (c) a more rapid onset, (d) a lack of topical activity, (e) both *a* and *b*, (f) both *c* and *d*.

29. A patient reports an allergy to procaine. Which of the following topical agents could be most safely used? (a) benzocaine, (b) tetracaine, (c) cocaine, (d) dyclonine.

CHAPTER 15: HISTAMINE AND ANTIHISTAMINES

1. Which of the following reactions is most characteristic of histamine release in humans? (a) vasodilation, decreased capillary permeability, and stimulation of exocrine glands, (b) vasoconstriction, bronchoconstriction, and stimulation of exocrine glands, (c) increased capillary permeability, bronchoconstriction, and stimulation of exocrine glands, (d) vasodilation, bronchoconstriction, and depression of exocrine glands.

2. Tissue histamine can be released by (a) allergic reactions, (b) physical trauma, (c) infection, (d) some drugs, (e) all of the above, (f) none of the above.

3. The best method of counteracting the effects of an acute release of histamine is by (a) physiologic antagonism, (b) specific antihistaminic medication, (c) use of adrenal steroids, (d) induction of emesis.

4. Which of the following antihistamines would be expected to produce the most sedation? (a) chlorpheniramine (Chlor-Trimeton), (b) tripelennamine (Pyribenzamine), (c) chlorocyclizine (Di-Paralene), (d) promethazine (Phenergan).

5. Which one of the following actions of histamine is not blocked by antihistamines? (a) vasodilation, (b) increase in gastric secretions, (c) itching, (d) increase in salivary secretions.

6. Antihistamines act by (a) inhibiting the release of histamine from mast cells, (b) competitively blocking histamine tissue receptor sites, (c) increasing the metabolic breakdown of histamine, (d) chelating histamine into an inactive complex.

7. The prolonged use of antihistamines may produce xerostomia. This results from their (a) anticholinergic action, (b) cholinergic action, (c) inhibition of histamine-induced salivation, (d) direct depression of salivary gland cells.

8. Which of the following antihistamines have been shown to have terato-

genic effects in laboratory animals? (a) chlorpheniramine and diphenhydramine, (b) tripelennamine and promethazine, (c) promethazine and meclizine, (d) meclizine and cyclizine.

CHAPTER 16: HORMONES AND RELATED SUBSTANCES

1-6. Match the pituitary hormone in column A with the letter representing the proper descriptive term or statement in column B. All items in column B will be used once.

Column A	Column B
1. Corticotropin	(a) Gonadotropins
2. MSH	(b) Growth hormone
3. FSH and LH	(c) ACTH
4. Somatotropin	(d) Stimulates the thyroid
5. Thyrotropin	(e) Stimulate melanocytes of the skin
6. Oxytocin and vasopressin	(f) From posterior pituitary

7. The sex hormones consist of estrogens, androgens, and progesterone. Which of the following effects are caused by *estrogens?* (a) control maturation and function of female sex organs, (b) promote water and nitrogen retention, (c) promote protein synthesis and glycogen deposition, (d) all of the above except *b*, (e) all of the above.

8. Testosterone is the most potent natural androgen. How does it differ from progesterone? (a) Only testosterone is anabolic. (b) Only testosterone promotes masculinizing effects. (c) Progesterone is more intimately involved in the female endometrial cycle. (d) Only *a* and *b* are true. (e) Only *b* and *c* are true.

9. The drugs propylthiouracil and methimazole are frequently used (a) against non–pituitary-induced hypermetabolic thyroid pathologic conditions, (b) against pituitary-induced hyperthyroidism, (c) as replacement therapy in non–pituitary-induced hypothyroidism, (d) as replacement therapy in pituitary-induced hypothyroidism.

10. Parathormone does *not* (a) increase bone resorption, (b) decrease intestinal absorption of calcium, (c) increase selective renal reabsorption of calcium, (d) do any of the above.

11. The alpha and beta cells of the islets of Langerhans produce respectively (a) insulin and glucagon, (b) glucagon and insulin, (c) only insulin, (d) only glucagon.

12. Which of the following reactions is (are) accelerated by insulin? (a) conversion of glucose to glycogen, (b) uptake and oxidation of glucose, (c) conversion of carbohydrate to fat, (d) protein synthesis, (e) all except *c*, (f) all except *d*, (g) all of the above.

13. Why is zinc contained in many insulin preparations? (a) to increase its potency, (b) to decrease its toxicity, (c) to aid in crystallization, (d) for all of the above reasons.

14. What is Lente insulin? (a) insulin combined with globulin, (b) insulin combined with protamine, (c) a microcrystalline suspension of insulin, (d) an acidified solution of animal pancreas.

15. Which of the following insulin preparations would least likely be used for daily home injections? (a) regular or amorphous, (b) protamine zinc, (c) globulin zinc, (d) neutral protamine Hagedorn, (e) Lente.

16. Aside from different routes of administration, what is the principal difference between insulin replacement therapy and the use of the oral hypoglycemics (sulfonylureas)? The sulfonylureas (a) are more effective, (b) only release endogenous insulin, (c) are less toxic, (d) are only effective in the young diabetic.

17. Although the place of glucagon in human physiology and its potentialities

as a therapeutic agent are largely unknown, we know that one of its basic functions is to (a) assure a continuous supply of glucose, (b) increase plasma amino acids, (c) decrease the formation of glycogen, (d) increase fat deposition.

18. Which of the following hormones are believed to affect body defense mechanisms? (a) secretin, (b) gastrin, (c) pancreozymin, (d) cholecystokinin, (e) prostaglandins, (f) all of the above except c and d.

CHAPTER 17: ADRENOCORTICOSTEROIDS

1. Which of the following principally affects electrolyte balance? (a) cortisone, (b) hydrocortisone, (c) desoxycorticosterone, (d) corticosterone.

2. The major impetus for the development of synthetic corticoids was to make agents available that (a) have more specific anti-inflammatory effects, (b) have more specific effects on carbohydrate metabolism, (c) are less expensive, (d) are more potent.

3. The glucocorticoids are basically catabolic agents; consequently, they (a) increase the utilization of glucose and decrease gluconeogenesis, (b) increase gluconeogenesis and decrease the utilization of glucose, (c) increase both, (d) decrease both.

4. You would expect excessive blood levels of corticosteroids to cause (a) hyperglycemia, (b) hypoglycemia, (c) no change in blood glucose.

5. Abnormally high levels of corticoids are *not* likely to cause (a) negative nitrogen balance, (b) a depression of growth, (c) impaired wound healing, (d) a decrease in the deposition of fat.

6. The corticoids, particularly the mineralocorticoids, act on the renal tubules to _____ sodium retention and _____ potassium excretion. (a) increase, decrease, (b) decrease, increase, (c) decrease both, (d) increase both.

7. Excessive levels of mineralocorticoids would most likely cause (a) dehydration and hypertension, (b) dehydration and hypotension, (c) edema and hypertension (d) edema and hypotension.

8. In Addison's disease you would expect to see a tendency toward (a) dehydration, hypotension, and hypoglycemia, (b) edema, hypotension, and hypoglycemia, (c) dehydration, hypertension, and hypoglycemia, (d) edema, hypertension, and hypoglycemia, (e) dehydration, hypotension, and hyperglycemia, (f) edema, hypertension, and hyperglycemia.

9. Which of the following effects would you expect might be induced by imbalances in corticoid levels? (a) inhibition of the activity of leukocytes, (b) altered mental function, (c) altered heart function, (d) inhibited bone formation, (e) all of the above except b, (f) all of the above except d, (g) all of the above.

10. By what mechanism can the therapeutic administration of glucocorticoids result in atrophy of the adrenal cortex? (a) by direct depression of cell growth within the cortex, (b) by causing a sclerosing effect on cortical interstitial tissues, (c) by depressing the secretion of most endogenous glucocorticoids, and some endogenous mineralocorticoids, (d) by depressing the secretion of corticotropin (ACTH), (e) by all the above mechanisms.

11. Many undesirable effects can result from the long-term use of the corticosteroids. These effects are extremely varied and occur frequently in one combination or another. Additionally, the rapid withdrawal of corticoid therapy after long-term use is most likely to cause symptoms of (a) withdrawal because of physical dependence, (b) withdrawal because of psychological dependence, (c) adrenal insufficiency, (d) adrenal hyperactivity.

12-15. Fill in the blanks.

12. An adrenal crisis can be precipitated by dental procedures. The basis of this crisis is that the patient is unable to make a physiologic adjustment to _____.

13. When used for replacement therapy, _____ is frequently used to alleviate the mineralocorticoid deficiency.

14. Individuals taking corticoids are likely to have a lowered resistance to _____.

15. The most frequently used method of administration of corticoids in dental practice is the _____ route.

CHAPTER 18: ANTINEOPLASTIC DRUGS

1. Antineoplastic agents may be used (a) as palliative therapy or as a primary treatment modality, (b) in conjunction with surgery and x-ray therapy, (c) when surgery or x-ray therapy is not curative, (d) in all of the above approaches to cancer therapy.

2. In the "cell cycle" theory (a) antimetabolites act in all phases, (b) antimetabolites act only in the mitosis stage, (c) alkylating agents act only in the synthesis stage, (d) alkylating agents act in all phases.

3. Allopurinol (Zyloprim) is sometimes prescribed with antineoplastic agents to (a) prevent hyperuricemia, (b) decrease liver toxicity, (c) inhibit alopecia, (d) accomplish all of the above.

4. An important but least frequently seen toxic manifestation of antineoplastic drug therapy is/are (a) suppression of bone marrow activity (leukopenia, thrombocytopenia, anemia), (b) gastrointestinal disturbances (nausea, stomatitis, vomiting, hemorrhagic diarrhea), (c) cutaneous reactions (erythema, exfoliative dermatitis, Stevens-Johnson syndrome), (d) hepatotoxicity and neurotoxicity, (e) renal tubular impairment, (f) immune deficiency (increased susceptibility to infection and second malignancy), (g) inhibition of spermatogenesis and oogenesis.

5. List six oral conditions often caused by the antineoplastic agents. (a) _____ (b) _____ (c) _____ (d) _____ (e) _____ (f) _____

6. The best oral rinses for patients receiving antineoplastic drug therapy are (a) pleasant-tasting commercial mouthwashes, (b) antibacterial mouthwashes, (c) 3% hydrogen peroxide, (d) warm saline rinses.

CHAPTER 19: CARDIOVASCULAR DRUGS

1. The treatment of mild hypertension is usually initiated with (a) reserpine, (b) hydralazine, (c) a thiazide diuretic, (d) a nonthiazide diuretic, (e) methyldopa.

2-5. Indicate the type of diuretic that the statement describes: (a) mercurial, (b) carbonic anhydrase inhibitor, and (c) thiazide.

2. Orally effective sulfonamides whose adverse effects include drowsiness, fatigue, gastrointestinal distrubances, paresthesias of the face and extremities, allergic dermatologic reactions, blood dyscrasias, and renal calculi.

3. The most potent diuretics that are usually administered intramuscularly.

4. Adverse potentialities include cardiac toxicity, allergic reactions, nephrotoxicity, stomatitis, gastric irritation, weakness, vertigo, and drowsiness.

5. Side effects are usually mild—hypokalemia caused in some patients.

6. What is (are) the principal differences between chlorothiazide and hydrochlorothiazide? Hydrochlorothiazide is (a) more potent, (b) less toxic, (c) more consistently effective, (d) more potent, less toxic, and more effective.

7-10. Indicate the sympatholytic agent that the statement describes: (a) guanethidine, (b) methyldopa, (c) *Rauwolfia* alkaloid, and (d) hydralazine.

7. Produces a prompt decrease of the norepinephrine content of post-ganglionic sympathetic nerve terminals.
8. Established side effects include nasal congestion, diarrhea, lethargy, fatigue, dreams, and psychic depression with suicidal tendencies.
9. Acts directly on the smooth muscle of peripheral arterioles to produce vasodilation and a decrease in blood pressure.
10. A potent antihypertensive that blocks efferent sympathetic nerve transmission.

11-16. Mark items true (T) or false (F) relative to nitroglycerin.
   11. Taken sublingually
   12. Effective prophylactically
   13. Produces coronary vasodilation
   14. Sometimes causes sudden hypotension
   15. Sometimes causes syncope
   16. Drug of choice for relief of anginal attacks

17-23. Mark items true (T) or false (F) relative to amyl nitrite.
   17. Taken by inhalation
   18. Has a bad odor
   19. Produces coronary vasodilation
   20. Sometimes causes sudden and severe hypotension
   21. Sometimes causes syncope
   22. Slowest acting form of nitrite
   23. Prone to produce headaches

24. Quinidine is one of the oldest and most commonly used drugs in the treatment of cardiac arrhythmias. Which of the following is (are) *not* decreased by quinidine? (a) myocardial excitability, (b) conduction velocity, (c) refractory period, (d) vagal influence on myocardium.

25-28. Are the statements true (T) or false (F)?
   25. The effect of procaine amide on cardiac muscle is similar to that of quinidine, including an anticholinergic effect.
   26. As an antiarrhythmic agent, lidocaine's greatest use is in patients recovering from cardiac surgery or after myocardial infarctions.
   27. When used as an antiarrhythmic, phenytoin does not appear to depress either cardiac excitability nor automaticity.
   28. As an antiarrhythmic, digitalis is most effective against ventricular arrhythmias.

29. Heparin is one of the most commonly used anticoagulants. It acts (a) by interfering with the interaction of thromboplastin with calcium ions, (b) as a vitamin K antimetabolite and thereby interferes with the hepatic synthesis of prothrombin, (c) as an antithromboplastin, and prevents the enzymatic conversion of prothrombin to thrombin, (d) by blocking the conversion of fibrinogen to fibrin.

30. Which of the following is *not* true of heparin? (a) It cannot be used orally. (b) It is expensive. (c) It has a slow onset. (d) It has a short duration of action.

31. The coumarins are commonly used oral anticoagulants. They act (a) by interfering with the interaction of thromboplastin with calcium ions, (b) as vitamin K antimetabolites and thereby interfere with the hepatic synthesis of prothrombin, (c) as an antithromboplastin, and prevent the enzymatic conversion of prothrombin to thrombin, (d) by blocking the conversion of fibrinogen to fibrin.

32. Relative to heparin, the coumarins are (a) less expensive, more convenient to administer, and have a slower onset, (b) more expensive, more convenient to administer, and have a slower onset, (c) less expensive, less convenient to administer, and have a slower onset, (d) more expensive, more convenient to administer, and have a faster onset, (e) less expensive, more convenient to administer, and have a faster onset.

CHAPTER 20: ANTIMICROBIAL AGENTS

1. Antibiotic sensitivity tests (a) determine in vivo potency, (b) differentiate between bactericidal and bacteriostatic effects, (c) do neither *a* nor *b*, (d) do both *a* and *b*.

2. The culture of fluid from a periapical abscess indicates the presence of beta-hemolytic streptococci. The use of an antimicrobial drug is determined to be necessary. You would continue therapy for at least (a) 48 hours after the symptoms of infection are absent, (b) 10 days, (c) 14 days after fever and tenderness are absent, (d) 20 days.

3. Sulfonamides are not considered to be antibiotics because they (a) only inhibit bacterial growth, (b) are semisynthetic chemicals, (c) are not produced by microorganisms, (d) are organic chemicals.

4. The principal difference between the potassium, procaine, and benzathine salts of penicillin G is their (a) toxicity, (b) potency, (c) duration of action, (d) antibacterial spectrum.

5. How many international units are in 125 and 250 mg of penicillin? (a) 100,000 and 200,000, (b) 200,000 and 400,000, (c) 300,000 and 600,000, (d) 400,000 and 800,000.

6. In relation to penicillin G, the penicillinase-resistant penicillins are generally (a) more effective against nonpenicillinase producers, (b) more toxic, (c) safer during pregnancy, (d) less allergenic.

7. Ampicillin differs from penicillin G in that it (a) has fewer toxic potentialities, (b) is less allergenic, (c) is resistant to penicillinase, (d) has a slightly broader spectrum.

8. Carbenicillin should be reserved for use against (a) sensitive strains of *Pseudomonas* and *Proteus*, (b) penicillinase-producing staphylococci, (c) group A beta-hemolytic streptococci, (d) all the above.

9. The most common side effects of erythromycin are _____ in nature. (a) gastrointestinal, (b) dermatologic, (c) auditory, (d) hematologic.

10. Which of the following cephalosporins would be most practical for dental use on an outpatient basis? (a) cephalothin, (b) cephalexin, (c) cephaloridine, (d) cephaloglycin, (e) cephazolin.

11. Which of the following is a true comparison of lincomycin and clindamycin? (a) Clindamycin has a slightly broader antibacterial spectrum and less gastrointestinal side effects. (b) Lincomycin is absorbed faster and is more effective against osteomyelitis. (c) Clindamycin is more potent but more toxic. (d) Lincomycin causes more gastrointestinal problems but is less allergenic.

12. Tetracyclines should not be used with methoxyflurane because of (a) cross-tolerance, (b) antagonistic effects, (c) additive hepatic toxicity, (d) additive nephrotoxicity.

13. However, they are notably ineffective for (a) acute necrotizing ulcerative gingivitis, (b) recurrent aphthous stomatitis, (c) prophylaxis against subacute bacterial endocarditis, (d) all of the above conditions.

14. The use of chloramphenicol is extremely limited because of its great toxicity. This toxicity manifests principally as serious and often fatal (a) blood dyscrasias, (b) liver damage, (c) kidney impairment, (d) cardiovascular effects.

15. Streptomycin is a toxic drug. Bacteria develop resistance to it quickly and frequently. Partly for these reasons its current use is principally in the treatment of (a) syphilis, (b) shigellosis, (c) typhoid, (d) tuberculosis.

16. Which of the following drugs has had the most significant use against

staphylococcal enterocolitis? (a) gentamicin, (b) kanamycin, (c) vancomycin, (d) all three of the above are equally effective.

17. The currently important topical antibiotics are all (a) toxic systemically,
(b) well absorbed orally, (c) of moderate allergenicity, (d) broad-spectrum drugs.

18. Nystatin is important in dental practice in the treatment of superficial
candidiasis. What drug would be used systemically against disseminated
candidiasis? (a) nystatin, (b) amphotericin B, (c) candicidin, (d) griseofulvin, (e) flucytosine.

19. Stevens-Johnson syndrome is associated with (a) most sulfonamides,
(b) long-acting sulfonamides, (c) less soluble sulfonamides, (d) topical
sulfonamides.

20. The following drugs are primarily used in the treatment of urinary tract
infections. Which one acts by releasing formaldehyde in an acidic urine?
(a) sulfisoxazole, (b) trimethoprim-sulfamethoxazole, (c) methenamine,
(d) nitrofurantoin, (e) nalidixic acid.

21. Tuberculin converters and reactors exposed to tuberculosis are usually
treated for one year with (a) streptomycin, (b) isoniazid, (c) ethambutol,
(d) rifampin, (e) aminosalicylic acid (PAS).

22. When is streptomycin used alone in the treatment of pulmonary tuberculosis? (a) When the case is mild. (b) When the case is severe. (c) In
both severe and mild cases. (d) It is seldom if ever used alone.

23-32. In questions 23 to 32 match the drug with its most appropriate description. Each drug and description will be used once.

Drug	Description
23. Idoxuridine	(a) An orally effective cephalosporin
24. Amatadine	(b) May produce an orange-red color in urine,
25. Rifampin	saliva, and sweat
26. Ethambutol	(c) Especially effective in the treatment of uri-
27. Nalidixic acid	nary tract infections caused by *Proteus*
28. Nitrofurantoin	(d) An antiviral agent that exerts its effect largely
29. Flucytosine	on DNA synthesis
30. Spectinomycin	(e) Has largely replaced PAS in the treatment of
31. Tobramycin	tuberculosis
32. Cephradine	(f) Especially active against *Pseudomonas*
	(g) A synthetic antifungal that has been suc-
	cessfully against mucocutaneous candidiasis
	(h) Effective against many common urinary tract
	pathogens
	(i) An antiviral agent having prophylactic effects
	against Asian (A2) influenza
	(j) Effective against gonococci

33. Which of the following presents the least problem relative to the development of bacterial resistance? (a) penicillin G, (b) penicillin V, (c) streptomycin, (d) tetracycline.

34. Allergic reactions are a more serious concern with which of the following
antimicrobial agents? (a) penicillin, (b) erythromycin, (c) tetracycline,
(d) lincomycin.

35. Assume that all the following drugs "hit" the pathogen involved in a particular infection. Which agent could most likely be used safely at several
times the usual dosage levels if necessary? (a) penicillin, (b) erythromycin, (c) tetracycline, (d) clindamycin.

36. Which of the following has the broadest spectrum? (a) penicillin G, (b)
erythromycin, (c) tetracycline, (d) ampicillin.

37. Bacterial resistance will develop less frequently and less quickly to (a) penicillin G, (b) ampicillin, (c) tetracycline, (d) streptomycin.

CHAPTER 21: ANTISEPTICS AND DISINFECTANTS

1. The following statements relate to distinguishing between agents defined as antiseptics and those defined as disinfectants. Which statements are true? (a) Antiseptics kill all bacteria, whereas disinfectants kill only pathogenic bacteria. (b) Both kill all bacteria. (c) Both only kill pathogenic bacteria. (d) Antiseptics can be safely applied to living tissue. (e) Disinfectants cannot necessarily be safely applied to living tissue. (f) All except *a* and *b* are true. (g) All except *b* and *d* are true. (h) All except *c* and *e* are true.

2-4. According to the Spaulding classification, indicate whether the actions of the disinfectants described provide (a) first-level, (b) second-level, or (c) third-level disinfection.
  2. Kills only vegetative forms of bacteria, fungi, and lipid-containing viruses.
  3. Produces sterility if time of contact is adequate.
  4. Kills vegetative forms of bacteria, fungi, lipid and nonlipid viruses, and tubercle bacilli, but not spores.

5-7. Again according to Spaulding, indicate whether the items listed generally require (a) first-level, (b) second-level, or (c) third-level disinfection.
  5. Items introduced beneath body surfaces.
  6. Items making contact with intact mucous membranes.
  7. Items not coming into direct contact with the patient.

8. First-level disinfection *cannot* be obtained with (a) ethylene oxide, (b) 2% alkalinized aqueous glutaraldehyde, (c) aqueous formaldehyde, (d) phenol.

9. Which of the following agents act by dissolving the lipid film around bacteria and then disrupting the normal function of the cell membrane? (a) isopropyl alcohol, (b) mercurials, (c) detergents, (d) oxidizing agents.

10. The halogens kill bacteria by (a) inhibiting cell membrane formation, (b) destroying cell membranes, (c) oxidizing chemical groups essential for microbial enzyme activity.

11. What is the advantage of mixing iodine with surface-active agents to produce iodophors? Unlike tinctures of iodine, the iodophors (a) release iodine more slowly, (b) are less irritating, (c) are nonstaining, (d) have all the above advantages.

12. How would you characterize hydrogen peroxide as an antiseptic? (a) harmless, but relatively ineffective, (b) harmless and relatively effective, (c) irritating and relatively ineffective, (d) irritating, but relatively effective.

CHAPTER 22: FLUORIDES

1. The average plasma fluoride level in normal humans is from 0.14 to 0.19 ppm and is not elevated above this range in people consuming water with up to _____ ppm of fluoride. (a) 1, (b) 1.5, (c) 2, (d) 2.5.

2. Acute fluoride poisoning is very rare. The acute lethal dose of sodium fluoride for an adult is (a) 2 Gm, (b) 3 Gm, (c) 4 Gm, (d) 5 Gm.

3-13. Mark items true (T) or false (F).
  3. Mottling of enamel associated with chronic endemic dental fluoroses is a hypoplastic defect that results from a disturbance in the function of ameloblasts during tooth development.
  4. Erupted teeth can develop mottling if exposed to sufficiently high concentrations of fluoride in drinking water.
  5. People living in an area with a high mean annual temperature will

have a higher fluoride intake than those in an area with a low mean annual temperature.

6. The accumulation of fluoride ions in the developing tooth occurs primarily at the external enamel surface.

7. The amount of fluoride incorporated in surface enamel can increase after eruption.

8. The surface layer of fluoroapatite is believed to impart caries resistance to teeth.

9. Protection afforded enamel during tooth formation is not lost if non-fluoridated water is consumed after eruption.

10. Fluoride levels of surface enamel increase throughout life in people who drink water containing 1 ppm or more fluoride.

11. The fact is generally conceded that neither the incidence nor the severity of gingivitis or other periodontal disease in a community is influenced by the fluoride level of its water supply.

12. The addition of sodium fluoride does not appear to have any adverse effect on the action of vitamin preparations and vice versa.

13. Part of caries reduction obtained from fluoride vitamins may result from the topical effect of chewable vitamins.

14. Why is the approach of using fluoride supplements combined with vitamins more advantageous than using fluoride tablets alone? (a) Parents are more likely to see that their children take vitamins prescribed for them than a fluoride tablet alone. (b) Vitamin preparations increase the absorption of fluoride ions. (c) Vitamin-fluoride preparations taste better. (d) All of the above are advantages of the vitamin-fluoride preparations. (e) None of the above is an advantage of the vitamin-fluoride preparations.

15. What is a disadvantage of the vitamin-fluoride tablet approach? (a) Vitamins decrease the systemic absorption of fluoride ions. (b) Vitamins decrease the topical adsorption of fluoride ions. (c) Only a small group of children who require vitamin supplementation should receive fluoride in this manner. (d) Vitamin-fluoride preparations are expensive. (e) All of the above are disadvantages.

16. Prenatal fluoride supplements should not be routinely prescribed for expectant mothers because (a) evidence of effectiveness is conflicting, (b) fluoride ions are suspected of having teratogenic effects, (c) fluoride does not cross the placental barrier, (d) all of the above reasons.

17. The most consistently beneficial results from the topical application of sodium fluoride consist of four applications of a 2% sodium fluoride solution made at 1-week intervals at 3, 7, 11, and 13 years of age. Why are these ages generally recommended? (a) They represent the times shortly after the usual eruption of groups of teeth. (b) Only because they represent adequately spaced times during critical calcification periods.

18. The first application of sodium fluoride is preceded by a prophylaxis. The teeth are thoroughly wetted with the 2% sodium fluoride solution and allowed to dry for _____ minutes. (a) 1, (b) 2, (c) 3, (d) 4.

19. How does sodium fluoride differ from stannous fluoride? (a) The taste of sodium fluoride is not unpleasant. Stannous fluoride has a most unpleasant taste. (b) Sodium fluoride is stable in solution and does not have to be mixed for each patient. Stannous fluoride should be mixed for each patient. (c) Stannous fluoride is normally applied once annually. (d) Stannous fluoride application need not be preceded by a prophylaxis. (e) All of the above are true except c and d. (f) All of the above are true except d. (g) All of the above are true.

20. An 8% stannous fluoride solution is applied to air-dried and isolated teeth a quadrant or a half mouth at a time. The teeth are continually wetted for _____ minutes. (a) 1, (b) 2, (c) 3, (d) 4.

21. The topical application of stannous fluoride is generally considered to be _____ effective than (as) sodium fluoride treatment. (a) more, (b) less, (c) as equally.

22. What is the difference between the application of acidulated phosphate solution (APF) and stannous fluoride? The APF (a) is applied as a gel in trays, (b) need not be applied to dried teeth, (c) is applied for only 2 minutes, (d) must be applied four times annually.

23-31. Give the letter below which indicates the agent or agents that are described by the statement (a) sodium fluoride, (b) stannous fluoride, (c) acidulated phosphate fluoride, (d) agents *a* and *b* only, (e) agents *b* and *c* only, (f) agents *a* and *c* only, (g) all three agents.
   23. Is effective in permanent teeth of children in nonfluoride areas.
   24. *Known* to be effective in deciduous teeth in nonfluoride areas.
   25. *Known* to be effective in fluoride areas.
   26. *Known* to be effective in adults.
   27. Requires a simple one-appointment procedure.
   28. Is stable in solution.
   29. Has a pleasant taste.
   30. Stains teeth.
   31. Can arrest existing caries.

32. What is the difference in effectiveness between stannous fluoride and sodium monofluorophosphate (SMP) dentifrices? The SMP dentifrices appear to be (a) more effective, (b) equally effective, (c) less effective, (d) ineffective.

33. All commonly used prophylaxis pastes are abrasive and remove significant amounts of enamel; thus fluoride in surface enamel is lost unless the prophylaxis paste contains fluoride. There is adequate evidence to indicate that prophylaxis pastes containing _____ are effective in reducing caries rate. (a) sodium fluoride, (b) stannous fluoride, (c) acidulated sodium fluoride phosphate.

34. A number of methods of self-treatment with topical fluorides have been discussed. What is (are) the principal disadvantage(s) of fluoride mouthwashes? (a) They have not been shown to be effective. (b) They are expensive. (c) The solutions pose a toxic potentiality in the home. (d) All of the above statements are true.

35. Although it is too early to draw absolute conclusions, *encouraging* results have been obtained when fluorides were added to (a) silicate cements, (b) amalgam restorations, (c) zinc oxide and eugenol cements, (d) zinc oxyphosphate cements, (e) all of the above materials.

CHAPTER 23: VITAMINS

1. A 50-year-old white woman is referred to you because of a severe glossitis characterized by a smooth-surfaced, slightly edematous tongue. The patient reports a burning sensation in the tongue. Clinical examination also reveals angular cheilosis, dermatitis, and erythema of the nasolabial folds. Dietary intake on the basis of a discussion of diet, appears to be adequate. The medical history indicates that the patient is in menopause and has been taking an antihistamine and a tetracycline for 4 days to combat an acute sinusitis. The patient was exposed to tuberculosis 6 months earlier and has been taking isoniazid daily since the exposure. Just on the basis of the preceding information, you would most likely suspect (a) pyridoxine inhibition by isoniazid, (b) deficiency of vitamin K due to tetracycline-induced reduction in intestinal bacterial flora, (c) generalized vitamin deficiency as a result of menopause, (d) a hormonal etiology not involving nutritional deficiencies.

2. Pyridoxine deficiency would most likely be seen in a (a) 16-year-old woman taking a tetracycline for acne, (b) 30-year-old, well-nourished male narcotic addict, (c) 40-year-old woman taking an oral contraceptive, (d) 6-year-old man taking digoxin for congestive heart failure.

3. Glossitis and angular cheilitis are *least* likely to be seen in a patient with a deficiency of (a) pantothenic acid, (b) thiamine, (c) riboflavin, (d) niacin.

4. Pellagra, characterized by the "3 D's" (dermatitis, diarrhea, and de-

mentia), is caused by a severe deficiency of (a) niacin, (b) thiamine, (c) riboflavin, (d) biotin.

5. Beriberi is caused by a severe deficiency in (a) niacin, (b) thiamine, (c) riboflavin, (d) biotin.

6. Water-soluble vitamins, except for vitamin C, function as (a) antioxidants in cellular respiration, (b) enzymes in oxidation reactions, (c) micro-chelating agents, (d) essential components of coenzymes.

7. Lean meats, liver, and poultry are good sources of (a) pyridoxine, (b) thiamine, (c) niacin, (d) riboflavin.

8. The amino acid tryptophan is metabolized in the body to (a) pyridoxine, (b) thiamine, (c) niacin, (d) riboflavin.

9. Why would eating uncooked egg whites reduce biotin absorption?

10. Pernicious anemia is a conditional cobalamin (B_{12}) deficiency caused by a lack of (a) extrinsic factor in the diet, (b) intrinsic factor in gastric mucosa, (c) both a and b, (d) neither a nor b.

11. Megaloblastic anemia caused by cyanocobalamin deficiency is indistinguishable from that produced by a deficiency in (a) biotin, (b) choline, (c) folic acid, (d) pantothenic acid.

12. Why cannot a deficiency of cynaocobalamin, secondary to pernicious anemia, be treated with the oral administration of cyanocobalamin?

13. Ascorbic acid is extremely important in wound healing. Its principal effect is on (a) epithelial proliferation, (b) collagen formation, (c) maturation of osteoblasts, (d) reduction of inflammation.

14. Scurvy is caused by a deficiency of vitamin (a) A, (b) B_1 and/or B_2, (c) C, (d) D.

15. The principal effect of vitamin A is in the maintenance of what tissues? (a) epithelial, (b) connective, (c) osseous, (d) vascular.

16. Nyctalopia, xerophthalmia, and keratomalacia are seen with a deficiency in vitamin (a) A, (b) B_2, (c) C, (d) D.

17. Liver disease is most likely to be related to deficiencies in vitamin (a) B complex, C, and D, (b) B complex only, (c) C, D, and folic acid, (d) A, D, E, and K.

18. The normal mineralization of bone and the homeostatic regulation of plasma calcium depends on an adequate supply of vitamin D. Its principal functions in this regard are to (a) stimulate intestinal absorption of calcium and promote mobilization of calcium from bone, (b) stimulate intestinal absorption of calcium and decrease the mobilization of calcium from bone, (c) decrease renal excretion of calcium and promote mobilization of calcium from bone, (d) decrease renal excretion of calcium and decrease mobilization of calcium from bone.

19. In children, vitamin D deficiency results in rickets, whereas in adults the disease state is _____.

20. Toxicity from excessive intake of vitamin D has been observed. This toxicity primarily manifests itself as (a) liver damage, (b) renal damage, (c) hypercalcemia, (d) all of the above.

21. Vitamin E (tocopherol) appears to prevent both the oxidation of essential cell constituents and the formation of toxic oxidation products. Severe vitamin E deficiencies in animals have been associated with degenerative changes in skeletal muscle and reproductive failure, sterility, and fetal death. The evidence that vitamin E is therapeutic against these changes in humans is (a) conclusive, (b) inconclusive.

22. Vitamin K is essential for the hepatic synthesis of prothrombin and blood-clotting factors VII, IX, and X. The usual causes of vitamin K deficiency are malabsorption syndromes and inadequate intake. Other causes include (a) liver disease, (b) prolonged use of antibiotics, (c) biliary obstruction, (d) all of the above.

23. Toxicity from hypervitaminosis will most likely be seen with vitamins (a) A and D, (b) B and C, (c) B_{12} and D, (d) E and K.

In questions 24 through 32 match the vitamin deficiency with the proper deficiency state.

Vitamin deficiency	Related deficiency state
24. A	(a) Hypoprothrombinemia
25. B_1 (thiamine)	(b) Reproductive failure
26. B_{12} (cyanocobalamin)	(c) Hypocalcemia
27. C	(d) Defective connective tissue formation
28. D	(e) Dermatitis, dementia, diarrhea
29. E	(f) Beriberi
30. Folic acid	(g) Megaloblastic anemia
31. K	(h) Defective vision
32. Niacin	(One of the above will be used twice)

In questions 33 through 44 list the three most significant clinical considerations in severe deficiencies of the vitamins indicated.
33. Pyridoxine (B_6)
34. Thiamine (B_1)
35. Pantothenic acid
36. Riboflavin (B_2)
37. Niacin
38. Biotin
39. Cyanocobalamin (B_{12})
40. Folic acid
41. Ascorbic acid
42. Vitamin A
43. Vitamin D
44. Vitamin E

CHAPTER 24: EMERGENCY DRUGS

1. There are only two instances in which epinephrine is indicated in dental office emergencies. These are (a) acute hypotension and respiratory arrest, (b) anaphylaxis and cardiac arrest, (c) respiratory arrest and extrapyramidal reactions to phenothiazines, (d) hypovolemia and myocardial infarction.

2. Epinephrine is *not* the drug of choice for the treatment of shock because its use may (a) further reduce venous return, (b) intensify highly undesirable renal ischemia, (c) precipitate ventricular fibrillation in the ischemic and irritable myocardium, (d) lead to all of the above.

3. The purpose of intravenous sodium bicarbonate in an emergency situation is to (a) counteract metabolic acidosis, (b) stimulate the vasopressor center, (c) increase oxygenation of hypoxic tissues, (d) all of the above.

4. Hydrocortisone sodium succinate (100 mg IV) is effective as a part of the management of cardiac arrest, anaphylactic shock, and acute adrenocortical insufficiency. The basis of its hemodynamic effects in these emergencies is that it (a) stimulates the vasopressor center, (b) stimulates the release of endogenous vasopressors, (c) potentiates vasopressors, (d) does all three of the above.

5. The intravenous use of 2 to 5 ml of 1% diphenhydramine will generally provide prompt relief from (a) severe allergic reactions, (b) minor dermatologic allergic reactions, (c) extrapyramidal reactions to phenothiazines, (d) all of the above.

6. Inhaled ammonia acts against syncope by (a) irritating the sensory end-

ings of the trigeminal nerve, (b) direct stimulation of the vasomotor center, (c) direct stimulation of the respiratory center, (d) both *b* and *c*.

7. When glyceryl trinitrate (nitroglycerin) is used against anginal pain, relief is normally obtained within (a) 30 seconds, (b) 1 minute, (c) 2 to 3 minutes, (d) 5 to 10 minutes.

8. A disadvantage of amyl nitrite relative to nitroglycerin as a coronary vasodilator is that amyl nitrite (a) is less potent, (b) causes more nausea and vomiting, (c) has a shorter shelf life, (d) is less potent and also has a shorter shelf life.

9. The principal reason for having morphine sulfate in a dental emergency kit is for early administration to a patient experiencing (a) an attack of angina pectoris, (b) acute myocardial infarction, (c) anaphylactic shock, (d) convulsions associated with severe pain.

10. An extremely important advantage of phenylephrine HCl over many other vasopressors is that it (a) has greater potency, (b) does not directly stimulate the heart, (c) is less toxic, (d) acts on both alpha and beta receptors.

11. What are the advantages of diazepam over thiopental sodium as an anticonvulsant for use in dental emergency kits? Diazepam has (a) less potential for cardiovascular and respiratory depression, (b) a greater versatility as to route of administration, (c) a shorter duration of action, (d) only *a* and *b* as advantages, (e) only *b* and *c* as advantages, (f) all of the above advantages.

CHAPTER 25: PHARMACOLOGY OF INTRAVENOUS SEDATION

1. The depressant effects of drugs on the central nervous system are due to actions on the reticular activating system (RAS), medulla, and cerebral cortex. Barbiturates produce sedation and hypnosis by acting on the RAS to depress ascending neuronal conduction. Doses that produce anesthesia do so by depressing (a) ascending neuronal conduction in the RAS, (b) excitatory pathways within the cerebral cortex, (c) both *a* and *b*, (d) neither *a* nor *b*.

2. Hypnotic doses of barbiturates depress respiration by depressing (a) neurogenic control in the higher brain centers, (b) chemical centers responsive to changes in blood pH and P_{CO_2}, (c) chemoreceptors responsive to hypoxic stimulation, (d) all of the above controls.

3. Higher anesthetic doses of barbiturates depress respiration by which of the mechanisms listed in question 2?

4. The effects of barbiturates on the cardiovascular system are (a) extremely serious because of the unpredictability of their effects, (b) serious because of the effects on medullary vasomotor tone, (c) mild and do not ordinarily constitute a hazard in clinical practice, (d) of no concern whatever.

5. What effect would you expect from heavy hypnotic doses of morphine or meperidine that you would not expect from thiopental? (a) euphoria and analgesia, (b) euphoria and respiratory depression, (c) analgesia and amnesia, (d) amnesia and respiratory depression.

6. The main differences between meperidine and alphaprodine are (a) chemical and physical properties, (b) potency and duration of action, (c) doses and routes of administration, (d) all of the above.

7. Fentanyl is chemically related to meperidine. It has an almost immediate onset of action and is the _____ narcotic analgesia available for use in intravenous sedation. (a) most toxic but most reliable, (b) least potent and least toxic, (c) most potent and shortest acting, (d) least toxic and longest acting.

8. The phenothiazines produce only sedation and not true hypnosis or general anesthesia because they (a) only block ascending neuronal projections in the RAS, (b) only block descending neuronal projections in the RAS, (c) affect cortical areas only, (d) affect the RAS and subcortical areas only.

9. Phenothiazines cause few side effects after single intravenous doses. The cardiovascular response to these drugs is minimal, but they are likely to cause (a) hypotension and reflex tachycardia, (b) hypertension and reflex tachycardia, (c) hypotension and reflex bradycardia, (d) hypertension and reflex bradycardia.

10. When used for intravenous sedation, diazepam produces (a) analgesia and some degree of muscle relaxation in 90% of patients, (b) tranquilization in all and neurolepsis in most patients, (c) euphoria in some patients and retrograde amnesia in approximately 50% of patients, (d) all of the above effects.

11. In neuroleptanalgesia, droperidol (Inapsine) is frequently used to provide the tranquilization component and fentanyl (Sublimaze) to provide the analgesic component (as in Innovar). Dissociative anesthesia is accomplished with (a) Innovar, (b) ketamine (Ketalar), (c) phencylidine, (d) all of the above.

CHAPTER 26: PARENTERAL SEDATION AND NITROUS OXIDE ANALGESIA

1. Which of the following are *advantages of oral sedation* relative to IM and IV administration? (a) safer, (b) provides more predictable degrees of sedation, (c) more rapid onset, (d) easier delivery, (e) greater patient acceptance, (f) cheaper, (g) *a, b, d,* and *e,* (h) *a, d, e,* and *f,* (i) all of the above.

2-7. Indicate which method of administration is more intimately related to the characteristic listed. Answer (a) for oral, (b) for IM, (c) for IV, (d) for both IM and IV, and (e) for all three methods.
   2. A principal hazard is overdepression of the cardiovascular, respiratory, and central nervous systems.
   3. It is the most effective method of ensuring predictable, adequate sedation.
   4. Safest.
   5. Poor patient acceptance.
   6. There is an inability to remove the drug if overdose of overreaction has occurred.
   7. Slowest onset.

8. You have inadvertently injected a barbiturate extravascularly. Your treatment is to inject up to 10 ml of a 1% solution of procaine HCl into the area. How is the procaine injection helpful in preventing tissue damage? (a) It dilutes the agent injected. (b) It causes vasodilation and thereby speeds absorption of the agent. (c) It tends to neutralize the alkalinity of the barbiturate. (d) It is helpful by all the above mechanisms.

9. Why would lidocaine HCl *not* be a good substitute for procaine HCl in question 8? Lidocaine would not (a) dilute the barbiturate well because of its spreading tendency, (b) dilate blood vessels as well as procaine, (c) neutralize the alkalinity of the barbiturate, (d) dilute, dilate, or neutralize as well as procaine.

10. The alcoholic will usually require increased doses of a barbiturate for parenteral sedation unless (a) liver disease is present, (b) he is under 50 years of age, (c) he is over 50 years of age, (d) both *a* and *b* are true, (e) both *a* and *c* are true.

11. This text describes the use of a 15 mg/ml pentobarbital solution for intravenous sedation. What is the percentage concentration of this solution? (a) 0.015%, (b) 0.0015%, (c) 0.15%, (d) 15%.

12. During intravenous sedation the patient's vital signs must be monitored at all times. The adult test dose of the solution mentioned in question 11 is 0.25 ml. If no adverse effects occur after the administration of this test dose, an additional 3.75 to 4.75 ml are injected slowly over a 30- to 45-second period. In a healthy patient, what is the minimum time you should wait before assuming that the full pharmacologic effect of the dose has manifested itself? (a) 30 seconds, (b) 60 seconds, (c) 2 minutes, (d) 4 minutes.

13. After the appropriate waiting time indicated in question 12, additional 15 mg (1 ml) doses are administered at 60-second intervals until the desired level of sedation is obtained. At this point sedative effects (a) are maintained by 15 mg doses every 15 minutes, (b) are maintained by 15 mg doses every 30 minutes, (c) may extend 30 to 60 minutes without further drug administration, (d) may extend 2 to 4 hours without further drug administration.

14. Why is a larger volume of a low concentration of the drug recommended as opposed to a smaller volume of a more concentrated solution? The larger volume at lower concentration (a) increases control over the depth of sedation obtained, (b) reduces chemical insult to the vein, (c) has the advantages of both *a* and *b*, (d) has neither of the advantages of *a* or *b*.

15. In the Jorgensen technique of using pentobarbital with meperidine, (a) the drugs are injected together to obtain "baseline" anesthesia; (b) the drugs are injected together throughout the procedure; (c) baseline sedation is obtained first with pentobarbital; (d) baseline sedation is obtained first with meperidine.

16. Which of the following effects is (are) *not* obtained with diazepam? (a) muscular relaxation, (b) amnesia, (c) analgesia, (d) respiratory depression, (e) neither *a* nor *b* is obtained, (f) neither *c* nor *d* is obtained, (g) none of the above effects is obtained.

17. Neuroleptanalgesia is a state of pronounced tranquility and profound analgesia. This is generally associated with the use of (a) meperidine, (b) diazepam, (c) diazepam and meperidine, (d) Innovar, (e) all of the above agents.

18. The objective of nitrous oxide–oxygen analgesia is to provide a relaxed but cooperative patient with adequate analgesia and some degree of amnesia with little or no depression of reflexes. This must be accomplished without entry into stage (a) II, (b) III, plane 1, (c) III, plane 2, (d) III, plane 3.

19. The use of the nitrous oxide–oxygen technique in combination with other sedative regimens (a) decreases the potential dangers, (b) increases the potential dangers.

20. Absolute contraindications to nitrous oxide–oxygen analgesia include (a) upper respiratory obstruction, (b) coryza, (c) emotional instability, (d) all of the above conditions, (e) none of the above conditions.

21. Nitrous oxide has little or no direct effect on organ systems other than the central nervous system. Important local effects are that it (a) stimulates nasal and pharyngeal secretions, (b) irritates mucous membranes, (c) does both *a* and *b*, (d) does neither *a* nor *b*.

22. Diffusion hypoxia after nitrous oxide analgesia is best prevented by (a) never using more than 60% nitrous oxide, (b) maintaining at least 30% oxygen in the system, (c) having the patient breathe 100% oxygen for 4 to 5 minutes after the procedure, (d) bringing the patient out of analgesia very slowly.

23. Although dental procedures cannot be accomplished while the patient is wearing a face mask, this piece of equipment should always be available (a) to obtain greater depths of analgesia, (b) for the application of posi-

tive pressure during emergency situations, (c) for use during emergence from analgesia, (d) for all of the above purposes.

24. During nitrous oxide–oxygen analgesia, at least _____% oxygen at a flow rate of no less than _____ liters per minute should be maintained at all times. (a) 25%, 2, (b) 25%, 4, (c) 50%, 2, (d) 50%, 4.

25. Which of the following statements is *false* relative to the patient under nitrous oxide–oxygen analgesia? He may (a) exhibit slurred speech, (b) relate a feeling of well-being, (c) be relaxed and cooperative, (d) have little or no response to local anesthetic injection, (e) have eyes open or easily opened by operator, (f) have pupils normal, (g) have respiration normal except if deep, (h) none of the above is false.

CHAPTER 27: PHARMACOLOGIC CONSIDERATIONS IN PATIENTS WITH SYSTEMIC DISEASE

1. Which of the following drugs is *least* likely to cause xerostomia? (a) nitroglycerin, (b) reserpine, (c) acetazolamide, (d) chlorothiazide.

2-11. Ten different patients list the conditions indicated below on their medical histories. Match their respective conditions with the drugs listed that they would be most likely taking. Each drug is used once.

Condition	Drug
2. Angina pectoris	(a) Indomethacin
3. Congestive heart failure	(b) Digitoxin
4. Hypertension	(c) Propantheline
5. Fluid retention	(d) Hydrochlorothiazide
6. Tuberculosis	(e) Nitroglycerin
7. Rheumatoid arthritis	(f) Methotrexate
8. Peptic ulcer	(g) Isoniazid
9. Hyperthyroidism	(h) Tolbutamide
10. Leukemia	(i) Deserpidine
11. Diabetes	(j) Isothiouracil

12. Orthostatic hypotension is *least* likely to occur in a patient who is taking (a) nitroglycerin, (b) digitalis, (c) reserpine, (d) hydralazine.

13. The oral manifestations of pregnancy gingivitis may be caused by (a) norethynodrel, (b) liothyronine, (c) polystyrene sulfonate, (d) salicylazo-sulfapyridine, (e) all of the above drugs.

14. Which of the following anticoagulants is (are) used parenterally? (a) sodium warfarin, (b) bishydroxycoumarin, (c) heparin, (d) all of the above, (e) none of the above.

15. Transplant patients would be most likely taking (a) antihistamines and bishydroxycoumarin, (b) prednisone and isothiouracil, (c) norethynodrel and levothyroxine, (d) phenylbutazone and methimazole, (e) azathioprine and corticosteroids.

16. Mercaptopurine, methotrexate, and chlorambucil are likely to cause or predispose to (a) bleeding tendencies, (b) infection, (c) oral candidiasis, (d) oral ulcers, (e) all of the above, (f) none of the above.

17. Chlorpropamide, tolbutamide, acetohexamide, and tolazamide are used in the treatment of (a) diabetes, (b) gout, (c) mental depression, (d) epilepsy.

CHAPTER 28: PHARMACOLOGIC MANAGEMENT OF CERTAIN COMMON ORAL DISEASE ENTITIES

1. Which of the following statements is (are) *false* relative to the pharmacologic management of acute necrotizing ulcerative gingivitis? (a) Oxygen-releasing mouthwashes are known to be more effective than saline rinses. (b) There is no convincing evidence that the vitamin preparations are routinely helpful. (c) Several antibiotics will improve the clinical course,

(d) The routine use of antibiotics is to be condemned. (e) Topical caustics should not be used on the lesions. (f) All of the above are false. (g) None of the above is false.

2. Which of the following statements is (are) false relative to the pharmacologic management of primary herpetic gingivostomatitis? (a) Antibiotics generally have little or no effect on the clinical course of the disease. (b) Antipyretic analgesics are usually indicated. (c) Topical caustics are usually helpful. (d) Corticosteroids should not be used. (e) All of the above are false. (f) None of the above is false.

3. Which of the following antibiotic regimens was reported effective against recurrent aphthous stomatitis? One teaspoonful (a) tetracycline syrup (125 mg/5 ml) is swished in the mouth for 2 minutes and then swallowed four times daily. (b) Tetracycline syrup (250 mg/5 ml) is swished in the mouth for 2 minutes and then swallowed four times daily. (c) Tetracycline suspension (125 mg/5 ml) is swished in the mouth for 2 minutes and then swallowed four times daily. (d) Tetracycline suspension (250 mg/5 ml) is swished in the mouth for 2 minutes and then swallowed four times daily.

4. The treatment of oral candidiasis with nystatin should continue for a minimum of 14 days and not be discontinued until two successive smears are negative or at least until ___ hours after the signs of infection have disappeared. (a) 24, (b) 48, (c) 96, (d) 120.

5. You have determined that a severe case of angular chilitis is caused by bacteria. Which of the following drugs in ointment form would you expect to be helpful? (a) nystatin, (b) bacitracin, (c) neomycin, (d) tetracycline, (e) a, b, and c, (f) b, c, and d, (g) all of the above.

6. The treatment of lichen planus is directed toward (a) obtaining a more physiologic hormonal balance, (b) determining and prescribing the antibacterial agent that will be effective against the etiologic agent, (c) improving the host response and the general nutritional state of the patient, (d) all of the above.

7. The use of a 0.5% sodium carboxymethyl cellulose aqueous solution as a rinse is effective in the treatment of (a) hypersensitive dentin, (b) xerostomia, (c) burning tongue syndrome, (d) lichen planus.

8. The use of local tetracycline prophylaxis to prevent alveolar osteitis ("dry socket") (a) should be instituted routinely in all extraction cases, (b) should be instituted routinely in third molar extraction, (c) may be indicated in third molar extractions when factors predisposing to infection are present, (d) is never indicated.

9. Hypersensitive dentin can be completely and predictably eliminated by (a) sodium or stannous fluoride applications by the dentist, (b) adrenal steroid applications by the dentist, (c) desensitizing toothpastes, (d) none of the above.

CHAPTER 29: DRUG INTERACTIONS

1. If two drugs that have the same actions are given together, the resulting effects may be a simple addition of their individual effects. On the other hand, if the two drugs have opposing actions, such as a sedative and a stimulant, their effects may be subtractive or antagonistic. In addition to this simple arithmetic relationship, one drug may accentuate or reduce the effect of another by more complex mechanisms. Can you name these mechanisms and give an example of each?

2. Certain divalent metal ions may impair the gastrointestinal absorption of (a) penicillin, (b) tetracyclines, (c) erythromycin, (d) nystatin.

3. What is the significance of drug binding to plasma protein? (a) Bound drugs are usually inactive. (b) Bound drugs are usually more toxic. (c) Both a and b are true. (d) Neither a nor b is true.

4. How could phenobarbital decrease the effect of a specific regimen of bishydroxycoumarin? (a) by decreasing the absorption of bishydroxycoumarin, (b) by forming inactive complexes with bishydroxycoumarin, (c) by inducing the formation of enzymes that metabolize bishydroxycoumarin, (d) by displacing bishydroxycoumarin from protein-binding sites.

5. How can aspirin increase the effects of coumarin derivatives? (a) by inhibiting the enzymes that metabolize coumarins, (b) by displacing coumarins from their plasma protein-binding sites, (c) by decreasing gastric pH, thereby increasing absorption of coumarins, (d) by all of the above mechanisms.

6. How might the use of a tetracycline reduce the effectiveness of concomitantly administered penicillin? (a) by reducing its absorption, (b) by increasing its renal excretion, (c) by reducing bacterial multiplication rate, (d) by increasing bacterial multiplication rate.

7. How could the long-term use of an antihistamine and an anticholinergic cause the loss of teeth? By an additive interaction that (a) decreases the inflammatory response in the periodontium, (b) increases the inflammatory response in the periodontium, (c) accelerates the demineralization of dentin, (d) produces prolonged xerostomia.

8. Acetaminophen enhances the effect of (a) barbiturates, (b) MAO inhibitors, (c) amphetamines, (d) coumarin anticoagulants.

9. Aspirin is antagonized by (a) phenylbutazone, (b) probenecid, (c) phenytoin, (d) orphenadrine.

10. Chloral hydrate antagonizes (a) probenecid, (b) coumarin anticoagulants, (c) chlordiazepoxide, (d) meperidine.

11. In an additive manner, propoxyphene appears to accentuate the toxic effects of (a) corticosteroids, (b) orphenadrine, (c) phenothiazines, (d) tolbutamide.

CHAPTER 30: DRUG ABUSE

1. The withdrawal syndrome is a combination of certain drug-specific symptoms that occur on sudden discontinuation of the drug. This syndrome is associated with (a) psychological dependence, (b) physical dependence, (c) the development of tolerance, (d) *a* and *b*, (e) *a*, *b*, and *c*.

2. Addiction is associated with the existence of (a) psychological dependence, (b) physical dependence, (c) tolerance, (d) *a* and *b*, (e) *a*, *b*, and *c*.

3. Generally speaking, which of the following best characterizes the morphine abuser? (a) satisfied, complacent, cooperative individual with suppressed hunger and reduced sexual desires, (b) satisfied, but uncooperative individual with suppressed hunger and increased sexual desires, (c) quarrelsome, uncooperative individual with increased appetite and sexual desires, (d) quarrelsome, dissatisfied, uncooperative individual with a reduced capacity to make a contribution to society.

4. Generally speaking, which of the following best characterizes the alcohol abuser? (a) satisfied, complacent, cooperative individual with suppressed hunger and reduced sexual desires, (b) satisfied, but uncooperative individual with suppressed hunger and increased sexual desires, (c) quarrelsome, uncooperative individual with increased appetite and sexual desires, (d) quarrelsome, dissatisfied, uncooperative individual with a reduced capacity to make a contribution to society.

5. In the morphine addict, tolerance does *not* develop to the (a) lethal dose, (b) constipatory action, (c) sedative dose, (d) respiratory effects.

6. Cross-tolerance develops between (a) morphine and heroin, (b) nar-

cotics and sedative hypnotics, (c) sedative hypnotics and alcohol, (d) all of the above drugs.

7. Withdrawal symptoms reach peak intensity between 48 and 72 hours after the last dose of heroin or morphine and, without treatment, disappear in about ___ days after the last dose. (a) 4, (b) 8, (c) 14, (d) 30.

8. What are the most significant side effects known from the long-term use of methadone? (a) blood dyscrasias, (b) liver damage, (c) bradycardia and hypotension, (d) impotence and constipation.

9. Which sedatives are the most subject to drug abuse? (a) barbiturates, (b) nonbarbiturate sedatives, (c) minor tranquilizers, (d) major tranquilizers.

10. The initial symptoms of withdrawal from central nervous system depressants consist of (a) muscular rigidity, hyperreflexia, salivation, and miosis; (b) abdominal cramps, blurred vision, xerostomia and tachycardia; (c) abdominal cramps, rapid respiration, and chills; (d) nausea, vomiting, weakness, anxiety, and perspiration.

11. The most serious problem related to the abuse of central nervous system stimulants in young people is the (a) development of nutritional disturbances, (b) loss of sleep, (c) induction of mental abnormalities, (d) effect on the heart.

12. Certain generalizations can be made relative to the response to psychedelics. Which of the following statements is not true? (a) Psychedelics affect perception by increasing or exaggerating the awareness of sensory input. (b) Senses of sight, hearing, taste, and smell are made more acute. (c) One sensory impression may be translated to another; music may appear as color, etc. (d) Judgment of reality is impaired and there is a loss of the sense of time. (e) None of the above is false.

13. In addition to its hallucinogenic activity, LSD causes (a) an increase in blood pressure, tachycardia, hyperreflexia, nausea, piloerection, and an increase in body temperature; (b) a decrease in blood pressure, bradycardia, hyperreflexia, xerostomia, and a decrease in body temperature; (c) only gastrointestinal effects; (d) only other psychological effects.

14-17. Indicate whether the statement applies more completely to LSD or to marihuana.
   14. The setting in which the drug is taken determines to a great extent the type of behavioral changes experienced.
   15. Tolerance develops within days and some physical dependence is believed to develop.
   16. Prolonged, high-level use may cause xerostomia.
   17. Produces more sympathomimetic actions.

ANSWERS TO BOARD REVIEW QUESTIONS

Chapter 1: Introduction
1-b 2-d 3-c 4-d 5-d 6-b 7-d

Chapter 2: General principles of drug action
1-a 2-a 3-a 4-c 5-a 6-d 7-c 8-a 9-c 10-b
11-b 12-a 13-b 14-d 15-b 16-reversible 17-d
18-see text 19-see text 20-c 21-b 22-c

Chapter 3: Adverse drug reactions
1-b 2-e 3-a 4-b

Chapter 4: Prescription writing
1-b 2-b 3-c 4-a 5-b 6-11-see text 12-b
13-b 14-c 15-b 16-e

Chapter 5: General anesthetics
1-a 2-b 3-c 4-c 5-b 6-c 7-d 8-b 9-e 10-d
11-a 12-a 13-d 14-c 15-c 16-e 17-a 18-i

Chapter 6: Sedative-hypnotic drugs
1-b 2-a 3-b 4-d 5-e 6-a 7-a 8-d 9-f
10-a 11-d

Chapter 7: Psychotherapeutic drugs

Chapter 8: Minor tranquilizers and centrally acting muscle relaxants
1-b 2-a 3-c 4-b 5-b 6-d 7-e 8-a 9-c 10-a
11-c 12-d 13-d 14-b 15-a 16-b 17-e 18-d
19-a 20-c 21-a

Chapter 9: Nonnarcotic analgesics

1-d 2-d 3-b 4-a 5-b 6-e 7-a 8-b 9-b 10-c
11-c 12-c 13-a 14-a 15-c 16-d 17-c 18-b
19-e 20-a 21-g 22-i 23-h 24-f

Chapter 10: Narcotics

1-b 2-h 3-a 4-e 5-a 6-b 7-c 8-b 9-c 10-d
11-d 12-a 13-b 14-a 15-d 16-e 17-b 18-c
19-e 20-d 21-a 22-c 23-a 24-b 25-d 26-d
27-a 28-b 29-f 30-a 31-d

Chapter 11: Central nervous system stimulants

1-e 2-b 3-c 4-e 5-b 6-f 7-a 8-a

Chapter 12: Anticonvulsant drugs

1-d 2-d 3-d 4-c 5-e 6-b 7-d 8-a 9-a 10-a
11-d 12-a 13-a 14-b 15-b 16-b 17-b 18-d
19-e

Chapter 13: Autonomic drugs

1-P 2-S 3-P 4-P 5-S 6-P 7-e 8-b 9-a
10-c 11-d 12-c 13-d 14-d 15-see text
16-see text 17-see text 18-e 19-c
20-a 21-a 22-c 23-a

Chapter 14: Local anesthetics

1-d 2-a 3-b 4-d 5-f 6-d 7-c 8-a 9-b 10-d
11-d 12-b 13-b 14-c 15-c 16-d 17-b 18-c
19-a 20-e 21-b 22-e 23-b 24-d 25-a 26-a
27-c 28-f 29-d

Chapter 15: Histamine and antihistamines

1-c 2-e 3-a 4-d 5-b 6-b 7-a 8-d

Chapter 16: Hormones and related substances

1-c 2-e 3-a 4-b 5-d 6-f 7-e 8-e 9-a 10-b
11-b 12-g 13-c 14-c 15-a 16-b 17-a 18-e

Chapter 17: Adrenocorticosteroids

1-c 2-a 3-b 4-a 5-d 6-d 7-c 8-a 9-g 10-d
11-c 12-stress 13-desoxycorticosterone 14-infection
15-topical

Chapter 18: Antineoplastic drugs

1-d 2-d 3-a 4-c 5-sensitive oral tissues,
mucosal ulcerations, gingival hemorrhage,
xerostomia, impaired taste sensation, candidiasis 6-d

Chapter 19: Cardiovascular drugs

1-c 2-b 3-a 4-a 5-c 6-a 7-c 8-c 9-d 10-a
11-T 12-T 13-T 14-T 15-T 16-T 17-T 18-T
19-T 20-T 21-T 22-F 23-T 24-c 25-T 26-T
27-T 28-F 29-c 30-c 31-b 32-a

Chapter 20: Antimicrobial agents

1-c 2-b 3-c 4-c 5-b 6-b 7-d 8-a 9-a 10-d
11-c 12-a 13-b 14-a 15-d 16-c 17-a 18-b

19-b 20-c 21-b 22-d 23-d 24-i 25-b 26-e
27-c 28-h 29-g 30-j 31-f 32-a 33-d 34-a
35-a 36-c 37-c

Chapter 21: Antiseptics and disinfectants

1-f 2-c 3-a 4-b 5-a 6-b 7-c 8-d 9-c 10-c
11-d 12-a

Chapter 22: Fluorides

1-d 2-d 3-T 4-F 5-T 6-T 7-T 8-T 9-F
10-T 11-T 12-T 13-T 14-a 15-c 16-a 17-a
18-d 19-f 20-d 21-a 22-a 23-g 24-d 25-b
26-b 27-e 28-f 29-f 30-b 31-b 32-b 33-b
34-c 35-e

Chapter 23: Vitamins

1-a 2-c 3-a 4-a 5-b 6-d 7-c 8-c 9-see p. 252
10-b 11-c 12-d 13-b 14-c 15-a 16-a 17-d
18-a 19-osteomalacia 20-c 21-b 22-b 23-a 24-h
25-f 26-g 27-d 28-c 29-b 30-g 31-a 32-e
33 through 44 see text

Chapter 24: Emergency drugs

1-b 2-d 3-a 4-c 5-c 6-a 7-c 8-b 9-b 10-b
11-d

Chapter 25: Pharmacology of intravenous sedation

1-c 2-a 3-d 4-c 5-a 6-d 7-c 8-d 9-a 10-c
11-b

Chapter 26: Parenteral sedation and nitrous oxide analgesia

1-h 2-c 3-c 4-a 5-d 6-e 7-a 8-d 9-b 10-a
11-c 12-b 13-d 14-c 15-c 16-f 17-d 18-a
19-b 20-d 21-c 22-c 23-b 24-a 25-h

Chapter 27: Pharmacologic considerations in patients with systemic disease

1-a 2-e 3-b 4-i 5-d 6-g 7-a 8-c 9-j 10-f
11-h 12-b 13-a 14-c 15-e 16-e 17-a

Chapter 28: Pharmacologic management of certain common oral disease entities

1-a 2-c 3-d 4-b 5-f 6-c 7-b 8-c 9-d

Chapter 29: Drug interactions

1-see text 2-b 3-a 4-c 5-b 6-c 7-d 8-d
9-a 10-b 11-b

Chapter 30: Drug abuse

1-b 2-e 3-a 4-d 5-b 6-a 7-b 8-d 9-a 10-d
11-c 12-e 13-a 14-M 15-M 16-M 17-L

Index